MATERNAL-CHILD NURSING

Maternal-Child Nursing

Violet Broadribb, R.N., M.S.
Formerly Assistant Professor of Pediatric Nursing,
University of Oregon School of Nursing,
Portland, Oregon

and

Charlotte Corliss, R.N., M.Ed.
Formerly Assistant Professor of Maternal-Child Nursing,
Arizona State University, College of Nursing,
Tempe, Arizona

J. B. Lippincott Company

Philadelphia   Toronto

Copyright © 1973 by J. B. Lippincott Company

Distributed in Great Britain by
Blackwell Scientific Publications
Oxford, London, and Edinburgh

ISBN 0-397-54140-6

Printed in the United States of America

 3 5 7 9 8 6 4 2

Library of Congress Cataloging in Publication Data

Broadribb, Violet.
    Maternal-child nursing.

    Includes bibliographies.
        1. Obstetrical nursing.   2. Pediatric nursing.
I. Corliss, Charlotte, joint author.   II. Title.
    [DNLM: 1. Obstetrical nursing.   2. Pediatric nursing.
WY157   B863m   1973]
RG951.B77   618.2   73-9784
ISBN 0-397-54140-6

Preface

The maternal-child nurse today comes to her assignment with responsibilities and goals that differ widely from those of the nurse who worked with mothers and children in the past. No longer can she think of the mother or the child as an isolated unit apart from the family as a whole. She has learned that a child's normal growth and development take place within the family unit, and that pregnancy has an impact on the entire family constellation (grandparents included). Family-centered maternal-child nursing means that the nurse considers all of the family members in giving care to the mother, infant or child.

Maternal-Child Nursing is written with a realization of the nurse's need to develop a broad and deep perspective of the meaning of family-centered maternal-child nursing. It endeavors to assist the nurse to catch a glimpse of the past in order to enable her to see where we are now, and how we arrived here. Having come this far, we must now consider what our present weaknesses are and where we still fail the families presently under our care. Because the student is the policy maker of tomorrow, what is she going to do to help solve these problems? What are our responsibilities concerning the future of today's mother and child?

This book includes the basic information necessary for the nurse to care for the mother throughout her pregnancy, labor, delivery and puerperium and to provide nursing care of the newborn, infant, child and adolescent. Material related to care of children has been taken from the second edition of *Foundations of Pediatric Nursing* by Violet Broadribb.

The authors believe that the student needs practical help as well as broad guidelines in planning her nursing care. Included in the text are suggestions concerning the day-by-day care of the mother and child in health and sickness. Some background concerning the effects of illness on the child is given in the belief that the nurse who understands the nature of the condition is better able to give the child the support and physical care necessary for his recovery. Emotional support for the hospitalized patient is extremely important; of equal importance is the physical care the patient receives. Frequently, the physical care given *is* the means by which emotional support is given.

No attempt is made in this book to delve deeply into the psychological aspects of child behavior. However, an introduction to the works of present day psychologists who have done so much to enrich our understanding of childhood has been included. It is hoped that the student will acquire a working knowledge in this area, become motivated to accept the child where he is, and go on from there.

An appreciation of the importance of a child's genetic heritage on his physical health and his personality is also necessary if he is to be cared for intelligently. A brief introduction to basic human genetics is therefore given.

It is also important that the nurse know the medications she administers to her patients. She should have a means for discovering what is the average dose, why the drug is given, its usual effects, and its possible adverse effects. A modified listing of drugs commonly used in maternal-child care, with their usual dosages and their effects is given in the appendix of this book.

Also included in the appendix are the answers to the study questions which appear after the various units in the book.

The major function of this text is to provide a foundation; to help the student lay a groundwork on which she can build to the depth and breadth she needs and desires. The emphasis is on getting started. If she can learn to put herself in the expectant mother's place for a short time, to think the hospitalized child's thoughts and feel his needs, to understand the family's fears and hopes, she will be well on her way toward becoming a successful worker with mothers, children and families.

Violet Broadribb
Charlotte Corliss

Acknowledgments

Grateful appreciation is expressed to the many persons who have assisted us with their encouragement and practical support.

We especially appreciate Miss Cynthia Tice's clear exposition of the Care of the Premature Infant in Chapter 19. We also thank Dr. Donald Broadribb and Dr. Rosemary Broadribb for their major participation in writing the section Psychological Aspects of Growth and Development in Chapter 25.

We thank Dr. C. Woolf of Arizona State University for his counsel and sharing of references on the subject of basic genetic inheritance. We also express appreciation to all those organizations and individuals who contributed generously with reference materials and illustrations and who gave their valuable time in putting together this book.

The Study Questions were contributed by Arizona State University Maternal and Child Nursing faculty.

We thank several illustrators for their excellent drawings and photographs; among whom are Carol Baldwin, Clarice Francone, Peter Whitney, David Poor, and Paul Miller. We are particularly grateful to Larry Kuriger, Medical Photographer at Good Samaritan Hospital in Phoenix, Arizona, and to his assistant, Mrs. Lola Parr, for the outstanding photographs taken in the maternity department.

We thank Mr. David Miller and Miss Mary Dennesaites for their support, advice, and encouragement.

Finally, we wish to express gratitude to those who worked so diligently typing the manuscript.

Violet Broadribb
Charlotte Corliss

Contents

x   *Contents*

Unit One: Introduction to Maternal-Child Nursing

History of Maternal and Child Care

1

FAMILY-CENTERED NURSING

Nursing has traditionally been concerned with the care of the sick. However, to *nurse* has a number of meanings, including "to take charge of or watch over; to promote the development or progress of; to take care of and wait on (as a sick person)."*

For too long a time nurses saw their function restricted to taking care of the sick. Only recently have we come to realize that we have a far more important role—that of helping those under our care to reach and maintain *optimal* physical, mental, and emotional health. Our role does indeed include promoting the development or progress of our fellow human beings.

What do we mean by *optimal* health? The word optimal means most desirable or satisfactory. Therefore maintaining a state of optimal health means far more than keeping free from disease. It means, rather, the ability to live at the highest possible level of physical, mental, and emotional well-being. It encompasses the entire life span, from conception onward. To help others (as well as ourselves) toward this goal is an enormous task we have assumed, but an eminently satisfying one.

In speaking of family-centered nursing we again become aware of a new and broadened concept. We can no longer feed and bathe Johnny, give him his "shots" ("Be a

good boy now and don't cry!"), and cheerfully go off duty feeling we have given adequate nursing care. How much do we know about Johnny? Is he just a young patient having his tonsils out? No person is ever just a patient; no child exists in a vacuum. He has parents, he belongs to a family, a community, a unique way of life. When we insist on separating him from his background, physically or in our thinking, we meet his needs in a most superficial manner, if indeed, we meet them at all.

The same is true for a woman who comes into the hospital to have a baby. She also comes from a family and is influenced by the community in which she lives. We as nurses can no longer just time her contractions in labor and get her into the delivery room on time. We need to consider how much support and comfort she would receive if her husband or someone close to her were at her side during this experience. We need to be aware that when a mother has a baby each member of the family is affected.

It appears then that even if our nursing takes place entirely inside the hospital walls, we are still concerned with family-centered care. Teaching maternal-child nursing as a unit acknowledges how inseparable the individual is from his family and environment. Whether we start with the beginning of the mother's pregnancy or with the beginning of the child's life probably does not matter greatly. In either case we are following a normal sequence.

*Webster's Seventh New Collegiate Dictionary. Springfield, Mass., Merriam Co., 1969.

1

THE PLACE OF THE FAMILY
IN TODAY'S CULTURE

It is generally conceded that the child holds the center place in today's society. But we wonder if perhaps we have become so child-centered in our thinking that we have encouraged the child to believe he is all-important. We have an uneasy feeling that we may have become too child-centered. If so, this is neither in his best interest nor in ours. Children need and want our guidance now as much as they ever did. Perhaps they need more, provided it is honest, thoughtful, and meaningful. But do we know how to give it? Have we become too confused, too uncertain of ourselves to serve as leaders?

If we can spend some time looking at the interrelationships of the child, the family and the community, we should be able to clear up some of our confusion. To get things in proper perspective let us look, briefly, at the past history of family life in society. Such an overview will show us the conse-

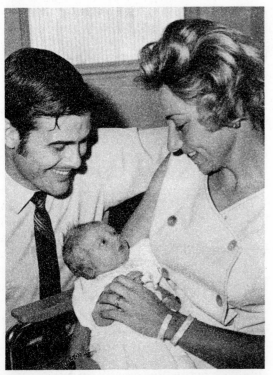

Figure 1-1. The new baby is ready to go home.

quences of certain practices which we can then judge as helpful or deleterious to society in general and to the individual in particular. We will also understand better why and how we arrived where we are. And perhaps we can understand better how to proceed.

The concept of family in any social structure has a distinct bearing on the patterns of child bearing and child rearing. The term extended family is used to denote a grouping of related persons. It may contain grandparents, aunts, uncles and cousins as well as the mother, father, and children. The term nuclear family refers to a smaller unit, that includes the marriage partners and their offspring.

It has been asserted that the nuclear family exists as a distinct and strongly functional group in every society, universally performing four fundamental social functions—sexual, economic, reproductive and educational.* However, the form of the family group has varied widely in different cultures, affecting in turn the manner in which the children are raised:

"Men and women will always go on loving one another, will always go on having children, whether they limit their numbers or give free rein to instinct, and will always go on guiding the first steps of those children. . . . The point is that the ideas entertained about these relations may be dissimilar at moments separated by lengthy periods of time."†

MATERNITY AND CHILD CARE
THROUGH THE AGES

Primitive Societies

Anthropology and archeology have taught us much about the concept of family life in various primitive cultures. Both of these disciplines can give us fascinating glimpses into life as it was lived long ago.

---

*Murdock, G. P.: Social Structure. New York, MacMillan, 1965.
†Aries, P.: Centuries of Childhood. p. 9. New York, Knopf, 1962.

We can also learn much by observing primitive tribes that still follow their old traditions. Inevitably, as contact with present western civilization proceeds, these people become caught up in the twentieth century and quickly discard old methods and beliefs.

The understanding of our own culture is greatly helped by this backward look. We often find that many customs we have discarded contained more than a grain of common sense. Quite frequently we find our scientists proving the value of some practice long ago discarded by Western nations. For instance, we know that when a woman was ready to give birth, she assumed a squatting position or sat on a special birth stool. Although our present-day practice places the delivering mother in a lithotomy position, we are beginning to realize that this works against nature. Thus, a semi-upright position is being advocated by some specialists today.

The kind of life people lead, their geographic location and its climate, and the ease in obtaining the necessities of life, all shape the culture of the society which in turn, exerts a major influence on patterns of child care in the community.

Children generally have been loved and treasured in all cultures, if for no other reason than their future value as members of society. Nomadic groups that had to move quickly from place to place were forced to place the safety and welfare of the group over consideration for any sick, weak, or deformed members. This practical aspect of survival for the tribe undoubtedly was the origin of the practice of infanticide, whereby certain young children were left to die in isolated, exposed places.

Abhorrent as such a custom seems to us, it was not repugnant to those who practiced it. In most primitive societies a child was not considered to be a person possessing a soul until he had received his name and had been presented to the spirits. Therefore, the death of a child before he was named had little significance. Even today, we debate the question of when a child becomes a living human being. Is it at his conception, or at the moment when his mother feels the quickening, or at his birth? And lest we laugh at the notion that the conferring of a name on a child gives him a personality, we must remember that we still have christening rites.

Life in the Ancient World

The people who eventually settled in fertile, well-watered lands developed cultures that gave thought to the welfare of their children. For example, in ancient Egypt children were valued highly, and infanticide was forbidden by law. Children were encouraged in healthful outdoor play, unhampered by restrictive clothing, and were sent to school to learn to read, to write, to figure, and to participate in athletic games.

The study of medicine in Egypt became such a fine art, that the Greeks in later times considered the Egyptians to be the founders of medicine. They were also known to have a collective health scheme and a form of socialized medicine. Much of our knowledge about medical practice in ancient Egypt comes from the Papyrus Ebers, which was written about 1500 B.C. and is a sort of encyclopedia of medical lore, a collection of writings dating from earlier sources. One section is devoted to the diseases of children.

The practice of obstetrics was more sophisticated in Egypt than among more primitive peoples. For instance, forceps were used for delivering babies, cesarean sections were performed on dead mothers, and podalic versions were done. (A podalic version is the process of changing the presenting part of the baby at birth so that the buttocks are born first instead of the head.) It is used infrequently in present day obstetric practice.

In ancient India, a clear, rational doctrine of pediatric medicine appeared during the second and third centuries B.C. Long before that, however, great stress was laid on personal cleanliness and the hygienic preparation of food as a means of maintaining health.

We know that the Greek culture while it fluorished greatly influenced the world and continued to exert its influence in the centuries that followed. The Greeks were a people who rejoiced in life, finding the world beautiful and delightful to live in. The famous Greek physician, Hippocrates (460–375 B.C.) in his voluminous writing, frequently mentioned conditions peculiar to children. In fact, he wrote an entire treatise on the subject of teething. His treatises on obstetric methods are the oldest records on the subject in the Western world.

During the period of Hippocrates normal obstetrical cases were handled by midwives, who were under the supervision of physicians. Abnormal labor and other complications were managed by members of the medical profession. To show how history repeats itself, it seems we might be heading in that same direction in the United States today. Of course, this is the pattern for maternity care now followed in some parts of the world.

We need to keep in mind that anatomy, medicine and the treatment of disease were not understood in ancient times as they are today. Many medications were mixtures of several ingredients in the hope that one would help. The microscope, x-ray machine, and all the present day scientific aids were far in the future. As for the treatment of children, in spite of the few pioneers who recognized that children had special needs, the general view was that children were simply small adults, and they were generally treated as such.

Family Life During the Middle Ages

During the middle ages, most of the enlightened progress made in previous centuries was lost. However, hospitals and nursing services were organized during this age, and history records that there were lying-in hospitals. Lying-in is an old-fashioned term which refers to childbearing. Women were confined during the latter months of pregnancy because it was considered unseemly for them to be seen in public. All they could do was to "lie in" and wait for the baby to arrive. Midwives performed most of the deliveries, and women gave birth on a special stool or obstetric chair. This practice persisted until the 19th century.

Children were considered to be infants until the age of five or six and then were abruptly treated as adults. There seems to have been little place for childhood. Infants were breast-fed by their mothers or by wet nurses for periods of two years and often much longer. (Shakespeare has Juliet weaned at the age of three.) At the age of six or seven when they were scarcely able to care for themselves they were absorbed into the world of adults. Paintings of the day show all young children dressed just like the grownups, all with adult faces. They look like tiny men and women; even the babies have old faces. Children were taught to behave with such formality and awe toward their fathers, that the familiarity we experience in the 20th century would have been unthinkable in the Middle Ages.

Country children were expected to do a man's share of work on the farms. In the towns, boys were apprenticed as young as seven or eight to live, work, and learn a trade in a stranger's house. Even sons and daughters of the nobility were frequently sent to be trained in the homes of others.

Education was practically nonexistent, except for boys going into church service. Even here, the required rituals and formulas were learned by rote, not by reading.

Unhygienic practices were responsible for a high mortality rate, particularly among infants. It is said that out of a family of 14 or 15, only three or four were likely to reach maturity. Parents dared not let themselves become attached to their children; the chances that they would live to grow up were too slim.

The Industrial Revolution

The Industrial Revolution established a pattern of life radically different from the preceding eras. Previously society had consisted of two classes, the rich and the poor. There now arose a middle class to separate the two extremes.

Even so, family customs change slowly. The father of the family remained the head of the household; his word was law and not to be disputed. He had almost unlimited legal rights over his children. The belief of the day was that children were born in sin and were naturally willfully disobedient, wickedly proud, and deceitful. According to this thinking the child's will had to be broken and beaten down by harsh punishment.

Although education was beginning to be valued for boys whose parents could afford it, more attention was paid to whippings and deprivation of privileges than to learning. Education was not thought necessary for girls, and it was said that teaching children of peasants and craftsmen did more harm than good.

Not all fathers, school masters, and employers were sadistic in their use of punishment. Many sincerely believed this was the way to bring up children.

The Industrial Revolution in Europe brought great numbers of poor farm workers and their families into the cities. Thousands of children from six to ten years of age worked in the mills and in underground mines. Many of these children were taken from workhouses and orphanages and worked a 12-hour day, coming in constant contact with all the vices and debaucheries of the period.

Dickens' novels give us a picture of life as a child saw it in schools, workhouses, prisons, and slums. Contemporary accounts show that he did not exaggerate. Undoubtedly he wrote from first-hand experience since he himself was apprenticed at the age of 12 in a shoe-blacking business and lived in a garret (attic) room, while his father was imprisoned for debt.

Industrialists, however, defended their brutal practices. At a hearing held early in the 1800's, one spoke for many mill owners when he testified, "The fingers of children at an early age are very supple, and they are more easily led into habits of performing the duties of their station." Again: "The work is full as well done by children, is better done by children."*

Perhaps we can better understand this state of affairs if we realize that infants and children of unmarried mothers, or of families too poor to care for them, were abandoned in large numbers in the streets of the cities. Unwanted young children thronged the cities and countryside, eating what they could find and sleeping where they could.

Beginnings of Reform in Europe

Throughout history there have always been compassionate people who have rebelled against the harshness of their times. Early in the 19th century, some of these people began to make their voices heard and their influence felt. No doubt there had been many more who were acutely uncomfortable about the hordes of homeless or ill-treated children. Perhaps such concerned people only needed a leader.

Investigation of child-labor practices in Britain was instituted early in 1800. About the same time a committee was appointed to "inquire as to the best means of preventing the destruction of the lives of children put out to hire by their parents."

Some attempts were made to gather at least a few of the abandoned children into shelter. Asylums under the care of the Catholic Church appeared in various cities. Some of the most noteworthy were founded

---

*Gaskell, P.: The Manufacturing Population of England. London, Baldwin and Craddock, 1833 (in the Ford Collection, New York City Public Library).

by St. Vincent de Paul in the early 17th century.

From the 17th through the 19th centuries, children's asylums were established, in several countries, either under religious or secular management. These were not, strictly speaking, hospitals but rather shelters for abandoned infants and children. Later, many of these asylums were converted into children's hospitals for both sick and well children. St. Vincent de Paul reorganized an asylum in 1670 into what is believed to be the first children's hospital. Two hospitals founded in the early 1800's and still functioning are the Hôpital des Enfants Maladies in Paris, and Great Ormond Street Hospital for Sick Children in London. But attempts to rescue impoverished and abandoned children were not always successful.

Children in the United States

In the 1800's the plight of children in the United States was no different from that of children in Europe. Concern over the hordes of homeless children brought about the formation of the Childrens' Aid Society in New York City in 1853. In 1876, the Society for the Prevention of Cruelty to Children (SPCC) was organized: incidentally, an organization to prevent cruelty to animals (SPCA) had been formed much earlier.

Enforceable laws regulating child labor came very late in the United States. Several federal laws were enacted, only to be declared unconstitutional. It was not until 1938 that the Fair Labor Standards Act became federal law, finally putting teeth into the laws abolishing a good portion of child labor.

However, little had been done in earlier years to lower the death rate of infants and young children. Preventive medicine was still in the future. Although no accurate statistics were kept, a study made as late as 1913 estimated that of 2,500,000 babies born each year in the United States, 300,000 died before their first birthday. This gave a ratio of approximately 124 deaths per 1000 live births.

Mothers did not have the most elementary knowledge about infant care, and small children in orphanages or infant homes received little care or attention. Public dismay mounted, and indignation grew.

A letter received by Miss Lillian Wald, founder of the Henry Street Settlement, triggered action in 1903. "Why is it," the writer asked, "so many children die like flies in the summer time? Is there anything I can do to help matters?"

On the same day the letter was received, Miss Wald read in the morning paper an item about the government's concern over the cotton crop. "If the government can have a department to take such an interest in the nation's cotton crop," she questioned, "why can't it have a bureau to look after the nation's crop of children?"*

Miss Wald was a woman of action. Presently she was able to interest President Theodore Roosevelt in her project, and together they worked to mobilize public opinion. The idea gained momentum, but it was not until 1912 that the Children's Bureau came into being.

The first job tackled by the newly formed Bureau was a nationwide study of the high infant mortality problem. After the fact-finding came wide dissemination of expert advice on child care, advice that was desperately needed. The Bureau eventually became the chief agency for dispensing financial and technical aid for the betterment of child welfare.

White House Conference

In 1909, while working actively for child welfare, President Theodore Roosevelt called a conference to consider how the nation could best serve its children. The recommendation of this *First White House Conference* was the formation of a Children's Bureau.

---

*It's Your Children's Bureau: Children's Bureau Publication #357, 1964.

White House Conferences have since been called every ten years by the President of the United States. The meetings provided useful opportunities for discussing child-related problems on a nationwide scale. Recommendations for action are carried back to the states by their representatives.

Some of the conferences have been especially noteworthy. The 1950 Midcentury White House Conference focused on the emotional development of the child. At this conference, the Pledge to Children was written (see page 8).

The Golden Anniversary Conference on Children and Youth in 1960 was attended by over 14,000 persons, including 1400 young people in the high school-to-college age group. Its theme: "To promote opportunities for children and youth to realize their full potential for a creative life in freedom and dignity."

MATERNAL AND CHILD CARE IN THE UNITED STATES IN THIS CENTURY

Looking back over the history of maternity care is like seeing a rerun of an old movie. Although many of our present day practices are similar to the way we did things in the past, some of the changes that have occurred in the past 50 years have led us to our present concept of family-centered maternity nursing. We can divide this 50-year period roughly into three phases.

During the first phase, which began at the turn of the century, most women delivered at home. Pregnancy and childbirth were regarded as a normal and natural biologic process. Women received *little prenatal care* and were delivered by general practitioners and midwives. People knew that there were certain risks involved but they felt that these were inherent in childbearing and no special care was necessary. The nurse had learned to give general care to the mother and baby, but most women depended on nonprofessionals for their nursing care.

During the second phase when more attention was given to prenatal care, the nursing of maternity patients took on a different character. Obstetricians and nurses with interest and experience in the field started maternity care as close to conception as possible and continued it until six weeks after the baby was born. Another trend was toward hospitalization for childbirth.

However, education in maternity nursing remained fixed at three months' training in routine techniques. The nurse's education was oriented toward pathological conditions rather than physiological development and function. It was attuned to complications and surgical techniques, ignoring the impact of the childbearing experience on the mother and on the family as a whole.

The nurse spent most of her time carrying out routines and administrative duties. She had only fragmentary contact with patients. Instead of offering comfort and care to the whole woman, she centered her attentions on the application of impersonal techniques. Her interest in efficient routines overshadowed her concern for patients as individuals.* However, her intentions were the best and she believed that she was providing good nursing care.

The third phase, which began fairly recently, has a striking similarity to the first phase in that we realized that we had almost forgotten the impact that pregnancy and a new baby have on the entire family. Now we are encouraging the husband and wife to share in the childbearing experience. We have found that in many instances husbands cannot be surpassed in giving comfort and support to their wives during labor and delivery, especially when the husband knows what to expect and how he can be of help to his wife.

Many modern hospitals today find that

---

*Corbin, H.: Maternal nurse education— yesterday, today and tomorrow. *Nursing Outlook.* 7:82–84, 1959.

PLEDGE TO CHILDREN

To you, our children, who hold within you our most cherished hopes, we, the members of the Mid-century White House Conference on Children and Youth, relying on your full response, make this pledge:

From your earliest infancy we give you our love, so that you may grow with trust in yourself and in others.

We will recognize your worth as a person and we will help you to strengthen your sense of belonging.

We will respect your right to be yourself and at the same time help you to understand the rights of others; so that you may experience cooperative living.

We will help you develop initiative and imagination, so that you may have the opportunity freely to create.

We will encourage your curiosity and your pride in workmanship, so that you may have the satisfaction that comes from achievement.

We will provide the conditions for wholesome play that will add to your learning, to your social experience, and to your happiness.

We will illustrate by precept and example the value of integrity and the importance of moral courage.

We will encourage you always to seek the truth.

We will provide you with all opportunities possible to develop your own faith in God.

We will open the way for you to enjoy the arts and to use them for deepening your understanding of life.

We will work to rid ourselves of prejudice and discrimination, so that together we may achieve a truly democratic society.

We will work to lift the standard of living and to improve our economic practices, so that you may have the material basis for a full life.

We will provide you with rewarding educational opportunities, so that you may develop your talents and contribute to a better world.

We will protect you against exploitation and undue hazards and help you grow in health and strength.

We will work to conserve and improve family life and, as needed, to provide foster care according to your inherent rights.

We will intensify our search for new knowledge in order to guide you more effectively as you develop your potentialities.

As you grow from child to youth to adult, establishing a family life of your own and accepting larger social responsibilities, we will work with you to improve conditions for all children and youth.

Aware that these promises to you cannot be fully met in a world at war, we ask you to join us in a firm dedication to the building of a world society based on freedom, justice, and mutual respect.

So may you grow in joy, in faith in God and in man, and in those qualities of vision and of the spirit that will sustain us all and give us new hope for the future.

their rooming-in units are in popular demand, particularly by couples who are having their first baby. This arrangement is flexible and natural for feeding, handling, and cuddling the new arrival. The parents can become better acquainted with their child before they take him home where professional help is not as readily available to help them make this adjustment.

Factors Influential in Changing the Concept of Maternity Nursing

First of all, due in large part to the G.I. bill which increased the number of college graduates in this country, there has been a narrowing of the educational gap between the professions and a large segment of the population. Thus more people are aware of the needs of both mother and child.

Today it is generally recognized that education for childbearing and parenthood is an indispensible part of maternity care.

Another factor influencing the concept of maternity nursing has been health and hospital insurance which has increased the number of people who are able to pay for health services. They have a strong voice in the care they receive. But more needs to be done in this area. For example, many young couples cannot afford the high costs of insurance or if they can, maternity benefits prove to be inadequate in many instances.

A third influence for change has been the development of psychosomatic medicine which has brought about a greater awareness of the influence of emotions on body function. There is increased recognition that the mother's emotional attitudes toward childbearing may influence the course of her pregnancy, labor and delivery, and postpartum period. Additionally, there is some evidence that the mother's emotions have an effect on her unborn child.* The quality of the childbearing experience and

---

*Montagu, A.: Life Before Birth. Chapter XI. New York, Signet Books, 1965.

the satisfactions derived from it may affect the development of maternal feelings and the postpartal interaction between the mother and child.

Changes in Children's Hospitals and Institutions

When institutions for child care first came into being, they were notorious for their unsanitary conditions, neglect, and ignorance of proper infant nutrition. Even up into the 19th century, mortality rates were commonly 50 to 100 per cent among institutionalized children, whether in asylums or hospitals.

Eventually, medical personnel in Europe and in the United States became concerned about these appalling conditions, particularly in the numerous foundling homes. As late as 1914 a report made by the New York State Department of Charities on 11 institutions gave a death rate for infants under two years of age at 422.5 per 1000 as against a rate of 87.4 per 1000 in the general population. Indeed, one such institution had a death rate of 100 per cent for all babies under two years of age.

It was known that a major cause of death in children's institutions was the intractable diarrhea which the majority of the children developed. When the simple practice of boiling milk and isolating children with septic conditions was instituted the incidence of diarrhea was lowered.

Once such practices were introduced, a new era began in the institutional care of children, both in hospitals and foundling homes. A period of strict asepsis and isolation began. Babies were placed in individual cubicles, and the nurses were strictly forbidden to pick the children up except when absolutely necessary.

Crib sides were draped with clean sheets, so an infant had nothing to do but stare at the ceiling. The importance of toys in a child's environment was not understood—besides, such objects could carry infection, or so it was reasoned. Visiting hours were limited to parents only, who could visit perhaps an hour or a half hour once a week. They were strictly forbidden to pick up their children under penalty of losing their visiting privileges.

Although aseptic techniques were practiced, the high mortality rate continued. One of the first to suspect the cause was Dr. Joseph Brennaman of Children's Memorial Hospital, Chicago. He reasoned that the infants suffered from a lack of stimulation. When writing in 1932 about the management of the infant ward in his hospital, he made a rule that every infant must be picked up and carried around several times a day. He also made a firm rule that no infant who could be cared for at home should be admitted to the hospital, and every infant should be discharged as soon as possible.

Other concerned specialists entered the fight. In the 1940's René Spitz published the results of studies which he believed proved his contention that deprivation of maternal care caused a state of dazed stupor in an infant. He believed this condition could become irreversible if the child was not returned to his mother promptly. He termed this state *anaclitic depression*. He also coined the term *hospitalism* which he defined as "a vitiated [weakened] condition of the body due to long confinement in the hospital." Later the term came to be used almost entirely to denote the evil effects of institutional care on infants. Another physician, Dr. H. Bakwin, found that infants hospitalized for long periods actually developed physical symptoms, which he attributed to insufficient emotional stimulation and feeding satisfaction.

Dr. John Bowlby of London, working under the auspices of the World Health Organization, thoroughly explored the subject of maternal deprivation. His report in 1951 received world-wide attention. His study concentrated on the results of the separation of the hospitalized child from his mother. His work, together with that of John Robertson, an associate, led to a re-evaluation of hospital visiting policies for children. Present day thinking has clarified and modified this thinking to some extent.

Recent Trends in Care of Children in Hospitals

One result of the studies and observations of the effect of hospitalization on children was a gradual change in hospital policies.

A slow, cautious relaxation of isolation practices for children who did not have infectious diseases *did not* result in cross-contamination as many had believed. Children were allowed to play together, and a few toys were provided and exchanged between them. For some time, however, a truly conscientious nurse carefully washed (or even soaked in a disinfectant) any toy that had passed from one child to another or had dropped on the floor.

If hospitalized children were to play together, they had to be out of bed. Here, too, progress was gradual. The new practice of getting adult patients up much earlier was cautiously tried with children. One didn't quite know whether this was safe — children play so hard and run fevers so easily! Besides, when they were up and about, they *did* get underfoot so! How much easier to care for a ward full of children each sitting quietly in his bed, staring listlessly at a well-worn picture book!

Unfortunately for the above concept but most fortunately for the children, it was found that children got well much faster when allowed up. Since it proved to be impossible to make them sit in chairs and be quiet, it became expedient to set aside a certain section of the department as a play area. This in turn called for a larger supply of playthings. Eventually, many hospitals provided playrooms which opened a few hours a day whenever volunteers were available to supervise the children.

The employment of "play ladies" or trained *recreational directors* on a part-time basis when hospitals could afford it was another step forward. In some instances this led to full-time employment of play

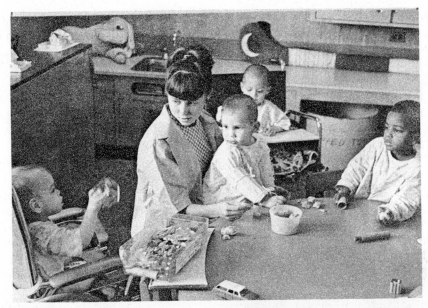

Figure 1-2.   In the children's ward of the hospital patients may play together.

leaders for children's departments. The play leader directs activities, supervises volunteers, and attempts to provide some interesting pastimes for children who must remain on bed rest. Unfortunately, their case loads are large and their administrative duties heavy. Closed playrooms and locked toy cupboards are still the rule when volunteer play ladies or helpers are not available.

Liberalized Visiting Hours

A great boon to hospitalized children occurred when visiting hours were extended. The majority of hospitals shifted from weekly or semimonthly visiting hours to daily periods of one or two hours in the afternoon. Visitors were still restricted to the child's parents or a parent substitute. The only times exceptions were made were just before a child went to surgery or when he had been officially designated as critically ill. Even these exceptions were hedged about with rules, at times with tragic results. For example one mother was not allowed to see her seriously ill child because the resident doctor failed to put the child's name on the "danger list." She returned home, only to receive a phone call informing her that her child had just died.

While some hospitals were liberalizing their visiting hours, hospitals for chronic or long-term illnesses still limited visiting hours to weekly or, frequently, monthly "visiting days" when parents could come during specified hours. The proponents of this policy argued that since these were regional hospitals, set up to serve an entire region of the United States, parents who lived far away could not get to visit their children frequently, perhaps coming only when the child was admitted or discharged. It was therefore argued that these children would suffer when they saw more fortunate children visited by their parents. The idea of *foster grandparents*, older women employed to visit children in hospitals and to cuddle and play with them, was still in the future.

Parents were still denied the right to care for their own children in the hospital. This extended even to changing a baby's diaper or giving a child a drink of water. Whenever possible, nursing procedures were carried out before visiting hours, thereby losing invaluable teaching oppor-

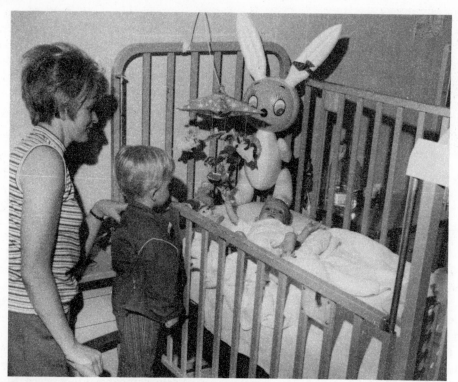

Figure 1-3. A visit from the family helps the small patient toward a speedier recovery. (Courtesy Good Samaritan Hospital, Phoenix.)

tunities which most parents would have welcomed. Whenever any nursing care had to take place during visiting hours, parents were promptly sent out of the room. No one seemed to realize that this removed the child's only emotional support. It is difficult to see the reason behind these regulations, beyond the obvious fact that the nurses might feel uncomfortable if the parents observed their actions. The child's comfort and emotional security were ignored.

Slowly, a new concept was accepted in a few children's departments. New, that is, to us in our culture, but actually as old as time. We actually were willing to let a few parents stay in the hospital with their children and participate in their care! This did indeed seem revolutionary. At the present time we have come to realize the wisdom of such a plan and, indeed, have gone far beyond this concept.

Recent Advances

To the child the nurse in her white uniform, or large white apron, with her strange looking white cap, was seen as a symbol of authority, thereby intensifying the child's fear of the strange hospital appearance and its frightening apparatus. When hospital administrators realized that this further threatened the child's adjustment to the hospital, a move was proposed to put pediatric nurses in colored uniforms, minus caps.

Eventually many schools adopted a plain, colored dress without apron or cap for their student nurses. In some medical centers where students came from many schools for their pediatric clinical experience, there was a veritable rainbow of colors. Canary yellow, peacock blue, light and dark green, and pink dresses brightened the wards.

That the severe appearance of the nurse

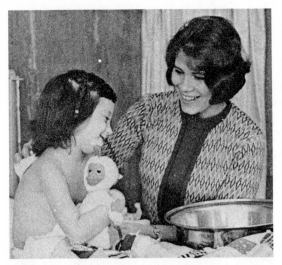

Figure 1-4. Parents can participate in their child's hospital care.

in white dress, footwear and cap did symbolize an unpleasant experience and an invasion of privacy, to some children at least, can perhaps be illustrated by the following amusing anecdote.

A group of students in ordinary street dress visited a classroom of deaf children. These children were being taught to read lips and to form words, so naturally the teachers seized every opportunity for teaching. One teacher had posted a picture of a nurse in uniform on the bulletin board in anticipation of the visit. "Now, children," she said when the nurses arrived, "we talked this morning about these young ladies. Who can point to the picture and tell us what they are?"

Jimmy thought he could. Going to the board he pointed to the picture of the uniformed nurse and said just one word— "Witch!"

CHANGING ATTITUDES TOWARD CHILDREN IN THE HOME

The strict authoritarian approach to childrearing continued on well through the first half of the 20th century. According to the philosophy of the day babies must be fed on a very strict schedule. If one were a conscientious mother, one did not dare feed her crying baby 15 minutes early. Who knew what harm she might do him! We can now feel pity for the poor baby who finally dropped off into an exhausted sleep, only to be shaken and slapped into wakefulness for the feeding denied him a short time earlier.

Mothers took the advice of writers on child care very seriously. They worked hard at molding their children into strict routines of eating, sleeping and early toilet training. It was considered of paramount importance to start a child, right from birth, on an impersonal, rigid routine. This would set the pattern for his future life and mold his character.

Babies were not to be picked up when they cried. This would soon teach them that they could not have their own way (the old concept of breaking the child's will). Mothers worked so hard at "bringing their children up properly" that they had little time to really enjoy their young children. (One suspects that the young children didn't enjoy life much either.)

Slowly, the tide began to turn. Parents and child-concerned specialists began to see children as individuals with developing personalities, who need opportunity and encouragement to develop and grow, each according to his own pattern. Dr. Spock's sensible advice to mothers, "Enjoy your baby" came as a welcome relief. His *Common Sense Book of Baby and Child Care* was just that, a guide toward common sense in child raising.

Trend Toward Unlimited Permissiveness

It appears to be a trait of human nature to go from one extreme to the other. Thus common sense in childrearing seems to have been forgotten and childhood was again viewed out of proportion. It was now believed that one must not discipline or thwart a child for fear of harming his ego and warping his personality. The fact that an immature child, unfamiliar with the world, needs and wants guidance was forgotten. The child's rights were paramount; parents' rights ceased to exist.

We are now unhappy with the results of such permissiveness. Strangely enough, such men as Gesell and Spock, who did so much to relieve the tyranny of authoritative parental control, are now accused of setting the stage for complete elimination of controls. Anyone who takes the trouble to read their writings will find this accusation to be untrue.

CHILDREARING CHANGES DURING THE PAST CENTURY*

1880's-1900's. Discipline was based upon authority with instant, unquestioning obedience expected. Training was directed toward "uprooting the evil in human nature."

The Society for the Prevention of Cruelty to Children was organized to attack cruel ways of treating children. Articles on the subject mentioned that children were given "whippings until bruised and sore," were "shut in dark closets until ill with fright," and were "depriv[ed] of food until emaciated and feeble."

School authorities expected instantaneous obedience, "no sulkers, laggards or independents." All students were to move "uniformly, quietly and instantly."

1900's-1920's. Discipline in schools was still a major issue. Sixteen out of eighteen schools questioned in a survey still reported the use of corporal punishment. Some qualified this by saying "as a last resort," or "never punish in anger." Advice was to "use a switch on legs or ruler on palm of hands, but never box the ears."

The first edition of *Child Care,* published by the Children's Bureau, recommended

pinning a baby's sleeve down over his hand to stop thumbsucking.

The writings of psychologists and educators such as Marie Montessori, John Dewey, and Sigmund Freud were beginning to be mentioned frequently in popular literature. A movement was started to give children "freedom to develop."

1920's-1940's. Although emphasis on the child and a "child-centered approach" appears often in the literature, rigid patterns of childrearing prevailed. No deviation from set schedules for feeding, sleeping, toilet training in early infancy was allowed. An objective viewpoint toward children prevailed; parents were advised to be "cool, detached and unperturbed."

Discussion of spanking as discipline continued among parents, but corporal punishment was decreasing in the schools.

1940's-1960's. Strict childrearing practices commenced to give way to flexible, permissive ways with children. Sibylle Escalona contrasted the past with the more recent thinking. "It is now thought that it is up to us as adults to meet the needs of the younger child, rather than to expect early adaptation from him." "We prize self-expression, sincerity of feeling and spontaneous interest above good manners, self-restraint or intellectual accomplishment."*

It seems inevitable that the tide would turn from the permissive practices of the 1960's toward a more limit-setting approach. In 1969, Bruno Bettelheim wrote "I consider it not at all startling that we encounter violence today on our campuses and on our streets. We are engaged in a process of removing inner and outer controls, and as long as the process is not reversed, ours will become a time of more violence still."†

*Freely adapted from Duvall, E. M.: *Family Development.* ed. 4, Philadelphia, J. B. Lippincott 1971.

*Escalona, S.: A commentary upon some recent changes in child-rearing practices." *Child Development,* 20:157, 1949.
†Bettelheim, B.: Children Must Learn to Fear, *New York Times,* April 13, 1969.

BIBLIOGRAPHY

Along the road to modern medicine. World Health Magazine. May, 1970.

Aries, Phillipe: Centuries of Childhood. New York, Knopf, 1962.

Bakwin, H.: Emotional deprivation of infants. Journal of Pediatrics, *35:*512, 1949.

Bullough, Vern L. and Bullough, Bonnie: The Emergence of Modern Nursing. ed. 2. New York, Macmillan, 1969.

Cianfrani, Theodore: A Short History of Obstetrics and Gynecology. ch. 1. Springfield, Ill., Charles C Thomas, 1960.

Duvall, Evelyn Millis: Family Development. ed. 4. Philadelphia, J. B. Lippincott, 1971.

Gaskell, P.: The Manufacturing Population of England. London, Baldwin & Craddock, 1833.

Murdock, George Peter: Social Structure. New York, Macmillan, 1969.

Spitz, R.: Anaclytic depression. Psychoanalytic Studies of Children, *2:*313, 1946.

————: Hospitalism. Psychoanalytic Studies of Children, *1:*53, 1945.

U.S. Dept. of Health, Education and Welfare. It's Your Children's Bureau. Washington, D.C., Government Printing Office, 1964.

Suggested Readings for Further Study

Bell, John E. and Bell, Elisabeth A.: Family participation in hospital care for children. Children, *17:*154, 1970.

Brown, Ivor: Dickens and His Time. London, Nelson, 1963.

Jameson, Edwin M.: Gynecology and Obstetrics, ch. 1. New York, Hafner Co., 1962.

National Geographic Society: Everyday Life in Ancient Times. Washington, D.C., National Geographic Society, 1963.

Queen, Stuart A. and Haberstein, Robert W.: The Family In Various Cultures. Philadelphia, J. B. Lippincott, 1967.

Present Day Trends in Maternity and Child Nursing 2

Much of our present day thinking about maternity and child nursing is the result of the work done by pioneers in recent years. However, we have modified some of their conclusions as we have progressed in our understanding of the relationship of each member to the family group.

No one will dispute the contention that deprivation of emotional support, especially in early childhood, has disastrous effects on a child. Certainly we believe that a child thrives best when he has a mother figure to sustain him, someone he can trust absolutely. He needs to know that someone is always there—to come to his defense, to shield him from harm, to comfort and sustain him.

We know now that a rejecting mother, a mother figure who does not give the child the security and support he must have, cannot possibly be meeting his needs. However, the mother who actually rejects her child in this manner should not be confused with the woman who in the early part of her pregnancy wishes that she were not pregnant. This is not a true rejection of the baby, because these feelings often disappear after the first three months of pregnancy. (See Chapter 6 for further discussion.) Thus if these feelings occur, the woman should not fear that she is going to reject her baby and be a bad mother.

NEW TRENDS IN MATERNITY CARE

Preparation for Hospitalization

Anyone old enough to understand has a right to be well informed about a forth-coming hospital experience. In this age of mass communication it might be expected that the general public would be well prepared for hospitalization. We know, however, that this is not the case. People tend to concentrate on the potentially painful aspects of unpleasant experiences. It is their way of preserving their self-respect, of

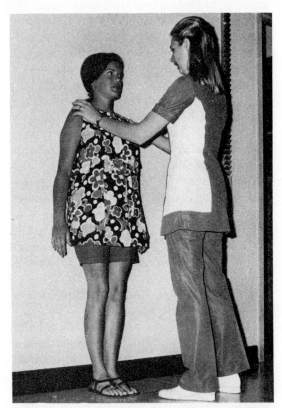

Figure 2-1. The instructor helps an expectant mother with her posture at a childbirth education class.

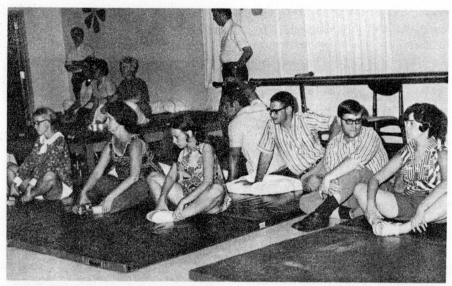

Figure 2-2. Expectant parents learn helpful exercises at a prenatal exercise class. (Courtesy Good Samaritan Hospital, Phoenix.)

proving to themselves that they really are brave in the face of danger or discomfort. Thus, expectant parents are frequently exposed to many horror tales about complications of pregnancy and difficult deliveries. To dispel these fears, it becomes especially important to prepare both parents for labor, delivery, and the hospital experience.

A woman going into the hospital to have a baby without any preparation as to what to expect has many fears, especially if this is the first time she has ever been in a hospital. This fact coupled with her lack of knowledge about what labor will be like and what will happen to her and her baby increases her apprehension. Programs which prepare couples for parenthood through reading, childbirth education classes, and tours of the hospital's obstetrical department aim at dispelling these fears.

Thus couples who are expecting a baby, especially their first child, are encouraged to attend parent education classes. The classes cover a wide range of subjects, from the anatomy and physiology of the male and female reproductive systems to relaxation techniques for the mother during labor.

One of the highlights of the class is a tour of the obstetrical department. During the tour the parents have an opportunity to see the nursery, the labor and delivery rooms, and the postpartum unit. The object of the tour is to remove some of the parents' fear by familiarizing them with the hospital environment. Some hospitals show movies which prepare the parents for what will happen to them from the time the woman is admitted to the hospital in labor until she and the baby are discharged. However, some movies with scenes of the woman in labor and delivery have been known to produce more fear than they dispel. Thus movies should be carefully selected and shown by a person who can adequately discuss questions raised by parents seeing the film.

Other means of preparing parents for parenthood are the Grantly Dick-Read method of "natural childbirth" and the Lamaze method of psychoprophylaxis for childbirth. (These two widely used methods in training for childbirth will be discussed in more detail in Chapter 7.)

Fathers in the Labor and Delivery Rooms

In many maternity departments the husband or a relative or close friend is encouraged to stay with a woman in labor. In this way she can derive comfort and reassurance from having someone she knows and loves with her during this sometimes trying and emotional experience. Being left alone in labor should not happen to any woman!

It is common practice to have fathers in the labor room with their wives, usually up until the time the woman is ready to be taken into the delivery room. Not only is the husband useful because of the emotional support he can give his wife, but if he has been prepared for his role he can also comfort his wife by rubbing her back (giving sacral pressure during contractions), reminding her to do the breathing and relaxation techniques she learned, doing pelvic lifts, helping her into a more comfortable position, and timing her contractions. Fathers are no longer merely tolerated in the labor rooms; in fact their efforts to assist their wives are welcomed by hospital staff. They are often an important member of the team (indispensible in their wives' opinions).

Now husbands and wives are asking to carry this togetherness one step farther; they would like husbands to be allowed into the delivery rooms. This request has met with a great deal of opposition from both doctors and nurses. Those who oppose the idea argue that the husband will probably faint, presenting the staff with another patient to take care of. Others think of the danger of a lawsuit. Some contend that the husband might introduce infection into the delivery room. Finally, others argue that if the delivery is complicated and something happens to the mother or the baby it would be an emotionally traumatic experience for the husband. However, there are no studies to support any of these arguments.

When promoting the idea of allowing fathers into delivery room the first principle is to allow the father to make the choice. He should be given the option of going with his wife if he wants to. He should not be excluded arbitrarily nor should he

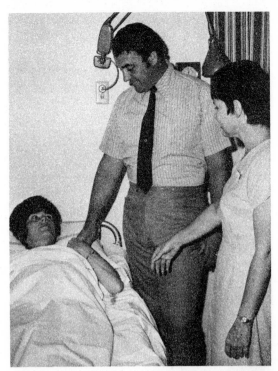

Figure 2-3. A husband gives emotional support to his wife in labor. (Courtesy Good Samaritan Hospital, Phoenix.)

be forced to go against his will or made to feel guilty if he does not want to.

Secondly, he should be prepared for the experience by attending expectant parents classes, by reading, or by learning from other instructional means. He should know that his role in the delivery room is to continue to support and encourage his wife in her efforts to deliver their baby. Therefore, he should be up at the head of the table—talking to her, holding her hand, wiping her face. He should not be down at the foot of the delivery table.

Some American hospitals which have allowed husbands and wives to be together in the delivery room have had good results. Now more and more hospitals, in response to demands by the expectant parents themselves or by other interested groups such as the ICEA (International Childbirth Education Association), are opening delivery rooms to fathers. One of the foremost champions of this policy is Dr. Robert Bradley, author of *Husband-Coached Childbirth.*

However, until the doctors, nurses, and other personnel in the labor and delivery room accept this philosophy and see the value of it, it will not work out successfully. As with the policy of rooming-in, the personnel must wholeheartedly understand, accept, and support the principle of having fathers in the delivery room if it is to work.

Visits by Children

Another trend in hospital maternity departments (less common than having husbands in the labor rooms) is to allow children to visit their mother while she is in the hospital. Some of the thinking behind this is that the children need contact with their mother and she with them. Instead of being mystified about where mother went suddenly, they can see her and, sometimes, their new brother or sister. This lessens the amount of separation-anxiety experienced by both the mother and the children. The children know where their mother is and are reassured that she has not gone off and left them as a sort of punishment for some real or imagined misdeed.

Trend Toward Continuity in Maternity Care

Author Anne Hilliard, in an article titled "New Horizons in Maternity Nursing," notes that we use an assembly-line approach in giving care to maternity patients. The different stations to which an expectant mother must go when she attends clinic for her prenatal care are described in Chapter 6. This method is employed for the sake of efficiency so that the most number of women can be seen in the least amount of time.

When the expectant mother comes to the hospital to have her baby, she is again processed through labor and delivery. The focus of attention is on her abdomen and the baby she is carrying and the progress of her labor. After she has delivered, she is taken to the recovery room where her abdomen and perineal pads are frequently inspected. Her baby also undergoes a series of inspec-

tions. If mother and child pass these examinations, the mother is sent to a postpartum unit and the baby, to a nursery. In each of these areas, labor and delivery, recovery room, postpartum, and the nursery, the mother must try to relate to different nursing personnel who often ask the same questions: "What baby is this for you?" and "Did you have a boy or a girl?" Sometimes they perform the most intimate kinds of physical care on the mother without adequate explanations. After a stay of two or three days, if the mother and baby both pass the various examinations and inspections, they are discharged from the hospital. As they leave, the mother is admonished by the hospital staff to return to the clinic in four weeks so the baby can be checked, and six weeks so she herself can be examined. No wonder that the mother feels like an object when she is treated in this manner.

One way to do away with this fragmented kind of nursing care would be to have the same nurse attend to the maternity patient throughout her hospital stay. Ideally the nurse would first meet the expectant mother in the prenatal clinic or doctor's office and get to know her there. The nurse would be with the mother through labor giving her and her husband physical care and emotional support. The nurse would go to the delivery room with the patient and continue her support and care there. She would then accompany the patient to the recovery room and in the following days care for the mother and baby until they are discharged from the hospital. If home visits are wanted (or needed) by the family, this same nurse would make the visits as frequently as necessary.

Is this kind of care feasible? In answer to this question we might note that this is how nurse-midwives are functioning now, particularly in other countries of the world, and in some nursing schools the learning experiences for student nurses in maternity nursing are planned along these lines. Not only would this approach provide a more satisfying experience for the mother and her family in most instances, but it would also be a more rewarding and challenging experience for the nurse.

Home Delivery Versus Hospital Delivery

There are many advantages for a woman having a baby at home. For one thing the emotional support offered by her husband and family is more readily available than in the hospital. Secondly, it is less expensive to have a baby at home than in a hospital. And thirdly, there is less danger of infections that may cause complications for the infant and the mother. For example, in the 1950's when certain strains of antibiotic-resistant staphylococci were prevalent in hospital nurseries it was dangerous to have a baby in the hospital. If an infant picked up this infection, the result could be serious illness and even death. If the baby had been born at home, during this period the danger would have been less.

The main disadvantage of home deliveries is the lack of services, sophisticated equipment and techniques, and trained personnel available in the hospital. For this reason most doctors in the United States refuse to do home deliveries. So for most women there is no choice. Hospital deliveries with the advantages of trained personnel, blood transfusions, medications, and emergency equipment are credited with the dramatic reduction of maternal and infant mortality rates in the United States.

In other countries where home deliveries are more commonplace, and where the emotional advantages to the mother are more highly regarded, the practice seems to work quite well. It would appear that the practice has a place in the United States also. However, it seems doubtful that home deliveries will become a major trend.

Nurse-Midwives in the United States

So far the United States has lagged behind other countries in the use of nurse-midwives. Even if a certified nurse-midwife were available and wanted to practice, it would not be legally possible for her to do so in those states which refuse to license nurse-midwives.

The opposition to nurse-midwives stems from the term midwife itself. People, including those in the medical professions, tend to associate it with "granny midwives," many of whom still practice in parts of the United States where there is a larger percentage of underprivileged and uneducated people. These women have learned their work by word of mouth or sometimes by watching unskilled or unscrupulous "granny midwives" deliver babies. Thus the term midwife has fallen into disrepute.

To remedy this situation members of the medical profession have suggested using titles such as obstetrical assistant or obstetrical technician. However, members of the American College of Nurse-Midwifery object to changing the title. Their reasoning is that it is a title which is understood internationally. Furthermore, the term midwife means "with woman," which they believe describes the essence of their profession.

While this debate rages, inadequate obstetrical care in the United States continues owing to our shortage of doctors. Even though the national birth rate is declining, the number of doctors available is declining more rapidly. Thus the need for clinically prepared and certified nurse-midwives is becoming more pressing.

The first use of professionally trained nurse-midwives in the United States was made by the Frontier Nursing Service in Wendover, Kentucky, in 1925 under the late Mrs. Mary Breckenridge. In the 1950's there were only five or six programs in the United States which prepared nurse-midwives for certification. There are now at least 12 such programs, which can be divided into two groups—those that prepare a registered nurse to become certified and those which lead to a master's degree and a certificate in nurse-midwifery. The training period for the former programs usually lasts from six months to a year; the latter lasts about 12 months to two years. Loans, scholarships, and financial aid now are

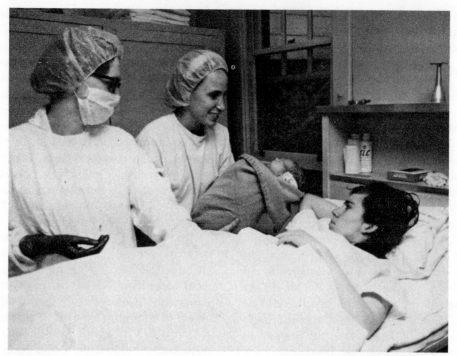

Figure 2-4.   Nurse-midwives show a mother her new baby. (Courtesy of Frontier Nursing Service, Wendover, Ky. Photograph by Vision Associates.)

available to those wishing to enter midwifery programs.

How does a nurse-midwife function? Much depends on whether she practices in an urban or rural area. The midwife in the city practices in hospital maternity departments and clinics. The patient on her first visit to the prenatal clinic is examined by both the nurse-midwife and the physician. If she appears to have no complications or abnormalities, she can decide whether she wishes the physician or the nurse-midwife to care for her throughout her pregnancy. If the nurse-midwife is chosen, she follows the patient throughout her pregnancy, supports her throughout labor, and delivers the baby. She observes the patient's condition throughout the immediate postpartum period and gives her emotional support. She also assumes a teaching role, such as helping the mother to learn to breast feed her infant. Throughout this entire period of pregnancy and delivery a doctor is available for consultation should any complications arise.

NEW TRENDS IN CHILD CARE

Preparing the Child for Hospitalization

Parents have an obligation to prepare their children for a hospital experience. In the past, adults frequently failed to consider a child's feelings or to view the world from the child's point of view. When their children misbehaved they often threatened to send for the policeman or the doctor. Doctors, policemen, even school principals were presented to the child as dispensers of punishment for disobedience.

Consequently, it was perfectly natural for the child, entering the hospital as a patient and seeing the array of mysterious, potentially punishing apparatus, to believe that his worst fears had been realized. He had been continually reminded of his badness at home; now he was about to receive the punishment so often promised. No wonder he was paralyzed with fear. When his parents prepared to go home and leave him, it is no wonder he cried out in terror, "Take me with you! I'll be good!"

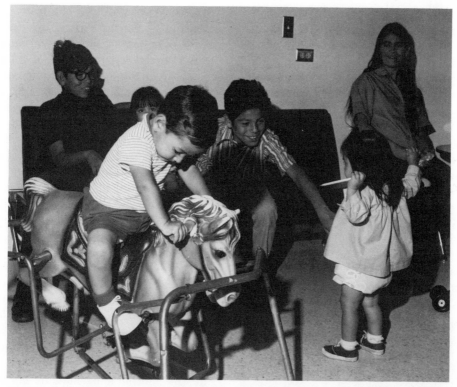

Figure 2-5. Hospitalized children play with their brothers and sisters in this playroom. (Courtesy of Maricopa County General Hospital, Phoenix.)

It is true that most parents feel as much apprehension about hospitals as their children do. But how much does the average parent know about the children's division of the hospital? Present day trends toward liberalizing visiting hours have been useful for the parent as well as for the child. A mother can see what is going on, and the child can find security in her presence. A few hospitals have set up special procedures similar to those for expectant parents for acquainting children and their parents with the hospital setting.

A group of young school children may be given a guided tour of a children's department. They are taken into a demonstration ward where they can experiment with the cribs, raising and lowering the sides and even climbing into one of the cribs to get the feel. They try out the call bell, examine bedside tables, and ask questions. They usually get a peep at the playroom, meet some of the nurses, and perhaps wind up the tour

with ice cream and cookies. All this does not mislead the child into believing that a hospital is entirely a fun place; he knows better. But it does help remove the strangeness.

When such a routine is not practical, the least that can be done is to encourage a parent to visit the department before her child is admitted. She can then relay her knowledge to him and play "going to the hospital" to give him some familiarity with the routine. In some children's departments, the prospective patient is allowed to make this visit with his mother. If he is to be admitted shortly, he is no more likely to bring infection into the department than he will on admission as a patient.

Rooming-in for Mothers and Children

Those hospitals which make provision for a parent to live in the hospital with the child are still in the minority. Some allow this only if a child has a private room or if he is under the age of three. Others keep some departments open to parents throughout the day and allow a parent to sit beside her child during the night if necessary. Still others provide sleeping accommodations for parents even when their children are in a ward.

Developing countries have generally taken it for granted that the child's mother (or other relatives) will live in the hospital with him. Today, in many countries the family of the patient is generally welcomed, except in those hospitals trying to adopt Western standards. Some nurses trained in the west see the patient as their only responsibility; others see the whole family as clients of the hospital and seize the opportunity to offer some teaching on

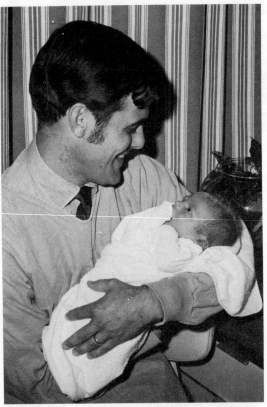

Figure 2-6. A father has an opportunity to get acquainted with his new baby in a rooming-in unit. (Courtesy Good Samaritan Hospital, Phoenix.)

health practices. "For children . . . regular continuing contacts with parents and relatives offer more psychological support than any contrived expressions of affection and concern, or any gift. . . . Participation of the family in hospital care is not an exotic curiosity, but a natural expression of family conviction strongly adhered to in three-fourths of the world. The practice is followed because it is a humane response to the rights of children."*

Rooming-in has a somewhat different connotation in the obstetrical department than it does in the pediatric department. There is a trend toward giving a maternity patient the option of rooming-in when she comes to the hospital to have her baby.

This is a flexible plan whereby the parents can see and care for their newborn infant as much as they desire. There are many different versions of rooming-in. Some plans have the baby with the mother 24 hours a day, and other plans have the baby at the mother's bedside at certain hours during the day. The point is that rooming-in is more a philosophy of care than a specific plan of care. The father is encouraged to handle and even to feed and bathe his infant provided he wears a hospital gown over his street clothes and washes his hands to minimize the possibility of infection.

It is interesting to see that even in more traditional obstetrical departments where babies are brought out to the mothers at scheduled intervals, there is a trend toward having the fathers present at feeding times.

Parent Care in the Pediatric Department

A plan for parents to take care of a hospitalized child was inaugurated in 1966 at the University of Kentucky Medical Center and has proved very satisfactory. Its originator, Dr. James, says, "In most parts

---

*Bell, J. E., and Bell, E. A.: Family participation in hospital care for children. *Children*, *17*:154, 1970.

of the world, parents care for their children in hospitals. Only in our culture do we turn the child completely over to professional personnel."*

An 18-bed department is set aside for the patients cared for by the Care by Parent Plan. "Mothers live in with their children and are taught to give them complete care. Unless the child needs specialized nursing care the mother gives her child his medicines, bathes him, collects specimens, gives treatments such as eye drops, etc., takes his temperature, and keeps precise records. Trained assistants are on duty in the department; a registered nurse comes from the adjoining clinic only if called. At night, the mothers are alone with their children and have access to an emergency call bell. Although the parent staying with the child is usually the mother, the father occasionally relieves her. This program has proved successful enough to have been started in several other medical centers.

Recreational Opportunities

In some forward-looking hospitals, considerable imagination is used in providing the hospitalized child with opportunities for play. We now understand that "play is the business of children," and that the child who is denied the right to play is deprived of the principal means for healthy development. We are beginning to realize how much we hinder the sick child by denying him the right to play in the hospital.

In one children's hospital, tricycles are being ridden up and down the corridor. Unless things get out of hand, no one is told to be quiet, or to "play in your room." One little fellow is apprehended by a friendly intern and presented with a traffic ticket, much to his delight.

Opportunity for active games is provided for those whose medical condition allows it.

---

*MD's new aid: mother. *Medical World News,* Aug. 20, 1970, p. 15.

Crafts, ceramics, and table games are available for those who must be quiet. A children's library is also handy.

Provision for play out of doors (or quiet observation) is a valuable aid toward restoring health. Few hospitals have broad tree-shaded lawns any more, but playgrounds are sometimes available. Failing these, the solariums and sun decks can be used as play areas to help take the emphasis off the institutional atmosphere.

Of course the active play described above presupposes that these children are dressed in daytime clothes. It is difficult to run around in poorly fitting pajamas, cloth slippers, and a dragging bathrobe. In fact it seems difficult to justify the use of night clothing for children who are up and about. Simple cotton suits and dresses are no more difficult to make and launder than hospital gowns and pajamas.

Mealtime

An encouraging trend is that of serving meals around a table, family style. Since eating is a social function, few enjoy eating alone. Yet we are apt to forget this when handing out trays to children, one by one. Since serving oneself from a serving dish is satisfying, a child is much more likely to eat what he has taken for himself than what is set down before him in ready-made plates.

Balanced diets are certainly desirable, especially for a sick child, but we have finally come to realize that wholesome food placed on a child's tray and returned to the kitchen uneaten does nothing for a child's nutrition. Another appetite booster is the newer practice, in some hospitals, of giving children menus to check. Of course, the menu items should be written in terms the child can understand. Beatrice Bachrach tells about the boy who enviously watched his neighbor enjoying a hot dog on a bun. He had not ordered one for himself because, he said, it was not on the menu. When shown the item "frankfurter on a bun," he said, "Oh, is that what a frankfurter is?" She also cites the children's interpretation of "molded Waldorf salad" as "It's moldy."*

Care at Home

A question about the necessity of putting small children in the stress situation of a hospital has nagged at the consciousness of some people for a long time. It is good to see that this concern is beginning to appear in print. One eminent child psychologist writes:

"If parents and physicians were willing to make an effort not to hospitalize children, many sick children might be nursed effectively at home. Much hospital equipment is portable: beds, crouptents, intravenous stands. With a visiting nurse as a daily consultant, the mother may be able to care for the child herself. Homemaker services— if available—might be called in to assume some of the household burdens while the mother is so occupied. . . . This assumes, of course, that these supporting services exist in the locality in sufficient quantity to be available when needed."†

Pediatric Nurse Practitioners

A fairly new field of great promise for the nurse is that of the nurse practitioner. The pediatric nurse practitioner or pediatric specialist finds a place waiting for her in the well-child conference, in pediatrics clinics, and in the community. She also acts as a consultant to the generalized pediatric nurse.

Such a nurse receives special preparation. She is able to furnish comprehensive care to well children of all ages and can identify acute and chronic childhood illnesses and refer them to the proper facilities for treatment. She can temporarily manage

emergency situations until medical help is available.

Programs for the preparation of nurse practitioners have been set up in several collegiate programs. A new venture of specialization on the baccalaureate level has been described in *Nursing Outlook.**

BIBLIOGRAPHY

Bell, John E.: The Family in the Hospital. Chevy Chase, Md., National Institute of Mental Health, 1969.
Bell, John E. and Bell, Elisabeth A.: Family participation in hospital care for children. Children, *17*:154, 1970.
Chioni, Rose Marie and Panicucci, Carol: Tomorrow's nurse practitioners, Nursing Outlook. *18*:32, 1970.
Haller, J. Alex, ed.: Hospitalized Child and His Family, Baltimore, Johns Hopkins, 1967.
Hilliard, A.: New horizons in maternity nursing. Nursing Outlook, *15*:33, 1967.
Markowitz, Milton and Gordis, Leon: A family pediatric clinic. Children, *14*:25, 1967.
M.D.'s New Aid. Medical World News, August 28, 1970.
Millar, T. P.: The hospital and the preschool children. Children, *17*:171, 1970.
Ruderman, Florence A.: Child Care and Working Mothers. chap. 12. New York, Child Welfare League of America, 1968.
Standards of Adoption Service, New York, Child Welfare League of America, 1968.

Suggested Readings for Further Study

Adams, Martha L. and Berman, Dorothy C.: The hospital through a child's eyes. Children, *13*:102, 1969.
Bettelheim, Bruno: The Children of the Dream. New York, Macmillan, 1969.
Scahill, Mary: Preparing children for procedures and operations, Nursing Outlook, *17*:36, 1969. June
Shope, Joanne: Parental involvement program. Nursing Outlook, *18*:32, 1970. April.
Storlie, Francis: Nursing and the Social Conscience. New York, Appleton-Century Crofts, 1970.

*Bachrach, B.: Pediatric menu terminology. *Hospitals,* 44:84, 1970.
†Millar, T. P.: The hospital and the preschool child. *Children,* 17:171, 1970.

*Chioni, R. M., and Panicucci, C.: Tomorrow's nurse practitioners. *Nursing Outlook,* 18:32, 1970.

Community Resources Available to the Family

3

With the increased emphasis on preventive nursing, the nurse must know what the community has to offer a family in its effort to achieve optimal physical, mental, and emotional health. The nurse who expects to pursue her career inside the hospital or in a doctor's office has as great an obligation to keep informed about community resources as does the nurse whose work takes her into the home. In fact, she has a greater obligation. She is the person who most often sees the family in distress over the illness of a child or acutely anxious about how they are going to manage with yet another new member. Since the family may turn to her for direction, she should make certain she does not misdirect them.

HEALTH SERVICES FOR CHILDREN

Foundations for the study and treatment of specific childhood diseases are numerous. Many are funded by private grants and donations from the public. Others receive money from state and federal grants. These foundations have done extensive and invaluable research into the causes and treatment of childhood diseases. They offer help to families who could not otherwise afford the expensive treatment necessary for their sick children. Other services include treatments and medications, instruction as to the methods of home nursing, and the loan of expensive apparatus for home treatment.

Parents of children with long-term or chronic illnesses are frequently unaware or inaccurately informed as to what services are available. The nurse may not necessarily know all the details of each service offered, but she should keep aware of what is available and know where to go for necessary information. A partial listing of nationally known maternal and child health services is given at the end of this chapter.

CHILDREN OF WORKING MOTHERS

Mothers working outside the home make up a large segment of our population. They work both to support their families and to fulfill their human potential.

No longer can we take it for granted that the great majority of mothers accept employment outside the home because of financial need. Many do, of course, because they are heads of households or the only source of income for the family. But today in American society mothers frequently work because they want to, because they enjoy it. Rather than grudgingly accepting this fact, we might note that there are positive aspects for both the parents and the child, especially if the child is afforded the opportunity of attending a child care center.

Day care centers or nursery schools can be valuable supplements (not substitutes) to the home, particularly in our crowded cities. Since increasingly smaller families provide fewer peer contacts for a small child, here is where a good day care center or nursery school can do much to help the

27

small child. More about day care centers and nursery schools in the chapter on normal growth and development.

There appears to be good evidence that children, including babies, can profit from the interest of more than one person. However, a real effort must be made to enrich the child's day both emotionally and physically. It is true that the young child needs more personalized and affectionate care than does the older child and that his need for environmental stimulation and for companionship is at least as great as that of the older child.

It seems fairly obvious that the infant can have his developmental needs better met in a professional setting where these needs are understood and respected than in the private day care home where he is fed and kept clean but left in his crib. This is not saying that all private day care homes fall short, or that all professional day care centers give emotional support to the young child or infant. At present the need is great for the right kind of care, under whatever sponsor is available to provide it.

Florence Ruderman states, "The conditions of contemporary life have created the need for a new institution: widely available, professional child care center. . . . [Day care should be] a program directed to optimal social and psychological health for the young child whose mother cannot care for him for some part of the day.*

HOMEMAKER SERVICE

In places where homemaker service is available, it has been of great help to families faced with difficult situations. In circumstances in which a mother is caring for an ill or handicapped child, the homemaker can relieve her of some of the routine housework, thus leaving her free to give her attention to the sick child's needs. In instances when a mother is ill or hospitalized,

*Ruderman, F. A.: Child Care and Working Mothers. Ch. 12. New York, Child Welfare League of America, 1968.

the homemaker takes over temporary day care for the children or, in some cases, lives in for a while.

The handicapped mother may also receive help from this service. For example, Mrs. C had lost her eyesight in adult life but was still anxious to care for her baby in her own home. With the help of a homemaker she became proficient in bathing, feeding, and otherwise caring for the child in a competent manner. Eventually, the homemaker only dropped in occasionally to visit and to answer any questions that came up.

Homemakers are recruited from various walks of life. They should have important qualities such as reliability, adaptability, kindness, maturity, and home-management skills. While training courses are offered in many cities, the supply is small in proportion to the demand.

CLINICS FOR MATERNITY AND CHILD CARE

Wherever maternity clinics as well as pediatric and well-child clinics have been established, we have seen marked reduction in mortality rates for women and children. Perhaps even more important, women have gone through childbirth with fewer complications and with better chances of producing healthy infants. Well-child clinics have been instrumental in reducing morbidity rates among the world's children.

WELL-CHILD CONFERENCES

The well-child clinic, frequently called the well-child conference, is one place where the nurse contributes to the effort to help children achieve optimal health. The nurse herself finds great satisfaction in the role she plays, because the well-child conference gives her the opportunity to use her knowledge and skills to the best advantage for parent and child. It has frequently been observed that mothers are inclined to talk much more freely to a nurse than to a busy doctor about everyday problems involved in child care.

In the well-child conference the nurse

has the major responsibility of interviewing and counseling parents. She takes the child's history, weighs and measures him, discusses nutritional needs and any other aspects of child care which she or the parent thinks necessary. The pediatrician examines the child during the first visit and thereafter whenever a medical evaluation is needed. At other times the nurse checks the child and gives necessary immunizations.

PEDIATRIC CLINICS

The pediatric clinic differs from a well-child conference in that it serves the sick child. Children with medical problems often may be spared the trauma of hospitalization through careful follow-up in the pediatric clinic. These clinics have traditionally been located in the hospital outpatient department. However, many have been established in other locations under the auspices of specialized organizations concerned with childhood diseases.

FAMILY-CENTERED CLINICS

In the family-centered clinic, an effort is made to improve the health of the entire family. The initial contact may be a child patient, or perhaps a prospective mother who attends a prenatal clinic. Thus a channel for helping with family-centered problems is provided.

The awareness of widening horizons in the nursing and medical professions is encouraging. However, one disappointment has been the poor response of the public, especially among those most in need of the services offered. Why are these facilities not used to their fullest potential? What can be done to encourage parents and prospective parents to use these facilities?

In a maternity clinic you can see women who do not come into the clinic for their first prenatal visit until the latter part of their pregnancies. Other women frequently break their clinic appointments even though they may have started to come to maternity clinics earlier in their pregnancies. In some areas it is not uncommon for a woman to come to a hospital in labor without having had any prenatal care.

The following is a partial list of the more common reasons why clinics are not used more extensively. Some suggestions to alleviate these problems are included. You may wish to conduct your own survey to find out some of the reasons patients give for not making better use of the facilities available.

Transportation Problems. The clinic may be located some distance from the area in which the patient lives. Public transportation is generally time consuming and inconvenient, frequently not available at all. Many families have no opportunity to use a private car, particularly during the husband's working hours.

It is important that clinics be accessible to those families who need them most. Smaller neighborhood clinics, sometimes called satellite clinics, can be set up within walking distance, as has been done in some areas. The evening hours can very well be utilized for clinic visits. This not only helps with a transportation problem, but relieves daytime congestion. Volunteer services for providing transportation offer another solution. This type of service needs to be greatly expanded.

Baby-Sitting Problems. Women who have other children at home often have difficulty finding someone to care for them while they are away. Often they are forced to bring all of their children along to the clinic. To accommodate these patients, some clinics have established playrooms for the children. While these playrooms are sometimes staffed by volunteers, they can provide an excellent opportunity for student nurses to observe normal child development.

Long Waiting Periods. Clinic hours begin at a set time, but little has been done to "stagger" examination times. The practice has been to tell all patients to be at the clinic at opening time. It may be considered too difficult to make individual appointments, but surely hours could be adjusted. Perhaps there could be a quota of patients for each hour. If a mother knows that when she comes to the clinic at 10 o'clock she stands a good chance of being out at 11 o'clock, she can plan intelligently. If she has school children coming home at noon, she can choose an earlier hour so as to be home in time to feed them.

Too often parents wait several hours before being seen by the doctor or nurse, and then they only spend a few minutes in the examining room. One possible solution is to utilize clinic visits by having the mothers get together to discuss their feelings and concerns and to learn about childbearing and childrearing.

Impersonal Treatment. Patients object very strongly to being treated as insensible objects. Unfortunately, we have a tendency to see them all as patients, rather than as individuals like ourselves. The intelligent mother who brings her baby in with "three-month colic" deeply resents being told "if you fed the baby properly there would be no problem," yet no attempt is made to find out how she *does* feed her baby.

Similarly, the prospective mother objects to being treated like an object on an assembly line. She may go to one place to have her blood pressure checked, another cubicle to be weighed, and a third area to present her urine specimen. Each time she is asked the same questions.

It is important for the clinic personnel to try to make the patients and their families feel that they are personally interested in them as people. It helps to call the patient by name, to introduce oneself, and above all, to listen. In some clinics it can be arranged for the same doctor or nurse to see the patient at each visit.

Fear. Some women in the maternity clinic fear being examined by the doctor and may be embarrassed, particularly if their modesty is not considered during a pelvic or breast examination. Careful explanations of what is going to be done and why may help to allay the expectant mother's fear of the examination. It may lessen the embar-rassment if the nurse points out that these examinations are routine for the doctor, that they are part of his work, and that his personal feelings are not involved. The nurse can also provide for the woman's modesty by draping her to minimize the amount of exposure necessary.

A fact equally obvious, but too often not considered, is the need which a child patient has for explanations he can understand. And how often do we give thought to the child's embarrassment over the invasion of his privacy?

Lack of Understanding of the Importance of Maternity and Well-Child Care. Some cultural groups believe that because pregnancy is a normal, natural event, maternity care is not important or necessary, so they only go to the clinic or see a doctor when they are ill. It also is very difficult to persuade a mother of the importance of periodic check-ups for her well children. Here is where the news media, as well as PTA meetings, schools, the Red Cross, and other organizations concerned with the health of the population can help by stressing the importance of good health care.

It is also important to use values and concepts which people understand and accept within the context of their culture when teaching them.

One word of digression here. Student nurses sometimes say, "Why tell me about the need for improvement? Hospital rules are set by the administration, what can I, a student, do?" Well, actually, a great deal. After all, you are the people who will soon be setting the pace and making the rules. If you calmly accept the status quo, nothing will be changed in the future. Even now it is encouraging to see the trend toward allowing—yes, even seeking—the opinions and constructive thinking of students. We need your fresh thinking.

MATERNITY CLINICS

A comprehensive approach to caring for maternity patients is to provide prenatal, postpartum, and family planning clinics.

Sometimes, if the number of patients warrants it, a special clinic for "high risk" maternity patients who might have a complication such as toxemia or diabetes is held. The purpose of a prenatal clinic is, of course, to provide prenatal care. A definition of prenatal care is the medical supervision and care given to pregnant women during the period between conception and the onset of labor.

HOMES FOR UNWED MOTHERS

A community agency which should be familiar to a nurse working with maternity patients is the home for unwed mothers. Two examples of homes for unwed mothers are the Catherine Booth Memorial Home, which is a branch of the Salvation Army, and the Florence Crittendon Home. The purpose of these homes is to provide a shelter for women and girls who are pregnant and unmarried and who do not want the community in which they live to know about their plight. Most of the babies that are born to these mothers are put up for adoption.

Generally, the unwed mother enters the home when her pregnancy begins to "show." While she lives there for the remaining months, she may do light housekeeping tasks, continue her schooling, or take classes to prepare for a vocation while she is in residence. She should have an opportunity to see a social worker so that she can make a decision about keeping the baby or giving it up for adoption. Some homes have facilities for delivering the patients right there; in others, the mother goes to a nearby hospital for delivery. An interesting book which gives the reader insight into how it feels to live in a home for unwed mothers is *House of Tomorrow* by Jean Thompson. It is a day-by-day account of the author's experiences. (See Suggested Reading at the end of this chapter.)

The nurse may find out about homes for unwed mothers by calling adoption agencies such as Family Service or Catholic Charities. These agencies often have a list of private homes where an unwed mother can live during her pregnancy in exchange for housekeeping or baby-sitting services. However, these private residences should be carefully investigated to make certain that the girl is not being exploited or only used to work.

Since there is less censure of pregnancy out of wedlock in today's American society, there are fewer girls and women who go to these homes to wait out their pregnancies. Also, the liberalized abortion laws in several states are decreasing the number of unwanted pregnancies.

FAMILY PLANNING CLINICS

Other community agencies to which the nurse can refer maternity patients are the family planning clinics. In this day and age when we hear so much about the population explosion, we realize that limiting the number of babies is important for the survival of the world. In most cities in the United States, family planning clinics are available as well as other clinics offered by the local health department.

An older, volunteer association which offers this service is the Planned Parenthood Association. This organization was started by the late Margaret Sanger, a public health nurse, who pioneered in the field of birth control. Many communities have Planned Parenthood clinics which offer a range of services, from helping couples prevent unwanted pregnancies to helping couples who want to have a baby but are unable to do so because of infertility. Fees at Planned Parenthood are on a sliding scale. Clients are accepted regardless of marital status, religion, and in some states, age. The third resource for family planning in a community is, of course, private physicians.

The nurse is in a position, when working with a family, to refer the members to the family planning resource which best meets their needs. For example, a Catholic couple who would only use the rhythm method of contraception would properly be referred to a clinic or physician who teaches this

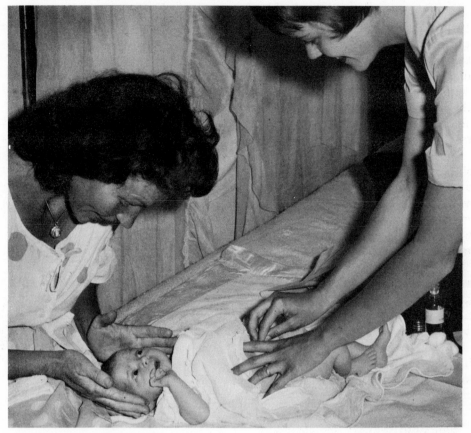

Figure 3-1.   A public health nurse shows a mother how to take care of the baby's umbilical cord. (Courtesy of Maricopa County Health Department, Phoenix.)

method. Some clinics offer only one or two methods of contraception, perhaps the "pill" and the diaphragm. If the woman wants to use an intrauterine device, the nurse would refer her to a clinic or physician who inserts IUD's. In other words, the nurse assists the couple in obtaining information about the contraceptive methods of *their* own choosing.

It should be kept in mind that one of the major reasons women give for not availing themselves of contraceptive methods is that they don't know where to get them. Some interested girls and women are too shy or embarrassed to ask. Therefore, the nurse should not assume that the patient knows about contraceptive methods because she doesn't ask.

PUBLIC HEALTH AND VISITING NURSE ASSOCIATIONS

A valuable resource in the field of maternal and child nursing is the public health nurse or visiting nurse who provides follow-up care after a maternity patient or sick child has been discharged from the hospital.

The function of the public health nurse is to teach and supervise health practices. She makes home visits but seldom gives physical care. She may make routine visits to antepartum and postpartum patients, to families who have mentally retarded or chronically ill children in the home, to mothers who have had premature babies, and to other families needing her services.

There is no charge to the family for home visits made by the public health nurse.

The visiting nurse may make home visits for the same kinds of patients the public health nurse sees. The main difference is that the visiting nurse gives more physical care to the patient than the public health nurse. Another difference is that the Visiting Nurses Association is a voluntary agency. Therefore, payment for services is on a sliding scale based on the patient's ability to pay. The visiting nurse will make return home visits as often as they are desired or needed by the patient.

It is a satisfying experience to make out referrals to these agencies since the person sending the referral will get a report back from the nurse who makes the home visit. It is usually very interesting to read the report and learn how the patient is getting along. It is helpful to the nurse who is making the home visit to have *complete* information on the referral about the patient and his hospitalization.

LA LECHE LEAGUE

Many communities have one or more groups of nursing mothers, such as the *La Leche* League which takes its name from the Spanish word for *milk*, la leche. One of the main goals of La Leche League is to give support and encouragement to a mother who is breast feeding her infant. The group is composed of lay women who are interested in promoting the "womanly art of breast feeding." (This is the title of their book.) When a woman is having difficulty nursing her baby, she can telephone a member of La Leche League for advice.

La Leche League has informal meetings at members' homes. Pregnant women who are planning or considering breast feeding as well as those who are already breast feeding their infants are welcomed to the meetings. It may be helpful to refer a mother who has decided to breast feed her baby to this organization. The nurse can tell her the purpose of the organization and give her

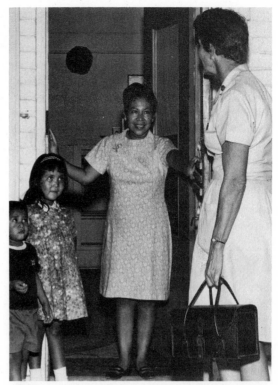

Figure 3-2. A public health nurse makes a home visit for child health supervision. (Courtesy of Maricopa County Health Department, Phoenix.)

the local phone number to call when she goes home from the hospital.

PARENT EDUCATION

The idea that couples should have an opportunity to learn together about childbirth and parenthood has received a great deal of emphasis in the past 25 years. Today many different organizations offer "education for parenthood" classes. In many communities a series of classes for expectant parents is taught in hospitals by members of the staff, such as a nurse, doctor, physical therapist, or a combination of all of them. Sometimes a small fee is charged by the hospital or the person teaching the classes.

Generally the person who teaches the classes has some experience and knowledge of maternal and child care. Ideally, the teacher should satisfactorily complete a course in teacher preparation for childbirth education prior to teaching these classes. The teacher should know how to work with a group in an unstructured situation. It is felt that if the parents can discuss their concerns and ask questions, it will be more valuable for them than attending a highly structured series of classes. However, certain subjects of general interest to most expectant parents should be covered, such as pregnancy, fetal development, labor and delivery, exercises and relaxation techniques, analgesia and anesthesia, and breast feeding and bottle feeding. The parents may also be taken on a tour of the hospital's obstetrical department. Throughout these classes the emphasis should be placed on the normal childbearing process rather than on all the things that could go wrong. After all, 96 to 98 per cent of pregnancies and deliveries are normal.

Besides hospitals, other groups sponsor these "education for parenthood" classes. One resource is the American Red Cross which offers classes free of charge. In most instances, the classes are taught by nurses and cover such practical points as how to bathe, diaper, and handle the new baby as well as many of the topics mentioned above.

The local chapter of the ICEA (International Childbirth Education Association, founded in 1960) is another resource for parent education. Since this is an organization for both lay people (parents) and professionals, the classes may be taught by the lay member or by doctors and nurses, or both. In addition to its classes for expectant parents, the Childbirth Education Association has a variety of other functions. It conducts regular regional conferences and groups for mothers who are breast feeding. It also serves as a good resource for up-to-date films, books, and pamphlets on family-centered maternal and infant care. For further information you can write to ICEA Executive Office, P.O. Box 5852, Milwaukee, Wisconsin 53220, or ICEA Supplies Center, 208 Ditty Building, Bellevue, Washington 98004.

While we have been placing emphasis on educating the expectant couple, it is just as important to educate the unwed mother. Some of the homes for unwed mothers have excellent preparation classes for their residents. Or special educational programs for unwed mothers may be offered by the Board of Education.

ADOPTION

Adoption is a matter of social concern and a responsibility for all child-concerned services. The number of adoptable children is said to be decreasing in Western countries as a result of new and varied methods of preventing unwanted pregnancies. Liberalized abortion laws, availability of contraceptives, and growing acceptance of sterilization procedures help limit the number of unwanted children.

However, at the same time, there is an urgent need for more adoptive homes for those children previously considered unadoptable. This need has been considered urgent enough to bring about a reexamination of adoption practices, resulting in the discard of a number of previously rigid requirements for adoptive parents.

Among the children urgently in need of homes are children of minority groups, children with medical, neurological, or orthopedic conditions, and children with personality problems. It has come as a surprise to many adoption agencies that would-be adoptive parents are eager to accept such children and the responsibilities they entail.

The Child Welfare League of America sets the standards for adoptive practices. These standards are accepted by adoption placement agencies as goals for the continuous improvement of services to children. They are directed to all who are concerned with improving services to children—the general public as well as professional groups.

The nurse needs to be aware of present day standards, whether or not she becomes directly involved in any aspect of adoption.

Present-Day Adoption Standards*

Infants should be placed in the adoptive home as early as possible. Early placement works to the advantage of the child, his natural parents, and the adoptive parents. Delaying adoption for additional months of study has not yielded any better basis for predicting future development. It is noted that many adoptive parents are ready to take the same risks as natural parents. They do not need guarantees of perfect babies. Delay, however, may be necessary if a parent, such as an unmarried mother, is not emotionally ready to give up her child.

In any adoption plan, the best interests of the child should be the determining factor. Other factors, such as racial background should not in itself be the basis for selecting or rejecting an adoptive home.

Lack of a religious affiliation or of a religious faith should not of itself bar applicants from adopting children. However, opportunity for religious, spiritual, or ethical development should be seriously considered.

Chronological age or marital status of the adoptive parents should receive consideration, but not necessarily determine their eligibility. In such cases, as in all others, consideration must be given to the circumstances that would best satisfy the individual child's physical, emotional, and intellectual needs.

Single parents, male or female, are considered as prospective parents provided they meet other criteria for adoptive parenthood. These include emotional maturity, positive feelings about children, motivation, and the ability to offer the child a reasonably happy and secure family life with love, happiness,

---

*Child Welfare League of America Standards for Adoption Service, New York, Child Welfare League, 1968.

and companionship. (In practice, the number of children adopted by single parents is a relatively small percentage.)

Financial stability and security are important in meeting the daily expenses of caring for a child and in providing for his future. The recommendation is made that when a family meets the other qualifications consideration be given to supplementing the family income when necessary.

Working mothers should not be barred from adopting children. However, they should be able to remain at home with the child as long as necessary to provide security and establish a method of adequate care. Foster parents should not be denied the opportunity to adopt children they have had in their care if they so desire. Parents with children of their own and couples who are childless should also be given an equal opportunity in adopting children.

The Nurse and Adoption

The nurse may encounter various situations involving adoption during her career. She may be working with either an unmarried or married mother who plans to give her baby up for adoption, or with an adopted child in a pediatric department, or she may be called upon in her off duty hours to answer questions about adoption. Thus the nurse needs to know what her role is in regard to adoption. For example, she should know that she does not take on the role of the social worker, or physician, or lawyer in handling the complexities of adoption proceedings. Nor should she attempt to tell a person what to do when the question of adoption comes up. She should find out what the person already knows and what he has done or would like to do, and help him to use problem solving methods to make *his* decision. For example, if the mother asks the nurse if she thinks she should give her baby up for adoption, the nurse could ask her "Why do you ask?" or "How do you feel about it?" The nurse may also refer the person to an agency or professional who is more qualified to help. The nurse should recognize her limitations and not be afraid to say "I don't know, but I'll find out for you" or "You can contact this person (or agency) for help." Some of the agencies which offer adoption services are Jewish Family Service, Catholic Charities, various children's homes, Florence Crittendon Home, Catherine Booth (Salvation Army), and public adoption and welfare agencies.

There have been some changes in the way certain commonly asked questions concerning adoptions are handled. These changes reflect the general trend of our society away from rigidity and punishment. One question is, should the mother see the baby she is giving up for adoption? Whereas before, an unmarried mother who was giving her baby up for adoption was not allowed to see it (or even ask questions about it), the belief now is that the mother should see and handle her baby if she so desires. In some instances the mother may even dress and turn over the baby to the adoption agency. It is felt that this gives her a sense of completion and a feeling that she has actively participated in the decision-making instead of passively allowing others to make decisions for her. On the other hand, if the mother requests not to see the baby (or doesn't want to talk about it) she should not be forced to do so.

As regards a question parents of an adopted child might ask—should the child be told that he is adopted—it is generally agreed that he should be told early in life, because it is less traumatic for the child to find out from his parents than from an outsider. However, if a nurse is asked how to tell a child he is adopted, she must realize that she cannot generalize since each situation must be treated individually. However, she should know to whom to send the parents to discuss this problem and also have references (books, articles) she could recommend should they be needed. (See suggested readings at the end of the chapter.)

The nurse will undoubtedly make her

own decisions about whether she wants to participate in private adoptions or getting an expectant mother to sign relinquishment papers (a document which states that the mother relinquishes all rights to her baby) prior to delivery. It is the author's opinion that the nurse is using good judgment in avoiding such legal entanglements.

In summary, the nurse can offer valuable assistance by being supportive to children and parents who have concerns about adoption. She should know her limitations in working with the legal and social complexities of adoption.

FOSTER HOMES

As we have become more sensitive to children's needs, we have begun to look for more and better foster homes for those who need their services. We have come to recognize the importance of a family setting and have come to believe that an institution, no matter how well organized and administered, cannot take the place of a warm, well-integrated home. However, not all foster homes supply the atmosphere that a child needs. Good foster homes are not easy to find. It takes a person with a true love of children and a sensitivity to their needs to provide a good foster home. It also takes broad vision and often a real sacrifice on the part of the foster parents to let these children go when they are ready to return home or be placed for adoption.

Many children in foster care go through the traumatic experience of being moved from one home to another, often many times. A most moving look into a little girl's heart has been portrayed in the story of one such child. She had gathered into herself all of the hurt and the criticism that she had received in her moves from one home to another, until she was afraid to respond naturally to anyone. Always she was the outsider. "In this home, do they want me to make my bed as soon as I get up, or will I be scolded for not letting it air? Should I offer to help with breakfast, or will I be in the way?" It took long, patient understanding and acceptance in a home where she was really wanted before her barriers could finally come down. For some children, it is too late.

All states require the licensing and the inspection of foster homes. Usually the number of children in a single home is limited, and the standards for hygienic practices and health measures are predetermined. Foster families must have a sufficient income to meet their living needs without the board payments on behalf of the child. Efforts to find foster homes in which handicapped or disfigured children can also receive loving physical care and emotional support are meeting with considerable success as concerned people become aware of the need.

NATIONAL AND INTERNATIONAL ORGANIZATIONS CONCERNED WITH MATERNAL AND CHILD CARE

Children's Bureau

In the United States the Children's Bureau is still the focus of concern for all children. It has worked actively in cooperating with international organizations such as UNICEF and WHO.

The Children's Bureau has been an organization within the U. S. Department of Health, Education and Welfare (HEW). Recent organizational changes have been made in HEW and the Children's Bureau is now a part of the new Office of Child Development (OCD). It maintains its role of leadership in instituting and coordinating child-and-parent programs, and it continues to investigate and report on all matters pertaining to the welfare of children.

The OCD now consists of three major branches: the Children's Bureau, the Bureau of Head Start and Child Development, and the Bureau of Program Development and Resources.

Social service programs for children and adults formerly located in the Children's Bureau are now located in the new Community Service Administration. Health programs formerly administered by the Children's Bureau have been transferred to the Health Services and Mental Health Administration (HSMHA), where they will comprise a new Maternal and Child Health Service.

The Children's Bureau has been publishing authoritative, up-to-date, practical pamphlets on nearly every aspect of child welfare since 1914. Among these are *Prenatal Care, Infant Care, Your Child from One to Six,* and *Your Child from Six to Twelve.* The bi-monthly periodical, *Children,* is published for professional personnel serving children.*

The United Nations Children's Fund

In 1946 the United Nations General Assembly established the United Nations International Children's Emergency Fund (UNICEF) on a temporary basis to assist needy children, primarily in war-devastated countries. Its charter came to an end in 1953, but the General Assembly voted unanimously to continue the agency indefinitely as the United Nations Children's Fund, although it retained the symbol UNICEF.

UNICEF is simply and completely concerned with the health and welfare of children and mothers. It works with any nation that requests service, without regard to race, creed, or politics. Assistance is provided when any country requests it and is a cooperative venture. Assisted governments spend approximately $2.50 for every dollar contributed by UNICEF, for materials, local personnel, and facilities.

UNICEF works in cooperation with WHO (World Health Organization), FAO (Food and Agricultural Organization), and UNESCO, (United Nations Educational, Scientific and Cultural Organization). A

*Subscriptions to *Children Today* can be made through the Superintendent of Documents, U. S. Government Printing Office, Washington, D. C. 20204.

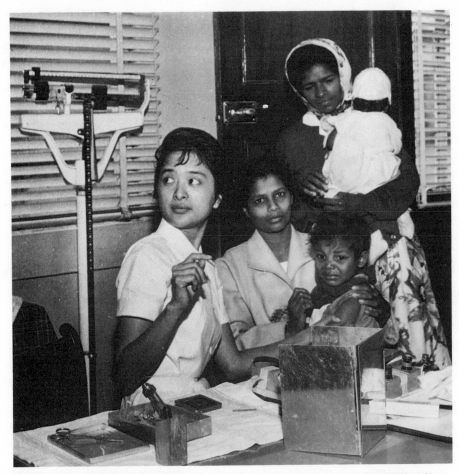

Figure 3-3. A Mauritius girl who studied nursing in Asia on a UNICEF fellowship has returned to her island home to help with public health programs. (Photo by Alastair Matheson, Courtesy of UNICEF.)

joint UNICEF/WHO committee on Health Policy (JCHP), has been very valuable in coordinating activities.

UNICEF puts great emphasis on assisting people to learn how to help themselves. As has been said, it is "one organization that works to put itself out of business," by training and educating persons within their own countries to take over the projects. More than one third of UNICEF's aid goes into training health personnel. The greatest number of trainees have been auxiliary and paraprofessional personnel. However, an attempt is made to achieve balance through training schemes that include nursing educators, as well as supervisory and medical personnel. For example, in India in 1970, 5000 nurses were trained, as well as 4000 auxiliary nurse-midwives. In addition, 400 medical officers received reorientation training.

UNICEF is well aware that special attention must be given to training personnel to fit local conditions. For example, health service personnel have to understand the special needs of people in rural areas who are rarely reached by health services.

Preventive medicine for children is one large area of UNICEF concern. Others are environmental, sanitation, family planning and general education. To carry out their educational aims, textbooks, manuals and teaching aids have been provided, as well as teacher training centers. A wide range of support for health services has been offered for several years. In 1970, such aid was provided in 85 countries.

UNICEF's work is financed entirely by voluntary contributions from governments, private groups and individuals. In the United States, the Trick or Treat for UNICEF Halloween Program is well known, and it receives hearty support from the nation's children. The sale of UNICEF greeting cards, calendars, children's books and games helps to sustain its program for needy children all over the world. UNICEF believes that the future of mankind depends on the well-being of our children. Its slogan is, "The child of today for the world of tomorrow." UNICEF has a proud record. It has received the commendation of every president of the United States since its inception, it receives active cooperation from the major religious faiths, and in 1965 it received the Nobel Prize for Peace.*

The World Health Organization

The World Health Organization (WHO) is one of the special agencies of the United Nations. Through this organization, which came into being in 1948, the public health and medical professions of more than 100 countries exchange their knowledge and experience and collaborate in an effort to achieve the highest possible level of health throughout the world. WHO deals with problems that can only be solved by the cooperation of all, or of certain groups of countries—the eradication of diseases such as malaria, and the control of diseases that affect or are a potential danger to many, such as most of the infectious and parasitic diseases, some cardiovascular disease, and cancer. In many parts of the world there is

need for improvement in maternal and child health, nutrition, nursing, mental health, dental health, social and occupational health, environmental health, public health administration, professional education and training, and health education for the public. Thus a large share of the organization's resources is devoted to giving assistance and advice in these fields and to making available—often through publications—the latest information on these subjects.

Many countries have well-developed maternal and child welfare programs that have lowered infant mortality rates and have raised child health standards to high levels. Among many of the developing countries, and among some of older cultures as well, conditions still prevail that are based on traditions difficult to overcome, and serious diseases with high mortality rates are common.

"Mankind must accept the challenge that this is one world, that however great the dangers of atomic destruction, there is the even greater danger of an unequally divided world that keeps on merely rolling along, some of its areas riddled with ignorance, poverty and disease."* These are the words of a physician who understands from personal observation and from practical experience what he is talking about.

The World Health Organization explains: "More than half the world's population—are victims of hunger or inadequate nutrition in one form or another. Over large areas of the world, people's everyday meals are insufficient; the children go without milk after they are weaned, and child mortality between the ages of one and five is often fifteen times higher than it is in places where people are able to get proper food. All this is nothing new. It is probable that the world has never in its history fed all its people adequately."†

---

*Additional information concerning UNICEF, its purpose, its scope and its functions, may be obtained from the United States Committee for UNICEF, United Nations, New York, or from one of the state United Nations Associations.

---

*World Health Magazine. p. 6. May, 1963.
†World Health Magazine. p. 5-6. March 1963.

WHO has worked in cooperation with UNICEF and with the FAO to prevent and treat deficiency diseases, particularly among children. As the UN agency charged with working for health improvement, WHO combats epidemics, trains health workers, and promotes research. Its campaign to eradicate malaria has been outstandingly successful in large sections of once-infested countries.

There are several WHO publications. *WHO Chronicle* (published monthly for the medical and for the public health professions) provides a record of the principal health activities undertaken in various countries with WHO assistance. The *Bulletin of the World Health Organization* contains technical articles in English or in French and is published monthly. *World Health* is an illustrated monthly magazine for the general public, and gives an idea of WHO activities throughout the world. It is published in English, French, Portuguese, Russian and Spanish editions. Other publications include a Monograph Series, a Technical Report Series, and Epidemiological and Vital Statistics Report, and others.* WHO Headquarters is located in Geneva, Switzerland.

International Social Service

International Social Service (ISS) is a voluntary, nonsectarian family and child agency with headquarters in Geneva, Switzerland. Founded in 1921, ISS presently has branches in 20 countries, with cooperating agencies in over 80 others.

Its branches are staffed and supported indigenously, providing individualized service and working closely with local social and welfare agencies.

Services for children include assisting the homeless child. Efforts are made to reunite the child with his family whenever

feasible. The organization works to "develop programs of foster care, and secure the passage of modern laws which place the needs of children first in adoption procedures."†

ISS also offers services to hospitals and health agencies, when treatment is requested for patients from another country. The following is an example of the kind of service rendered:

From Greece, the parents of a five-year-old boy who had been severely crippled wrote to a hospital in the United States, pleading for the boy's admission for treatment. The hospital requested ISS to investigate the case and get full medical and social information. ISS arranged for a social worker to visit the family in their Greek mountain home and to consult with a local clinic that had given the boy initial care but could not provide extended treatment. After receiving the social worker's report, the hospital accepted the boy as a patient. ISS then helped the boy's mother to complete travel arrangements for him and herself. Through funds provided by American and Greek donors, accommodations were found close to the hospital. As several surgical procedures were recommended, ISS mobilised community resources, including social agencies, to help the mother find her way in a large city where the language and the customs were strange. An interpreter was provided to explain medical instructions. The mother was introduced to the Greek community and arrangements made for her son to attend Greek nursery school in between hospitalizations. Meanwhile, the worried mother's letters to her husband in Greece could not offer him much encouragement; but the Greek social worker kept in touch with the father and, as the months passed, reassured him with information received from the hospital through ISS. Eventually the boy, vastly improved, returned home with his mother.‡

Adoption Services of ISS

ISS acts in the belief that a child's best interests are served when he can grow up in his own country among familiar surround-

---

*WHO publications, or information concerning them, may be obtained in the United States through the American Public Health Association, Inc., New York, N.Y.

†Nobody's Child: the Story of WAIF. [pamphlet] The Children's Division of International Social Service, American Branch.
‡International Social Services to Hospitals and Health Agencies. [pamphlet] New York, International Social Service, American Branch, Inc.

ings. Adjustments to a new culture, language and way of life are difficult and add to a homeless child's insecurity. However, there are thousands of homeless children for whom no satisfactory homes can be found in their own country. ISS has been successful in assisting in the adoption of several of these children. They make the claim that "most of these inter-country adoptions have been successful largely because the families who adopted these children have a remarkable capacity for love, patience and understanding. For people with such qualities, inter-country adoption can be deeply satisfying and rewarding."*

WAIF, Children's Division of ISS, American Branch, gives information on inter-country adoptions. Statistics indicate that it is the older child, the child of mixed parentage, or the child with a physical handicap who is most in need of an adoptive home outside his own country. At present those children are from the following countries.

Korea. These are Korean-Caucasian, Korean-Negro and fully Korean children, ranging in age from 1 to 14 years.

Hong Kong. Preference is given to Chinese families if available. Japan has a few older children of mixed parentage who need homes.

Vietnam. At present only a limited number of children are available for adoption. Most of the children in orphanages have relatives who hope to reclaim them when conditions improve.

Europe. In Europe, a few children of mixed parentage need placement abroad. ISS also assists families who wish to adopt children of relatives or children they know who are living in other countries.

Persons wishing to adopt children from other countries should contact their state adoption or welfare agencies for preliminary planning. ISS works with local agencies in selecting children, helps complete necessary documents, and assures that the child is properly escorted and cared for on his way to the new country. Detailed information is available from the agency.

WAIF personnel point out that there are many children in the United States in urgent need of secure homes. WAIF works closely with the Adoption Resource Exchange of North America (ARENA), which is an agency specializing in bringing together families and adoptable children from different states or communities, when no adoptable children are available locally. (Addresses for these and other social service agencies are given below.)

RESOURCES AVAILABLE FOR MATERNAL AND CHILD CARE

American Academy of Pediatrics, P.O. Box 1034, Evanston, Ill. 60204

American Cancer Society, P.O. Box 5590, Grand Central Station, New York, N.Y. 10017

American Dental Assn. Bureau of Health Education, 211 E. Chicago Ave., Chicago, Ill. 60611

American Diabetic Assn., 18 E. 48th St., New York, N.Y. 10017

American Foundation for the Blind, Box FH, 15 W. 16th St., New York, N.Y. 10011

American Heart Assn., 44 E. 23rd St., New York, N.Y. 10010

American Medical Assn., 535 N. Dearborn St., Chicago, Ill. 60610

American Red Cross, 17th and D St. N.W., Washington, D.C. 20006 (See local chapters)

ARENA — Adoption Resource Exchange of North America, 67 Irving Place, New York, N.Y. 10003

Bureau of Product Safety. Medical Review and Poison Control Branch, 200 C St. N.W., Washington, D.C. 20204

Center for Disease Control, Office of Information, Atlanta, Georgia 30333

Child Guidance Clinics. See local address

Child Study Assn. of America, 9 East 89th St., New York, N.Y. 10028

*When You Adopt a Child from Abroad. [pamphlet] WAIF/ISS, American Branch.

Child Welfare League of America, 67 Irving
Place, New York, N.Y. 10003
Council on Family Health. Dept. FH, 201 E.
42nd St., New York, N.Y. 10017
Easter Seal Society for Crippled Children
and Adults, 2023 W. Ogden Ave., Chicago,
Ill. 60612
Epilepsy Foundation of America, 733 15th
St. N.W., Washington, D.C. 20005
Hemophilia Foundation, 25 W. 39th St.,
New York, N.Y. 10018
Homes for Unwed Mothers, Florence
Crittenden's Homes, Salvation Army
Booth Memorial Homes (see local ad-
dress)
International Childbirth Education Assn.
(ICEA), P.O. Box 5852, Milwaukee, Wisc.
53220
International Social Service (ISS), American
Branch/WAIF, 345 E. 46th St., New York,
N.Y. 10017
Maternal and Child Health Service, Office of
Information, Parklawn Bldg., 5600
Fisher's Lane, Rockville, Md. 20852
Maternity Center Assn., 48 East 92nd St.,
New York, N.Y. 10028
Medic Alert Foundation, Turlock, Califor-
nia, 95380
National Society for the Prevention of
Blindness, Public Information Dept., 79
Madison Ave., New York, N.Y. 10016
National Assn. of Hearing and Speech
Agencies, 919 18th St. N.W., Washington,
D.C. 20006
National Cystic Fibrosis Research Foun-
dation, 202 E. 44th St., New York, N.Y.
10017
National Foundation—March of Dimes,
Public Education Dept., Box 2000, White
Plains, N.Y. 10602
National Society for the Prevention of
Blindness, Inc., 79 Madison Ave., New
York, N.Y. 10016
Planned Parenthood Assn., Box S, 810 7th
Ave., New York, N.Y. 10022

Play Schools Assn., 120 W. 57th St., New
York, N.Y. 10019
Project Head Start, Office of Economic
Opportunity, 1200 19th St. N.W., Wash-
ington, D.C. 20006
Public Affairs Committee, 381 Park Ave. S.,
New York, N.Y. 10016
Shriners Children's Hospitals. Check local
address
Sex Information and Education Council of
the U.S. (SIECUS), 1855 Broadway, New
York, N.Y. 10023
United Cerebral Palsy Assn., 321 W. 44th
St., New York, N.Y. 10036
United States Department of Health,
Education, and Welfare, Office of Child
Development, Children's Bureau, P.O.
Box 1182, Washington, D.C. 20013
United Nations Children's Fund (UNICEF),
331 E. 38th St., New York, N.Y. 10016
World Health Organization (WHO), Avenue
Appia, 1211, Geneva 27, Switzerland

BIBLIOGRAPHY

Against Hidden Hunger, World Health Maga-
zine. p. 12. March, 1963.
Branham, Ethel: One parent adoptions, Chil-
dren, *17*:103, 1970.
Industry: Babyfood: Health, World Health Maga-
zine. p. 6. May, 1963.
Nobody's Child—The Story of WAIF, New York,
Children's Division of International Social
Service (American Branch).
When You Adopt a Child from Abroad. New
York, Children's Division of International
Social Service (American Branch).

Suggested Readings for Further Study

Franklin, David S. and Massarik, Fred: The
adoption of children with medical conditions.
[Three parts.] Child Welfare, *58*:459, 533,
595, 1969.
Gallagher, Ursula M.: The adoption of mentally
retarded children. Children, *15*:17, 1968.
Thompson, Jean: The House of Tomorrow. New
York, Harper and Row, 1967.

Maternal and Child Morbidity and Mortality

4

MORTALITY RATES

The purpose of this unit is to compare maternal and infant mortality rates on a state, national, and international basis. A look at the national rates should emphasize the socioeconomic difference between those who fare well and those who do not in this the most affluent of all nations. The "disadvantaged" who fall into this latter category are those mothers in the low socioeconomic group, a large proportion of whom are non-white.

Before comparing statistics it is essential to define some common terms.

Maternal mortality—any maternal death resulting from childbirth and complications of pregnancy, labor and delivery, and the postpartum period. (An expectant mother who dies in an automobile accident is not considered to be a maternal mortality.)

Maternal mortality rate—the number of mothers who die, according to the above definition, per 100,000 live births.

Note: It is important when looking at statistics to be aware of the number of live births which is being used as a base. In previous statistics 10,000 live births was the base used in reporting maternal mortality rates. However, because the rate has dropped considerably in the past 50 years, in order to avoid the use of fractions or decimals, the standard base number has been changed to 100,000. For example, instead of reading that 0.6 mother per 10,000 live births died in 1970, you will read that 6 mothers per 100,000 died.

Fetal death—the death of a fetus weighing 500 grams or more (usually after the twentieth week of gestation) or a baby who is stillborn.

Abortion—the termination of pregnancy before the period of viability.

Viability—the ability of the fetus to sustain life outside the uterus. This usually occurs between the twentieth and twenty-eighth week of gestation.

Infant death—an infant who dies within the first year of life (or prior to his first birthday).

Stillborn—a newborn infant who has no signs of life such as heartbeat, respirations, muscular activity (other than those produced reflexly), or pulsation of the cord.

Neonatal death—an infant who has died in the first four weeks of life.

Perinatal death—fetal and neonatal deaths combined. (This number is obtained by adding the two numbers together.)

Perinatal death rate—the combined number of fetal and neonatal deaths per 1000 live births. Because of the higher proportion of babies who die as compared to mothers, the base 1000 live births is frequently used in reporting neonatal, perinatal, and infant mortality rates. However, some statistics do express the ratio of these deaths per 10,000 and 100,000 live births.

Maternal Mortality

The term high-risk maternity patient refers to a woman who either has a physical condition which threatens her pregnancy or is faced by life conditions which may adversely affect the course of her pregnancy and its outcome. For example, if a woman becomes pregnant out of wedlock or in her early teens (under the age of 17) she may become a high-risk maternity patient. The same is true if she has diabetes, toxemia, or a history of several miscarriages. In fact, the three leading causes of maternal mortality are hemorrhage, toxemia, and infection.

In spite of the fact that high-risk maternity patients exist, the United States has an excellent record for making the course of pregnancy and delivery safe for women. Internationally, the United States shares second place with Denmark, the United Kingdom, and Norway, while Sweden ranks first with the lowest maternity mortality rate. In the last 30 years in the United States, maternal mortality declined about 90 per cent thanks to better prenatal care, better trained hospital personnel, the

availability of blood transfusions, and the use of antibiotics.

Although the per cent of reductions in maternal deaths among the white and nonwhite mothers in the United States is approximately equal, the relative difference between the two groups has increased. Thirty years ago the nonwhite mortality rate was approximately twice the white rate. In 1967, the rate was 19.5 for white and 69.5 for nonwhite (see Table 4-1).

Consistent with the changing patterns of infant mortality is the fact that in cities of 500,000 or more, the maternal mortality rate is 37 per cent higher than the national rate. Among 21 cities in this group, only seven had rates below the national average. Cities with maternal death rates which were 70 per cent or more in excess of the national average were Detroit, Washington, D.C., New York, and St. Louis. The highest maternal mortality rates are now in cities of 500,000 or more and in the rural parts of nonmetropolitan counties.

Table 4-1.   U. S. MATERNAL, FETAL, NEONATAL, AND INFANT DEATH RATES BY COLOR: 1940–1967*

	1940	1945	1950	1955	1960	1965	1966	1967
†Maternal								
deaths	376.0	207.2	83.3	47.0	37.1	31.6	29.1	28.0
White	319.8	172.1	61.1	32.8	26.0	21.0	20.2	19.5
Nonwhite	773.5	454.8	221.6	130.0	97.9	83.7	72.4	69.5
§Fetal								
deaths	N.A.	23.9	19.2	17.1	16.1	16.2	15.7	15.6
White	N.A.	21.4	17.1	15.2	14.1	13.9	13.6	13.5
Nonwhite	N.A.	42.0	32.5	28.4	26.8	27.2	26.1	25.8
Neonatal								
deaths	28.8	24.3	20.5	19.1	18.7	17.7	17.2	16.5
White	27.2	23.3	19.4	17.7	17.2	16.1	15.6	15.0
Nonwhite	39.7	32.0	27.5	27.2	26.9	25.4	24.8	23.8
Infant								
deaths	47.0	38.3	29.2	26.4	26.0	24.7	23.7	22.4
White	43.2	35.6	26.8	23.6	22.9	21.5	20.6	19.7
Nonwhite	73.8	57.0	44.5	42.8	43.2	40.3	38.8	35.9

*Source: United States Bureau of the Census, Statistical Abstract of the U. S. 1970. 91st edition, Washington, D.C., 1970 p. 55, 57.
†Per 100,000 live births from deliveries and complications of pregnancy, childbirth, and the puerperium.
§Per 1000 live births.
N.A.: not available.

Perinatal Mortality Rates

The peak incidence of perinatal infant death in this country occurs during the period of delivery. From the thirty-sixth week of pregnancy to the fourth week of life 3.5 per cent of the infant population dies. This is a little less than 10 per cent of the deaths in the United States at all ages and from all causes. The association of perinatal mortality with selected demographic factors has been well established. The following are factors associated with high perinatal mortality rates:

Very young and old mothers: Statistically, the years between 20 and 30 seem to be the best for childbearing. Women over 30 and teenage girls have the highest perinatal mortality rate.

First and high parity births: The mother with no previous pregnancies or the mother with a high number of previous births also has a high perinatal mortality rate.

Prematurity: Prematurity is one of the leading causes of death among the deaths categorized under the heading of perinatal mortality. The prematurity rate for twin births is significantly higher than for single births.

The mother's previous reproductive loss: Mothers who have had one or more previous losses experience another loss more frequently than do mothers who have had no previous losses.

Low socioeconomic levels: There is an inverse relationship between the number of perinatal deaths and the socioeconomic level of the mother (i.e., the higher the number of deaths, the lower the economic status). Countries which have very low perinatal mortality rates, Sweden, for example, have very few slums and poor people.

Illegitimacy: The woman who becomes pregnant out of wedlock tends to delay going for prenatal care; she usually eats a poor diet and may deny or try to hide her pregnancy.

In contrast to maternal mortality rates, reduction in perinatal mortality rates has proceeded slowly.

Infant Mortality Rates

How does the United States compare with other countries of the world? With all of the affluence in medical, physical, and professional resources, the United States ranks behind 12 other countries who have lower infant mortality rates. Furthermore, the United States is moving backward from the sixth place it held in the period from 1949 to 1951.

The countries having fewer deaths than the United States are listed below in order of increasing death rate.*

1. Sweden (lowest)	7. Switzerland
2. Finland	8. New Zealand
3. Holland	9. Australia
4. Norway	10. United Kingdom
5. Denmark	11. East Germany
6. France	12. Japan
	13. United States

On a worldwide basis, the infant mortality rates (among recording countries) range from 200 or even 500 per 1000 live births in some segments of the population down to 12. Moreover, in some countries many births and deaths are not reported. In the United States the infant mortality rate decreased from 100 in 1915 to 21.7 in 1968, with the greatest decrease occurring during the early part of the 20th century. Beginning in 1950 the decrease slowed considerably and then reached a plateau.

According to Falkner† there is an incorrect assumption both here and abroad that the major reason for the high infant mortality rate in the United States is that twice as many black babies die as compared to white babies. However, if blacks (who compose 15 per cent of the population) were excluded from the rates the infant mortality rate in the United States would only have been two points lower for 1967 — 20 instead

---

*Reported by the National Center for Health Statistics, United States Department of Health, Education, and Welfare, 1967.

†Falkner, F.: Infant mortality, an urgent national problem. *Children, 17:* No. 3, 1970.

of 22. There are, in fact, some indications that poor white families in some areas may have higher infant mortality rates.

Racial factors and their socioeconomic ramifications are the least of the problems as far as the high overall infant mortality rate is concerned. It is important to attack not only the environmental, social, and economic problems associated with infant mortality but also the biological problems.

What are the leading causes of deaths among infants? Low birth weight (of full-term and premature babies) heads the list of causes. Other high ranking causes of death are congenital malformations, birth injuries, and respiratory disorders.

What can be done to reduce the infant mortality rate? This calls for (1) predicting which infants will be high risks, and (2) providing highly skilled care for the mothers and infants during the birth process and in the immediate postnatal period. The following points should be taken into consideration in attacking the problem of high infant mortality.

1. Deaths in the first week of life account for two thirds of all infant deaths. Since a large percentage of the babies who die weigh under 2500 grams (5 lb. 8 oz.), prematurity and low birth weight are fundamental issues in any attempt at reducing the infant mortality rate. It is interesting to note that births of premature and low-birth weight babies have increased by 8 per cent in the United States since 1950.

2. The cause of premature birth should be explored further. Many factors such as the social, economic, and environmental conditions in which the baby is conceived and carried should be considered. Also, some of the biological factors concerning the mother such as the interval between her pregnancies, her age, and the state of her nutrition should be further investigated.

3. The relief of social and economic disadvantage would have a major effect on infant mortality. Poor nutrition, lack of sanitation, and inadequate health education, all stem from poverty. Thus if the nutrition of poor families could be improved,

there might be a reduction in the incidence of low-birth weight babies.

4. Provisions for staff to carry out high quality services to both mothers and babies is needed. Not only should more people be trained for the health services, but those currently serving on the health team should be trained in new ways. These health team members would provide primary prevention through highly skilled prenatal care, and secondary prevention through highly skilled, intensive neonatal care.

5. Better family planning programs would reduce infant mortality. The better spacing of children promotes and protects family health. Family planning would reduce the number of pregnancies among very young girls and women beyond the peak childbearing years. Both of these groups, as we have seen, have a high incidence of low-birth weight babies.

6. Further research into the key factors which contribute to infant mortality is needed. While research is being carried out on such problems as respiratory distress in newborns, little research has been done on certain important problems such as the effect of malnutrition on fetal development.

MORBIDITY AND MORTALITY AMONG CHILDREN

Mortality

Vital statistics reports for 1969 show that accidents continue to be the number one killer of children in the United States. Table 4-2 shows some interesting comparisons as to the cause of death among children, adolescents, and young adults between 1968 and 1969.

Although there was a decrease in most diseases in 1969, notable was the slight increase in influenza and pneumonia.

The largest decreases in deaths from any cause occurred in the 1 to 4 age group, down 7.4 per cent from 1968, and in those children under 1 year, down 4.8 per cent.*

---

*Differentiation in specific diseases between the two age groups is not available at this time.

Table 4-2. DEATH RATES FOR SPECIFIED CAUSES, BY AGE GROUPS OVER 1 YEAR: UNITED STATES, 1968 AND 1969*

Cause of Death	Year	All Ages	1–14 Years	15–24 Years
Malignant neoplasms, including neoplasms of lymphatic and hematopoietic tissues	1969	160.1	6.6	7.7
	1968	159.6	6.6	7.8
Malignant neoplasms of digestive organs and peritoneum	1969	46.4	0.1	0.3
	1968	46.8	0.1	0.5
Malignant neoplasms of respiratory system	1969	32.7	0.0	0.2
	1968	32.2	0.1	0.2
Malignant neoplasm of breast	1969	14.5	–	0.0
	1968	14.6	0.0	0.1
Malignant neoplasms of genital organs	1969	20.1	0.1	0.8
	1968	20.9	0.1	0.9
Diabetes mellitus	1969	18.5	0.1	0.7
	1968	19.2	0.2	0.6
Major cardiovascular diseases	1969	499.7	1.2	4.4
	1968	511.0	1.6	4.5
Diseases of heart	1969	364.1	0.7	2.3
	1968	372.9	0.7	2.4
Cerebrovascular diseases	1969	102.0	0.5	1.6
	1968	104.8	0.7	1.7
Cerebral hemorrhage	1969	21.8	0.1	0.4
	1968	23.1	0.2	0.5
Cerebral thrombosis	1969	29.0	0.0	0.1
	1968	30.6	0.1	0.1
Arteriosclerosis	1969	16.7	–	–
	1968	16.7	–	–
Influenza and pneumonia	1969	34.7	3.4	2.7
	1968	34.9	3.1	2.7
Bronchitis, emphysema, and asthma	1969	15.6	0.3	0.5
	1968	16.6	0.4	0.4
Cirrhosis of liver	1969	15.0	0.2	0.8
	1968	14.5	0.1	0.5
Accidents	1969	56.0	22.0	68.9
	1968	55.8	23.7	67.4
Motor vehicle accidents	1969	26.8	9.9	47.7
	1968	27.0	10.0	48.3
All other accidents	1969	29.2	12.1	21.2
	1968	28.8	13.7	19.0

(Based on a 10 per cent sample of deaths. Rates per 100,000 population in specific group.)
*Monthly Vital Statistics Report: Annual Summary for the United States, vol. 18, no. 13, October 21, 1970.

Comparison with the adolescent and young adult group shows a marked increase in motor vehicle accidents, with proportionately few deaths from other accidents.

Communicable Disease

Deaths from the common, uncomplicated communicable diseases of childhood are rare in the United States, except in the case of congenital rubella. However, complications may be serious. Table 4-3 presents statistics on the number of reported cases in 1969–1970 of the most common and well-known communicable diseases.

Rubeola. Rubeola is endemic in most communities, assuming epidemic proportions about every other year. In areas, such as the Arctic, where there are long intervals between outbreaks fatality rates may be high.

Table 4-3. CASES OF NOTIFIABLE DISEASES IN THE UNITED STATES FOR 1969–1970*

	1969	1970
Diphtheria	207	436
Encephalitis (arthropod-borne)	1,295	1,544
(postinfectious)	308	367
Measles	24,786	46,775
Mumps	86,983	100,461
Poliomyelitis	18	31
Rubella	54,739	54,885
Aseptic meningitis	3,458	6,091

*Morbidity and Mortality Weekly Report (for the week ending 26 December, 1970).

Pertussis. Mortality rates from pertussis in the United States have shown a marked decline, but in many less developed countries pertussis is among the most lethal of the common communicable diseases of childhood.

Diphtheria. Once a common cause of death in families in the United States, diphtheria has been considered to be nearly extinct in this country. However, recent outbreaks in certain states have shown that vigilance cannot be let down without disastrous effects.

Poliomyelitis. "In the United States and Canada, in Australia and New Zealand, the reduction of cases can be considered to be a thousandfold in 1969, compared with the averages for 1951–55."* In Europe the annual poliomyelitis incidence has dropped markedly since polio vaccine was introduced.

However, the World Health Organization reports that "in Africa, as in Central and South America and in Asia, the frequency of outbreaks is increasing and countries there may have to face extensive epidemics at any moment."† (See Table 4-4.)

*World Health Organization Magazine, July 1970, p. 35.
†Id.

Table 4-4. CASES OF POLIOMYELITIS FROM MAJOR REGIONS OF THE WORLD*

	Average annual number of cases		Annual reports of cases
	1951–55	1961–65	1969
Europe	28,359	6,665	475
U.S.A., Canada, Australia, New Zealand	44,378	851	21
Africa (34 countries)	3,660	3,932	3,726
Central and South America (20 countries)	4,639	3,903	1,527
Asia (17 countries)	4,718	4,647	758

*World Health Organization Magazine, July, 1970.

Infectious Hepatitis. Infectious hepatitis is a disease most prevalent among children and young adults. Although the disease may last a long time, the fatality rate is less than 1 per cent.

Tuberculosis. Tuberculosis has shown a downward trend in numerous countries throughout the world. Prevalence of pulmonary tuberculosis is now low in the age group under 20 years.

Infectious Mononucleosis. This disease is widespread among children and young adults throughout the world. It appears to be a mild infection, but more research is needed.

Venereal Disease. Venereal disease has become a serious problem among children and young people in the United States and elsewhere. Gonorrhea has assumed epidemic proportions. The serious effects of syphilis and gonorrhea are discussed in Chapters 21 and 44.

Other Diseases. Diseases such as smallpox, plague, cholera, and malaria are still present throughout the world. *Smallpox* is slowly yielding to an eradication program of the World Health Organization (WHO). The only known case in the United

States since 1949, occurred in 1962, when a young boy traveling with his family from Brazil passed through New York City after he had become ill. Upon his arrival in Canada his illness was diagnosed as smallpox. All known contacts were urged to report for vaccination. No transmission of this case occurred.

Malaria has essentially disappeared in many countries, due to WHO's program of eradication. In certain countries where the program has been interrupted due to war or other causes, it is again on the increase. In 1970, some cases in the United States developed among heroin users, presumably from infected needles.

BIBLIOGRAPHY

Around the world. p. 35. World Health Magazine. July, 1970.

Falkner, Frank: Infant mortality, an urgent national problem, Children, *17*:83, 1970.

Hunt, Eleanor: Infant mortality trends and maternal and infant care, Children, *17*:88, 1970.

Monthly Vital Statistics Report: Annual Summary for the United States, vol. 18, no. 13, Oct. 21, 1970.

Statistical Abstract of the United States Bureau of the Census, ed. 91. Washington, D.C. 1970.

Anatomy and Physiology of the Reproductive System

5

THE FEMALE REPRODUCTIVE SYSTEM

In the female the reproductive system has two basic functions: to prepare the body for conception and gestation and to house and maintain the fetus during gestation. The structure of the reproductive system is divided into external and internal organs, many of which are analogous to those found in the male.

External Genitalia

The external organs of the female are called the vulva and consist of the mons veneris, labia majora, labia minora, clitoris, hymen, vestibule, and various glands (Fig. 5-1). Sometimes the word vulva has been used to refer only to the labia majora and labia minora. Labia means lips.

Labia Majora. The labia majora are

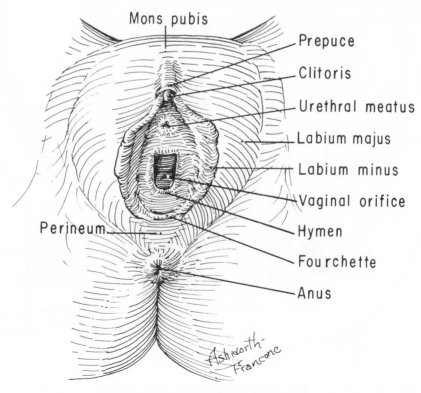

Figure 5-1. External female genitalia.

the two fatty, fairly thick folds of skin that serve as a protection for the more delicate underlying structures. From adolescence on their external surface is covered with pubic hair, whereas the internal surface consists of mucous membrane. The labia majora in the female are analagous to the scrotum in the male.

Labia Minora. Lying between the two labia majora are the thinner more delicate structures of the labia minora, the outer surfaces of which consist of mucous membrane. They too serve as protection to the underlying structures.

The labia majora and labia minora join anteriorly at the prepuce, or hood of the clitoris. Posteriorly, they meet to form the fourchette. There is a firm pad of adipose tissue, called the mons pubis or mons veneris (mons means mountain), which

overlies the symphysis pubis and is covered by pubic hair.

Clitoris. The clitoris is a small round organ which is situated under the prepuce and is the seat of sexual excitement in the female. When stimulated in sex play it becomes engorged with blood and hence more erect. The many tiny nerve endings become increasingly sensitive to erotic stimulation and may produce an orgasm. Hence, the clitoris in the female is analogous to the male glans penis.

Vestibule. A roughly almond-shaped area, bordered anteriorly by the clitoris, posteriorly by the fourchette, and on each side by the labia minora, is called the vestibule. There are four different kinds of openings on the vestibule, including the vaginal opening. Beneath the clitoris usually about midway between the clitoris

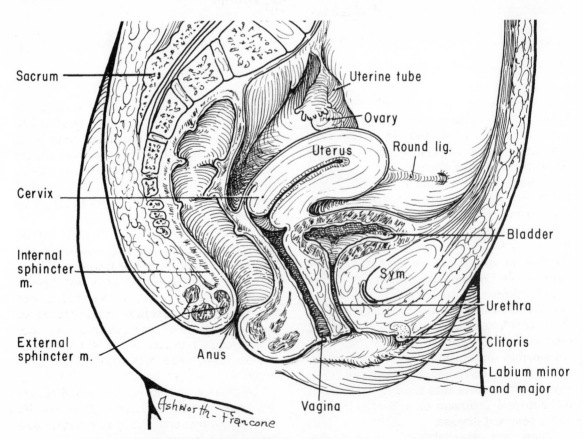

Figure 5-2. Midsagittal section of the female pelvis and the internal reproductive organs.

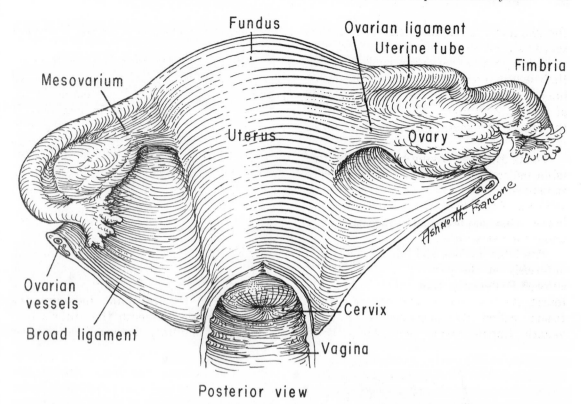

Posterior view

Figure 5-3. Internal female reproductive organs.

and the vagina is a small dimplelike opening—the urinary meatus. Its location may vary somewhat and, in a few rare instances, has even been found in or near the anterior wall of the vagina.

Glands. On either side of the urethra are the Skene's glands, which are analogous to the prostate gland in the male. Bartholin's glands are two glands situated in either side of the vagina. Their function is to lubricate the vagina with a mucoid material to prepare it for sexual intercourse. If these glands become infected and fill up with pus the formation is called Bartholin's cyst. When this happens, the labia may be greatly distended and painful. Sometimes the responsible organism is the gonococcus which causes gonorrhea. However, not every patient who comes into the hospital for an incision and drainage of a Bartholin cyst has a venereal disease.

There are other glands located in the external genitalia such as the apocrine or sudoriparous glands. These glands become more active during pregnancy and may create offensive odors. There is also a cheesy substance called smegma which may collect in the folds of the labia. This is why careful cleansing of the external genitalia is so important.

Hymen. The hymen is a thin elastic membrane which partially occludes the vaginal opening. It is the traditional symbol of virginity. However, it is well known today that the absence of the hymen does not necessarily preclude virginity. Some girls are born with practically no evidence of a hymen. Then too, an accident or strenuous sports activity may have caused it to rupture.

In girls or women who have had sexual intercourse or have borne a child usually only the remnants of the hymen remain and are called carunculae myrtiformes.

If the hymen completely covers the vaginal opening with a thick, tough membrane, then a rare condition called imperforate hymen exists. In such instances, an opening is made surgically (hymenotomy) so that the menstrual flow is released and sexual intercourse can take place.

Vestibular Bulb. There is a group of veins beneath the mucous membranes on either side of the vagina called the vestibular bulb. If not properly repaired in childbirth they can hemorrhage.

Internal Reproductive Organs

The internal organs of female reproduction are the vagina, uterus, uterine (fallopian) tubes, and ovaries (Figs. 5-2 and 5-3).

Vagina

The vagina connects the internal and external genitalia and serves as the excretory duct for the uterus, as the female organ of copulation, and as a part of the birth canal. The area between the vagina and the rectum is called the perineum.

The healthy vagina has a pH of between 4 and 6. It lies in folds known as *rugae* and is capable of great softening, stretching, and distension in childbearing. The vagina is about three to five inches in length and is lined with mucous membrane which becomes thicker during pregnancy. For more information about the vagina during pregnancy see Chapter 6.

Uterus

The uterus is a hollow pear-shaped organ which is about the size of a fist and is covered by peritoneum and lined by mucous membrane. It is divided into three parts: the *fundus,* or top of the uterus; the *corpus,* or body of the uterus; and the *cervix* or neck of the uterus (Fig. 5-3).

The main function of the uterus is to house the products of conception. During pregnancy it increases in weight from one ounce to two pounds, as its capacity and its length increases. Not only do the muscle cells enlarge, but a greater number of new cells are formed because of the tremendous growth that takes place in this organ.

The muscles of the uterus are composed of circular, longitudinal, and figure-of-eight fibers. They contract involuntarily in childbirth, that is, they are not under the conscious control of the mother. An important fact to know is that these muscles run in all directions. If they are well contracted following delivery, they will occlude the open blood vessels at the site at which the placenta was attached, thereby preventing hemorrhage.

The three layers of the uterus are the *parametrium,* which is that portion of the uterus not covered by peritoneum; the *myometrium,* composed of the muscles which have just been referred to; and the *endometrium,* which is the lining of the uterus.

During pregnancy the endometrium is called the *decidua*. For purposes of description, the decidua has been divided into three parts. The part that lies directly under the implanted ovum is called the decidua basalis. The part which encloses or is pushed out by the growing ovum is called the decidua capsularis. And the remainder of the decidua, which is not in contact with the ovum, is known as the decidua vera.

Fallopian (Uterine) Tubes

The fallopian tubes are about seven to fourteen inches long. They appear somewhat like a horn in shape and consist of three parts—the *isthmus,* which is the point of insertion into the uterus; *the ampulla,* which is the slender midportion; and the *fimbriated end,* which is fingerlike in appearance.

The tubes are lined with cilia (fine hairs) and have a peristaltic action (like the intestinal tract). When ovulation takes place the ovum enters the fimbriated end of the fluid-filled tube. It is swept along toward the uterine cavity by the cilia which are set into motion by the peristaltic movements.

Ovaries

The ovaries are two almond-shaped organs which develop and expel a mature ovum each month and produce the hormones, estrogen and progesterone. They store thousands of undeveloped follicles, which have been present since birth. It is fascinating to think that at the time of birth a female child has *all* of the potential ova from which she will produce her offspring.

The ovaries, which are analogous to the testes in the male, are located near the fallopian tubes embedded in the broad ligaments. In addition they are supported by three other ligaments called the suspensory, meso-ovarian, and ovarian ligaments.

Muscles of the Pelvic Floor

The muscles which form a sling for the pelvis are mainly the coccygeus, the levator ani, and the perineal body. Since these muscles run in different directions they are capable of giving good support to the pelvic organs. However, they offer resistance to the descent of the presenting part of the baby during childbirth. The main muscle

of support is the *perineal body*. It is composed of the superficial transverse muscle, the bulbocavernous, and the external sphincter ani. The perineal body is frequently cut in an episiotomy or torn during childbirth. If it is not repaired subsequently, there is a tendency for the organs such as the uterus to prolapse into the vagina.

Pelvic Ligaments

Ligaments or bands of fibrous and connective tissue are essential in holding the internal female reproductive organs in place. There are four such ligaments.

The broad ligaments extend on either side of the uterus to the pelvic wall (Fig. 5-3). They divide the pelvic cavity into anterior and posterior compartments.

The *round* ligaments are attached on either side of the fundus just below the fallopian tubes. They extend forward and attach in the upper part of the labia majora. Their function is to maintain the normal anteflexion of the uterus.

The *uterosacral* ligaments help support the cervix by extending from the lower part of the uterus near the cervix to the sacrum.

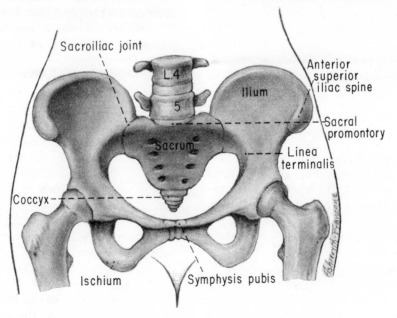

Figure 5-4. The female bony pelvis.

The *cardinal* ligament is the lower portion of the broad ligament and is firmly united to the supravaginal portion of the cervix. Acting with the perineal body, it prevents prolapse of the uterus.

Blood and Nerve Supply

The blood supply to the internal reproductive organs goes through the uterine and ovarian arteries which are branches from the hypogastric arteries.

There is central nervous system control of the reproductive system. The sympathetic nervous system maintains vasoconstriction and muscle tone, whereas the parasympathetic system causes vasodilation and inhibits contractions. Hence the two systems are antagonistic to each other and usually achieve a balance.

The Pelvis

The female reproductive organs are contained within the pelvis (pelvis means basin). A knowledge of the parts and dimensions of the female pelvis is necessary if labor is to be understood, for the baby must pass through this structure in order to exit into the world.

The Bony Pelvis

Four bones make up the pelvis: two innominate (or hip) bones which are irregularly shaped, wide, and flaring; the sacrum which is a wedge-shaped bone; and the coccyx, which is a small triangular bone attached to the sacrum (Fig. 5-4).

The innominate bone is made up of three separate bones, the ilium, the ischium, and the pubis, which are fused together in the adult in such a way that it is impossible to tell that it was formerly divided. Fusion of these bones is completed around age 20 to 25.

The largest division is the *ilium* which forms the upper and back part of the pelvis. The crest of the ilium is the part of the hip bone that you can feel as you press on the sides of your abdomen. The *ischium* is the lower part below the hip joint. The tuberosity of the ischium (or ischial spines) is a landmark used in obstetrics to determine the degree of descent of the presenting part (known as station) of the baby during labor. It is the part of the anatomy on which we sit. The pubis is the front part of the hip bone. The anterior articulation of the two pubic bones is called the symphysis pubis or pubic arch.

The two bones, the sacrum and coccyx, which are located in the posterior part of the pelvis, are both important in obstetrics. The sacral promontory (the junction between the sacrum and the last lumbar vertebra) can create difficulty in delivery if

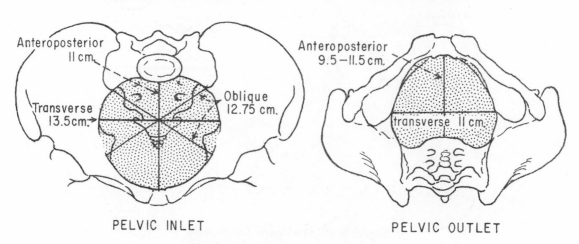

Figure 5-5. Pelvic outlet and inlet.

it is too prominent. Or if the coccyx is fixed and immovable, this too can cause problems.

For obstetrical purposes the pelvis is conceived as being divided into two parts, the false and true pelvis. The false pelvis is the wide, flaring upper part which contains the reproductive organs. The true pelvis has more significance obstetrically because during labor this is the narrow part of the bony basin through which the largest diameter of the baby's head must fit.

For descriptive purposes, the true pelvis can be divided anatomically into an inlet, a cavity, and an outlet.

Pelvic Inlet. The true pelvis can be separated from the false pelvis by drawing an imaginary line called the linea terminalis around it. In a woman with a normally shaped pelvis, the inlet, or brim, is heart-shaped because of the protuberance of the sacral promontory. The widest diameter is from side to side (transverse diameter) and the narrowest is from front to back (anteroposterior) (Fig. 5-5).

In labor the widest diameter of the baby's head turns so that it will accommodate itself to the widest part of the pelvis. Since the widest dimension of the baby's head is anteroposterior, it enters the transverse diameter of the inlet.

Pelvic Cavity. This is the cylindrical part of the true pelvis between the inlet and the outlet. It is shaped somewhat like an inverted stovepipe. The top is fairly straight, but the bottom is curved forward (toward the birth canal). Not only must the baby turn sideways to accommodate itself to the irregularities of the pelvis, but it must take a curved route as well. This adds to the difficulties of being born.

Pelvic Outlet. The boundaries are the symphysis pubis anteriorly, the coccyx posteriorly, and the sides of the two ischial tuberosities. It is significant that the normal female pelvis has a wide pubic arch rather than a narrow one as is found in the male pelvis.

The largest diameter in the pelvic outlet is the anteroposterior (from front to

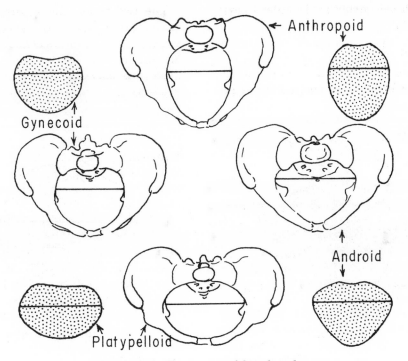

Figure 5-6.   Four types of female pelves.

back) which is the opposite from the pelvic inlet (the transverse diameter being the largest). Therefore, the baby's head must rotate 90 degrees in order for its largest diameter to pass through the largest diameter of the outlet.

Types of Pelves

No two pelves are exactly alike. Usually, however, there are only slight variations from one person to the next. Because of these differences, it is routine to check pelvic measurements when the pregnant woman makes her first prenatal visit. There is always a chance that some abnormality of the pelvic passageway may exist.

There are several reasons why a woman's pelvis could be inadequate in size or shape. She might have inherited a small pelvis, or had rickets or tuberculosis in childhood, or been in an accident. Any of these factors could cause a permanent deformity of the pelvis which might require delivery by cesarean section.

Female pelves have been classified into four different types. The first, called the gynecoid pelvis is the best one for childbearing. The other three types, known as the anthropoid, platypelloid, and android pelves, may produce obstetric difficulties (Fig. 5-6).

A brief description of each of the classifications follows:

Gynecoid: the pelvic inlet is heartshaped, the pubic arch is wide and shallow. It is lighter and more commodious than the male pelvis.

Anthropoid (ape-like): the inlet is deep and increased in the anteroposterior diameter.

Platypelloid (flat): the inlet is flat with a decreased anteroposterior diameter.

Android (male): the pelvic inlet is wedge-shaped and angular. It is heavier and more confining.

Even though the android, anthropoid, and platypelloid types of pelves are less suitable than the gynecoid type, other facts will determine if the birth will terminate

vaginally or by cesarean section. The size of the baby, the strength of the contractions, and the condition of the mother, as well as the type of passageway should all be considered.

Pelvic Measurements and X-Ray Pelvimetry

There are three different ways of measuring the pelvis. One is to use a pelvimeter which is an instrument that looks like a calibrated set of ice tongs and can be used to obtain external measurements, such as the distance between the iliac crests. Since most of these external measurements concern mainly physicians and not nurses, discussion about them will be omitted. If you are interested in reading about them see the bibliography at the end of the chapter.

A second way the physician obtains pelvic measurements is during a vaginal examination, while the patient is in a lithotomy position with her feet in stirrups. The following pelvic measurements are the most important for the nurse to know about.

Diagonal conjugate: distance between the sacral promontory and the lower margins of the symphysis pubis. The average is around 12.5 cm. or above.

True Conjugate (conjugate vera): distance between the sacral promontory and the posterior aspect of the symphysis pubis. To obtain this estimated measurement the physician subtracts 1.5 to 2 cm. from the diagonal conjugate. This is the smallest diameter through which the baby's head passes. The true conjugate should be about 11 cm.

Transverse diameter of the outlet: the distance between the two ischial tuberosities as measured by a pelvimeter (other names are the biischial diameter or the intertuberous diameter). Average measurement is about 8 cm. or above.

The third way, and also the most accurate way, of measuring the pelvic dimensions is x-ray pelvimetry. Often the physician will wait until the last trimester starts

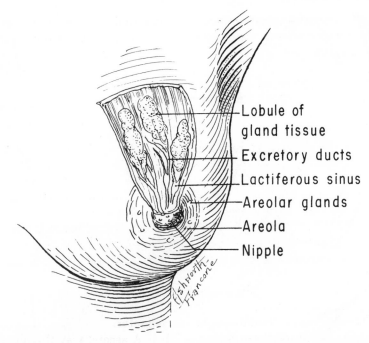

Lobule of
gland tissue

Excretory ducts

Lactiferous sinus

Areolar glands

Areola

Nipple

Figure 5-7. The female breast with the skin partly removed to show the under-lying structures.

to use this method. Then if there is any indication that the baby is large, or that there are twins, or the progress of labor is poor, or the presenting part has not engaged in a primigravida at term, the physician will order x-ray pelvimetry. The results of the x-ray complete with measurements are usually returned to the labor and delivery department. It is always interesting if you yourself look at the x-rays and check the various measurements, comparing them to normal.

The Breasts

The breasts are considered to be accessory organs of reproduction. They are composed of glandular, fibrous, and adipose tissue and rest on a foundation of connective tissue. The glandular tissue of the breasts forms 15 to 20 lobes which are arranged radially around the nipple (Fig. 5-7).

Each lobe is divided into several lobules, each of which contains numerous *acini,* the cells that produce milk. The nipple is a small, cylindrical body which projects slightly from the center of each breast. It is composed of erectile tissue which responds to tactile stimulation. The tip of the nipple is perforated with 15 to 20 minute openings of the lactiferous ducts.

The blood supply to the breasts comes by way of the thoracic branches of the axillary, intercostal, and internal thoracic arteries. There are many cutaneous veins, which follow the same course as the arteries. During pregnancy and lactation, when the blood flow increases, the cutaneous veins may become distended and blue, giving the chest wall a characteristic "road map" appearance. Observe for it when you are helping a mother who is breast feeding.

Colostrum is a thin yellowish fluid composed of colostrum corpuscles, watery fluid, and fat globules. Colostrum contains more protein, but less fat and sugar than mature human milk.

Following delivery colostrum continues to be secreted until about the third day postpartum when the breast milk "comes in." Breast feeding during this time stimu-

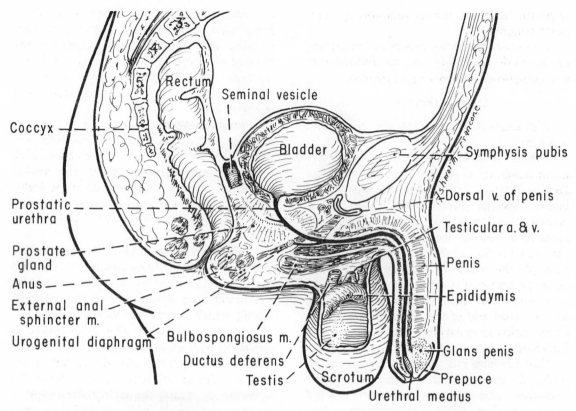

Figure 5-8. Midsagittal section of the male pelvis and external genitalia.

lates lactation and satisfies the infant's urge to suck.

Prior to parturition the high levels of estrogen and progesterone inhibit the release of prolactin from the anterior pituitary gland. Because of the rapid decrease in the hormone levels following delivery (the placenta which produces them has been removed), this lactogenic hormone is now released, bringing about the production of milk.

Another hormone oxytocin from the posterior lobe of the pituitary gland stimulates the expression of milk from the lactating breasts. This is called the let-down reflex, which is found in both animals and humans. It is initiated by the infant nuzzling or sucking at the breasts. This sends a nerve impulse to the brain to signal the release of oxytocin into the bloodstream.

It is believed that oxytocin causes the alveoli to contract, thus forcing the milk into the ducts. The milk then flows into the lacteriferous sinuses which lie beneath the surface of the areola. Hence, one can see the importance of getting not only the nipple but also the areola into the infant's mouth, so that the sucking action of his jaws will compress the lacteriferous sinuses.

After the let-down reflex is established other stimuli in addition to sucking can release or inhibit it. Sounds of the infant crying may produce it. Fright, pain, or emotional stress may inhibit it.

For additional material about the changes in the breasts during pregnancy see Chapters 6 and 8.

THE MALE REPRODUCTIVE ORGANS

The main functons of the male reproductive organs are to produce sperm (spermatogenesis), to perform the sex act, and to regulate the male sexual function by various hormones.

As in the female the reproductive organs of the male (Fig. 5-8) can be divided into two categories; external and internal.

External Genitalia

The external organs are the penis and scrotum.

Penis. The penis is a cylindrical organ made up of spongy cavernous bodies. During sexual excitement the cavernous bodies become filled with blood which causes the penis to become erect and capable of sexual intercourse. Otherwise, the organ is flaccid. The urethra runs down through the center of the penis and opens near the center of the *glans penis*. The glans is a somewhat enlarged conical structure at the distal end of the penis; in uncircumcized males it is covered with a *prepuce* or foreskin.

The urethra has a dual purpose in the male. It carries both urine and sperm. However, there is an automatic cutoff valve so that during intercourse when ejaculation takes place only semen can be released into the vagina.

Scrotum. The scrotum is a loose pouch which contains the testicles. The reason the testicles must be outside of the body is that higher body temperatures destroy the sperm. From adolescence on, the scrotum and the area surrounding the penis is covered with pubic hair.

Internal Genitalia

The internal organs are the testes, canal system, and accessory structures.

Testes. The testes, or testicles, are divided into wedges. Each wedge contains convoluted (twisted) seminiferous (sperm-producing) tubules called the rete testis. The seminiferous tubules combine to form the epididymis. The sperm remain there for 18 hours, when they become motile and capable of fertilizing an ovum. The testes manufacture a very important male hormone, testosterone, which is responsible for

secondary sex characteristics such as a deep voice, characteristic pattern of hair growth, etc. Human spermatogenesis begins at the age of puberty and continues through life. However, there is a decline with advancing age due to degenerative changes.

Canal System. The canal system is made up of the epididymis, the vas deferens, the ejaculatory duct, and the urethra. This is the system through which the viable sperm are carried to the outside of the body. At the time of sexual intercourse there are from 300 to 500 million sperm released in a single ejaculation.

Accessory Structures. The accessory duct system in the male consists of: the two seminal vesicles which are located behind the bladder on either side of the prostate gland, which contribute to the production of semen (the fluid in which the sperm is carried); the prostate gland which surrounds the urethra and ejaculatory duct and secretes an alkaline secretion into the semen to neutralize the acidity of the vagina so that the sperm will not be destroyed; and *Cowper's gland* which provides a mucoid secretion into the urethra.

PHYSIOLOGY OF MENSTRUATION

Menarche is the term used for the onset of menstruation. It is caused by a gradual increase in gonadotrophic hormone secreted by the pituitary gland. The menarche usually begins between the ages of nine and 13. However, in some girls it does not occur until the ages of 16 to 18. Its onset depends on nutritional status, heredity, climate, and a number of factors. For example, the onset of menstruation tends to appear earlier in girls who are well nourished and girls who live in warm climates. In fact the average age for the start of menstruation has decreased by six months in the last decade. The average age is now 11.5 years. Experts attribute this to better nutrition and, hence, an earlier maturation.

The menarche is characterized by anovulatory cycles. This means that ovulation fails to occur. In almost all girls the first few cycles immediately after puberty are anovulatory. Since ovulation does not occur there is no development of the corpus luteum. Consequently, there is no secretion of progesterone during the cycle so that the rhythm of the cycle is often disturbed. Hence, another characteristic of the onset of menstruation is the irregularity of the cycles.

Once the menstrual cycle is established it is characterized by monthly rhythmical changes in the rates of secretion of the sex hormones with corresponding changes in the sexual organs themselves.

The range of the cycle in completely normal women may be as short as 20 days or as long as 45 days. The usual range is 28 days. Some women do not realize that there may be a normal variation in the menstrual cycle of a few days, in which case the cycle is still considered to be regular. For example, it may be 27 days one time, 29 days the next, 31 the next and so on.

There are two significant results of the menstrual cycle: (1) it normally causes a single mature ovum to be released from the ovaries each month, and (2) it prepares the endometrium of the uterus for implantation of the fertilized ovum. If the ovum is not fertilized, the menstrual flow takes place, during which approximately

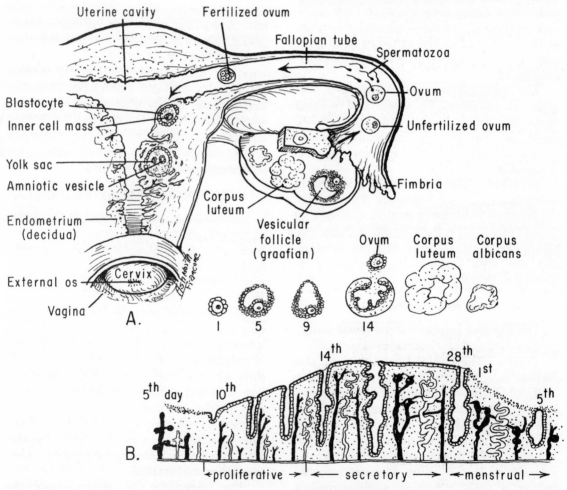

Figure 5-9. (A) Physiologic processes of the ovary and uterus, showing ovulation, fertilization and implantation; (B) cyclic menstrual changes in the uterine endometrium.

35 cc. of blood, 35 cc. of serous fluid, along with desquamated tissue, are lost on an average.

The Phases of the Menstrual Cycle

Menstrual Phase. The first day of menstruation is considered to be day 1 of the menstrual cycle. This phase is caused by the sudden reduction in estrogen and progesterone. Because estrogen acts as an endometrial vasodilator, when it is suddenly withdrawn vasospasm occurs. As a result, beginning necrosis of the endometrium, especially of the blood vessels, takes place. Hemorrhagic areas appear all over the uterus and separate the necrotic endometrium from the uterus. The desquamated tissue and blood initiate uterine contractions which expel the uterine contents. This phase usually lasts around five days with three to seven days being the normal range.

The menstrual blood is normally nonclotting because fibrinolysin is released along with the necrotic endometrial tissue. If excessive bleeding occurs there may not be enough fibrinolysin to prevent clotting.

Proliferative Phase. The proliferative phase, around 11 days in length, is also known as the estrogen phase. The endometrium increases in thickness due to the growth of stromal cells, endometrial glands, and blood vessels. This occurs during the first two weeks of the cycle. Then ovulation takes place. There is a degeneration of the outer cells of the follicle, and fluid leaks out increasing the tear in the follicle. The ovum surrounded by granulosa cells is expelled into the abdominal cavity. It is then picked up by the beckoning fimbriated ends of the fallopian tube.

Secretory Phase. The secretory phase lasts around 12 days and may be called the progesterone phase. During the latter half of the menstrual cycle both estrogen and progesterone are secreted in large quantities by the corpus luteum.

Progesterone, acting with estrogen, causes considerable swelling of the endometrium. The glands become more tortuous (twisted) and begin secreting. Blood vessels also become highly tortuous. There are lipoid (fat) and glycogen (sugar) deposits in the stromal cells. The endometrium has become thick and velvety–a perfect bed for the fertilized ovum. If fertilization does not take place, the whole process repeats itself (Fig. 5-9).

Hormonal Control of the Menstrual Cycle

The pituitary gland, or master gland, plays an essential part in the hormonal control of the menstrual cycle. It secretes three different hormones necessary for full functioning of the ovaries. These are: FSH or follicle-stimulating hormone, LH or luteinizing hormone, and LTH or luteotropic hormone. This last hormone also helps to promote the secretion of milk by the breasts and is known by the names *lactogen, prolactin,* or *lactogenic hormone.* Cyclic variations (increase and decrease) in the amounts of these hormones each month cause the cyclic ovarian changes.

FSH. FSH is responsible for follicular growth. The primordial follicles which are present at birth grow and mature when stimulated by a large quantity of FSH. First the ovum enlarges, followed by an increase of granulosa and theca cells. These cells secrete follicular fluid.

The secretion of LH increases and with FSH causes more rapid growth of follicles. During each monthly cycle about 20 or more primordial follicles develop, but ordinarily one follicle far outgrows the others. It becomes known as the graafian follicle. The growth of the follicles is associated with an increased secretion of estrogen.

LH. LH is necessary for the development of vesicular follicles (more mature primordial follicles) and ovulation. The developing vesicular follicles that do not ovulate, atrophy either before or immediately after ovulation occurs.

The Corpus Luteum. After the expulsion of the ovum the follicle undergoes luteinization, and the mass of cells becomes the corpus luteum. It has a distinctive yellow color, so it is sometimes called the yellow body. Sometimes blood is expelled into the abdominal cavity shortly after ovulation which irritates the peritoneum and causes pain. This pain is called "mittelschmerz" which is German, meaning pain in the middle (of the month).

The corpus luteum then involutes (or undergoes retrogressive changes) approximately 12 days following ovulation. It becomes the corpus albicans or white body. This further degenerates and is replaced by connective tissue. While it is active the corpus luteum secretes large amounts of both estrogen and progesterone. If pregnancy occurs the corpus luteum persists and becomes the corpus luteum of pregnancy.

In studying the menstrual cycle one is impressed with the beautiful balance and interplay between the hormones secreted by the pituitary and those secreted by the ovaries. It is a delicate balance, and it is amazing that it operates so smoothly much of the time.

Effects of Female Hormones on Sex Organs and Pregnancy

A discussion of female hormones would not be complete without describing other effects that they have in addition to regulating the menstrual cycle.

Effects of Estrogen on the Sex Organs.

1. Causes an increase in size of the fallopian tubes, uterus, and vagina.

2. Causes deposit of fat on the mons pubis and labia majora. Produces enlargement of the labia minora.

3. Changes vaginal epithelium from cuboidal to stratified type, which is more resistant to trauma and infection.

4. Produces changes in the endometrium (as described previously). Following puberty, the size of the uterus increases about two times.

5. Has the same effect on the lining of the fallopian tubes as it has on the uterine endometrium.

6. Causes the number of ciliated epithelial cells in the tubes to increase. The cilia help propel the fertilized ovum toward the uterus.

7. Causes fat deposits in the breasts. Initiates the growth of breasts and milk-producing glands and ducts but does not complete the job. (Large quantities of estrogen secreted during pregnancy will completely inhibit milk formation.)

Other Effects of Estrogen.

1. Effect on bones
   a. Causes an increase in osteoblastic activity with a rapid rate of growth at puberty.
   b. Causes early uniting of the epiphysis with the shafts of the long bones. Growth of the female usually stops earlier than the male.

2. Makes the skin smooth and soft.

3. Broadens the pelvis.

4. Causes more fat to be deposited in breasts, buttocks, and thighs, giving the female rounded "curves."

5. Causes characteristic hair distribution in pubic region.

Effects of Estrogen in Pregnancy.

1. Causes a marked increase of cells of the decidua.

2. Causes enlargement of the uterus, breasts, and genitalia.

3. Relaxes pelvic ligaments (along with the hormone "relaxin").

4. Causes retention of calcium, phosphorus, and sodium.

Note: Estrogen increases 50 to 60 times during pregnancy.

Effects of Progesterone on Sex Organs.

1. Promotes secretory changes in the endometrium, as previously stated.

2. Inhibits contractions of the uterus.

3. Produces same changes in the fallopian tubes as it does in the uterus.

4. Promotes final development in the breasts. Cells proliferate and become secre-

tory in nature. (It does *not* cause the alveoli to secrete milk.)

5. Causes breasts to feel full and heavy.

Functions of Progesterone During Pregnancy.

1. Promotes secretory changes in the decidua.

2. Decreases contractility of the pregnant uterus.

Note: Progesterone increases 10 times during pregnancy.

The Menopause

As a part of the degenerative changes that accompany the aging process, the production of hormones gradually decreases due to atrophic changes in the ovaries. This brings about a cessation of menstruation, known as the menopause, which usually begins between the ages of 45 and 50. Among American women, 47 is a usual age.

The following characteristics accompany the menopause. The menstrual cycles become irregular and the duration of the period may be shorter with a smaller amount of flow. (Of course, this varies greatly among individuals.) Ovulation fails to occur in many cycles. In a few months to a few years the cycle ceases entirely.

A woman who is going through the menopause may have other generalized symptoms, such as depression or irritability.

She may experience a phenomenon called "hot flashes" which occurs without warning. A red flush spreads up from the neck and over the face, followed generally by profuse perspiration. It is easy to see how these symptoms can be emotionally trying and embarrassing.

Because at the time of the menopause the quantity of estrogen decreases rapidly and no progesterone is secreted after the last ovulatory cycle, hormones may be prescribed by the doctor to alleviate these unpleasant symptoms. It is interesting to note that in general the menopause tends to occur earlier among women who had a late menarche, and later among women who had an early menarche!

BIBLIOGRAPHY

Davis, M. E., and Rubin, R.: DeLee's Obstetrics for Nurses. ed. 17. Philadelphia, W. B. Saunders, 1962.

Eastman, N. J., and Hellman, L. M.: William's Obstetrics. ed. 13. New York, Appleton-Century-Crofts, 1966.

Fitzpatrick, E. *et al.*: Maternity Nursing. ed 12. Philadelphia, J. B. Lippincott, 1971.

Jacob, S., and Francone, C.: Structure and Function in Man. ed. 2. Philadelphia, W. B. Saunders, 1970.

The Mammary Glands and Breast Feeding. Ross Laboratories. Nursing Education Service, No. 10 of a series.

Remov.
Ahead
draina.
seal off.
Arm exercises.
+ active a.

...all down

...umonectomy - either

...VS q̄ 15' - shock

Coughing & deep breathing -
        splint, breathe deep, exhale
        then cough

The First Trimester of Pregnancy 6

Someone has said that pregnancy begins at that unfelt, unknown moment of time when a single, wiggling sperm penetrates a mature ovum. Even though this momentous event of fertilization occurs without notice, the changes which take place within the mother's body in the next nine months are undeniable and amazing.

In order to understand the many different aspects of pregnancy, the nine months will be divided into three trimesters. Since pregnancy lasts approximately 280 days, 40 weeks, 10 lunar months, or nine calendar months, it is convenient to divide it into the first, second, and third trimesters. Each trimester covers a three-month span of time.

A way of determining the approximate expected date of confinement (E.D.C.) is to take the first day of the woman's last normal menstrual period, add seven days, subtract three months, and add one year. For example, if the woman told you that her last menstrual period began on June 14, 1971, you could make the calculation in the following manner:

$$
\begin{array}{r}
6 \ / \ 14 \ / \ 71 \\
-3 + \ 7 + \ 1 \\
\hline
3 \ / \ 21 \ / \ 72
\end{array}
$$

You would be correct in telling her that the approximate date she could expect her baby would be on March 21, 1972.

In each of the trimesters we will be concerned with the following aspects:

1. Growth and development of the fetus

2. Physiological changes in the expectant mother
3. Common discomforts and emotional changes
4. Aspects of health protection and promotion
5. Danger signs for which the parents, especially the mother should be alert
6. How the family can be included as part of the pregnancy.

FETAL GROWTH AND DEVELOPMENT

Fertilization

Pregnancy is much more interesting if one understands how conception takes place. Male sex cells (spermatozoa or sperm) enter the upper vagina by the millions when the man ejaculates during the sexual act. These cells are much smaller than the ova and move by lashing their long slender tails. Within 10 to 20 minutes they swim through the cervix into the uterus and up through the fallopian tubes. If there is an ovum in either of the two tubes a spermatozoon will usually succeed in fertilizing it by entering it and combining with it. Fertilization usually occurs in the outer third of a fallopian tube. But conception cannot take place if the sperm is late in arriving, since the ovum can be fertilized for only about 12 hours after it has been expelled from the ovary into one of the fallopian tubes.

Implantation

Implantation or the attachment of the embryo to the uterine wall, is essential in the development of the fetus and placenta. There is a total interval of some seven days between ovulation and implantation. By the time the embryo has reached the uterus it has so developed that it is now ready to imbed itself into the uterine wall. At the same time, the lining of the uterus has reached its greatest succulence and thickness.

The embedding of the embryo is done by the outer "foraging" layer of cells, the trophoblasts. These cells are able to digest or liquefy the tissues with which they come in contact. In this way, the cells not only burrow into the uterine lining and eat out a nest for the embryo but also digest the walls of the many small blood vessels that they encounter beneath the surface. Thus, the mother's blood stream is tapped, and soon the embryo is surrounded by tiny pools of blood. Finger-like projections sprout from the trophoblasts and extend into the blood-filled spaces. These finger-like projections become known as chorionic villi. They contain blood vessels connected with the fetus and are very important because they are the sole means by which oxygen and nourishment are received from the mother and by which waste products are disposed. Thus,

there is *no direct* communication between the maternal blood stream and the blood stream of the fetus. The placenta is formed by the infiltration of the chorionic villi into the decidua basalis.

Development of the Placenta

The placenta plays an essential part in the well-being of the fetus. As previously described, the lining of the uterus grows thick with small, active cells called trophoblasts that come from the fertilized egg. These foraging cells grow in size to form the placenta. They form tiny projections something like the roots of a plant and have a similar function; they reach out and bring nourishment to the fetus. The placenta connects the fetus to the uterine wall and is the organ which carries on the nutritive, respiratory, and excretory functions of the fetus.

Not only does the placenta carry on all of these functions for the fetus, but it also acts as an endocrine organ. It produces chorionic gonadotropin, estrogen, and progesterone and takes over the function of the corpus luteum in pregnancy. No wonder that it is considered to be a most amazing and fascinating organ! The placenta is composed

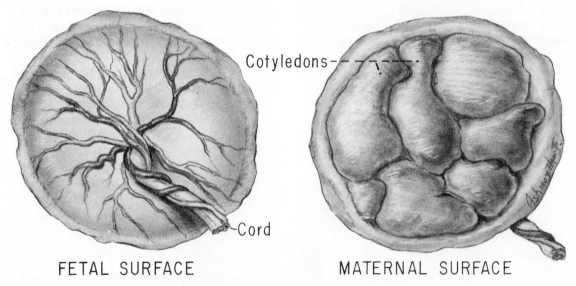

FETAL SURFACE   MATERNAL SURFACE

Figure 6-1. The human placenta.

of a fetal portion and a maternal portion. The decidua basalis is the portion directly beneath the implanted ovum. It is from the decidua basalis that the maternal portion of the placenta is developed. The decidua basalis contains large numbers of blood vessels. The arteries pursue a spiral course and penetrate the entire thickness of the decidua. Many of the veins become markedly dilated and form large sinuses. These small vessels, after pursuing their course through the superficial layer of the basalis, open into the intervillous spaces of the developing placenta.

On the fetal side of the placenta there are two membranes, the amnion and the chorion. The thinnest membrane, the amnion, lies closest to the fetus. As the sac enlarges with amniotic fluid the amnion lies in close proximity to the outermost membrane called the chorion, which forms the amniotic sac. Amniotic fluid fills the sac and maintains a constant temperature for the fetus as well as cushioning it against possible injury.

The fetus is attached to the central part of the placenta by the umbilical cord (Fig. 6-1), which contains three blood vessels: two arteries and one vein. The two arteries carry blood loaded with waste products and carbon dioxide from the fetus to the placenta. The vein carries pure oxygenated blood to the fetal circulation. The placenta, cord, and membranes are structurally completed by the end of the first trimester of pregnancy.

The mature placenta is a circular organ which is about eight inches in diameter and one inch thick and weighs approximately one pound. The fetal side is smooth and glistening, beneath which can be seen many large blood vessels. In contrast, the maternal surface is irregularly rough and reddish gray and composed of many irregularly shaped lobes called *cotyledons* (Fig. 6-1). After delivery, the placenta becomes detached and is known as the afterbirth.

The First Month

During the first four weeks of pregnancy some amazing changes take place. The single cell which is the result of the combined sperm and ovum is called a *zygote*. As the zygote travels down the fallopian tube it divides into 2, 4, 8, 16, 32, 64, 128, cells, and so on. The process of cell division takes place in spurts with periods of rest lasting several hours. The mulberrylike appearance of this round ball of cells at this stage of development gives rise to the name *morula*. It organizes into two layers at the time of implantation as described earlier. During the next couple of weeks the embryo, as the developing zygote is called for the first 8 weeks of life, is arranged into three layers: (1) the ectoderm or outer layer which becomes the future skin and nervous system;

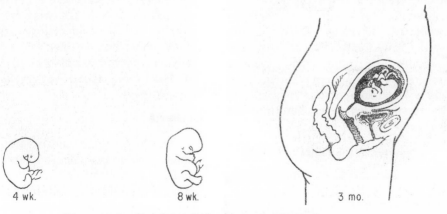

Figure 6-2. Fetal development in the first trimester.

4 wk. 8 wk. 3 mo.

(2) the endoderm or inner layer which will be the mouth, throat, and digestive system; and (3) the mesoderm or middle layer which is the future supporting tissues, skeleton, and muscles.

At the end of four weeks the embryo is a quarter of an inch long with one third taken up by the head. It now has a tail and rudiments of eyes, ears, nose, and a future digestive tract. Incipient arms and legs are represented by small buds (Fig. 6-2). Recognizable traces of all organs exist as the cells have become differentiated. The tube that will form the heart has formed; it pulsates regularly and propels blood through microscopic arteries.

The Second Month

Four weeks later (at the end of the second lunar month) the embryo has become a *fetus* (Fig. 6-2). It is now one inch long and weighs one thirtieth of an ounce. At this time it begins to assume a human form with an unmistakably human face. There are arms and legs with fingers, toes, elbows, and knees. The external genitalia become apparent but one cannot tell the sex yet. At the end of this time the tail undergoes retrogression.

The Third Month

At the end of 12 weeks the fetus is over three inches long and weighs almost one ounce (Fig. 6-2). The sex can now be distinguished. Fingers and toes have become differentiated and the finger- and toenails appear as fine membranes. Early in this third month, buds for temporary teeth are present. There are rudimentary kidneys which secrete a small amount of urine into the bladder (which escapes into the amniotic fluid). Movements also occur, but they are too weak to be felt by the mother.

Dangers to the Fetus

During the first trimester of pregnancy because of the tremendous growth, development of organs, and differentiation of cells there are certain dangers to the fetus.

Drugs

Some drugs have been found to have a teratogenic effect on the fetus. A teratogen is a substance which can produce serious malformations or deviations from the normal structure. A drug which the mother takes can pass to the fetus through the placenta which links the maternal and fetal circulations and serves as the source of nutrition for the fetus. The mechanism by which drugs reach the fetus is probably the same as that for the passage of other nutrients. It has been found that drugs, like nutrients, cross the placenta by the process of osmosis. In this process, the concept of the *placental barrier* plays an important part. In general, the higher the molecular weight of the drug, the lower is the rate of transfer, and vice versa. An example of a drug of low molecular weight that crosses the placental barrier freely is nitrous oxide.

Some drugs which are known to have teratogenic effects as a result of either animal experiments or clinical experience with humans, are tranquilizers, steroids, antibiotics, anticoagulants, and chemotherapeutic agents. The classic example is thalidomide, a tranquilizer that caused congenital malformations of the limbs in countless babies in the early 1960's.

Because of the possible teratogenic effects of drugs the nurse should tell a woman who is contemplating pregnancy or one who is pregnant to avoid self-medication. Since the teratogenic effects of a number of drugs are unknown it is not wise for a pregnant woman to take even aspirin unless it has been prescribed for her. If, however, she needs medications which have been ordered for her by her doctor, she should not avoid taking them.

X-Rays

There is some controversy over how much risk exists for the fetus when the mother is x-rayed during her pregnancy. Most of the information that is available has been extrapolated from animal studies. However, most authorities agree that x-rays should only be done when absolutely necessary with as low a dose of radiation as possible when the woman is in the first trimester of pregnancy. In some animals, radiation is lethal to the fetus in the first three weeks and produces gross abnormalities at three to six weeks. Hazards of radiation are decidedly less in the later part of pregnancy. Therefore, the nurse in discussing this subject with a pregnant woman could point out that only x-rays which are essential should be taken in the early weeks of pregnancy. Dental x-rays, diagnostic x-rays, and x-rays taken to see if there are twins, should be postponed if possible.

Rubella

Certain diseases constitute a danger to the fetus because the virus can pass through the placenta and affect the fetus. An example of this is German measles or rubella. This disease, if contracted during the first months of pregnancy, can pass from the mother to the embryo and disrupt the structural ordering of the cells, thus causing deformity. If an expectant mother knows she has been exposed to German measles she should contact her doctor or the clinic right away. A nurse could suggest to a pregnant woman that she avoid exposure to this disease as much as possible. Other diseases which could be teratogenic are those which produce a high fever, such as pneumonia and typhoid fever.

PHYSIOLOGICAL CHANGES IN THE MOTHER

Amenorrhea

If the woman has previously had fairly regular menstrual periods one of the first noticeable signs of pregnancy is cessation of menstruation. This is known as amenorrhea. The reason menses ceases during pregnancy is that high levels of estrogen and progesterone are maintained after fertilization has taken place to sustain the rich lining of the uterus into which the embryo will be implanted. During the normal menstrual cycle in which fertilization has not occurred,

the levels of estrogen and progesterone drop rapidly causing the endometrium (the lining of the uterus) to degenerate and slough off in the menstrual flow.

However, cessation of menstruation, although it is highly suspect as being one of the first signs of pregnancy, may occur for other reasons. An endocrine dysfunction (such as hypothyroidism) may cause amenorrhea, as may acute or chronic disease (such as tuberculosis). Emotional factors may also cause disturbances in menstruation. For example a woman who is worried that she might be pregnant may indeed have a delayed menstrual period. Or students who are under pressure at examination time may miss a menstrual period. Extremes in climate have also been known to cause either a delay in or an absence of a menstrual period (sometimes more than one). Consequently, when menstruation ceases in a girl or woman whose periods have previously been regular it is considered to be a presumptive rather than a positive sign of pregnancy.

Breast Changes

Another commonly noted change is enlargement of the breasts, often with some tingling, fullness, and even soreness. In a woman who has never been pregnant before, the pigmentation of the nipple and areola, which is the area surrounding the nipple, becomes more extensive and darker. This pigmentation change varies with the hair and skin color of the individual. For example, brunettes have a more striking change than either blonds or redheads.

The tiny glands of Montgomery, which are enlarged sebaceous glands, are scattered throughout the areola and become prominent during pregnancy. There may even be a small amount of colostrum, a watery precursor of milk, secreted as early as the first trimester.

However, because the breasts may enlarge before a menstrual period and because the other breast changes described may be present in a multipara (a woman who has had a previous pregnancy), these changes are not considered to be a positive sign of pregnancy.

Other Signs of Pregnancy

Many other physiological signs occur during pregnancy, some of which are named after the physician who first described them. The change in color of the mucous membranes in the genital tract (vagina), which become bluish or violet owing to the increased blood supply to the area, is called Chadwick's sign. However, because this change can be found in other conditions which result in pelvic congestion, such as when tumors are present, it is not considered to be a positive sign of pregnancy.

A second change, known as Goodell's sign, is a softening of the cervix due to increased vascularity. Normally, the cervix feels hard like the end of a person's nose. However, when a woman becomes pregnant, the cervix feels like the lips.

A third change (Hegar's sign) is a softening of the portion of the uterus called the lower uterine segment which is located between the fundus (top of the uterus) and cervix (neck or opening of the uterus). To determine this change the examiner must do a bimanual examination in which he inserts two fingers into the vagina and then palpates the woman's abdomen with his other hand. If the examiner can easily compress the lower uterine segment between the fingers palpating the abdomen and those in the anterior or posterior fornix of the vaginal canal, this is called a positive Hegar's sign.

During pregnancy, the uterus changes in shape, size, and consistency; about the eighth week of pregnancy it becomes symmetrical and globular in shape. As the uterus changes in shape during the first trimester, painless intermittent contractions occur which enable the muscles of the uterus to enlarge to accommodate the growing fetus. These contractions are referred to as Braxton-Hicks contractions. The expectant mother may be aware that her abdomen becomes more firm at intervals, but these contractions usually do not cause her any pain or discomfort.

As pregnancy progresses, the pelvic joints and the symphysis pubis become relaxed due to a hormone called relaxin which interacts with estrogen and progesterone. As a result of this change, the woman walks with a "pride of pregnancy" or a waddling gait.

Vaginal secretions become more profuse, thick, and white, with lactic acid present in the secretions. The presence of glycogen in the vaginal epithelium increases the acidity of the vagina to protect it against invasion by pathogenic organisms.

A mucous plug forms in the cervix and serves as protection against pathogenic organisms. The cervical canal gradually becomes filled with thick tenacious mucous and remains this way until the onset of labor when the mucous plug is discharged.

In some women there is an increase in saliva called pytalism. For some unknown reason the mouth secretions become highly acidic, stimulating the salivary glands to produce large quantities of saliva. This can contribute to nausea and vomiting in pregnancy.

Some women experience pica which is a craving for certain unnatural foods. This may be caused by psychological or social factors or by certain nutritional requirements which the body needs. Many of us are familiar with stories of the pregnant woman who craves pickles (even with ice cream) or wakes her husband at 2:00 a.m. one January morning to go out and get her some fresh strawberries. Some women eat great quantities of starch or even dirt due to local or family custom. It is possible for a woman to eat such large quantities of the substance she craves that she does not get a nutritionally balanced diet. This is when intervention is necessary.

Pregnancy Tests

None of the aforementioned signs and symptoms are proof that a woman is pregnant. Sometimes, when it is important to know before the second trimester whether the woman is pregnant or not, pregnancy tests which make use of animals (rabbits, mice, or frogs) may be performed, or chemical tests may be run in the laboratory.

These tests are based on the fact that the chorionic gonadotropic hormone which is secreted by the trophoblasts (cells within the placenta) is present in the blood and urine during pregnancy. A sample of urine from the woman is injected into the test animal; if the animal is female and ovulation takes place the test is considered to be positive; if a male animal is used and sperm is released the test is also positive.

These tests are considered to be accurate 95 to 98 per cent of the time. However, they can be falsely positive when other conditions, such as tumors, exist. They can also be falsely negative if they are run early in pregnancy or late in pregnancy, the reason being that chorionic gonadotropin reaches maximum production about the sixtieth day of pregnancy and then rapidly decreases, until by the hundredth day it reaches a level which is maintained during pregnancy.

Besides the animal tests, which are expensive and rather time-consuming (it may take a couple of days to get the results), there are several other kinds of pregnancy tests, such as the Gravindex and Pregnosticon which are immunological tests that have the advantage of giving speedy results within two hours.

In another test of pregnancy, some physicians give female hormones to their patients for about three days. When the woman has stopped taking the hormones for a few days if she is not pregnant she will start having her menstrual period. It should be emphasized to the woman that giving her hormones or Prostigmine if she is pregnant will *not* cause bleeding.

Another diagnostic technique which has been reported in the literature is the use of ultrasound. The main uses seem to be in diagnosing multiple pregnancies or molar pregnancies or determining fetal measure-ments or abnormalities. Since the technique is being more widely used at this time, if you would like to pursue this topic see the references at the end of the chapter.

COMMON DISCOMFORTS

There are certain symptoms that a pregnant woman may experience which will cause her annoyance and discomfort and, in some instances, make her quite miserable. Because they are experienced rather frequently and are related to the physiological changes which are occurring rather than to any pathological condition, they are often referred to as common discomforts. They are often transient and self-limiting, with some being more characteristic of one trimester than another. However discomforts may overlap throughout the trimesters. For example, constipation is a discomfort which is more commonly experienced in the second and third trimesters because of the enlarged uterus pressing on the bowel. However, some women have difficulty with constipation in the first trimester.

Remember that some women will experience few if any of these discomforts. However, it is helpful for a pregnant woman to know about them so that if they do occur she will not become frightened, will understand why they are occurring, and may know what measures to take to try to relieve them. In some instances she may be able to prevent them from occurring.

In the first trimester the main discomforts are nausea and vomiting, fatigue, breast soreness, and urinary frequency.

Nausea and Vomiting

Nausea and vomiting usually begin shortly after the first missed menstrual period and disappear at the end of the first trimester. Although the cause of nausea and vomiting in pregnancy is not known it is believed to result from a combination of physiological and psychological factors.

One theory which supports the physiological basis contends that the high levels of estrogen, progesterone, and chorionic gonadotropin may trigger nausea and vomiting. Supporters of this theory note that the same side-effects occur in women taking birth control pills which contain estrogen and progesterone.

On the side of the psychological theory it is contended that many women (perhaps as many as 80 per cent) may have ambivalent feelings about being pregnant, especially in the beginning of pregnancy. Vomiting then may be an unconscious way of expressing their desire to reject the pregnancy by "vomiting up the fetus" and ridding themselves of the pregnancy. Both of these theories, however, have yet to be proven.

Because the nausea and vomiting frequently occur in the morning when the expectant mother first arises it is often referred to as "morning sickness." It should be kept in mind that often there is no characteristic pattern as to the time of occurrence or to the amount; it can vary from none to almost constant vomiting (see hyperemesis gravidarum). It should also be noted that at least 50 per cent of women have no nausea. It is also interesting to note that some husbands suffer "morning sickness" along with their wives, out of sympathy.

To relieve this discomfort the nurse can make several suggestions. She can explain that eating smaller, more frequent meals may help, since it is felt that if the stomach is not allowed to become completely empty there will be less nausea and vomiting. The nurse can also suggest that the expectant mother try to eat foods high in carbohydrates a half hour before arising. Foods such as dry toast or crackers left beside the bed may prevent nausea and vomiting. The reason why this measure might help is that the blood sugar tends to be low throughout pregnancy, and a disturbance in the metabolism of carbohydrates may cause the nausea and vomiting. The nurse might also suggest drinks such as ginger ale or cola which may help to settle the stomach. If cooking odors of certain foods bother the expectant mother, enlisting her husband's help in cooking these foods or even the entire meal may ease the situation. And finally, if these measures are not effective, the nurse should direct the expectant mother to tell her physician. There are several different medications the physician can prescribe to control the nausea and vomiting.

It is not uncommon for women to lose two to three pounds in the first trimester, particularly if they have been troubled by nausea and vomiting. In many instances once the woman is past the first trimester she overcomes this discomfort.

Fatigue

Many women feel fatigued and lethargic in the early months of pregnancy, because the basal metabolic rate gradually falls to a low of approximately −10. When the basal metabolic rate begins to rise, the development of the placenta is completed and the mother has adjusted to the implantation of the embryo into the uterine wall. She usually regains her former energy and may feel better during pregnancy than at any other time.

In the meantime, she may feel better (and less guilty) to know that she needs more sleep and rest at night and one or two naps during the day if possible. If she is working she should have at least two 15-minute periods during the average eight-hour working day, when she can sit down, put her feet up, and relax and rest.

Breast Soreness

As explained earlier, the breasts enlarge and may be sore as they gradually prepare for lactation. The reason for this is the increased amount of female hormones, progesterone and estrogen. In order to alleviate this discomfort, the nurse should encourage the expectant mother to wear a good supportive brassiere with wide comfortable shoulder straps. Since the bra and cup size may be about two sizes larger than the size she ordinarily wears, she should know about this before she buys any new brassieres.

If she is bothered by tingling in the nipples, which occurs more commonly in cold weather, she can pad the inside of her bra with a soft material such as cotton or lamb's wool.

Urinary Frequency

Another common occurrence in the first trimester is a need to urinate more frequently. Because the urinary bladder is located anteriorly to the uterus, the enlarging uterus exerts pressure on the bladder giving rise to this discomfort. There is no nursing intervention other than to tell the expectant mother that she may want to limit fluid intake during the evening so that she won't have to get up so often during the night. It may be helpful for her to know that as the uterus rises out of the pelvis into the abdominal cavity, this annoyance will usually cease by the end of the first trimester.

EMOTIONAL CHANGES

Most women experience fairly characteristic emotional changes during the first trimester of pregnancy. However, many people tend to know less about the emotional changes than the physical changes.

Mood Swings. The expectant mother may have mood swings, feeling happy one minute and sad or depressed the next. To her and her husband and other members of her family, these rapid changes in moods may be puzzling and upsetting. Over a trivial remark that her husband makes about what she served him for supper, she may burst into tears. If the family and the woman herself are prepared to expect these mood swings as a normal accompaniment of pregnancy, they can better understand and tolerate her behavior. On the other hand, the husband and other family members can make a more conscious effort to be tactful. Of course, her high spirits and happy moods will usually tend to benefit the family and the marriage.

Ambivalence. Another troubling emotion for the mother is ambivalence. The expectant mother frequently finds that she has conflicting feelings in the early months of her pregnancy. As Reva Rubin expresses it,

a woman faced with the probability of being pregnant, frequently wonders "Who me?" and "Now?"*

There may be many reasons—social, financial, and psychological—why a woman may not wish to be pregnant. Maybe she is working while her husband is going to school, or maybe her own schooling or career may be interrupted, or possibly the baby will be born at a time when the family has made other plans. There are many reasons and countless examples, even when the pregnancy is planned and the child wanted, as to why the pregnancy may be occurring at an awkward time.

Nurses, when dealing with this situation, can explain to the prospective parents that it is normal for the expectant mother to feel this way, that she need not feel guilty, and that it is good for her to talk about her feelings. Also, nurses should be sensitive to the mother's feelings. A mother who gives the information that she has just found out that she is pregnant will find it more helpful if the nurse asks how she feels about it. The nurse who automatically replies "How wonderful!" may be expressing her own views rather than allowing the mother to express her feelings.

It has been said that a mother will often reject the pregnancy but not the child. This means that as pregnancy progresses, the expectant mother has a chance to adjust to the idea of having a child, and as she begins to experience changes, such as feeling the baby's movements, the pregnancy becomes more real to her. Thus many women lose these feelings of ambivalence by or during the second trimester.

Sexual Desires. The expectant mother may have a change in her sexual desire during pregnancy. Some women experience a lessening of desire if they feel, for example, that the main purpose of sexual relations is for procreation. On the other hand, some women experience a desire for more frequent sexual intercourse and have climaxes

---

*Rubin, R.: Cognitive Style in Pregnancy. Am. J. Nurs., *70*:502, March, 1970.

more frequently. Once the fear of pregnancy is removed the woman may feel freer to enjoy sexual relations, especially if she no longer has the responsibility of using contraceptives. Whatever her response may be, her husband should be informed about these possible changes. If his wife's sexual desire decreases, he should know that this is temporary, and he may need to find other activities in which to sublimate his sexual drives. The paradox may be that his wife needs extra love and affection during pregnancy so that she can build up an "emotional bank account" to give the baby. It takes an understanding husband to give this extra amount of love and affection when he may be feeling that his sexual needs are not being gratified as often or as fully as he might wish.

Couples should be encouraged to discuss this change in sexual desire, since it can lead to serious marital problems. Just because a couple may be too shy to bring up the subject doesn't mean that they don't want to discuss it. Thus it is important to include this topic in prenatal teaching or even earlier as a part of sex education.

Passiveness. Another emotional change which may manifest itself in the first trimester is a tendency on the part of the expectant mother to become introverted and passive. By introverted is meant that she spends more time thinking about herself than others. By passive is meant that instead of being more active and aggressive, making her own decisions, doing for others, she sits back and lets others make the decisions and do things for her. This change becomes more pronounced as pregnancy advances into the second and third trimesters.

HEALTH PROTECTION AND PROMOTION

It is vitally important that the pregnant woman keep herself in a good state of health both physically and mentally throughout her pregnancy. One obvious reason for this is that there are two individuals to consider instead of just one. Since it is a role of the nurse to help protect and promote the health of the mother and growing fetus, we will consider various aspects that should be included in health teaching. They are nutrition (including weight gain), sleep and rest, exercise, and the importance of prenatal care.

Nutrition

Good nutrition is highly significant during pregnancy, because this is the period when the most rapid rate of growth known to medicine takes place. Many people have the false idea that the fetus develops at the expense of its mother. The truth is that the infant as well as the mother will suffer if the mother has a poor prenatal diet. A study done at Chicago Lying-In Hospital proved that: (1) there is a highly significant relationship between the protein intake of the mother and the condition of the baby; (2) the incidence of abortion is confined almost entirely to those mothers having the lowest intake of protein; and (3) the incidence of prematurity rises sharply among women with a low-protein and low-calcium intake.

Prematernal Nutrition

Fewer complications in pregnancy, fewer premature births, and healthier babies result when the mother is well nourished prior to conception. Experiments which were carried out during war years when food was rationed revealed that babies born during that time were smaller and lighter. Animal studies show that severe congenital malformations involving the skeleton, the central nervous system, the cardiovascular system, and the excretory system can be produced in the fetus when the mother's diet is deficient in nutrients such as vitamin A or riboflavin.

Many women do not enter pregnancy in a satisfactory nutritional status. One fourth of all first pregnancies occur in teenage girls, who are known to have the least satisfactory diet of any age category because they succumb readily to social pressures, are overly concerned about having slender figures, and indulge in food fads.

Prenatal Nutrition

Studies which have analyzed and rated the diets of pregnant women note the following results: (1) women who follow a poor or very poor diet during pregnancy have a large percentage of premature, congenitally defective, or stillborn infants; (2) women with good to excellent diets almost invariably have infants in good physical condition; (3) few cases of eclampsia are noted in those women receiving excellent or good diets; and (4) a good percentage of those receiving poor or very poor diets develop toxemia of varying degrees of severity.

Calories. The need for an increase in calories is small during the first half of pregnancy. It depends on the mother's size and age and whether she is active or inactive. In the literature, a range of from 1800 to 2100 calories is given for a 5′4″, 128 lb., moderately active, 24-year-old woman.

Protein. The diet must contain the essential amino acids to maintain the mother's tissues and build new tissues for the developing fetus. Protein allowance is satisfactory when 20 gm. of protein are added to normal daily allowances of 1 gm. per kg. of body weight. Good food sources are meats, fish, poultry, eggs, cheese, peanut butter, and legumes (dried peas and beans).

Minerals

Calcium and Phosphorus. In the fetus the first set of teeth begins to form during the eighth week of gestation. Therefore, it is advisable to increase calcium and phosphorus early in pregnancy. The best source of calcium is milk, although other important sources are American and cheddar cheese, cottage cheese, eggs, oatmeal, and vegetables. Instant dry nonfat milks, which are cheap, can be substituted for these foods. Since some people may object to the taste, you can suggest adding vanilla, almond extract, or some such substance.

Since one quart of milk daily is recommended to the pregnant woman, it is usually suggested that she drink two glasses and use the rest in her cooking. However, since milk is not used in sufficient quantities in cooking, it may be helpful for her to know what foods and what amounts of them are equivalent to an 8-ounce glass of milk. For instance, 1½ oz. cheddar-type cheese, or 1½ cups cottage cheese, or 1 lb. cream cheese, or 1 pt. ice cream each contains calcium equivalent to that of an 8-ounce glass of milk. If the mother does not like milk or dairy products she can supplement her diet by taking calcium tablets.

Iron. In the beginning stages of pregnancy iron is transferred from the mother to the fetus in moderate amounts. Thus adequate quantities of iron are required if iron deficiency anemia is to be prevented in the mother. Throughout the pregnancy, 700 to 1000 mg. iron must be absorbed and utilized. Of this amount, 240 mg. are released because of the cessation of menstruation. The remainder of the iron needed must be made up by the diet. A daily increase of 3 mg. will provide sufficient iron except for women who are anemic. Important food sources of iron are egg yolks, red meats (liver once a week is a good source of iron as is beef hearts), green leafy vegetables, fruit, and whole grain cereals. Often iron pills are given to pregnant women to supplement their diet. If a woman is taking iron pills the nurse should tell her not to become alarmed if her stools turn black or tarry. In some people iron medications produce some gastrointestinal disturbances, constipation or its opposite, diarrhea—all the more reason to have an adequate intake of iron by eating the right foods!

Iodine. It is important to have sufficient amounts of iodine in the diet to protect against the incidence of goiter in the mother and infant. The best food source is iodized salt.

Vitamins. Thiamine (vitamin B) and niacin allowances are increased in proportion to the caloric increase in pregnancy.

Riboflavin (vitamin B_2) allowances increase according to the higher protein requirement during pregnancy.

Vitamin D allowances increase in order to facilitate the greater amounts of calcium and phosphorus. A good food source is milk fortified with vitamin D.

Ascorbic acid (vitamin C) amounts are considerably increased because of its vital role in tissue structure. The simplest and least expensive way to increase ascorbic acid intake is to include two portions of citrus fruit daily.

To determine if the expectant mother is eating an adequate diet, the nurse or other appropriate person should sit down with her and write down what she eats for breakfast, lunch, dinner, and between meal snacks. In this way the strengths and weaknesses of her daily diet can be analyzed in reference to a recommended diet during pregnancy. Since culture, religion, and ethnic background play such an important part in our dietary habits, foods which fit into the aforementioned considerations as well as those which meet the mother's specific nutritional needs should be recommended. The foodlikes and dislikes of the woman should be taken into consideration as well as those of her family, since she will most likely be cooking for her family and not just for herself. Taking into consideration the cost of the recommended food item is essential too. Meal planning and marketing on a tight budget can be a challenging task.

Weight Gain

Most physicians recommend that a woman gain between 18 to 25 pounds during her pregnancy. During pregnancy the average total weight gain is 24 pounds. As previously stated women sometimes lose 2 or 3 pounds during the first trimester due to nausea and vomiting. However, the average weight gained is 2 pounds in the first trimester, 10.8 pounds in the second trimester, and 11.2 pounds in the third trimester.

What constitutes the weight gain of the mother?

infant	7½ pounds
placenta	1 pound
amniotic fluid	1½ pounds
breasts	3 pounds (average)
uterus	2–3 pounds
Total	15.5 pounds

The rest of the weight gain is presumably due to protein storage outside the uterus (4 pounds), and water retention, including blood water (about 3 pounds). Limiting

Table 6-1.   PATTERN FOR A GOOD DAY'S MEALS

Food	For the Nonpregnant Woman	For the Expectant Mother	For the Teenage Expectant Mother	For the Nursing Mother
Milk	2 cups	3 or more cups	4 or more cups	4 or more cups
Meat, fish, eggs, poultry or substitute	2 servings	2 to 3 servings	2 to 3 servings	2 to 3 servings
Vegetables and fruits	1 serving high in vitamin C; 1 serving high in vitamin A; 2 servings other vegetable or fruit	2 servings high in vitamin C; 1 serving high in vitamin A; 2 servings other vegetable or fruit	2 servings high in vitamin C; 1 serving high in vitamin A; 2 servings other vegetable or fruit	2 servings high in vitamin C; 2 servings high in vitamin A; 2 servings other vegetable or fruit
Bread and Cereal	3 to 4 servings	3 to 4 servings	3 to 4 servings	3 to 4 servings

weight gain during pregnancy has been a way of preventing toxemia.

Now experts are proposing that a weight gain of from 18 to 25 pounds should *not* be advocated for *all* pregnant women without considering their prepregnancy weight. Eastman and Jackson have found that a woman who weighs under 120 pounds before pregnancy could gain 30 pounds or more and thus reduce her chances of having a low-birth weight baby.*

In summary, the importance of getting off to a good start nutritionally cannot be overemphasized. "We are what we eat" applies to the pregnant woman and the growing baby inside her. Members of the health team have been fairly successful at putting across the idea to the public that a pregnant woman need not eat for two (meaning twice as much). Experts are de-emphasizing weight restrictions as an overall rule for every pregnant woman. The trend seems to be to look more at the individual needs of the woman and adjust advice to her circumstances. Table 6-1 may be a useful guide in determining if nutritional needs are being met.

Sleep and Rest

Fatigue has been discussed as being one of the common discomforts of the first trimester. It was pointed out that getting a sufficient amount of sleep and rest is necessary for the pregnant woman.

Depletion of nerve cell energy results in fatigue, which in turn results in irritability, apprehension, and restlessness. All the body processes such as walking, studying, working, or playing use up nerve cell energy. When the energy is used up, the only remedy is rest and sleep, which recharges the nerve cells. However, it is easier to prevent fatigue than to recover from fatigue.

Even though the pregnant woman feels fatigued and would like nothing better than to sleep, she often finds herself caught up in

---

*Eastman, N., and Jackson, E.: Weight gain in pregnancy—a new view. *Briefs.* Jan. 1969.

a busy schedule particularly if she has other small children to take care of or has a job or other responsibilities that make demands on her time.

Therefore, it is good anticipatory guidance to have her plan and carry out an earlier bedtime hour and planned rest periods during the day. When she is doing household jobs she can find ways to do them more easily. For example, she could try to prepare vegetables and peel potatoes sitting down rather than standing at the sink, or she might learn to iron sitting down.

Exercise

A pregnant woman should exercise daily as a means of maintaining good muscle tone and circulation. Exercise can offer many other benefits, such as helping to alleviate constipation, a common problem during pregnancy. If the woman decides to exercise by walking a mile or two daily (which is one of the best and least expensive ways to exercise) it offers her the opportunity of getting out of the house into the fresh air. And if she can persuade her husband to walk with her, she can enjoy sharing more of his time and company.

Pregnant women frequently wonder how much exercise to get, what kinds to avoid, and whether they need to exercise additionally if they hold a job and do housework. A general rule of thumb is that the exercise done should not overtire or strain the woman. Therefore, she is normally the best judge of whether or not she is exercising too strenuously. The same kinds of sport activities can be carried out after pregnancy as before. For example, if a woman is accustomed to swimming the length of a swimming pool several times, there is no reason why she cannot continue to do so after she becomes pregnant. The amount of physical activity that her job or housework requires should be considered before recommending any additional exercise. Some jobs, for example, are sedentary, so that if she sits all day she would need exercise just as much as someone who is unemployed. On the other hand, a housewife who is physically active with a small child at home may not need any additional exercise.

Exercises which are taught to prepare a woman for childbirth will be considered in the chapter on the second trimester of pregnancy.

The Importance of Prenatal Care

Ideally, a pregnant woman should go for her first prenatal visit during the first trimester of her pregnancy. The main purpose of prenatal care is to ensure a healthy outcome for both the mother and baby. Regular visits can help detect any deviations from normal and institute prompt measures of treatment. The emphasis should be on *prevention*. In other words, the mother and fetus should be carefully observed or monitored, the mother should be taught certain health practices, and immunizations should be carried out in order to prevent complications.

Expectant parents should know what constitutes good prenatal care so that they can decide whether or not the mother is receiving it. For example, if the fetal heart rate is not checked on each visit (once the heart beat becomes audible), the mother should know that an important aspect of her prenatal care has been omitted.

In health teaching, the nurse can stress the importance of *regular* visits to the clinic or doctor's office, and what to expect on the initial visit and subsequent visits. She should explain routine procedures and laboratory work and why each one is important.

Initial Visit

The first visit is usually the most time-consuming, because a history, a physical examination, including a pelvic examination, and laboratory tests are done.

History. The following information will be needed for the history: the patient's name, address, age, and parity (number of children she has borne). The patient is also asked when the first date of her last menstrual period occurred. From this date the expected date of confinement is calculated. Then a family history is obtained to determine if there is any hereditary disease or

evidence of tuberculosis or multiple pregnancies which could have an effect on this pregnancy.

If the patient has had any previous pregnancies and labors, this information is included. The date of deliveries, length of the labors, and size of the infants would be helpful information in predicting the outcome of this pregnancy. If, for example, the woman previously had a difficult labor, a large baby, and a cesarean section, she might need another cesarean section this time. In addition, a history of her present pregnancy is obtained to see if she has experienced any difficulty to date.

Physical Examination. The woman's weight and blood pressure are taken to establish baselines for future determinations. Also, any abnormality in weight and blood pressure which become apparent at this time should receive prompt attention. A record of the woman's weight before she became pregnant is also kept. Excessive weight gain and elevated blood pressure are often associated with toxemia, a complication of pregnancy. This will be considered at a later time.

In continuing the physical examination, the woman's teeth and throat are inspected. The condition of her teeth is important because infected teeth may become foci of infection which could be harmful to the mother and fetus. Similarly her throat is inspected for signs of infection. At the same time the size of her thyroid gland is noted. An enlarged thyroid gland may be indicative of thyroid disease which can be treated.

Next, the woman's heart is examined by auscultation (listening with a stethoscope), and her lungs are examined by percussion (thumping on a finger which is placed over the body part being examined). The purpose of these procedures is to detect any abnormality of the heart or lungs which may have an influence on the pregnancy.

Following this, the woman's breasts are examined for lumps which could be tumorous. The breasts and nipples are assessed for nursing the infant. If a woman has very small breasts she can be reassured that the size will not prevent her from nursing. However, if she has an inverted nipple, which is rare, it may be difficult or impossible for her to nurse her baby.

And lastly, the mother's abdomen is examined by palpation (applying the hands to external surfaces of the body to detect evidence of disease in the various organs) and auscultation. The uterus is felt to determine if its size and the height of the fundus are consistent with the date given for the woman's last menstrual period.

Pelvic Examination. The woman is then prepared for a vaginal examination. The nurse or assistant places her in a lithotomy position on the examining table. In the lithotomy position the woman is lying on her back with her buttocks at the edge of the table and her feet up in stirrups. She has been draped so that her abdomen and legs are covered and so that there is adequate exposure of the genitalia. It is more comfortable for the woman if she has had an opportunity to empty her bladder prior to having a vaginal examination. The nurse or other female assistant should stay with the woman during the examination if the doctor is a man. She can help the woman to relax by telling her to breathe deeply through her mouth and to try to keep her pelvic area as relaxed as possible. Diverting the woman's attention through conversation may help also.

Using a gloved hand, the doctor will examine the woman to find out if there are any abnormalities of the vagina (birth canal) and also to observe the various signs of pregnancy as explained earlier. A vaginal speculum will be used to better visualize the vagina and cervix. Another reason for the vaginal examination is to measure the diagonal conjugate (explained in Chapter 5). This is one of the important measurements in determining if the woman's pelvis is of adequate size to deliver a full-term infant.

Laboratory Tests

Papanicoulau Smear. A cancer screening test is usually done at the first visit. During the vaginal examination, after the vaginal speculum has been inserted, the physician will collect some material from the cervix by using a specially designed wooden spatula. This material is spread onto a glass slide and sent to the laboratory for examination. This is called a Pap smear. Sometimes the slide is placed in a 95 per cent alcohol solution before being sent to the laboratory. Other times it is dried and sent in an envelope.

In the laboratory the slide is stained and examined microscopically. It is then classified according to the type of cells which are seen. A denotation of Class I and Class II means that the cells are normal and that there is no evidence of malignancy. Classes III, IV, V mean that the cells are suggestive of malignancy or are actually malignant. The early detection of cancer of the cervix is important so that prompt measures can be taken to treat it successfully. The Papanicoulau test is one of the main ways to diagnose cancer of the cervix and uterus at an early stage and thus reduce the number of women who die from this disease. In women the cervix and uterus are among the most common sites for cancer to occur.

Urine Examination. On the first visit for prenatal care and on each subsequent visit a urine specimen is routinely tested for albumin and sugar. A major reason for testing for albumin is that this is one of the signs of toxemia in pregnancy. Although it is true that toxemia does not develop until the latter half of pregnancy, it would be possible to pick up albumin in the urine prior to this time, thereby indicating the presence of another complication such as kidney or bladder infection.

Of the various methods of testing for albumin, the easiest is to dip the end of a specially treated piece of paper into the urine. Wait a few seconds and then match the color that the paper turns to the color scale on the container. If no albumin is present then the test is negative. If albumin is present, the amount may be from trace (a slight amount) to 1+, 2+, 3+, and 4+ (the last number showing the greatest amount).

A similar test is done for sugar in the urine. This test has become routine for each prenatal visit because if a woman is prediabetic or diabetic, it may show up for the first time when she is pregnant. Various ways to perform this test are described in the chapter on diabetes. Occasionally during the latter part of pregnancy, lactose (or milk sugar) will spill over into the urine, giving a positive test. Therefore, a positive test for sugar does not necessarily mean that the pregnant woman is developing or has diabetes mellitus.

Blood Tests. A variety of blood tests are done at the initial prenatal visit. Some of these may be repeated later in pregnancy whereas others need be done only once.

Hemoglobin and Hematocrit. This test is done to determine if the mother is anemic. Of course, a pseudoanemia may develop because one of the physiological changes which may occur as pregnancy advances is an increase in the proportion of fluid in the bloodstream. If the hemoglobin is 10 gm. or below, diet teaching should be done and the woman's iron intake supplemented by medications. This test is repeated at least once during the latter half of pregnancy or as often as necessary.

Blood Type and Rh Factor. Because of the necessity of knowing the mother's blood type and Rh factor in case she needs a blood transfusion during the intrapartal period these tests are carried out at the initial visit and do not need to be repeated. One reason for doing an Rh factor is to determine if the woman is Rh negative. If so, then the blood type and Rh factor of the father of the child would be significant. (See discussion of erythroblastosis fetalis in Chapter 21.)

Serology. A blood sample is drawn from the vein to test for syphilis. Because the fetus can acquire syphilis from the mother in utero, this test is necessary so that the disease can be detected and the mother and fetus treated. Early and adequate treatment of the mother may prevent the infant from being born with congenital syphilis. Various tests for syphilis may be performed, such as an STS, a Kahn, or Wassermann. If the test result is negative then there is no disease. A positive result means that the person has syphilis. However, some positive results are inaccurate due to other diseases or conditions. The test may be repeated during the later months of pregnancy. However, if the incidence of venereal disease is low in the community, it may not be repeated.

Smears from the cervix and vagina may be taken during the pelvic examination to test for gonorrhea. This has not been a routine procedure in all prenatal clinics or private physicians offices, but with the increased incidence of venereal diseases in recent years, especially among teenagers, it would seem to be a good practice.

Chest X-Rays

In some areas—again depending on the incidence of tuberculosis in the community—routine chest x-rays are taken of all pregnant women. These may be postponed until after the first trimester because of the danger of taking x-rays during the fetus's most highly formative period. If a woman has not had a chest x-ray for a year or two and if it is not part of the routine practice where she lives, she may want to have an x-ray taken while she is receiving prenatal care.

Immunizations

Since pregnant women are considered to be more susceptible to communicable diseases, it might be advisable for them to receive immunizations. Then, too, some of the antibodies that the mother develops as a result of these immunizations may give the infant a temporary immunity. If the mother has not received polio vaccine, it is given to her at intervals during her prenatal visits. A woman may also be encouraged to receive influenza vaccine, since a pregnant woman may be more susceptible to the disease, and since flu can cause serious complications. Other immunizations, such as measles vaccine or smallpox may be contraindicated during pregnancy.

Dental Care.

Good oral hygiene and dental care are important during pregnancy. The gums tend to bleed as pregnancy advances, and dental caries and other problems tend to crop up. Regular toothbrushing, use of dental floss, and visits to the dentist every six months will help to keep the teeth, gums, and mouth in good condition. The old saying, "for every child a tooth," is not necessarily true if good nutrition and hygiene practices are followed. Many dentists are using fluorides on the teeth, if the water supply does not contain adequate amounts to prevent tooth decay. If extensive dental work needs to be done and requires long hours in the dentist's chair, the woman should have it done as early as possible in her pregnancy before she becomes uncomfortable due to her large size. As stated earlier x-rays of the teeth should be postponed until after the first trimester if at all possible. If x-rays must be taken, the woman's abdomen should be shielded with a lead apron to protect the reproductive organs from radiation.

DANGER SIGNS IN THE MOTHER

The nurse can alert the mother to certain danger signs which should be reported immediately to the doctor or the clinic. In the first trimester of pregnancy the main complication which occurs is spontaneous abortion (miscarriage). Therefore, if the mother-to-be notices any abdominal cramping similar to menstrual cramps or if she notices any vaginal spotting or bleeding, she should report these symptoms right away. Prompt measures may prevent the loss of the pregnancy.

THE EXPECTANT FAMILY

Pregnancy is a shared responsibility of the husband and wife. As such the husband should be included as much as possible in the event. In the first trimester a husband frequently feels left out because there are no visible signs as yet that his wife is pregnant. The expectant mother should let her husband know that it is his baby, too, and that she needs his understanding and support more than ever during this time. It is amazing how much comfort a husband can be!

There are some concrete ways husbands can help their wives. They can encourage them to get sufficient exercise, eat wisely, and practice good general health habits. They can be understanding of the emotional changes which occur such as the mood swings. And they can be tolerant of the changes in sexual desire that their wives may possibly experience at this time.

On the other hand, the expectant mother should make every effort to see that her husband still feels like a husband and father-to-be and not an outsider. She can discuss her preferences with him, such as where to go for prenatal care, what to name the baby, and what additional purchases should be made for herself (clothing) and the baby. If it is at all possible the husband can accompany his wife to the doctor's office or clinic. Many husbands would like to go but are not invited!

The same consideration holds true for any children or other members of the family. In general, the parents should start early to prepare their children for a new baby. They can draw them into any plans they make and should show them that they are still very important to both of them. They can tell them that the new baby will take their time but there will still be time for all. By including the children from the start, parents may be able to help prevent unhappiness in the future.

BIBLIOGRAPHY

Brecher, R., and Brecher, E.: A Guide to a Healthy Pregnancy. Redbook, February, 1964.

Eastman, N., and Hellman, L.: William's Obstetrics. ed. 13. New York, Appleton, 1966.

Fitzpatrick, E., et al.: Maternity Nursing. Philadelphia, J. B. Lippincott, 1971.

Ginott, H.: Between Parent and Child. New York, MacMillan, 1965.

Liley, H. M.: Modern Motherhood. New York, Random House, 1967.

Prenatal Care (Children's Bureau, U.S. Department of Health, Education, and Welfare). New York, MacMillan, 1965.

Rubin, R.: Cognitive style in pregnancy. Am. J. Nurs., *70*:502, March, 1970.

Schaefer, G.: The expectant father. Nursing Outlook, *14*:46, September, 1966.

Weight gain in pregnancy—a new view. Briefs, 33:6, 1969.

Wiedenbach, E.: Family-Centered Maternity Nursing. ed. 2. New York, Putnam, 1967.

Williams, S.: Nutrition and Diet Therapy. St. Louis, C. V. Mosby, 1969.

Suggested Readings for Further Study

How a Mother Affects Her Unborn Baby. Woman's Day, *33*:12 July, 1970.

Taylor, E.: Ultrasound diagnostic techniques in obstetrics and gynecology. Am. Jour. Obstet. Gynec., *90*:655, 1964.

The Second Trimester of Pregnancy

The middle three months of pregnancy are usually the most comfortable for the expectant mother. Often she has recovered from the fatigue and nausea and vomiting which were distressing her in the first trimester. She has a sense of well-being and increased energy, and indeed some women say they feel better during pregnancy than at any other time. In appearance, they may "bloom" and have a nicer complexion and a fuller bustline than usual. Because the breast size increases during pregnancy, women who have small breasts are usually quite pleased with this change.

FETAL DEVELOPMENT

Fourth Lunar Month

By the end of the fourth month the fetus is six inches or more in length and weighs approximately four ounces (Fig. 7-1). External genitalia have developed to the extent that his sex is clearly visible.

During the fourth month the fetus becomes active. This month is most remarkable because of the behavior the fetus exhibits. His movements vary from mild twitches to tonic contractions. His entire skin is sensitive to stimulation. At first he moves his upper lip, then his lower lip. Finally he is able to open and close his mouth and swallow amniotic fluid. He is able to rotate his head in the so-called oral (feeding) reflex. His arms and legs move occasionally. He is also able to move and bend his arms and open and close his hand, even moving his thumb independently.

During this month *lanugo* appears. Lanugo is the fine downy hair that is seen on

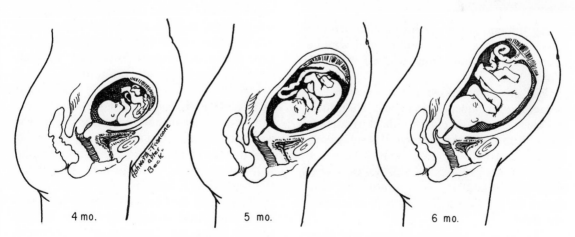

Figure 7-1. Fetal development in the second trimester of pregnancy.

85

the face, shoulders, back, and other skin surfaces. It is frequently seen in premature infants.

Fifth Lunar Month

During the fifth lunar month, the fetus grows to about ten inches in length and weighs about a half pound. His appearance is very much what it will be at full term. His face has an individual, human look (Fig. 7-1).

The most important changes that take place during this month are "quickening" and the appearance of a fetal heartbeat which can be detected with a stethoscope. Quickening refers to the fetal movements. Although the fetus has been active for a month or more the mother usually cannot feel the movements until about the middle or end of the fifth lunar month. The term "quickening" originated from the belief that fetal movement, felt by the mother, marked the moment when the fetus came to life.

The baby now goes through the motions of eating. He also exhibits primitive, widely spaced breathing movements. If he were born now he would try to breathe but would die because of the immaturity of his respiratory system. On the other hand, he has his full quota of nerve cells, and the cortex of his brain has differentiated into layers.

Sixth Lunar Month

By the end of the sixth lunar month the fetus is about a foot in length and weighs approximately one and a half pounds. (Fig. 7-1).

His skin is wrinkled and red because he is lacking in subcutaneous fat. Therefore, the blood vessels lie close to his skin surface giving him a red appearance. His sebaceous glands begin to operate and produce a cheesy white substance which is called *vernix caseosa*. This is a protective substance for his skin as he floats in the amniotic fluid.

The fetus is now able to open and close his eyes. Close inspection reveals that his lashes and eyebrows are developing. His breathing has developed to the extent that he has regular but shallow breathing movements. Sometimes he hiccoughs. These hiccoughs can be felt by his mother.

His digestive system has begun to work. Enzymes have formed, and his stomach muscles are motile. *Meconium*, the black tarry stool of the newborn, forms in his small intestine.

Other systems and organs begin to function too. His endocrine system, particularly the pituitary, thyroid, and pancreas, are coming into action. His liver and kidneys are partly functional. After the sixth lunar month his growth is a matter of increase in size, complexity, and organization. No new organs emerge.

PHYSIOLOGICAL CHANGES IN THE MOTHER

Between the third and fourth months, the growing uterus rises out of the pelvis and can be felt (or palpated) above the symphysis pubis. It rises progressively and by the sixth month reaches the umbilicus or slightly above.

Of course there is abdominal enlargement about this time, and along with it the umbilicus is pushed outward. The effect of this distention of the abdominal wall will cause a *diastasis recti* which is a separation of the rectus muscles in the midline. To give a comparison the rectus muscles act as "nature's girdle" if they have good tone. If you imagine the midline where the two muscles join together as a "zipper," then you can picture how this becomes "unzipped" to allow for expansion as the uterus enlarges.

As an abdominal organ the uterus may be felt as a soft fluid-filled sac. Ballottement can now be performed, whereby the person who is examining the abdomen of the expectant mother can push the fetus around and it will bounce back. Usually it is the head of the fetus that is ballotted.

There are certain changes in skin pigmentation that frequently occur in the second trimester. Deposits of a brownish pigment on the forehead, nose and cheeks, known as *chloasma,* or mask of pregnancy, may be noticeable. It is due to the increased hormones, estrogen and progesterone, and it is sometimes a side-effect seen in women who are taking birth control pills. It disappears when pregnancy ends. The nurse may suggest to the mother that if she goes out in the sun without shielding her face, it may tend to accentuate the pigmentation.

Another change is the development of *striae gravidarum* or the so-called stretch marks of pregnancy. These marks are caused by hyperactivity of the adrenal cortex* and by stretching of the skin. These streaks may appear on the breasts, thighs, abdomen, and buttocks and may vary in color from a pinkish, red hue to a purplish hue. After the woman has delivered they will fade in color and take on a silvery whiteness of scar tissue. Even though they get smaller and fade in color they never entirely disappear. Because these striae are caused by hormonal changes and by stretching of the skin, there is nothing the woman can do about them. However, it may make her feel better psychologically to rub cocoa butter or other creams or lotions on them, and it won't do any harm.

The *linea nigra,* a narrow line of brownish pigmentation, may be noticeable from the midline of the umbilicus to the symphysis pubis. This will fade but not entirely disappear when pregnancy is over.

Another change is the appearance of *vascular spiders* on the face, neck, upper chest, or arms, which probably is the result of large quantities of estrogen in the mother's tissues. Erythema of the palms may occur for the same reason.

PHYSICAL DISCOMFORTS

Heartburn

Heartburn is one of the common discomforts which often appear in the second trimester of pregnancy. It is a neuromuscular

*Ziegal, E., and Van Blarcom, C.: Obstetric Nursing. New York, Macmillan, 1964.

phenomenon in which the stomach contents are regurgitated into the esophagus. It occurs because there is a reduction in hyrdochloric acid during pregnancy that in turn causes a decrease in gastric motility. This causes an irritation of the lining, resulting in a burning sensation which occurs behind the lower part of the sternum and often radiates up along the esophagus. Although called heartburn, it really has nothing to do with the heart. Nervous tension and emotions may be a cause, with worry, fatigue, and improper diet contributing to its intensity. To help reduce its effects, little or no fat should be included in the diet. Strangely enough, though, taking a pat of butter or a tablespoon of cream before meals can prevent it as fat inhibits the secretion of acid in the stomach. It will not help if the woman already has heartburn.

Home remedies, such as soda bicarbonate, should not be used, because the sodium will tend to promote water retention which is undesirable during pregnancy.

If the usual measures do not work, the woman can report this to her doctor. He may wish to prescribe some of the aluminum compounds such as Amphojel or Creamalin.

Constipation

A woman may suffer from constipation at any time during her pregnancy. Since it is due largely to impaired peristaltic motion of the intestine caused by pressure from the enlarging uterus, it commonly occurs in the second trimester. To alleviate this problem the nurse can teach the woman about good bowel habits, adequate fluids, and an appropriate diet. Having a regular time each day to go to the bathroom may aid elimination.

In mild cases of constipation the woman can try a diet of fruits, vegetables, dark breads, coarse foods, and several glasses of water each day. She should *never* use enemas, laxatives, or cathartics unless they are prescribed by her doctor, the reason being that they could bring about premature labor by increasing the irritability of the uterus through their action on the intestinal tract.

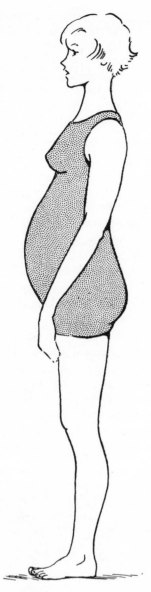

Figure 7-2. Good posture prevents backache during pregnancy.

Flatulence, the formation of gas in the gastrointestinal tract, is common and disagreeable. The nurse can suggest eating small amounts of food and chewing it thoroughly to prevent this. As flatulence frequently accompanies constipation, regular daily elimination is important. Also, the nurse can remind the woman to avoid such foods as beans, parsnips, corn, sweet desserts, fried foods, and cake and candy, as they tend to form gas.

Backache

During pregnancy backache is due to poor posture and incorrect body mechanics. The expectant mother's posture changes to compensate for the weight of her growing uterus and the shift in her center of gravity. Some helpful measures which the nurse can suggest are appropriate shoes, a supporting girdle, and strict attention to posture. Appropriate shoes give support and do not have high, narrow heels. Obviously tennis shoes or thongs are not suitable since they do not give proper support.

An excellent exercise to help alleviate backache is the *pelvic rock* which can be done standing, lying down, or on all fours. A description of the pelvic rock can be found in the following section on teaching prenatal exercises. Another help for backache is to remind the expectant mother to take rest periods, since standing or working for long periods can contribute to or cause a backache.

The nurse can demonstrate good posture to the woman by having her stand against a flat wall. She should pull her abdomen up and in and line her spine, shoulders, and head against the wall as much as possible. Instruct her to distribute her weight on the outer borders of her feet. Have her stretch her body tall, but not hold it rigidly. She should separate her feet to broaden the base supporting her body (Fig. 7-2).

Muscle Cramps

Pregnant women may feel painful, spasmodic muscular contractions in the legs, possibly as a result of fatigue, chilling, tense body posture, and *too much* milk consumption. Immediate relief may be obtained by forcing the toes upward and by causing pressure on the knee to straighten the leg. This is one occasion when the husband can help by carrying out the procedure for his wife. Elevating the feet and keeping the extremities warm are preventive measures.

The reason that drinking large quantities of milk may produce leg cramps is that too much phosphorus may be absorbed which predisposes to the muscular cramps. The remedy for this is to have the expectant mother take aluminum hydroxide with milk to remove some of the phosphorus and hence cut down on the pain. Another suggestion is to cut down on milk consumption and take calcium pills to compensate for it.

EMOTIONAL CHANGES

Some of the emotional changes of pregnancy result from hormonal and general metabolic variation. The presence of certain hormones in the blood influences the mood of the pregnant woman. One such hormone, progestin, may be related to the general *introversion* and *passivity* of the pregnant woman as well as to her narcissistic behavior which is demonstrated by her tendency to spend more energy thinking about herself than others. Increased introversion and passivity constitute one of the most characteristic changes of pregnancy and increases gradually until it reaches a peak about the seventh or eighth month. As a result the expectant mother has an increased need for love and affection; she wishes to receive instead of to give. Her husband can meet her needs if he demonstrates his love not only by words and kisses but by helping her around the house. He should understand that she is not exploiting her pregnancy; there has simply been a switch in her emotional situation.

The mood swings which are so prominent during pregnancy have no relation to external factors and do not seem to occur for any reason. They are evidenced by an increase in emotional lability, irritability, and sensitivity. As indicated earlier the husband and family will need to understand and accept these changes, in order to maintain the family equilibrium.

By the end of the second trimester the woman's body image is changing due to her bulging abdomen, which might make her feel large and very unattractive. If she feels that her husband married her because of her attractive physical appearance, this can be very upsetting. The nurse can explain to the woman that her perception of herself may not be anything like the perception her husband has of her. He may think she looks more attractive than ever. It would help if he would pay her compliments and take her out in public to show her he is proud of her appearance.

HEALTH PROTECTION AND PROMOTION

Prenatal Care

It is important for the nurse to stress to the mother that she should continue her prenatal care on a regular monthly basis. After the first visit the mother may feel that there isn't as much being done for her because the actual time she spends with the doctor is very brief. She may tend to conclude that these visits are not very important. The nurse can assure her that indeed these visits are very important for both her own health and safety and the baby's.

As with the first prenatal visit, these visits consist of weighing the expectant mother, taking her blood pressure and analyzing her urine for sugar and albumin. The reason her weight and blood pressure are checked is that rapid weight gain and increased blood pressure are early signs of toxemia. An abdominal examination is also carried out to check the height of the fundus and the position of the fetus and to listen to the fetal heart tones. During these visits the woman should be encouraged to ask the doctor and nurse any questions that may be of concern to her.

Care of the Breasts

The expectant mother may notice that enough colostrum is being secreted to necessitate wearing a pad to protect her clothing. The secretion may form a crust on the nipple, making the skin tender. If the crust is allowed to remain until the baby arrives and begins to nurse, the skin is likely to crack and infection could occur. Nipples that are kept clean and dry usually do not cause this problem.

The expectant mother should bathe her breasts daily. Using a clean washcloth and warm water (soap is drying), she should begin cleaning each breast by washing the nipple thoroughly in a circular motion. When she is certain that all the dried material is removed, she should gradually continue washing away from the nipple in a circular fashion until the entire breast is washed. Then she should dry with a clean towel.

The doctor may recommend some type of nipple cream if she plans to nurse. The second trimester is not too early for the expectant mother to begin to prepare her breasts for breast feeding. She should be instructed to first place a small amount on the thumb and first finger and then grasp the nipple gently between them. With a rolling type motion she can work the cream into the tiny creases found on the surface of the nipple. The position of the thumb and finger should be shifted around the entire nipple until a complete circuit has been made. This process should be limited to about 30 seconds on each breast. If the woman who desires to breast feed prepares her breasts this way in the antepartal period, she will usually find that her nipples are "toughened up" and will not be sore or crack in the early period of nursing.

Another suggestion for toughening the nipples is to massage them daily with a washcloth, gradually working up to a turkish towel and then to a soft toothbrush.

Diet

Since the nausea and vomiting of the first trimester have usually subsided by this time, the expectant mother should be encouraged to stay on a well-balanced diet. If her appetite has increased, she should not allow this to lead her into eating improper meals or excessive calories.

Exercise

Exercise usually means diversion. It steadies the nerves, quiets the mind, and stimulates the appetite; all of which are valuable aids to pregnant women. An expectant mother can usually maintain her normal work and play activities, but they should be of shorter duration. In addition, she should try to avoid standing for too long. Lifting or moving heavy objects, overreaching, or any activity which might involve sudden jolts or a change of balance that could result in a fall or the likelihood of physical trauma should be avoided.

The more strenuous sports (horseback riding, skiing, etc.) should be discussed by the pregnant woman with her doctor. If she is used to these sports she will probably be allowed to continue in moderation until such time as it becomes uncomfortable for her or hazardous to the baby.

Rest and Recreation

During the second trimester the pregnant woman should be reminded to get enough rest. Since she usually feels better and has more pep and energy, she may have a tendency to overdo. The nurse can suggest that she rest whenever possible. If she has trouble sleeping she can try one of the progressive relaxation techniques or the side-lying position of comfort (Fig. 7-6). If there is no opportunity to take a nap, she may be able to just sit down and put her feet up for a few minutes.

Recreation is as vital to her emotional well-being as rest is to her physical well-being. A change of pace or environment with a chance to socialize and have a good time is important to the pregnant woman's mental health. It gives her a chance to recharge her batteries, so to speak. Her husband can show his understanding of her need to get out and away from the four walls of home by taking her out to dinner, or the movies, playing cards, dancing, bowling, or any of the activities they might enjoy together.

Maternity Clothing

Many women wonder about when they should start buying and wearing maternity clothing. Generally, their waistlines have expanded enough by the second trimester to dictate loose fitting clothing. A woman who is really excited about having a baby (usually her first) may start to wear maternity dresses or tops sooner than is needed because she wants the whole world to know she is pregnant.

In discussing maternity clothing with the woman a nurse could suggest some guidelines. The mother should avoid wearing any tight constricting garters which impair circulation in her legs. However, maternity garter belts and girdles can be worn. A girdle may be more comfortable and ease her backache as pregnancy advances. She should learn to put on the girdle lying down in bed before she gets up in the morning. That way the abdominal organs will have fallen into place and the girdle will give better support. Some members of the health team feel that wearing a girdle habitually makes the abdominal muscles lazy. Therefore, if the woman keeps her abdominal muscles toned by good posture and exercise she shouldn't have to rely on a girdle.

Shoes for a pregnant woman should provide good support, especially to the arches, for the feet must bear the extra weight that she gains. They should have sensible heels to prevent backaches and accidents.

There are many attractive maternity clothes on the market, found in specialty shops or in department stores. A woman can spend a great deal of money purchasing them or can economize by making her own. However, attractive clothing is a great morale booster. Her husband should understand that, in most instances, she won't be able to get by merely by letting her waistband out on her clothes a little or by lengthening her hemline. The purchase of maternity clothing is usually considered a part of the expense of having a baby.

Teaching Prenatal Exercises

Since it is the nurse's role to teach an expectant mother (or a group of expectant mothers) the exercises and other techniques that may be helpful during pregnancy and labor, the more common ones will be dis-

cussed here. Exercises for the postpartum period will be found in Chapter 14.

You may ask why it is necessary to teach exercises to pregnant women. The answer is that many women are "out of shape" because they have not been getting regular exercise. As a result their muscles have lost their flexibility and tone. Labor is so named because it is hard work. Since one would not expect an athlete to be in a sports event without preparing for it, neither should a pregnant woman be expected to go through the work and exertion of labor without preparation. For example, since women have been taught to sit with their legs crossed since they were little girls, one of the prenatal exercises, tailorsitting, promotes gradual stretching and flexibility of the thigh muscles. At the time of delivery when her legs are put up in stirrups, the woman will be more comfortable if these muscles have been limbered up.

The nurse may decide to demonstrate the exercises herself and then have the mothers practice while she helps each one individually as necessary. One of the principles in teaching exercises is that they should be done slowly, calmly, and smoothly. It defeats the purpose if they are done hurriedly or with jerky movements. Regularity in doing them, which means practice every day, is necessary for beneficial results. Because most expectant mothers have housework to do, it is a good idea to teach them ways to incorporate the exercises into their household activities. For example, they may do the pelvic rock while standing at the sink doing dishes.

Expectant mothers should be taught the purpose of any exercise. For example, they should know that abdominal breathing lifts up the abdominal wall from the uterus so that there is less discomfort during a contraction. When to use the exercises or breathing and relaxation techniques should also be stressed. This kind of information helps to motivate the woman to practice the exercises.

Another principle to emphasize is that the pregnant woman should not do the exer-

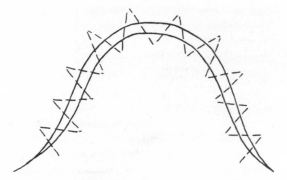

Figure 7-3. Application of abdominal breathing to a contraction during labor. The curved line represents the duration of a contraction. The dotted line represents the number of breaths.

cises to the point of becoming overtired. And last but not least, make the exercises fun. The nurse can suggest that maybe the whole family would like to learn and do them.

The nurse may explain the exercises as follows:

Breathing Exercises

Abdominal Breathing. To be used in the first stage of labor after contractions are well established (Fig. 7-3).

Lie on back with pillows under head and knees bent up. Place both hands on tummy above umbilicus. Breathe in through nose and lift abdominal wall up. Breathe out through relaxed lips and unclenched teeth, and your abdominal wall will sink down. Do about six breaths per 30 seconds.

Costal Breathing. To be used in the transition phase of the first stage of labor when you can no longer do abdominal breathing.

Lie on back with pillow under head and knees bent up. Place your hands at sides of ribs. Breathe in through nose and feel your ribs move sideways against your hands. Breathe out through relaxed lips and unclenched teeth, and feel your ribs move away from your hands. Do about six breaths per 30 seconds.

Panting. To prevent too rapid delivery of the baby and tearing of the birth canal.

Lie on back with a pillow or two under head, with knees bent up. Let your lips just part, your teeth unclench, and your tongue lie loosely on the floor of your mouth; head should be "heavy." Place the fingers of one hand over your breast bone. Breathe in and out at a more rapid rate, using the top of your chest in breathing. This breathing is similar to a dog's panting.

Bearing Down. To aid in expelling the baby and placenta.

Lie on your back with head and shoulders elevated. Pillows may be used. Bend your knees and separate your legs. Draw up your legs against your abdomen in a squatting position, holding your legs with your hands. Raise head. Take a deep breath and blow it out. Breathe in as quickly and deeply as you can: then hold your breath. In labor, this held breath will help to fix your diaphragm so that your abdominal wall will make more effective downward pressure on the uterus and baby. During practice *do not actually push.* You will be able to do so in labor.

Take catch breaths as needed. A catch breath is a short breath that may be taken whenever you can no longer hold your breath comfortably. Try to take no more than two or three catch breaths in each 60 to 65 seconds of breathing pattern.
(1) Maintain the pushing position.
(2) Exhale, moving head back.
(3) Take in a quick, deep breath.
(4) Tilt your head forward and hold your breath.

You can practice holding your breath a couple of times and then relax completely, take a deep breath and sigh it out.

Exercises to Strengthen Pelvic Muscles

Squatting

Keep back and knees apart. Squat down to floor. Practice this position to relax inner thigh muscles. Use this position when lifting, i.e., bend knees rather than back.

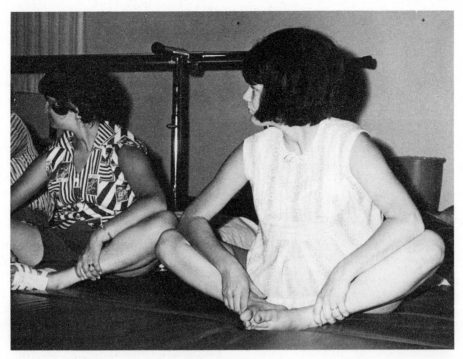

Figure 7-4. Expectant mothers practice "tailorsitting" at a prenatal class. (Courtesy of Good Samaritan Hospital, Phoenix.)

Control of Sphincter Muscles in Pelvic Floor. To control anal sphincter.

Lie on side. Contract sphincter as if controlling a bowel movement. Do not contract the buttocks. Relax.

When this can be accomplished you can learn to control the vaginal sphincter: Contract the sphincter as if to control urination without contracting the inner thigh muscles. To practice, start and stop the flow of urine once or twice as you urinate. You can practice this exercise anywhere. No one will know you are doing it.

Tailorsitting. To help stretch thigh and pelvic floor muscles (Fig. 7-4).

Sit with your legs crossed and your feet drawn toward you. Comfortably extend your knees downward toward the floor. Sit in this position as much as possible, when you are sewing or reading for example. Use a bed, sofa, large chair, or the floor for this exercise.

Exercises to Help Relieve Backache and Strengthen Abdominal Muscles. Can be done during pregnancy and labor.

Pelvic Tilting

Lying on back with one leg crossed over the other, pull in tummy, tuck seat under so that hollow of back flattens against the floor. Squeeze tops of thighs together. Pull up pelvic floor muscles as if controlling bladder. Hold to the count of five. Do five or six times a day.

Humping and Hollowing (Fig. 7-5).

Pull tummy and tuck head and seat down. Then slowly hollow back and bring head and seat up. This can be done about five or six times a day.

Pelvic Rocking. (standing)

Stand erect. Tighten your abdominal wall, pulling up and in, and tuck in buttocks. Slowly relax your abdomen and but-

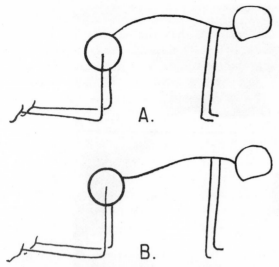

Figure 7-5. Humping (A) and hollowing (B) exercises are recommended for pregnancy.

tocks, allowing the hollow of back to return. Avoid hyperextension of lumbar spine. Breathe out as front of pelvis is rocked up; and breathe in as the pelvis is relaxed and dropped. Repeat the exercise five or six times, in a slow, rhythmic motion.

Relaxation Exercise. To help you rest or get to sleep. Used in later part of pregnancy and labor.

Lying in a Side Relaxation Position (Fig. 7-6).

Lie on side that feels most comfortable (for the purpose of illustration, we have assumed the right side). Your right arm and leg should be behind you, your left arm and leg in front of you. Place a pillow diagonally under your head, left breast, and left shoulder. Need for additional height may be the cause of pressure on your abdomen, right breast, or right shoulder: if so, a second pillow placed horizontally under the first should be used. Allow your abdomen to rest on the bed. If necessary, you may place a small pillow or folded towel under your abdomen for support. You may use a pillow to support your left leg, if it increases back or abdominal comfort.

Progressive Relaxation

Lie on side with underneath arm tucked right under behind you. First tense all mus-

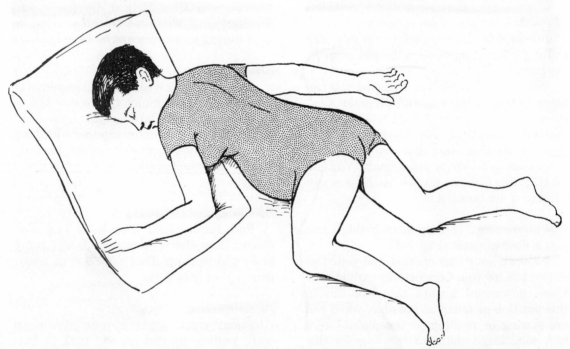

Figure 7-6. One relaxation position for the expectant woman is the side-lying position.

cles and then relax to feel the difference. Start by first contracting the muscles in the hand, then relax. Then tense the arm muscles, relax. Next go to face, then neck. Continue from the head toward the feet until all muscles have been tensed and then relaxed.

Later, progress to relaxing completely without tensing up first. You may use a pillow under forward knee also if more comfortable.

Prenatal Classes

During the second trimester, the woman and her husband may be interested in attending childbearing preparation classes. Much of the misunderstanding, fear, and apprehension of labor and delivery can be overcome by learning about the birth process. Increasing emphasis is being placed on the fact that there is an "emotional labor"

along with physical labor. In other words, the attitude that the woman has toward labor will have a considerable influence on the ease or difficulty of her labor. She can start now to establish the best possible physical condition and mental attitude for her labor.

If she chooses so-called natural childbirth she should realize that it does not have to be accomplished without medication to be rewarding. Fitzpatrick* says a woman should keep in mind that even if she requests medication or requires it, in no way has she "failed" to accomplish delivery by the "natural childbirth" method. The connotation of "painless" childbirth that has been associated with this method is by no means correct, for there is no painless labor

---

*Fitzpatrick, E. *et al:* Maternity Nursing. Philadelphia, Lippincott, 1971.

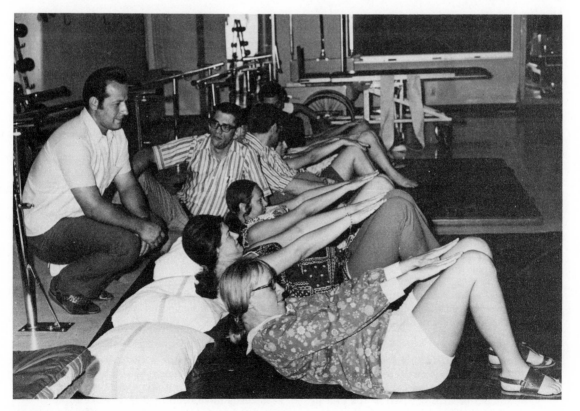

Figure 7-7. These husbands are encouraging their wives to do prenatal exercises. (Courtesy of Good Samaritan Hospital, Phoenix.)

or delivery unless nerve pathways have been destroyed or severed.*

It should be emphasized that the proponents of "natural childbirth" have never claimed that childbirth should be conducted without anesthetic aids or that it can be made devoid of pain. A person's response to pain is individual. "The only real measure of success lies in the satisfactions that the mother derives from being able to cooperate with the natural processes of labor to the best of her ability."*

The natural childbirth program has as a fundamental part of it a family-centered approach to maternity care. This program provides an opportunity to help both parents gain more knowledge and the satisfaction of mutual participation throughout pregnancy, labor, and delivery.

"The natural childbirth program is designed to eliminate fear. Facts concerning the anatomy and physiology of childbearing and appropriate care of the mother are taught."* The parents learn how labor progresses, what sensations are likely to accompany it, and ways of working along with them. The exercises are designed for the muscles the woman will use in labor as well as those which will promote the wellbeing of her body. She will learn breathing techniques which will help her relax during the first stage of labor and which will teach her how to work effectively with muscles used in delivery. Also, information about the baby's growth and development is included.

Another consideration of this program according to Fitzpatrick is "to help the expectant mother help herself so that her

---

*Fitzpatrick, E. *et al:* Maternity Nursing. Philadelphia, Lippincott, 1971.

Table 7-1.   COMPARISON BETWEEN THE READ METHOD AND THE LAMAZE METHOD

Read Method	Lamaze Method
Called natural childbirth	Called psychoprophylactic childbirth
Developed by Dr. Grantly Dick-Read (English obstetrician)	*Developed* by Drs. Nicolaiev and Velvovsky (Russian physicians)
Proponents: Drs. Thoms and Goodrich (New Haven, Conn.); Maternity Center Association, N. Y.	*Proponents:* Dr. Fernand Lamaze, French physician; Marjorie Karmel in the U. S.; American Society for Prophylaxis in Obstetrics (A.S.P.O.)
Theoretical Basis: Fear produces tension, tension produces pain. Educate the pregnant woman to eliminate fear and thus break the cycle	*Theoretical Basis:* Pavlov's theory of conditional reflexes (the substitution of a positive conditioned response for a negative one)
Exercises: to improve posture, body balance, increase muscle strength and flexibility used in childbirth and post-partum restoration	*Exercises:* to strengthen abdominal muscles and relax the perineum
Relaxation and Breathing Techniques: 1. Abdominal or "complete" breathing (used in the first stage of labor). 2. Costal or sternal breathing (used at the end to the first stage and in the second stage of labor).	*Breathing Techniques:* 1. Slow deep intercostal breathing (early labor) to 2. Rapid panting (end of first stage of labor). Breathing patterns have been modified, since rapid breathing may lead to hyperventilation.

pregnancy will be a healthy, happy experience and at the time of labor she will be better able to participate actively in having the baby."

The husband is shown how he can support his wife during labor. He is taught techniques to help relieve the pressures she experiences during labor. He learns how to time contractions, do pelvic lifts, and apply sacral pressure. Finally, he learns the importance of giving his wife the personal attention she may desire (Fig. 7-7).

Methods of Childbirth Education. There are two main methods of natural childbirth which are being taught in the United States at the present time: the Read method and the Lamaze method. Of course, individuals and groups have modified and made their own interpretations of these methods. Teachers of the Lamaze method are certified after they have completed a program in how to teach these classes.

Both methods are based on the following principles:

1. Fear leads to an increase in pain in labor. Education reduces fear.

2. Tension leads to increased pain in childbirth. If the woman in childbirth has a calm, pleasant atmosphere with supportive people caring for her, this will diminish her tension.

3. Relaxation and breathing techniques lessen the pains of labor and delivery.

4. Both aim to have the mother remain in conscious control during labor and delivery.

Table 7-1 compares the differences between the two methods. For further information about either of these methods of childbirth education, see the suggested readings at the end of the chapter.

DANGER SIGNALS

The major complications that can occur during the second trimester of pregnancy are symptoms of toxemia, antepartal bleeding, and premature labor. Therefore, the expectant mother should know what the danger signs are, and she should report to the doctor or clinic immediately if she notices any one of them.

Toxemia. The symptoms of toxemia are as follows: (1) a persistent headache that is not relieved by the usual remedies; (2) dizziness; (3) swelling of hands and feet; and (4) blurred vision or spots before her eyes.

Antepartal Bleeding. Antepartal bleeding manifests itself by a sudden gush or trickle of bright red bleeding from the vagina. Abdominal pain or cramps may or may not accompany it.

Premature Labor. A sudden gush of amniotic fluid from the vagina with or without abdominal cramps signals premature labor. Also, some bloody show may be present.

THE EXPECTANT FAMILY

It is important that the expectant mother and her husband keep communication lines open. Since the woman is now visibly pregnant her husband will probably be more aware of her pregnancy and be solicitous and attentive to her. He may want to attend childbirth education classes or make visits to the prenatal clinic or doctor's office with her. It is as important to prepare the husband for fatherhood as the mother for motherhood! He can show his love and affection for his wife by taking on some of the household tasks which may have become too difficult for her, such as heavy cleaning, moving and lifting furniture, etc.

The expectant mother should share her feelings with her husband in regard to the emotional changes she is experiencing, and both husband and wife should discuss sexual matters, financial responsibilities, and how the new baby is going to change their lives. The expectant mother can include her husband and other members of the family by sharing the progress she is making—telling them what the doctor or nurse said when she went for her visit, letting them feel the baby move in her abdomen, and asking them to help her do her exercises. The family members will be more likely to co-operate if they know why certain advice has been given to the expectant mother concerning diet, health, and hygiene measures. All members of the family will feel more a part of the pregnancy if they are consulted about decisions and sense that their feelings and opinions are listened to.

BIBLIOGRAPHY

Caplan, G.: Concepts of Mental Health and Consultation. Washington, D. C. U.S. Government Printing Office, 1959.

Fitzpatrick, E., *et al.:* Maternity Nursing, ed. 12. Philadelphia, J. B. Lippincott, 1971.

Ginott, H.: Between Parent and Child. New York, Macmillan, 1965.

Liley, H.: Modern Motherhood. New York, Random House, 1969.

Preparation for Childbearing. Maternity Center Association, New York, 1970.

Preparation for Labor: Breathing and Relaxation Techniques, Minnesota Dept. of Health, Minneapolis, 1967.

Psychophysical Preparation for Childbearing: Guidlines for Teaching. ed. 2. Maternity Center Association, New York, 1965.

Wiedenbach, E.: Family-Centered Maternity Nursing. ed. 2. New York, Putnam, 1967.

Williams, B.: Sleep needs during the maternity cycle. Nurs. Outlook, *15*:53, 1967.

Ziegal, E., and Van Blarcom, C.: Obstetric Nursing. NewYork, Macmillan, 1964.

Suggested Readings for Further Study

Dick-Read, G.: Childbirth without Fear. New York, Harper and Row, 1959.

Goodrich, F.: Preparing for Childbirth. Englewood Cliffs, Prentice-Hall, 1966.

Karmel, M.: Thank You, Dr. Lamaze. Philadelphia, J. B. Lippincott, 1959.

Thoms, H.: Childbirth with Understanding. Springfield, Ill., Charles C Thomas, 1962.

Vallay, P., *et al.:* Childbirth without Pain. New York, E. P. Dutton, 1960.

The Third Trimester of Pregnancy 8

To most women the last three months of pregnancy seem to be the longest and most wearisome. The expectant mother begins to tire of her size and of carrying the extra weight around with her. During the final weeks she becomes impatient to get it over with—to have her baby. Questions from her friends such as "Are you still around?" or "Haven't you had that baby yet?" make her feel worse. Of course, there are some women who feel fine throughout pregnancy and are never troubled by the pressure symptoms, awkwardness, or discomforts that can characterize the third trimester.

FETAL DEVELOPMENT

The last trimester of pregnancy is the period of greatest fetal weight gain and maturation of all body systems (Fig. 8-1).

Seventh Lunar Month. The fetus has grown to 15 inches and weighs two and a half pounds. He may have a poor to fair survival rate if born.

Eighth Lunar Month. The fetus is 16½ inches long and weighs about four pounds. He has an average to good chance of survival if born.

Ninth and Tenth Lunar Months. The fetus fills out rapidly and gains close to a half pound a week. The red color of his skin fades to pink as he develops subcutaneous tissue. He begins to shed lanugo and may suck his thumb. Born at nine lunar months, he has an excellent chance of survival.

PHYSIOLOGICAL CHANGES IN THE MOTHER

By the end of pregnancy the uterus becomes a thin, soft-walled muscular sac

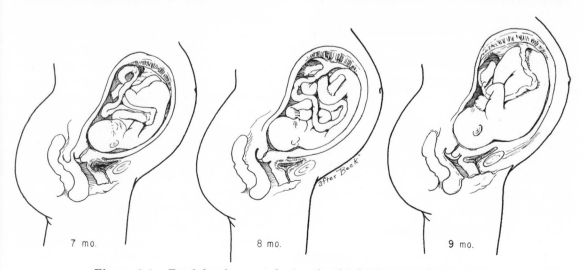

7 mo.   8 mo.   9 mo.

Figure 8-1. Fetal development during the third trimester of pregnancy.

which yields to the movements of the fetus. An examiner can easily palpate the fetus through the thin walls of the abdomen and uterus. By the ninth month the top of the uterus (fundus) is at the level of the xyphoid process of the sternum.

In most primigravidas, a phenomenon called lightening occurs from two to four weeks before term. Lightening means that the uterus settles down into the pelvic cavity thus relieving pressure on the diaphragm and lungs. In a multipara, lightening may not occur until the onset of labor.

The increased cardiac output declines to the nonpregnant level during the last weeks of gestation. However, the woman may experience palpitations of the heart during the last trimester. These are not uncommon and are caused by the intra-abdominal pressure of the enlarged uterus.

From the seventh month on marked changes take place in the placenta which becomes progressively *senile.* Some calcification occurs on the maternal surface. Occasionally infarcts (areas of ischemia caused by a lack of blood) may be seen in the placenta at the time of delivery. These changes reduce the efficiency of the placenta's exchange mechanism. Since they are progressive, it is thought that the aging of the placenta may be an important factor in limiting the period of intrauterine life.

The amniotic fluid undergoes changes too. The amniotic fluid which increased from 1000 to 1500. cc at the end of the sixth month gradually diminishes after the seventh month, reaching a level between 700 to 1000 cc. at term.

When the physician or nurse is listening for the fetal heartbeat with a stethoscope, other sounds can be heard in the abdomen. Occasionally a *funic souffle* may be heard, which is a soft, blowing sound of blood as it flows through the cord in synchrony with the fetal heartbeat.

PHYSICAL DISCOMFORTS

As in the first trimester, urinary frequency occurs, caused by the pressure of the enlarged uterus on the bladder, particularly after lightening takes place. There is nothing that the expectant mother can do about it except to wait patiently. It will, of course, disappear when the baby is born. She should continue to keep up her fluid intake of from six to eight glasses daily.

Some women are bothered by *dyspnea* which is shortness of breath or difficulty in breathing. Dyspnea results from pressure being exerted on the diaphragm by the enlarged uterus. It may be sufficient to interfere considerably with the pregnant woman's sleep and comfort during the last weeks of gestation. Unfortunately, it cannot be wholly relieved until after the birth of the baby, when it disappears spontaneously. Most expectant mothers find that shortness of breath is most troublesome when they lie down. It might be helpful to suggest that the mother use two or more pillows to prop herself up in bed. Also, good body mechanics and posture may help. The nurse may recommend an exercise called the rib cage lift, which involves raising the arm on the affected side, curving it over the head, and bending toward the unaffected side. This increases the space between the ribs and relieves discomfort.

Braxton-Hicks contractions which began in the early month of pregnancy may produce discomfort in the third trimester. Although they are usually painless, they gain strength and momentum in the last few months. Occasionally they come with such force that the expectant mother may mistake them for labor pains. These contractions are thought to contribute to the pulling up of the muscle fibers that surround the internal cervical os in the lower uterine segment. They often cause the cervical canal to be almost entirely effaced (thinned out) before labor begins. This is particularly true of primigravidas in whom effacement of the cervix is usually complete before dilatation begins. In multiparous mothers only partial effacement of the cervix occurs before the onset of labor. If Braxton-Hicks contractions are causing the pregnant woman discomfort the woman can try abdominal breathing for relief.

Other problems that may show up during the third trimester are *varicose veins* and *hemorrhoids*. Varicose veins usually occur in the legs though they are sometimes seen in the vulva and pelvic region. By definition a varicose vein is an enlargement in the diameter of the vein due to stretching and thinning of its walls. These distended areas occur at intervals along the vessel and give it a knotted appearance. In pregnancy, they are caused by pressure of the enlarged uterus on the large abdominal blood vessels which interferes with the return of blood from the lower extremities. To treat this (and prevent it) the pregnant woman should avoid wearing clothing that causes constriction. If varicosities develop she can lie in bed with her legs extended at right angles to her body, and her buttocks and heels resting against the wall. This can be done for two to five minutes several times a day. In addition, support stockings may be recommended. Or the doctor may advise her to wrap her legs daily with ace bandages. It is a good idea for all pregnant women to sit with their legs elevated whenever possible.

Hemorrhoids are varicose veins around the lower end of the rectum and anus. They may protrude through the anus and cause rectal bleeding. Hemorrhoids can be prevented by treating constipation promptly.

If the hemorrhoids protrude they can be pushed back in place in the following manner. The woman may either lie with her hips elevated or assume a knee-chest position. Once in position, she should gently and carefully push the hemorrhoids back into place with a finger well lubricated with oil. She may also apply an ice bag or cold witch hazel compresses for relief.

Edema (swelling) of the lower extremities is a common discomfort of the third trimester. It is prone to occur in hot weather or at the end of the day, particularly if the pregnant woman has been on her feet for long periods of time. Often it can be relieved by resting frequently during the day or by elevating the feet or assuming the right-angle position. Since edema can be a sign of pre-eclampsia, if the expectant mother notices that swelling occurs in her face and hands or that her ankles are swollen early in the day, she should immediately report these signs to her doctor. In fact any prolonged discomfort should be brought to the doctor's attention.

EMOTIONAL CHANGES

The mood changes and the introversive and passive behavior described in the second trimester reach their peak during the third trimester. Added to this are the normal fears that occur as full term approaches.

It is not unusual for the pregnant woman to fear that she might die from the analgesics or anesthetics which might be administered during labor and delivery. Then too, even though she knows that childbirth is much safer than it used to be, she is aware that there are still some women who die in childbirth. Stories she has heard from other women about bad experiences they had in childbirth increase her fears for her own safety. Usually after she has had one or more babies this fear is not as pronounced as during her first pregnancy. And with each subsequent pregnancy her fears lessen since she feels that she knows what to expect. Many times the fear of delivery is counterbalanced by her wish to have and see the baby.

Another fear is concerned with labor itself and how she will behave. She may have heard stories about other women screaming or saying "terrible" things while in childbirth. She may be afraid that she will not be able to cope with the pain, and she may lack confidence in the relaxation and breathing techniques she has learned. Another worry is that she will lose control of herself or look "silly" in front of her husband. To set her mind at rest, the nurse can assure her that these are normal concerns for a pregnant woman to have and that hospital personnel in the obstetrical department are accustomed to a variety of behavior from women in labor and are not shocked or offended by it.

It is also normal for the expectant mother to have fears for her child. There are justified uncertainties about what the baby will look like and whether it will have any abnormalities. The most frequent fears are: fear of losing the baby and fear of having a malformed or abnormal baby.

Fear of losing the baby is apt to arise if the pregnant woman has had any previous miscarriages, abortions, or stillbirths, if she has any complications, or if close friends or relatives have had such experiences.

Fear of having a malformed or abnormal baby sometimes arises from guilt feelings, superstitions, or lack of scientific understanding. Generally these fears are groundless.

What can the nurse do to alleviate the woman's fears? First, by understanding that these are normal, common occurrences in the latter part of pregnancy, she can reassure the expectant mother that many mothers share the same fears. It is often a great help for the mother to know that she is not different from others. Secondly, encouraging her to talk about her fears to others, such as the doctor, the nurse, her husband, or anyone who is a sympathetic listener, will help her considerably. She should not keep her thoughts bottled up inside; it will give her relief to express them.

There are two other emotional changes characteristic of the third trimester. One is that the pregnant woman may have fantasies and dreams about her unborn child. Often these fantasies are concerned with its appearance and sex and her ambitions and aspirations for it. The other is that the pregnant woman's id lies closer to the surface of consciousness than at any other time, causing her to express thoughts and feelings which she usually keeps hidden.

HEALTH PROTECTION AND PROMOTION

Prenatal Care

By the third trimester of pregnancy, the expectant mother is reporting more frequently for prenatal care. Her visits may occur about every two weeks during the eighth month and every week during the last month. The reason for this is that complications are more likely to occur toward the end of pregnancy. Also, the doctor will want to examine the woman for signs that she is ready to start labor. Since prenatal care is vital to the safety and well-being of both the mother and baby, the nurse should encourage the pregnant woman to keep her appointments regularly.

At these visits the nurse or doctor checks the expectant mother's weight, blood pressure, and urine and the fetal heart tones. The doctor will check the height of the fundus and the position of the fetus and will see if the presenting part of the fetus has engaged (settled into the pelvic inlet). During the last few visits he may perform a vaginal or rectal examination to determine if the cervix is "ripe" (soft, and partially effaced or dilated).

The doctor or nurse will ask the woman about any symptoms she may be having relative to the start of labor or any discomforts, or complications. If necessary she may receive final instructions regarding dietary restrictions. The doctor will probably want her to keep her weight gain to around 0.8 pound per week.

Nutrition

Nutrition is very important again in the third trimester because this is the period when the woman gains the greatest weight. She may need some additional reminders that will help her keep her weight down. She should avoid foods that are high in calories such as rich desserts, fried and starchy foods, gravies, potato chips, and buttered popcorn. Other high but "empty" calorie foods are doughnuts, jam, honey, candy, oil, mayonnaise, soft drinks, and alcoholic beverages.

If she has a tendency to retain fluid in her tissues, as evidenced by edema or rapid weight gain, she should cut down on her intake of salt. Some of the foods which have a high sodium content are ham, pork, crackers, potato chips, and lunch meats. She may also be advised to use salt sparingly in her cooking and to leave the salt shaker off the table.

In any case, the pregnant woman should continue to eat a well-balanced diet. Recent studies have indicated that the future mental abilities of the child may be influenced by the fact that the mother has proper nutrition throughout the third trimester of pregnancy.

The fetus stores large amounts of the following substances during the last trimester:

Calcium. Five sixths of the amount required is laid down at this time with half of it deposited in the last month. This amount is actually twice as much as the mother retains during the last month of her pregnancy. The same holds true for phosphorus.

Iron. Five sixths of the amount present in the baby is deposited during this last trimester. A large part of it is stored in the fetal liver, possibly in anticipation of the shortage of iron in the mother's milk.

Nitrogen. Two thirds of the total amount needed is acquired now, with half of it deposited in the last month.

Therefore, it is a good idea for the expectant mother to eat foods that are high in these substances, in addition to taking the vitamins prescribed by the doctor. Good food sources of iron are egg yolk, stem vegetables, and yellow or green leafy vegetables, lean meat (especially liver), fruits such as raisins and apricots, and whole grain cereals. Calcium is best derived from milk, cheese, eggs, oatmeal, and vegetables.

Exercise

The expectant mother does not have to restrict her activities in the third trimester unless her doctor has so indicated. Daily walks are still very good for her unless they cause fatigue. She should, of course, heed advice not to overdo (activities, housework). The point is that she needs to conserve her energy for labor and will not be in the best condition for it if she is overtired physically or mentally beforehand.

Rest

Rest is important all through pregnancy but especially during the last six weeks. The nurse can remind the pregnant woman to sit whenever she can and to rest or sleep when she feels the need or when she has a chance.

At this stage of pregnancy the expectant mother may find that she is becoming increasingly tired from her large size. The full-term pregnant uterus and its contents weigh about 12 pounds. Carrying this weight around all day may seem almost too much for her. In addition she may have trouble sleeping. Some of the discomforts, such as shortness of breath or urinary frequency may keep her from getting the rest and sleep she would like—in fact, needs.

Perhaps some of the following suggestions may be of help. During the last months of pregnancy lying on one side with a small pillow to support the abdomen can do much to relieve the discomfort that is common during this period.

The pregnant woman may also find it most relaxing to lie on her back with a small pillow under her head and a large pillow under her knees to provide support and prevent strain on her leg muscles. Her hips and knees should be comfortably flexed so that her abdominal wall is relaxed. The side-lying position described on page 94 can be used as an alternate to this position.

Sitting in an armchair is relaxing if the body is well aligned. Small pillows may be used to support the back and head, and a footstool may be used for support if the feet do not touch the floor. The woman should sit with her legs slightly apart to prevent tension on her enlarged abdomen. The progressive relaxation techniques described in Chapter 7 can be used to good advantage.

In order to get the most out of relaxation the mother should have a quiet and peaceful environment. Stimulation such as loud noises and bright lights should be kept to a minimum.

Sexual Relations

By the seventh or eighth month sexual desire may again diminish, and most women find that they cannot participate in coitus in the usual positions. The couple can be encouraged to experiment with positions, perhaps a side-lying one, which allow the wife to be more passive. Thus, the husband can be satisfied and not feel deprived, and his wife can feel that she can still contribute to his gratification and happiness.

The doctor will usually advise abstinence from intercourse during the last weeks before term in order to avoid possible premature labor or infection. However, some doctors tell their patients that intercourse is permissible up to the time that the baby is due, provided the husband is gentle, the wife is comfortable, and the movements during intercourse are not too vigorous. In the case that the wife has been advised to abstain from intercourse it is important for the husband to know the reasons why. Good communications between husband and wife and frank discussions of these matters are necessary to avoid feelings of hurt or rejection which could harm their relationship.

Bathing and Douching

Tub bathing may become increasingly awkward for the mother-to-be in the last trimester. She may find it difficult to get in and out of the bathtub because of her large size. Because there is an increased danger of her falling and injuring herself, it is recommended that during the last few weeks of pregnancy she take showers or sponge baths instead. Since her glands are more active during pregnancy and since she is perspiring more freely to get rid of the fetal waste products as well as her own, she will ordinarily want to bathe or shower daily to eliminate offensive odors and remove waste products. Feeling clean and fresh is a morale booster for many women, pregnant or not.

It is recommended that douching be kept to a minimum during pregnancy. Douching, in general, has received less emphasis in recent years. It is de-emphasized even more so in pregnancy because an unclean douche nozzle can introduce infection into the birth canal. And if the solution is too hot or if it runs into the vagina at too great a pressure it is possible to cause premature rupture of the membranes.

However, douching is permissible and may be advised under certain circumstances such as excessive vaginal secretions or a monilia or trichimonas infection of the vagina. It is often the nurse who teaches the woman how to carry out this procedure at home.

The following are general instructions for douching:

1. The douching equipment should be clean and the douche nozzle washed in hot water prior to using.
2. If douching equipment is to be purchased the nurse can recommend the "gravity flow" type because there is less pressure employed than when the "bulb syringe" type is used.
3. The woman should mix the solution using accurate measurements and warm water. Hot water should *never* be used.
4. She should wash the external genitalia from front to back before douching to prevent infection.
5. She may sit on the toilet seat if it is too awkward for her to lie in the bathtub. It is not necessary to undress.
6. She should introduce the douche tip only about two to three inches into the vagina and either hold or hang the bag not more than two feet above the vaginal opening. In this way the solution will slowly run in and out under low pressure.
7. She should slowly rotate the douche nozzle and at intervals compress the vulva around it so that the solution distends the vagina and reaches all surfaces. She should then release the vulva and allow the solution to run out. She will perhaps alternately compress the vulva and release the solution four to five times while she is douching.
8. The equipment should be rinsed or dried after using.

The whole procedure should require only five to ten minutes.

DANGER SIGNALS

Since danger signals are the same as for the second trimester, please refer to page 97.

THE EXPECTANT FAMILY

Preparing Children in the Family

The third trimester is a time when it is very important for the mother-to-be to make sure that she is including her children in her pregnancy. Regardless of how many children there are, each child needs to feel that he is a part of things and that his parents love him very much. The mother's leaving for the hospital can be a very threatening and anxiety-producing experience for a small child. It is compounded by the fact that when she returns she will bring with her a new member of the family, requiring that he share his parents with another being. Much anxiety and jealousy can be averted if he is adequately prepared and has felt that he has been a part of the pregnancy.

If a child is to be moved to another room (or bed) when the baby comes, he should be moved early in the third trimester so that he becomes accustomed to his new quarters. If the child is to share the same room with the new baby, his parents could let him help them to prepare the room. However, it is important that he has a place all of his own.

The Expectant Father

The husband too is probably having his problems. Not only is a husband inclined to worry when his wife has a baby but there are also other facts he has to face. Since the newest member will change the group composition, he probably wonders how much and in what way. Also, he will have another mouth to feed, adding to his responsibilities. This is a sobering thought and could perhaps lead to resentment. However, if he really feels involved with the pregnancy his reaction is much more likely to be one of joy when the new baby arrives. He will be more likely to feel that "This is our baby. We gave it life! Now I want to take care of that life." There will probably be a closeness that otherwise would be missing.

Since changes in the house and its arrangements certainly will involve the father, his suggestions and preferences should carry weight.

He should also understand something about babies. If he has some experience and knowledge about how to feed a baby or give him a bath, he can relieve his wife from time to time. He can also get more fun and fellowship with the newborn than an occasional chin tickling will bring.

The husband and wife should reach a sensible balance. Between the extremes of the men who help all the time and those who never help, there is the father who helps some of the time. He may offer to baby sit while his wife gets her hair done, now and then he might get up once during the night or early morning to feed the baby, or he might take over for her on a weekend morning or afternoon. He should also spend some time playing with the baby and their other child(ren).

ADDITIONAL INFORMATION THE PARENTS SHOULD KNOW

Breast or Bottle Feeding

The third trimester is a most opportune time for the nurse to discuss breast or bottle feeding with the mother-to-be. Since the husband may have definite opinions he may want to be included in the discussion too. Psychologically this is a good time to discuss the subject because the woman is beginning to make plans for the baby's arrival, and the whole idea of having a baby has become more real to her. If the woman is not given an opportunity to discuss breast or bottle feeding during her pregnancy, when she goes into labor she may suddenly find herself being asked, "How are you going to feed your baby?" without having given the question much thought.

If the mother-to-be does not bring up the subject herself the nurse should initiate the discussion. The nurse should not advocate one method over the other unless the woman has indicated a preference. The discussion will most likely center around the advantages and disadvantages of each method. Presently there is controversy over which is the "best" method. Frequently people have strong feelings concerning what they think is the "right" way. Everyone from grandmothers on down will have definite opinions and will try to influence the expectant mother. No wonder she is bewildered by all the advice! Therefore she will appreciate an opportunity to get factual information from the nurse who is not as emotionally involved in trying to persuade her to use a particular method. (See pages 256-260 for a discussion of breast feeding and bottle feeding.)

Analgesics and Anesthetics

The expectant mother is often very interested in knowing what analgesics and anesthetics may be administered during childbirth. In fact, she may select her doctor because she has heard he gives his patients a certain anesthetic for delivery. As with other subjects it is important that she have an opportunity to discuss various types of analgesics and anesthetics ahead of time with the doctor or nurse.

If she has a preference, this should be respected if at all possible. However, she should understand that circumstances may occur which warrant the use of a certain analgesic or anesthetic. If this happens, then of course, it is the doctor's decision.

Because many of the women's magazines have articles about obstetric analgesics and anesthetics and because it is a subject a woman would discuss with her friends, the expectant mother may have misconceptions or questions. The nurse should be able to give her factual information to clear up misconceptions and answer her questions.

If you don't know the answer, admit it, and tell the patient that you will find out. (For a discussion of analgesics and anesthetics in labor see Chapter 10.)

Preparation for Labor and Delivery

The prospective parents should be prepared for the hospital experience. The mother-to-be in particular will feel more at ease and will be more likely to have a positive, satisfying experience if she knows what to expect.

A visit to the maternity floor at the hospital where she plans to deliver will help to acquaint the couple with the physical setting of the hospital, will familiarize them with the strange looking equipment, and will give them a chance to meet some of the hospital personnel.

It is also a good idea for the parents to note the distance between their home and the hospital, the quickest route to take, and the parking facilities available at the hospital. They may also want to inquire about visiting regulations, rooming-in facilities, admission procedures, and financial arrangements. The expectant mother will want to discuss with her doctor at what point she should go to the hospital, after labor begins. She should also be instructed about the signs and symptoms of labor. For a multipara a review of the signs may be all that is necessary since she probably remembers what they are from her last baby. However, a primigravida usually needs more information.

About four to six weeks before the baby is due the mother should pack a suitcase with things that she and the baby will need during their stay in the hospital and on their retun home. Doctor's offices, clinics, and hospitals will often supply lists of suggested items to take.

Hospital Routine

The prospective parents will want to know what to expect during the hospital stay. When they arrive at the hospital all sorts of things happen. The mother-to-be is whisked into a labor room to be prepared for delivery. The husband is sent to the admitting office to fill out forms and make financial arrangements.

The expectant mother will undress and put on a hospital gown. A nurse or other staff member in the labor and delivery department will take the woman's temperature, pulse, respirations, and blood pressure.

She may also be weighed and be asked for a urine specimen. Her contractions are timed, and the fetal heart tones listened to. The woman is then examined vaginally or rectally. All of these procedures are done to see if everything is normal and to determine how far along she is in labor.

She may then be "prepped": the nurse or attendant shaves off most or all of the pubic hair. This is done for the sake of cleanliness during and after delivery and to prevent infection, especially if the woman requires "stitches" in the perineal region. (However, at some hospitals prepping is not done.) The procedure for a shave prep will be included in Chapter 10.

After being "prepped", the woman may be given an enema to clean out the lower intestinal tract so that there is more room for the baby to descend and less chance of soiling when the mother is pushing with contractions at the time of delivery. An enema is less of a routine than the prep and is usually ordered by the doctor if the woman needs it.

Of course, the woman may decide that she prefers to do these things herself at home (with her husband's help), so that it won't be necessary when she gets to the hospital.

Once the prepping and enema are done, the husband (or whoever has brought the mother to the hospital) will most likely have completed the admission procedure and can rejoin her in the labor room.

During the time that she is in labor her vital signs (blood pressure, temperature, pulse, and respirations), the baby's heartbeat, and the contractions will be checked at intervals by the nursing personnel and doctors. Vaginal or rectal examinations are performed and medications may be given to relieve the discomfort. Backrubs, ice chips, assistance in breathing and relaxation techniques will likely be used to make her more comfortable. Depending on the hospital (or how busy they are) nursing personnel may stay with the mother continuously or check on her frequently during labor.

Then when the baby is ready to be born she will be taken in her bed or on a cart into the delivery room. Depending on the hospital, her husband may or may not accompany her. The people in the delivery room with her are the doctor, the nurse or nursing personnel, possibly an anesthetist or anesthesiologist and, if it is a teaching hospital, a student nurse and an intern or resident. So she will have plenty of attention.

Once she is on the delivery table, her legs will be elevated in stirrups and she will have metal hand grips to hold on to which may aid in pushing. Her legs will be strapped into the stirrups with cloth straps, and her wrists may be strapped also. This is to prevent her from inadvertently touching sterile drapes which cover her abdomen and legs during delivery.

The husband can be a tremendous help and support to his wife in labor. He can provide emotional support by encouraging her and keeping up her morale. He can offer physical support by giving her ice chips, rubbing her back, and placing a cool cloth on her forehead.

Knowing that his wife will normally "turn inward", as labor progresses will help the husband to understand her response to him. Almost all of her concentration and energy is directed toward her contractions and the delivery. Even though she may not talk to him much, or even seem to be aware that he is there, she still appreciates his presence. By remembering that pregnant women are extremely passive and vulnerable, he will be aware that his wife is highly sensitive. Thus, she will be receptive to both positive and negative suggestions. She will readily accept the help that he has been taught to give during labor, but he should talk about her contractions, *not pains*. If the word pain is used with its negative connotation it will affect her adversely. By being with his wife during labor and delivery the husband has a chance to be an active participant in their baby's birth.

The baby will be placed in a warm incubator as soon as it is born. Bands will be placed on the baby's wrist and ankle and an identical band will be placed on the mother's wrist with identifying information so that there is no danger of a mix-up in babies. This is always done in the delivery room before the mother and infant are separated.

Usually the mother spends about an hour in the delivery room. If the husband has been sent to a waiting room he should be aware of this so that he will not be overly anxious. After the placenta has been expelled, and the episiotomy repaired (if there is one) the mother, baby, and father are reunited in the hospital corridor or perhaps in a room.

If the hospital has a recovery room for maternity patients the mother will spend from two to eight hours under close observation by the nursing staff. They will examine her uterus and her vaginal discharge and stitches and check her vital signs frequently, usually every 15 minutes to a half hour. If the mother desires, she can usually eat and drink in the recovery room. It's difficult to sleep, however, because of the frequent interruptions. Her husband may be with her also. She can expect similar postpartum care even if the hospital does not have a postpartum recovery room.

In the meantime the baby goes to the nursery to be weighed, measured, and examined. He is kept warm, and after his temperature has stabilized, he may be bathed, dressed, and brought to his mother for her to inspect and become acquainted with.

Then the mother is moved to a postpartum area where she stays for one to three days following delivery. Both the mother and baby may want to sleep for several hours, and the baby may not be brought to her again for his first feeding until about 12 hours after birth. The mother can be reassured not to worry about him, that he is being watched and cared for by the nursing personnel.

Her days in the hospital will be busy ones from early in the morning until 10 or 11 P.M. at night. She will be feeding her baby every three to four hours except possibly at night. Mealtimes for her may be at 7:30

A.M., 11:30 A.M., and 5:30 P.M. She will probably take a shower the first or second postpartum day and will be instructed in how to give special care to her perineum. Walking around the first or second day after the baby is born will help her regain her strength and restore body functions. Her days will be filled with receiving visitors, answering telephone calls, sending birth announcements, and learning how to care for herself and her baby.

When it is time for the mother and baby to be discharged, hospitals usually give the new mother a 24-hour supply of formula to take home if she is bottle feeding her baby, so that she will not have to prepare formula right away. She will be given instructions as to when she and the baby should return to the doctor or clinic. The baby is usually brought back in four weeks, and the mother returns for her check-up in six weeks.

Postdelivery Arrangements

For approximately two weeks after returning home the new mother will need some help. If she arranges for this at an early date she will feel easier, particularly if she plans to hire someone. In case she hasn't thought about it, the nurse can mention it to her in the third trimester.

Unless she has twins or triplets, the best helping hand for her will be someone who takes care of everything *except* the baby. It is primarily the mother who should care for the baby. The person who is there to help does the cooking, the dishes, the shopping, the cleaning, and anything else associated with the housework. Many times relatives will help, but if the new parents are hiring someone to help, that person should have had a recent chest x-ray and a clean bill of health from a doctor, and the parent should be prepared to pay for it if necessary.

It is well for the mother to remember that many a husband has been a more comforting source of help than an employee or a relative. If he is not able to stay home from work when she has the baby, he can often help with the baby, the house, or the other children in the evenings and weekends. If the husband is not particularly interested in doing this, the wife should not force the issue. It is far better for a new father to get used to his baby gradually than to suddenly feel burdened with diapers, bottles, and laundry. His wife will want him to feel proud of his new offspring and not a slave to him.

Diaper Service. Diaper service is a tremendous help. It is best if the mother-to-be selects a service ahead of time and lets them know if she wants them to supply the diapers. Of course, the service supplies a diaper pail. Even if she only has diaper service for a short time it saves her strength and energy in the early postpartum weeks and provides her with diapers (and other baby clothes) that are softer and cleaner than those done at home.

Baby Layette and Equipment. Many department stores (in the infant department), doctors' offices, clinics, and hospitals provide lists of what is needed for a newborn. A layette is considered to be the basic clothing, blankets, bedding, and towels, that the infant uses. It is wise to purchase larger sizes than will actually be needed at first, since the infant will rapidly grow into them. Here again, creativity in making garments and furnishings will afford the parents satisfac-

tion and save them money. Remember, even an orange crate or dresser drawer can be used by the infant as a crib at first. It should also be remembered that some cultural groups do not believe in preparing for the baby ahead of time.

BIBLIOGRAPHY

Bonica, J.: Principles and Practice of Obstetric Analgesia and Anesthesia. Philadelphia, F. A. Davis, 1967.

Caplon, G.: Concepts of Mental Health and Consultation. Washington, D. C., U. S. Government Printing Office, 1959.

Davis, M., and Rubin, R.: DeLee's Obstetrics for Nurses. ed. 17. Philadelphia, W. S. Saunders, 1962.

Fitzpatrick, E., *et al*: Maternity Nursing. ed. 12. Philadelphia, J. B. Lippincott, 1971.

Ginott, H.: Between Parent and Child. New York, Macmillan, 1965.

Marlow, D.: Textbook of Pediatric Nursing. ed. 3. Philadelphia, W. B. Saunders, 1969.

Wiedenbach, E.: Family-Centered Maternity Nursing. ed. 2. New York, Putnam, 1967.

Williams, S.: Nutrition and Diet Therapy. St. Louis, C. V. Mosby, 1969.

Suggested Readings for Further Study

Eastman, N.: Expectant Motherhood, ed. 5. Boston, Little, Brown, 1970.

Maternity Center Association: A Baby Is Born. ed. 2. New York, The Association, 1960.

Complications of Pregnancy *9*

ANTEPARTAL BLEEDING

Bleeding during the antepartal period poses a serious threat to both the mother and fetus. There are two kinds of bleeding: bleeding which occurs in the earlier part of pregnancy from causes such as abortion, ectopic pregnancy, and hydatidiform mole; and bleeding in the latter half of pregnancy, most frequently caused by placenta previa and abruptio placentae.

Abortion

Bleeding in the first trimester of pregnancy is most often indicative of abortion. Abortion is defined as the termination of pregnancy before the fetus has attained viability. This is generally regarded as before the twentieth week of gestation or at any time when the fetus weighs less than 400 grams.

There are two types of abortions: spontaneous and induced. In spontaneous abortion, the fetus is lost through natural causes. The lay term for this kind of abortion is miscarriage. In fact, a nurse or doctor, inquiring of the patient or relatives about losses of previous pregnancies, should use the term miscarriage. Lay people frequently associate the term abortion with a criminal act. An induced abortion is one which is artificially brought about and may include therapeutic and criminal abortions.

Spontaneous Abortions

Spontaneous abortions may fall into numerous categories. A *threatened abortion* is characterized by spotting or bleeding in the first trimester. Along with the bleeding the woman may have cramplike contractions and a backache. The cervix remains closed, and the bleeding may stop, so she may continue to carry the pregnancy to full term and have a normal, healthy baby.

In an *imminent abortion* there is more bleeding, and blood clots are frequently passed. The woman has severe cramps, and the cervical canal dilates. Usually the products of conception are passed in about two hours.

The characteristic signs of an *inevitable abortion* are rupture of the membranes and dilatation of the cervix. Part of the uterine contents may be protruding through the cervix. Inevitable means that there is no way to stop the process.

In an *incomplete* abortion there is profuse bleeding so that the patient may be in shock. Part of the products of conception have already been expelled, but part, usually the placenta, remains in the uterus. A *complete* abortion means that all of the products of conception have been passed.

In a *missed* abortion the fetus is retained in the uterus after it has died. It is designated as a missed abortion if the fetus is retained two months after death. The fetus undergoes degenerative changes, and the uterus gets smaller instead of larger. The breast changes which accompany pregnancy disappear, but the woman may continue to have amenorrhea.

Women who have three or more consecutive spontaneous abortions are called habitual aborters. A frequent cause of *habitual abortion* is an incompetent cervix. This is a cervix that begins to dilate usually during the second trimester of pregnancy. Because of an inherent weakness in its structure, the woman is unable to carry a pregnancy to term. Other causes of habitual abortion are thyroid dysfunction, a deficiency of progesterone, and congenital abnormalities of the reproductive system, such as a bicornuate (double) uterus.

If the cause is an incompetent cervix, a surgical procedure, called a Shirodkar operation, may be done to correct it. The operation, performed when the patient is pregnant, involves suturing a band of Dacron or fascia around the cervix to keep it closed. When the woman reaches full term, she may be delivered vaginally (the band must be snipped first) or by cesarean section.

Induced Therapeutic Abortion

There has been a marked change in attitudes toward therapeutic abortions in the United States. Other countries, such as Sweden and Japan, have had more liberal views for a longer period of time.

In the United States our abortion laws varied from state to state, until a recent Supreme Court ruling established a more liberalized outlook by making abortion a matter to be decided by a woman and her doctor. This has been a subject of much controversy because of moral and religious implications.

Methods of performing a therapeutic abortion have changed in the last few years. One method is to suction out the uterine contents with a suction curet. This method is often used during early pregnancy. The other method, referred to as salting out, involves introducing a hypertonic solution of

sodium chloride into the amniotic sac, thereby bringing about abortion of the fetus. Usually labor ensues spontaneously in a day or two. This procedure is more frequently used when pregnancy is further advanced because surgical procedures become more hazardous to the patient.

If the patient has been admitted for a therapeutic abortion, she may be admitted to either the obstetrical or gynecologic services. Teenage patients often prefer to be placed in a room with girls their own age, whereas an older patient may want to be alone.

When taking care of a patient who is having a therapeutic abortion, the nurse should reflect a nonjudgmental attitude and regard her as any other patient who has come to the hospital for medical treatment and nursing care. The nurse should examine her own feelings about abortion, and if she feels that taking part in an abortion or taking care of the patient goes against her religious and moral convictions, she should discuss this with her immediate supervisor. In other words, both the convictions of the nurse as well as the rights of the patient are to be respected.

Criminal Abortion

Criminal abortion is defined as any abortion that is done illegally outside of the hospital or clinic without proper medical supervision. One danger of a criminal abortion is that it is likely to be done by someone who is untrained and unskilled and who does not use aseptic technique. It is estimated that around 1 million American women a year, most of them married, have criminal abortions.

The most common method used to perform a criminal abortion is to introduce a foreign object into the uterine cavity. Or the woman may swallow drugs such as quinine, castor oil, or ergot. However, these drugs are not effective unless taken in such large doses that they damage the woman as well.

The major complications that bring the

woman to the hospital following a criminal abortion are infection and hemorrhage. If the patient has a septicemia or is in deep shock from blood loss, she may be one of the sickest patients the nurse will ever have to take care of. Unfortunately, some of these patients come to the hospital when it is too late. A somewhat less serious aftermath, perhaps, of criminal abortion is that the woman may be permanently sterile. This can be psychologically disturbing if she wants to have children.

Nursing Care in Abortion

The patient is usually admitted to a gynecologic service, but if she is further along in her pregnancy, she may be admitted to the obstetrical department. If she has been admitted because of a threatened abortion, she is probably very apprehensive and needs a great deal of emotional support. This means reassuring her about her condition without giving her false hopes about the outcome of her pregnancy. The nurse should maintain and encourage bed rest. The patient should be as quiet as possible and should not get up to go to the bathroom. Sedatives may be given to keep the patient relaxed and sleepy.

All clots and tissue passed, as well as all perineal pads, should be saved for inspection. Clots and tissue can be saved in a jar filled with normal saline solution; the pads can be saved in a paper bag. Vital signs should be taken every 15 minutes when the patient is first admitted or if she is bleeding heavily. If her temperature starts to rise, it should be taken every four hours.

The patient may be getting intravenous fluid with Pitocin added to bring about the expulsion of the products of conception, or she may be receiving IV fluids or blood as replacement therapy. In any case the nurse should monitor the IV carefully and keep it open unless otherwise ordered by the physician.

It is important to adhere to principles of medical asepsis because the patient is more susceptible to infection when she has lost a lot of blood. The patient should not have any cathartics or enemas; they might stimulate more bleeding. She is usually given a soft, light diet, or if she is being prepared for surgery, she may not be allowed anything by mouth (N.P.O.).

The doctor may order a hormone such as progesterone to be given to relax the irritable uterine muscle if the patient is threatening to abort. Prior to discharge the patient should be instructed about what signs to watch for and about saving any tissue or clots passed. The patient is often advised not to have sexual relations for a couple of weeks.

If the patient is losing the pregnancy and is bleeding heavily, she may go to the operating room for a dilatation and curettage (D and C). This is a surgical procedure in which the cervix is dilated and the contents of the uterus are scraped out. The main danger of a D and C is perforation of the wall of the uterus with a sharp instrument. As you recall, the uterine wall becomes softer during pregnancy.

It is recommended that Rh negative mothers receive Rhogam within 72 hours after the products of conception are expelled, because such women are liable to become sensitized and sensitivity could affect the next baby.

Spontaneous abortions can be emotionally upsetting to parents who are anxious to have a child. However, they often do represent nature's way of getting rid of a defective fetus. In a high percentage of spontaneous abortions when the embryo or fetus is examined, the abnormalities are gross ones which are incompatible with life. Thus an abortion, even though it saddens the couple, may be a blessing in disguise.

Ectopic Pregnancy

An ectopic pregnancy is a pregnancy located outside of the uterine cavity. Ectopic pregnancies most commonly occur in the fallopian tubes. Because fertilization normally takes place in the outer portion of the fallopian tube, a narrowing of the lumen of the tube may prevent its descent into the uterine cavity. If this happens, the fertilized ovum begins to grow and develop within the tube.

Symptoms. The tube has only limited elasticity; when it reaches its maximum, it ruptures, producing the signs and symptoms characteristic of a ruptured ectopic pregnancy:

1. Severe abdominal pain which radiates to the shoulder.

2. Faintness and shock: The shock may be out of proportion to the external bleeding, but there may be a great deal of bleeding internally in the abdominal cavity.

3. Change in the menstrual cycle: The woman may have missed one or two menstrual periods, and now she begins vaginal bleeding or spotting. This is caused by the rapid drop in hormones after the tube ruptures.

4. Vaginal tenderness: By far the most common physical finding is extreme tenderness, especially when the cervix is moved during a vaginal examination.

When the physician examines the woman, he finds her uterus to be enlarged to about six to eight weeks gestation, with a tender mass in the adnexae. He may do a culdocentesis, which is the aspiration of material from the cul-de-sac of Douglas (the blind pouch between the vagina and the rectum). If the space contains blood which does not clot, the diagnosis is probably ectopic pregnancy. If the woman has a history of infertility or pelvic inflammatory disease, this also helps him to make a diagnosis.

The incidence of ectopic pregnancies has increased by about 30 per cent in the past 25 years. This goes along with the increased amount of pelvic inflammatory disease and the treatment of salpingitis with antibiotics. An exudate or adhesions form in the tubes narrowing the lumina.

Although 95 per cent of ectopic pregnancies occur in the tubes, occasionally one will start to develop in the ovary. In rare instances the fertilized ovum ruptures out of the end of the tube and continues on to develop into a full-term pregnancy in the abdominal cavity. The fetus is then delivered through an abdominal incision.

Treatment. The patient should be kept flat in bed at all times. An intravenous infusion is started with a large needle, and the patient is typed and cross-matched for large amounts of blood. Usually no time is lost in sending the patient to the operating room for an emergency laparotomy. Sometimes the entire tube is removed (a salpingectomy) or the pregnancy is removed and the tube repaired. Despite modern methods of treatment, the maternal mortality rate from this complication is alarmingly high— 1 in 12 or 1 in 20, according to various reports.

Hydatidiform Mole

Although this is a rare condition in the United States, it is worthy of mention because it is most unusual and can cause bleeding in the early part of pregnancy. It is sometimes simply called a mole or a molar pregnancy. It is a benign neoplasm of the chorion. For some unknown reason the fertilized ovum deteriorates and instead of developing into a fetus and placenta, the chorionic vessels seem to go wild and grow in profusion, filling up the uterine cavity.

Symptoms. The patient's uterus enlarges more rapidly than it does in a normal pregnancy. For example, at two months gestation the uterus may be the size expected at around three and a half to four months. There are no fetal heart tones, and when an x-ray is taken, there is no evidence of a fetal skeleton.

Hyperemesis gravidarum, or excessive vomiting of pregnancy, may be present, and intermittent vaginal bleeding may occur. In addition chorionic vessels, which have a typical grapelike or tapioca pudding appearance, may be passed. There may also be symptoms of toxemia. This is the only time that toxemia appears in the first part of pregnancy. The woman may also have anemia and an infection.

Treatment. The uterus is evacuated

either by giving the patient a Pitocin drip or by doing a D and C. Antibiotics and blood transfusions are used as adjunctive therapy. The follow-up treatment is important because a certain small percentage of patients develop a malignancy after having a molar pregnancy. If it is untreated, it may metastasize to the lungs and other areas of the body. The malignant tumor is called a choriocarcinoma.

It is of utmost importance that the patient not become pregnant for one year. The reason is that the blood levels of chorionic gonadotropin are checked frequently. If they become positive (and it is certain that the woman is not pregnant), then this indicates the development of a malignancy which would probably necessitate a hysterectomy. Fortunately it has been found that spreading choriocarcinomas can be cured by the use of anticancer drugs such as methotrexate.

Placenta Previa

Sometimes the placenta is implanted in the lower uterine segment, thereby overlapping the internal os of the cervix. When Braxton-Hicks contractions occur, as they do more frequently and with greater intensity in the latter part of pregnancy, the placenta may be torn loose, with resultant bleeding.

If the placenta completely covers the internal cervical os, it is called a total placenta previa (also placenta praevia). A partial placenta previa impinges partially on the internal os (Fig. 9-1); and a low implantation means that the placenta cannot be palpated closer than 3 cm. from the center of the cervical os.

Symptoms. The patient experiences bright red, *painless* vaginal bleeding in the third trimester. It occurs quite suddenly, and she may awaken to find herself lying in

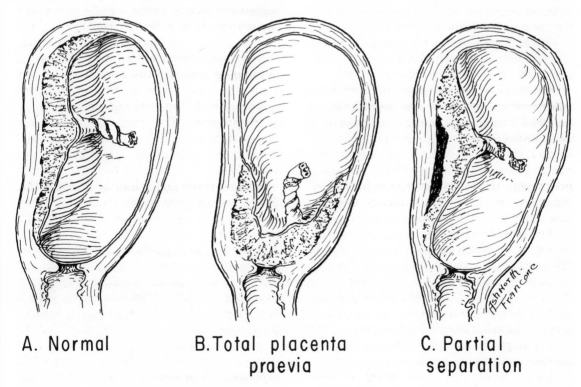

A. Normal　　B. Total placenta praevia　　C. Partial separation

Figure 9-1. (A) Normal implantation of the placenta. (B) The placenta completely covers the cervical os (placenta praevia). (C) Partial separation of the placenta (abruptio placentae).

a puddle of blood. About 50 per cent of patients have more than one episode of vaginal bleeding.

Blood loss may be considerable, and yet the fetal heart tones are good and strong. Since it is sometimes difficult when questioning the patient to get an accurate estimate of how much blood has been lost, the doctor frequently looks at the soles of her feet. If there is blood on them, it is indicative of a substantial blood loss.

Abnormal presentations of the fetus are associated with placenta previa. Presumably there is less room in the lower uterine segment for the fetus's head. X-rays, called placentograms, are used to confirm the diagnosis of low placental attachment.

Treatment. Treatment depends on the type of placenta previa and the condition of the fetus. If the patient is not at full term and if bleeding is minimal, the doctor may adopt a policy of watchful waiting. The patient usually stays in the hospital for a few days on bed rest. If bleeding stops, she is sent home, hopefully to carry the infant to full term. In the case of a low implantation of the placenta, she will most likely be able to deliver vaginally.

When the patient is admitted to the labor room with third trimester bleeding, no vaginal or rectal examinations or enemas should be given. Any of these procedures would be dangerous because they could cause increased bleeding. It may be necessary, however, for the doctor to examine the patient vaginally to determine accurately how much the placenta impinges on or occludes the cervical os. The vaginal examination is done in the delivery room under a "double set-up." This means that the delivery room personnel have set up the room and made preparations to do either a regular vaginal delivery or a cesarean section if the patient starts to bleed profusely. The anesthetist is there, two pints of blood are in readiness, and other necessary equipment is at hand.

When the diagnosis of a total placenta previa is made, the treatment of choice is delivery by cesarean section. However, in the case of a partial placenta previa, the woman can sometimes be delivered vaginally if bleeding is well controlled. This is a fine judgment which is made by the doctor. Although a placenta previa occurs by chance, it is seen more frequently in multiparas. The prognosis is excellent for the mother, but the fetal mortality rate is between 15 and 20 per cent.

Abruptio Placentae

Another cause of bleeding in the third trimester is the premature separation of a *normally* implanted placenta, called abruptio placentae. For some unknown reason the placenta, although implanted in the correct spot, either gradually or suddenly separates from the uterine wall (Fig. 9-1). All of it may detach (complete separation) or part may remain attached (partial separation).

The cause of abruptio placentae is not known, but it is frequently associated with toxemia and hypertension. Physical trauma plays a minor part.

Symptoms. A cardinal symptom of abruptio placentae is pain in the presence of vaginal bleeding. When bleeding occurs behind the placenta, it builds up a great deal of pressure, and the uterus becomes rigid and painful. If the patient is in labor, the uterus feels tense and hard all of the time instead of alternately contracting and relaxing.

Vaginal bleeding may be dark or in the form of clotted blood. Bright red bleeding indicates fresh bleeding, whereas dark blood is old. This is explained by the fact that it takes a longer time for the blood to reach the vaginal introitus than in the case of placenta previa. In some patients there is no vaginal bleeding, but the uterus increases in size. The hemorrhage can be concealed or visible. The patient may be in shock out of proportion to the amount of visible bleeding. Bleeding or clotting abnormalities, such as hypofibrinogenemia, frequently develop.

Fetal heart tones may be present early; but often they become irregular and then disappear entirely, as the fetus dies from lack of oxygen. Also, the fetal outline cannot be felt because of the tenseness of the uterus.

The patient may have albuminuria, oliguria (decrease in urine output), or anuria (absence of urine).

Treatment. The patient is started on intravenous fluids and typed and cross-matched for blood transfusions. If the patient is in shock, whole blood is given rapidly under pressure. Clot observation tests are done, and if necessary fibrinogen may be given to combat the hypofibrinogenemia. The height of the fundus is measured to determine the rate of bleeding.

If the patient is not in labor, the doctor will induce labor by rupturing the membranes, and he may give Pitocin intravenously. Vital signs, fetal heart tones, and urinary output are closely monitored. If the patient does not deliver soon, a cesarean section is done.

Occasionally a Couvelaire uterus develops. The pressure of the blood backs up behind the placenta to such an extent that blood is forced into the walls of the uterus, turning the uterus a deep purple color. Unfortunately, a hysterectomy must be done.

Prognosis. The maternal mortality rate is low, but the fetal mortality is between 30 and 60 per cent owing to hypoxia and prematurity.

Marginal Sinus Bleeding

A marginal sinus is a hollow structure around the periphery of the placenta. If the marginal sinus is torn, bleeding similar to that of placenta previa occurs.

Studies indicate that rupture of the marginal sinus accounts for about one third of the patients who experience bleeding during the third trimester. However, the bleeding is less severe than in placenta previa.

Nursing Care of the Patient with Antepartal Bleeding

These patients are quite a challenge to take care of, and the nurse must learn to "keep her cool" in order to be able to manage an emergency situation smoothly and efficiently. Because the patient is likely to be apprehensive, the calm manner of the nurse will be reassuring to her. The nurse can also reassure the patient in other ways. If the patient's vital signs and the fetal heart tones are good, the nurse can mention this to the patient. She can also keep the husband and relatives informed about the patient's progress and condition (and the baby's) in order to allay their fears.

The patient is *never* given an enema when she is admitted, nor is a rectal or vaginal examination done by the nurse. However, the patient is prepped (shaved) for delivery as usual. Do not give her anything by mouth because of the possibility that surgical intervention and the administration of an anesthesic might be indicated. A record of her intake and output should be kept. Because she will be receiving intravenous fluids and perhaps blood transfusions, and because a low output of urine may be a serious warning sign, accurate recording of intake and output is an important nursing responsibility. An accurate estimate of blood loss also should be made by making a pad count. If the patient bleeds heavily, the hip pads, Chux, and sheets should be saved, if possible, to show to the physician.

The patient should be given good physical care; she should be kept as clean and dry as possible. However, it may be more desirable to keep her quiet so that bleeding is not activated.

If she was not in labor when she came to the hospital, watch for signs of labor such as regular uterine contractions or rupture of the membranes. Labor may be rapid, especially if the patient has a premature separation of the placenta.

Immediately report any change in the patient, such as: (1) increased bleeding; (2) drop in blood pressure (A systolic blood pressure below 90 indicates shock, but if the patient has been hypertensive, she may be in shock with a higher systolic blood pressure reading.); (3) change in the fetal heart tones (Remember, the normal range is 120 to 160 beats per minute. Distress is also related to irregularity of the F.H.T's and meconium in the amnioitic fluid in a vertex presentation.); and (4) severe abdominal pain.

TOXEMIAS OF PREGNANCY

Toxemias of pregnancy occur in gestation or in the early puerperium (48 hours postpartum) and are characterized by hypertension, edema, and proteinuria. They represent one of the most serious complications of pregnancy because they are among the three leading causes of maternal mortality. The plural form of the word is used on purpose as there are different forms of the disease. They usually occur after the twenty-fourth week of pregnancy, except when they are caused by a hydatidiform mole.

The American Committee on Maternal Welfare has classified toxemias into three major categories: acute toxemia, chronic hypertensive vascular disease with pregnancy, and unclassified toxemia. This section will be concerned with acute toxemia because the majority of cases fall into this category.

Acute toxemia is further broken down into two kinds, pre-eclampsia and eclampsia, depending on the severity of the disease.

Pre-eclampsia. A patient who is in the pre-eclamptic stage of the disease has the following signs and symptoms:

If she has *mild* pre-eclampsia, her systolic blood pressure is increased by 30 mm. and her diastolic blood pressure by 15 mm. above the usual level. Thus, if her normal blood pressure is 100/70, she would be considered to have an elevated blood pressure if a reading of 130/85 is obtained. Another distinction is that the blood pressure must be elevated over a six-hour period. This removes the possibility that the patient was just excited when her blood pressure was checked. Another indication of the mild form of the disease is edema of the hands and face. The patient may notice that her face is puffy in the morning and her eyes are

swollen or that her rings are too tight. A third sign is that she has a small amount of albumin in her urine (a trace to 2+) on two successive days.

A sign of severe pre-eclampsia is blood pressure elevated to 160/110 or above when the patient is on bed rest. She also has marked albumin in the urine, spilling about 5 gm. in a 24-hour period. Pitting edema of the ankles of 3+ or 4+ is sometimes seen. (This means that when you press on the edematous skin surface, indentations from your fingers remain afterwards.) Scanty amount of urine, under 400 cc. in 24 hours, is a serious sign. The patient may also complain of headaches, spots in front of her eyes, temporary blindness, and epigastric pain. Thus, the disease can advance to the severe stage by the time the patient notices that anything is wrong.

Eclampsia. The next stage of the disease as it increases in severity is called eclampsia. The distinguishing feature is that the patient has had a convulsion. One of the most frightening aspects of the disease is the rapidness with which the patient may pass from a mild stage of pre-eclampsia to eclampsia. This is particularly true of young primigravidas.

Contributing Factors. Factors besides a first pregnancy and youth contribute to the development of acute toxemia. They are: anxiety, low socioeconomic status, malnutrition, family history of hypertension or toxemia, and excessive or unusual distension of the uterus (as with twins).

Treatment and Nursing Care

In the interest of preventing toxemia it is the nurse's job to urge women to seek early and regular prenatal care, because warning signs of the disease are not always noticeable to the woman herself. If the expectant mother does notice swelling of her feet and ankles on arising in the morning, it should be investigated. She should be taught the symptoms of pre-eclampsia so that she can report them promptly if they occur. It is wise to restrict the salt intake during the last trimester in those pregnant women who are known to be predisposed to toxemia as a result of chronic hypertension, obesity, diabetes, or multiple pregnancy. Weight restriction, too, may be necessary.

Some patients with mild symptoms of pre-eclampsia are treated at home. They should get plenty of rest and may be given a mild sedative such as phenobarbital to calm them. Diuretics are also given to decrease the edema. However, ambulatory treatment is not very successful and is a common reason for failure to forestall convulsions.

When the patient is admitted to the hospital, she is often put on complete bed rest. Medications are ordered to relieve the hypertension, reduce edema, and decrease central nervous system irritability. To maintain the urinary output, fluids are encouraged, up to 2500 to 3000 cc. daily.

A diet low in sodium and sometimes high in protein is given. An increase in protein may be necessary if the patient is losing large amounts in the urine. A low-sodium diet requires that salt be omitted from the diet and that foods high in sodium content be restricted. Beer and carbonated beverages should also be restricted because of their sodium content. Salt substitutes can be used and herbs such as bay leaves or thyme may be added as a flavorful seasoning. A diet high in protein should contain lean meat, an egg, and a quart of milk a day. Low-sodium milk can be substituted and can be made more palatable by adding chocolate, vanilla, or sugar. If the patient is on diuretics such as acetazolamide (Diamox) or chlorothiazide (Diuril), there is always a possibility of potassium depletion. Therefore, a glass of orange juice or citrus fruits should be included in the daily diet to replace this important electrolyte.

The patient is weighed at the same time every morning to see how much edema is being lost and to gauge the effectiveness of medications.

The severe pre-eclamptic patient should be admitted to a private, darkened room with a quiet atmosphere. Bright lights or noise could stimulate a convulsion. A *No Visitors* sign is placed on the door. There is even some question if the patient's husband should be allowed to visit, because his presence could tend to excite her. The nurse could refer him to the doctor for permission.

A pre-eclamptic tray is often taken into the patient's room in case it is needed in a hurry. It contains the following items: padded tongue blades or mouth gags, syringes, sterile water for mixing medicines, a tourniquet, alcohol sponges, and drugs— magnesium sulfate, aminophylline, sodium amytal (amobarbital), caffeine sodium benzoate, nikethamide (Coramine), and calcium gluconate.

Other safety precautions include padded side rails, which are kept up, and a mouth gag taped to the head of the bed. These are to prevent injury if the patient has a convulsion.

A foley catheter is inserted after magnesium sulfate and sedation has been given (this makes the insertion of the catheter less stressful). The foley catheter is used so that the urinary output can be measured with the utmost accuracy.

Imagine for a moment how the woman may feel finding herself alone in a dimly lighted room, with the side rails of her bed up. It must be a very frightening sensation. Remember that a woman with toxemia is going to have a baby; so watch for signs of labor and check the fetal heartbeat. Once labor starts it may progress rapidly. If the patient is unconscious, the nurse may notice that she becomes restless at regular intervals. On palpating the fundus, the nurse will probably observe that uterine contractions correspond to the intervals when the patient is restless! It's also a good idea to check for bloody show.

Medications

The patient will probably be rather heavily sedated at first. Magnesium sulfate is given because it acts as a central nervous system depressant, a vasodilator, and a mild diuretic. Large doses of 50 per cent solution of magnesium sulfate are injected deep within the gluteal muscle, with a special 3-inch needle. Since these shots are quite painful, a small amount of procaine is drawn up into the same syringe, so that the injection doesn't hurt the patient quite so much.

Before administering magnesium sulfate, a doctor should check the patient's knee jerk reflexes. Disappearance of this reflex is associated with high blood levels of the drug which could result in respiratory depression. It is also important to check the patient's respirations; if they are below 16, check with the doctor about giving the drug. The antidote for magnesium sulfate is calcium gluconate 10 per cent (or some form of calcium). Check and make sure it is on hand.

Blood pressure should be checked frequently when any antihypertensive drug is administered. If the patient has a convulsion, the nursing care and observations are the same as for a child with epilepsy or a febrile condition.

Preparation for Labor

Once the baby is delivered, the patient often makes a rapid recovery. However, preparation for labor is usually not begun until toxemia is under control.

The nurse should be careful not to give the patient too much information at one time. Her goal is to give realistic information without frightening the patient. Examples are: how to pant and push, information about contractions, what induction is and why it is done, and what procedures to expect (see Chapter 10).

Postdelivery

Observe the patient closely for convulsions in the first 24 hours. Severe preeclampsia predisposes the patient to another complication, postpartum hemorrhage, so be on the alert.

One of the main goals of nursing care is to insure rest. Keep the patient as calm and relaxed as possible. Sedation may be given three times a day and again at bed time to promote rest and sleep.

Follow-up care is very important. The mother should be encouraged to report for her postpartum checkup so that blood studies and kidney function tests may be done to make sure there is no permanent damage.

For her own safety, it is best that she postpone her next pregnancy for at least a year. She can be taught about contraception before she is discharged, or she can be referred to a family planning clinic or private doctor.

COMMON VAGINAL INFECTIONS

Pregnant women are more susceptible to vaginal infections because of the altered pH of the vagina and the increased amount of glycogen in the vaginal tissues. Although there is normally an increased amount of white mucoid secretion called leukorrhea from the vagina during pregnancy, if the discharge becomes cream-colored or yellow and causes itching around the vulva, it should be investigated. The two most common infections are *Trichomonas vaginalis* and *Candida albicans*.

Trichomonas

Trichomonas vaginalis is found in 20 to 30 per cent of women during antepartal exams. The symptoms are annoying and consist of a bubbly leukorrhea which is cream-colored or yellow and causes irritation and itching of the vulva and vaginal opening. The causative organism is a tiny parasitic animal called a trichomonad.

Trichomonas is not a venereal disease. However, it may be harbored by the male and transmitted to the female during sexual intercourse. The diagnosis is quick and easy to make. A hanging drop slide is prepared from the vaginal secretions, and the parasite can be seen under a microscope. Occasionally cultures are done to make the diagnosis.

Oral medications such as Flagyl have completely changed the outlook of this distressing condition. The patient takes the drug for 10 days, during which time it is carried in the bloodstream to areas that are not accessible to drugs applied topically. In addition, douches may be prescribed which promote the return of the vagina to its normal acidity. (Refer to the procedure on vaginal douching during pregnancy on page 104). If the source of infection is the male partner, he can also be treated with oral tablets.

Candida Albicans

Sometimes referred to as a monilia or yeast infection, candidiasis is quite common among women at term because of the increased glycogen in the vagina during pregnancy. The symptoms are a cheesy white vaginal discharge which may be very irritating. Sometimes there is edema of the external genitalia (quite extensive in some women). The diagnosis is made by stained smears or cultures. A new oral antibiotic called nystatin has been effective in curing it. If vaginal applications of the drug in cream form is prescribed, it is important to carry out the treatment for the length of time recommended, otherwise the condition may recur.

It usually subsides at the conclusion of gestation. However, if the mother has a monilia infection at the time of delivery, the baby can pick it up as he passes through the birth canal. This is the usual way for a newborn baby to pick up thrush, a monilia infection of the mouth.

HYPEREMESIS GRAVIDARUM

During the early months of pregnancy, about half the women experience some nausea and vomiting, the so-called morning sickness which is mild and transient, disappearing usually by the second trimester. In hyperemesis gravidarum, excessive vomiting of pregnancy, the woman vomits most if not all of her oral intake throughout gestation, which can lead to severe consequences of starvation and dehydration if untreated. It is uncommon today for mild

nausea and vomiting to progress to the extent that it produces systemic effects such as marked weight loss and acidosis. Complaints of nausea and vomiting should not be regarded casually because a mild case can progress into this serious complication if not treated with understanding and judgment. The patient who has hyperemesis should be admitted to the hospital for intensive treatment and nursing care. Symptoms severe enough to warrant hospitalization occur with a frequency of less than one in 300 and recovery is usually prompt.

Causes. Although the etiology is not definitely known, there are two possible theories that explain its cause. One is related to the tremendous physiological changes which occur in pregnancy—the increased hormonal production, the metabolic changes, and the decrease in the motility of the stomach.

The other theory claims that a neurotic factor produces the excessive vomiting. Because pregnancy is a crisis period in a young woman's life, it is understandable that she may be emotionally upset. In the early part of gestation, she may be uncertain about whether she is pregnant; her thoughts may go back to early childhood fears about being pregnant or becoming a mother. She might also be concerned about the changes which the responsibility of a child might have on her life and her relationship with her husband. Any person who is experiencing emotional tensions or upheavals may react by becoming nauseated, since the stomach is very sensitive to human emotions. Unpleasant sights and repellent odor, real or remembered, may trigger the response of nausea and vomiting.

Signs and Symptoms. "Morning sickness" in early pregnancy persists for four to eight weeks or longer. The woman vomits several times a day and is unable to retain any liquid or solid foods. If this continues, symptoms of dehydration and starvation appear. When dehydration is present, the patient's skin is dry and there is a decreased output of urine. Rapid pulse rate and a mild fever may be present. The patient may show symptoms of starvation by a weight loss varying from five to as much as 20 to 30 pounds.

The body has been forced to burn its reserve stores of fat to maintain body heat and energy. As a result some of the incompletely burned products of fat metabolism are found in the urine and bloodstream of the patient. This is why acetone is frequently found in the urine of patients who are vomiting excessively during pregnancy. Besides other evidence of fluid and electrolyte imbalance, vitamin starvation, particularly of vitamin B, is regularly present.

Treatment and Nursing Care

The principles of treatment are to (1) combat the dehydration through the administration of intravenous fluids; (2) combat the starvation with intravenous glucose and thiamine chloride injections, (In some cases, nasogastric tube feedings of a high vitamin liquid diet are instituted.); and (3) to combat the neurotic factor by isolating the woman from the family members and her husband, removing her to a different environment, and giving her psychotherapy, if indicated.

During the first 24 hours of hospitalization, it is customary to withhold food and fluid by mouth in order to give the patient's stomach as complete a rest as possible. Intravenous fluids, usually 10 per cent glucose solution, is given up to 3000 cc. or more in 24 hours. A very careful record of the patient's intake and output is kept, as well as the quantity of vomitus. Usually, the patient is allowed no visitors, and even phone calls are discouraged. The patient is kept sedated with injections of sodium luminal, 1 to 2 gr. every four hours.

After 24 hours, the patient may receive small frequent feedings of dry toast or crackers every two to three hours. These are alternated with small amounts of fluids (not over 100 cc. at a time); hot tea, ginger ale, or lemon soda may be tolerated. If the patient shows improvement, her food intake may be

gradually increased so that she is on a soft, high-calorie diet. Foods should be served in an attractive and appealing way; hot foods should be served steaming hot, and cold foods, icy cold. The emesis basin, or anything that could suggest vomiting to the patient, should be out of sight. When the patient's fluid intake is good, intravenous fluids are discontinued.

Usually, the patient shows rapid improvement on such a regime, but if she does continue to vomit, tube feeding may be indicated. A Levin tube is often used for the tube feeding, and large amounts of high-calorie, high-vitamin food may be given via the stomach tube. The liquid should be administered slowly at about 50 drops per minute. The secret of success lies in the slow but constant introduction of food into the stomach.

The nurse's attitude toward the patient is also very important. She should have a positive attitude that the patient will succeed in conquering this complication. Letting the patient know that there are "no failures" in this treatment may help the patient psychologically. Be an understanding and sympathetic listener. Allowing the patient to talk about fears associated with pregnancy, financial problems, or marital problems may be therapeutic.

The intravenous feedings, isolation, tube feedings, and injections which comprise the treatment may induce the patient psychologically to make a rapid recovery. In any event, most of them do.

TUBERCULOSIS

All pregnant women should be given skin tests for tuberculosis and subsequent chest x-rays if they have a positive reaction. Newly discovered tuberculosis may be treated by drugs such as streptomycin, isoniazid, and PAS (para-aminosalicylic acid) without special hazard to the mother or fetus. Termination of the pregnancy because of tuberculosis is rarely necessary or helpful, although steps may be taken to avoid prolonged labor. Once the baby is born, the infant should be removed from contact with the mother if she is still bacteriologically positive. A woman may be allowed to become pregnant after the disease has been inactive for two years, but she should be examined regularly for possible reactivation before becoming pregnant, then during the second trimester, and again after pregnancy.

Nursing Care

Long-term planning is essential for the adequate rest and supervision of a mother who has tuberculosis. Arrangements must be made in advance for the care of the baby, as the mother will not be able to care for it until the disease is arrested.

During labor, the woman will likely have a low forceps delivery to shorten the second stage of labor. Excessive sedation and inhalation anesthesia are to be avoided because they might suppress the cough reflex. Good emotional support and the use of comfort measures by the nurse will cut down on the need for analgesics and anesthetics.

After delivery, the nurse should promote drainage of lung secretions to prevent them from accumulating in the bronchi. Because there is a danger that the baby will become infected and because of the added physical strain, the mother will not be able to breast feed or care for the baby. Both the mother and baby may suffer emotionally from this deprivation.

HEART DISEASE

The two most common cardiac complications of pregnancy are damage to the mitral valve from rheumatic heart disease and congenital heart disease. The patient should be closely supervised throughout her pregnancy by both her cardiologist and obstetrician. Because pregnancy imposes an added work load on the heart, which is already damaged, the patient needs to be careful and use good judgment not to become overtired. The chances of heart failure are usually greatest during (1) the last trimester of pregnancy, when there is an increase in the volume of blood circulated, and (2) during labor and delivery.

Rest is probably the most important aspect of prenatal care. The expectant mother should avoid strenuous activities and great excitement, and she should protect herself from infections as much as possible.

The nurse, as well as the woman, should know the signs and symptoms of heart failure: increased dyspnea, tachycardia, and cough or a smothering sensation when coughing. During labor and delivery, the mother should be in a semiupright position or elevated on pillows, so that she can breathe more easily. She may be given oxygen, and she should avoid the exertion of pushing during the second stage of labor. A low forceps delivery will probably be done.

In the postpartal period, the danger of heart failure is greatly reduced. The nurse may be able to suggest ways by which the mother can conserve her energies when she goes home, — such as organizing her housework or using labor-saving devices.

DIABETES MELLITUS

This is a disease which affects both the mother and the infant. Until recent years, infertility was a major problem for these women because they had difficulty in becoming pregnant. Now that diabetes is so well controlled by diet and medications, more of these women are having babies. However, there is a sizeable group of women in whom diabetes only becomes evident when they are pregnant; these are so-called gestational diabetics.

What effect does pregnancy have on diabetes mellitus? Pregnancy increases the severity of diabetes throughout gestation. Apparently, there is an insulin antagonism, perhaps by the placenta, which raises the insulin requirement to as high as four times the amount needed when the woman is not pregnant. Thus, the insulin requirements can fluctuate a great deal during pregnancy. The woman is more likely to become hyperglycemic as pregnancy advances, and diabetic acidosis may ensue. In this event there is increased danger to the fetus. Also, complications due to toxemia and hydramnios are more frequent.

What effect does diabetes mellitus have on the pregnancy? Diabetes affects the cardiovascular system by producing premature arteriosclerosis; it has a similar effect on the blood vessels of the placenta: it creates placental insufficiency which causes the placenta to age prematurely. It has become a common practice to deliver the baby at around 37 weeks gestation because there is increased danger of the baby dying after that time. The woman will come to the hospital to have labor induced, and if induction is not successful, a cesarean section is done. When the mother has diabetes, there is an increased incidence of congenital malformations of the fetus and a higher number of spontaneous abortions and miscarriages.

Because babies tend to be large, there is a greater incidence of mechanical difficulties in labor and delivery. Also, there are more frequent birth injuries and, as stated earlier, a higher proportion of cesarean sections.

If the mother's diabetes is well controlled and if she follows the basic principles of good prenatal care, there is no reason why she cannot go through pregnancy very successfully and have a healthy baby. Many of the complications such as toxemia, hydramnios, and even a large baby may be lessened or eliminated if the woman takes good care of herself. Throughout her pregnancy the woman should be under the care of both a specialist in internal medicine to manage her diabetes and an obstetrician. And she should be seen more frequently, usually every two weeks. (See Chapter 40 for a discussion of the infant of a diabetic mother.)

BIBLIOGRAPHY

Abortion. Amer. J. Nurs., 70:1919, 1970.
Cianfrani, T., and Conway, M. K.: Ectopic pregnancy. Amer. J. Nurs., 63:93, 1964.
Donnelly, J.: Toxemias of pregnancy. Amer. J. Nurs., 61:98, 1961.
Hellman, L., and Pritchard, J.: Williams' Obstetrics, ed. 14. New York, Appleton-Century-Crofts, 1971.
Hogue, C., and Couch, K.: Care of the patient with toxemia. Amer. J. Nurs., 61:101, 1961.
Rodman, M., and Smith, D.: Pharmacology and Drug Therapy in Nursing. Philadelphia, J. B. Lippincott, 1968.
Slatin, M.: Extra-protection for high-risk mothers and babies. Amer. J. Nurs., 67:1241, June, 1967.
Willson, J.: Management of Obstetric Difficulties. ed. 6. St. Louis, C. V. Mosby, 1961.
Ziegel, E., and VanBlarcom, C.: Obstetric Nursing, ed. 5. New York, Macmillan, 1964.

Suggested Readings for Further Study

Garnet, J.: Pregnancy in women with diabetes. Amer. J. Nurs., 69:1900, 1969.
Hershey, N.: Abortion and sterilization. Status of the law in mid-1970. Amer. J. Nurs., 70:1926, 1970.

UNIT STUDY QUESTIONS

1. The morula or "mulberry mass" is:
   a. a small solid mass of cells.
   b. two layers of cells, the inner mass or formative cells and the outer layer or trophoblast.
   c. three layers of cells, the ectoderm, the endoderm, and the mesoderm.
   d. none of the above.

2. An expectant father can be most helpful to his wife during pregnancy by:
   a. supervising her diet and activities.
   b. protecting her from responsibility and problems.
   c. keeping her so busy she won't become too introspective.
   d. accepting the fact that her attention has been temporarily withdrawn from him.

3. The pregnant woman may be faced with conflicting emotions concerning her pregnancy. The nurse may be helpful by:
   1. being a good listener.
   2. giving factual information with adequate explanation.

3. working closely with the physician and knowing what his instructions have been.
4. recognizing her own limitations and referring the patient to the correct sources for help if she honestly doesn't know or isn't sure of the correct answer.
   a. 1, 2 and 3
   b. 1, 3 and 4
   c. 1, 2, and 4
   (d.) All of the above
   e. None of the above

4. The hormone responsible for a positive pregnancy test is?
   a. luteotrophin.
   (b.) chorionic gonadotropin.
   c. estrogen.
   d. progesterone.

5. Although the exact date of delivery for an expectant mother cannot be predetermined, if her last menstrual period began on March 8, when would you estimate her due date to be?
   a. November 15.
   b. December 1.
   (c.) December 15.
   d. December 28.

6. In talking with an expectant mother you would advise her to keep her appointments with the doctor so that he would be able to:
   a. check her for signs of abnormalities.
   b. check on the growth of the baby.
   c. teach her the danger signs.
   (d.) help her to maintain a state of good health.

7. The placenta is formed by the end of the:
   a. first month of gestation.
   (b.) third month of gestation.
   c. fifth month of gestation.
   d. seventh month of gestation.

8. In which position would you place a woman in order to measure most pelvic diameters?

a. Dorsal recumbent
b. Sims'
c. Trendelenberg
(d.) Lithotomy
e. Knee-chest

9. Local changes which occur as a result of pregnancy are:
1. The cervix, vagina, and vulva become softer and more elastic.
2. There is an increase in the vascularity of the cervix, vagina, and vulva.
3. There is a softening of the lower uterine segment.
4. The corpus luteum of pregnancy is present in one ovary.
   a. 1, 2, and 3
   b. 1, 2, and 4
   c. 2, 3, and 4
   (d.) All of the above

10. If a patient in the antepartal clinic complains of a sudden pain in the calf of her leg as she lies on the examining table, which of the following would nurse do?
    a. Massage the muscle
    b. Check for round garters and remove them immediately if she is wearing them
    (c.) Use one hand to force the toes upward, dorsiflexing the foot, while the other presses the knee downward to extend the leg
    d. Notify the doctor immediately

11. The hormone responsible for the development of the secondary sexual characteristics in the female is:
    a. progesterone
    (b.) estrogen
    c. luteinizing hormone
    d. follicle-stimulating hormone

12. Milk is produced in the:
    a. tubercle of Montgomery
    b. lactiferous sinus
    (c.) acini
    d. areola

13. An abortion in which the fetus has been

expelled and the placenta retained is typical of:
- a. an incomplete abortion
- b. a missed abortion
- c. an inevitable abortion
- d. a threatened abortion

14. Mrs. Erickson is in her early twenties. She comes to the prenatal clinic after having missed two menstrual periods, and states this is her first pregnancy. The best way for the nurse to establish rapport with Mrs. Erickson initially, is to:
- a. introduce her to the other patients.
- b. ask her if she has any questions.
- c. ask her how she feels about pregnancy.
- d. explain to her what will take place during the clinic visit.

15. Which of the following functions are present in the normal fetus before birth?
1. respiratory movements
2. swallowing
3. urination
4. thumb sucking
- a. 1, 2, 4
- b. 2, 3, 4
- c. all of the above
- d. none of the above

16. The most common cause of spontaneous abortion is:
- a. inherent defects in the products of conception.
- b. German measles
- c. severe acute infections
- d. endocrine dysfunction.

17. A serology is a test for:
- a. syphilis
- b. gonorrhea
- c. blood type
- d. Rh factor

18. The region between the vaginal orifice and the anus is called the:
- a. clitoris
- b. vestibule
- c. peritoneum
- d. perineum

19. As a nurse you should be aware of the cardinal signs of toxemia in order to help plan your nursing care. They are:
- a. weight gain, headache and proteinuria
- b. edema, hypertension, and proteinuria
- c. cerebral edema, oliguria, and diplopia
- d. excessive weight gain, edema and convulsions
- e. hypertension, oliguria, and vomiting

20. The nurse staying with an eclamptic patient notes that she is having periods of restlessness that seem to occur at regular intervals. The nurse should suspect that the restlessness:
- a. indicates an impending convulsion
- b. indicates a need for additional sedation
- c. has no significance
- d. indicates possible uterine contractions

21. A patient who is threatening abortion is given progesterone to:
- a. help thicken the decidua
- b. maintain blood pressure levels
- c. stop uterine bleeding
- d. produce muscular relaxation

22. A low roughage soft diet probably will be ordered for a patient who is threatening abortion:
- a. to prevent constipation
- b. to promote peristalsis
- c. to prevent straining at stool
- d. because she would be inactive for 2 or 3 days

23. Instructions to a patient who has just had an hydatidiform mole should include reliable contraceptive advice because:
- a. another pregnancy is contraindi-

cated until the possibility of choriocarcinoma has been ruled out.
  b. new pregnancy would cause a rise
in gonadotropin levels.
  c. new pregnancy might lead to er-
roneous suspicion of choriocarcinoma.
  d. all of the above.

24. Encircling an incompetent cervix, during pregnancy, with a Dacron "gauze"
strip is a method of treatment that was
introduced by:

a. Shirodkar.
b. Lash.
c. Scanzoni.
d. Lamaze.

25. The first sign of excessive blood levels of
magnesium sulfate is:
  a. disappearance of the knee jerk
reflex
  b. cardiac arrhythmias
  c. respiratory depression
  d. ringing in the ears

The Labor Experience   *10*

TERMINOLOGY

The following terms are often used in describing pregnancy, labor, and delivery. Although many of them have been used throughout the preceding chapters, they are included here for quick, easy reference. Some of these terms are used rather loosely and may have slightly different meanings in various settings where obstetrical care is given. The suffixes -*gravida* and -*para* are terms often used to describe the total number of pregnancies and previous pregnancies carried to viability.

Gravida: any pregnant woman; also refers to the number of pregnancies regardless of their duration.

Primigravida: a woman who is pregnant for the first time

Primipara: a woman who has delivered one viable child

Para: refers to past pregnancies that have gone to the period of viability

Multipara: a woman who has had two or more children.

Intrapartal: occurring at any time during labor and delivery

Labor: series of processes by which the mature, or almost mature, products of conception are expelled from the mother's body

Parturient: bringing forth; pertaining to childbearing; a woman in childbirth.

Engagement: passage of the largest diameter of the presenting part of the fetus into the pelvic brim

Dilation or dilatation: enlargement of the external cervical os from a few millimeters to an opening large enough to allow the passage of the fetus

Effacement: shortening of the cervical canal which is 1 to 2 cm. long to a circular opening with almost paper-thin edges

Crowning: when the largest diameter of the presenting part is encircled by the vulvar ring

Station: the numerical determination of the degree of descent of the presenting part of the fetus in relation to the ischial spines of the mother. If the presenting part is above the spines it is a −3 cm., −2 cm., −1 cm. station. When it is at the level of the spines it is called 0 station. As it descends past (below) the spines in coming through the birth canal it is +1 cm., +2 cm., +3 cm. (At +3 cm. the baby is being born.)

Attitude: the relationship between the fetal parts. The most common attitude is complete flexion in which the fetus's chin touches its chest, its arms are folded across its chest, and its legs are flexed on the abdomen. The fetus occupies the smallest possible space and conforms to the shape of the uterus. If the neck is extended, then the baby is said to have a "military" attitude.

Lie: relation of the long axis (spine) of the mother to the long axis of the fetus. This is either longitudinal or transverse. The fetus cannot be delivered vaginally in a transverse lie.

Position: relationship between a specific yet arbitrary point on the presenting part (of the fetus) to the four quadrants of the maternal pelvis. The specific yet arbitrary points on the fetus are vertex (occiput), face or chin (mentum), breech (sacrum), and shoulder (scapula). The four quadrants of the mother's pelvis are the right and left sides and the anterior and posterior portions of the pelvis. Thus, if the back of the fetus's head (*occiput*) lies in the *left* side of the *anterior* part of the mother's pelvis, the fetus is in the left occiput anterior or LOA position, the most common position for the fetus to be in. Similarly, ROA (right occiput anterior) means that the back of the fetus's head (*occiput)* lies in the *right* side of *anterior* part of the mother's pelvis; LSP (left sacrum posterior) designates that the sacrum of the fetus lies in the *left* side of the *posterior* part of the mother's pelvis; and LMA (left mentum anterior) indicates that the chin (*mentum)* of the fetus lies in the *left* side and *anterior* part of the mother's pelvis.

Presentation or presenting part: that part of the fetus's body which lies nearest to the internal os. Thus we speak of a vertex (head) presentation, or a foot or brow presentation. It is that portion felt first when the examining fingers are introduced into the cervix.

WHAT CAUSES THE ONSET OF LABOR?

Labor generally begins when the fetus is mature enough to cope with extrauterine conditions but not yet large enough to cause mechanical difficulties in labor. The cause of the onset of labor is not known. It seems strange that in this age of scientific advancement the reason why labor begins is still undetermined. However, there have been theories advanced to explain this phenomenon.

One can speculate that a combination of factors may be responsible. The following are some theories which seem highly plausible.

Progesterone Deprivation Theory. There is a balance during pregnancy between the stimulating effect of estrogen on the uterus and the relaxing effect of progesterone on the uterus. The belief is that the level of progesterone drops, and labor begins. However, there is no proof, because studies do not show a decrease in blood levels of progesterone at term.

Oxytocin Theory. Supporters of this theory believe that higher blood levels of oxytocin hormone initiate labor by increasing the sensitivity of the uterus to the hormone's stimulating effect. Oxytocin is used to induce labor but is only successful under certain conditions.

This theory fails to explain the *cause* of the increased sensitivity of the uterus to the hormone. Moreover, experimental animals have normal labors when the area of the brain which produces oxytocin is removed:

Uterine Stretch Theory. Any hollow organ such as the bladder or bowel tends to contract and empty itself when distended to a certain point. The myometrium of the uterus reacts to stretch in exactly the same manner, that is, with increased irritability.

It may be due to the growth of the fetus alone; or it may be that pressure on the placental site with the decrease of blood flowing through the placenta is also a factor. In support of the uterine stretch theory it might be noted that a woman who is carrying twins generally delivers earlier than a woman carrying a single fetus.

Placental Degeneration Theory. Near the eighth lunar month, thrombosis begins to take place in many of the venous sinuses of the placenta. Because of the impaired circulation, the placenta becomes senile and incapable of providing the fetus with sufficient nourishment. Advocates of this theory, which dates back to the time of Hippocrates, believe that pregnancy terminates as a result of these changes in the placenta.

PHYSIOLOGY OF LABOR
Duration

There is some degree of variation in the duration of labor. The average duration of first labor is 12 to 18 hours. If the labor lasts

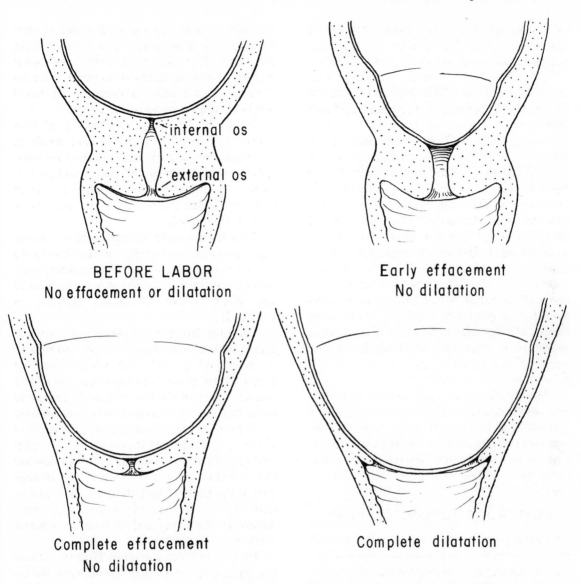

internal os

external os

BEFORE LABOR
No effacement or dilatation

Early effacement
No dilatation

Complete effacement
No dilatation

Complete dilatation

Figure 10-1. There are several stages in cervical effacement and dilatation.

14 hours, then the first stage lasts about 12½ hours, the second stage, 1 hour and 20 minutes, and the third stage, 10 minutes.

The average duration of multiparous labors is approximately 6 hours shorter than first labors. That is, 7 hours and 20 minutes in the first stage, 30 minutes in the second, and 10 minutes in the third. If the patient has been in active labor for 20 to 24 hours, the physician should be notified.

Stages of Labor

There are three stages of labor. The first stage of labor, the dilating stage, begins with the first true contraction and ends with complete dilatation of the cervix.

The second stage, the stage of expulsion, begins with complete dilatation of the cervix and ends with delivery of the baby.

The third stage, the placental stage, begins with delivery of the baby and ends with the birth of the placenta.

The First Stage of Labor

The dilatation of the cervix is brought about by a combination of physical, physiological, and mechanical factors (Fig. 10-1). The process starts with the contractions of the uterus. There is a difference in the contractility of various parts of the uterus. Ordinarily, the top section contracts most strongly, the midportion contracts with intermediate intensity, and the lower section hardly contracts at all.

There is a change in the character of the uterus too. During labor it is divided into two distinct parts: an active upper part made up of the fundus and body and a passive lower part made up of the isthmus (lower uterine segment) and cervix. A physiologic retraction ring separates the actively contracting fundus from the relatively passive lower uterine segment.

There is retraction of the musculature of the upper segment of the uterus following a contraction. Instead of returning to their original length when the fundus relaxes, the muscles remain fixed at a shorter length. As a result of the retraction the size of the uterine cavity decreases. The upper uterine segment becomes progressively thicker. In compensation for this, there is an increased relaxation and lengthening of the muscle fibers in the lower uterine segment. This causes the walls to become thinner and the area to become larger. It enables more of the uterine contents (the fetus and amniotic fluid) to fill it.

The uterus pulls forward with each contraction, causing the long axis of the fetus to be aligned with the long axis of the birth canal. The contractions of the round ligaments, which are extensions of the uterine muscle fibers, augment this alignment. The uterus lengthens and narrows with each contraction. This results in the fetus's spinal column being straightened out. Thus the presenting part is forced deeper into the mother's pelvis. At the same time the longi-

tudinal muscle fibers of the uterus are pulled taut. This causes the lower uterine segment of the uterus and cervix to be pulled up over the presenting part.

Contractions exert pressure on the bag of waters. Membranes bulge into the cervix in a pouchlike fashion, resulting in dilatation in the manner of a wedge. If the membranes are ruptured, the pressure of the presenting part has a comparable effect.

The Second Stage of Labor

The contractions of the uterus are aided by strong sustained contractions of the abdominal muscles which are under voluntary control. The mother participates actively by bearing down and pushing with each contraction.

The baby begins to leave the uterus and starts its descent into the birth canal. The upper uterine segment increases greatly in thickness and forces the presenting part through the fully dilated cervix with each contraction. When the head finally rests on the mother's perineum, less than half of the baby is in the upper segment of the uterus.

The mother's desire to push with each contraction is increasingly compelling, and her pushing efforts must be coordinated with contractions to be effective.

The head comes into view at the vaginal introitus (opening). As the head becomes more and more visible, the posterior portion of the pelvic floor is pushed downward and forward. The muscles are subjected to tremendous stretching, and finally the pelvic floor is converted into a thin-walled tubular structure through which the baby passes as it is born.

The vaginal opening, as well as the cervix, will dilate. Many doctors wish to spare the patient the extra time in labor required for the vaginal opening to fully dilate. They prefer to cut the vaginal opening before it fully dilates to expedite delivery.

The Third Stage of Labor

As soon as delivery is complete the uterus becomes a solid mass of muscle, with

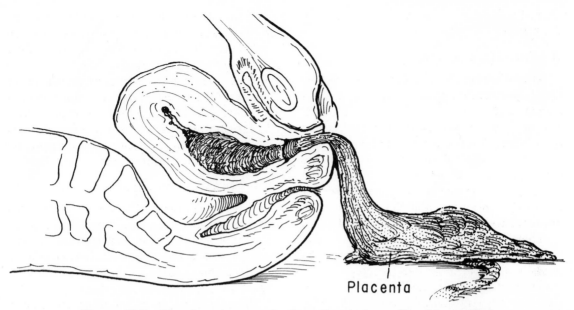

Figure 10-2. The placenta separates from the uterine wall and is expelled.

the fundus lying just below the umbilicus. Because the uterus is diminished in size, there is a correspondingly decrease in the size of the placental site. The placenta thickens to accommodate itself to the smaller area. Its elasticity is minimal, and it buckles on itself. The resulting tension causes the spongy layer of the lining of the uterus to give way, and the placenta separates from the uterine wall.

Pressure is exerted by the uterine walls, causing the placenta to slide down into the lower uterine segment or upper part of the vagina (Fig. 10-2). The mother may be able to push it out, but because she is lying on her back manual pressure from an attendant is usually necessary.

The placenta is expelled by one of two mechanisms (methods): the Schultz method or the Duncan method.

The *Schultz method* is the most common method of delivery. The placenta slips into the vagina through a hole in the amniotic sac. The smooth fetal surface appears first at the vulva with the membranes trailing behind. Blood from the placental site pours into the inverted sac, so usually none escapes until after the placenta is expelled.

In the Duncan method the placenta slides down the uterine wall sideways and the rough maternal surface appears first. This method is accompanied by a continuous trickle of blood because bleeding occurred between the membranes and the uterine wall as soon as the placenta started to separate. This is called a *retroplacental* hemorrhage.

MECHANISMS OF LABOR

By mechanisms of labor is meant the adaptation of the smallest diameters of the baby's presenting part to the irregular shape of the pelvis. The movements occur in sequence.

The exact mechanism of a particular labor depends on the position of the presenting part as it enters the pelvic inlet. Thus labor in a breech presentation would differ from labor in a vertex presentation. Vertex presentations are most common and will be the kind discussed here.

In thinking about the mechanisms of labor you have to use your imagination to picture the movements of the fetus as it adapts to the irregularities of the mother's bony pelvis.

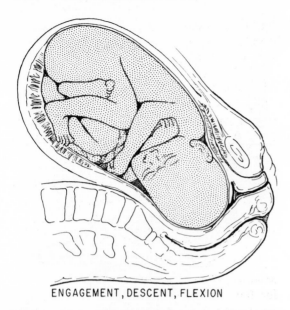

ENGAGEMENT, DESCENT, FLEXION

Figure 10-3. The first mechanisms of labor following engagement are descent and flexion.

Descent. The first mechanism is called descent. Descent first occurs when engagement takes place (Fig. 10-3). It is said to be continuous, but it really only occurs with contractions. During relaxation, the pre-

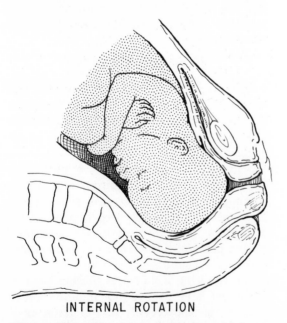

INTERNAL ROTATION

Figure 10-4. The third mechanism of labor is internal rotation.

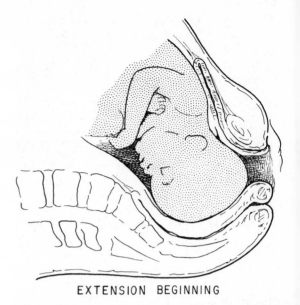

EXTENSION BEGINNING

Figure 10-5. The fourth mechanism of labor is extension during which the occiput passes out of the pelvis.

senting part recedes. There are two reasons for this: (1) it relieves pressure on the mother's soft parts and (2) it restores circulation to the fetus temporarily cut off by contractions. When the vertex is the presenting part, it usually enters the pelvis in the transverse position.

Flexion. The second mechanism is flexion. This means that the fetus's chin rests on its sternum. It is caused by the head encountering resistance. The reason that flexion is so important is that the narrowest diameter of the head must present at the pelvic outlet. This mechanism may take place at the brim of the pelvis or it may not occur until the head reaches the pelvic floor.

Internal Rotation. The third step is internal rotation whereby the occiput rotates 45 degrees to the left and lies beneath the symphysis pubis (Fig. 10-4). This involves twisting the neck.

Extension. Next is extension in which the occiput passes out of the pelvis and is arrested (stopped) under the pubic arch (Fig. 10-5). The head is born during extension (Fig. 10-6).

Restitution. As soon as the head passes

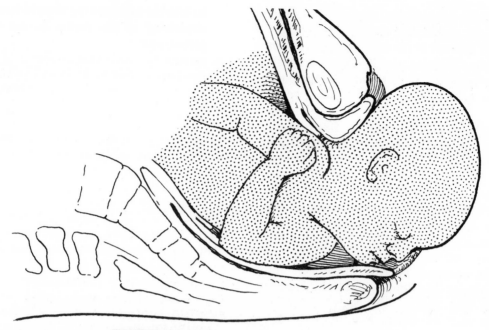

EXTENSION COMPLETE

Figure 10-6. The head is delivered during extension.

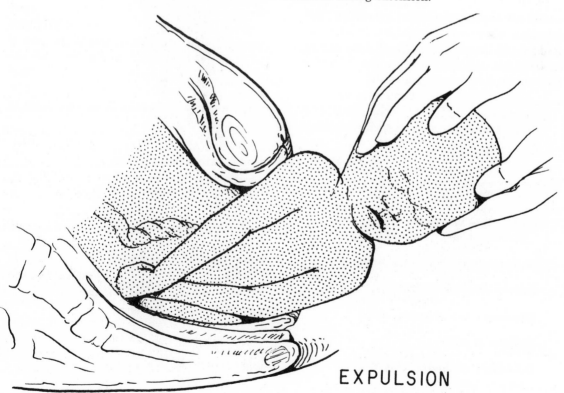

EXPULSION

Figure 10-7. The last mechanism of labor is external rotation and expulsion.

through the vulvovaginal ring, the neck untwists and restitution occurs. The occiput turns 45 degrees to the original position. In observing a delivery you can tell what position the baby was in in utero from the position the baby's head turns to during restitution.

External Rotation and Expulsion. Finally, external rotation and expulsion occur (Fig. 10-7). As the anterior shoulder meets resistance of the pelvic floor, the shoulders are brought into the anteroposterior diameter of the outlet and cause the head to rotate 45 degrees more to the left, in what is known as external rotation. For the birth of the shoulders, the anterior shoulder emerges under the pubic arch, and the posterior shoulder is born by lateral flexion. The rest of the body, which is smaller than the head, then follows in the final step called expulsion.

PAIN IN LABOR

Of all the physiological muscular contractions of the body, only those of labor are painful. Although the cause of pain during labor is not definitely known, the following hypotheses have been suggested:

1. anoxia of compressed muscle cells
2. compression of the nerve ganglia in the cervix and lower uterine segment

by tightly interlocking muscle bundles
3. stretching of the cervix during dilatation, and
4. stretching and displacement of the peritoneum due to direct pull and shifting of the underlying muscle fibers.

SIGNS AND SYMPTOMS OF LABOR

During the last few weeks of pregnancy a number of changes indicate that the time of labor is approaching. One of them, lightening, has already been discussed (see p. 100). The relief brought by lightening may be followed by such signs of pressure as shooting pains down the legs, increase in the amount of vaginal discharge, and greater frequency of urination.

The woman may also experience "false labor" three to four weeks before she actually goes into true labor. Table 10-1 compares the difference between false and true labor. The contractions which occur in false labor are merely an exaggeration of the Braxton-Hicks contractions which have occurred all along. They occur at irregular intervals, are confined to the lower part of the abdomen and groin, and do not increase in intensity, frequency, or duration. They do not effect cervical effacement and dilatation as true labor will. Also, they may be relieved by walking.

Table 10-1. COMPARISON OF TRUE AND FALSE LABOR

True Labor	False Labor
Contractions are regular and increase in strength, duration, and frequency.	Contractions are irregular. No increase in frequency, strength, or duration.
Is progressive and has a pattern	No pattern and no progression.
Activity—increases labor	Activity—produces no change.
Effacement and dilatation occur	No dilatation, some effacement.
Evidence of show	No show
Discomfort of radiating pain from back to front	Discomfort centered in abdomen.
Medications have no effect.	Will stop with medication

In true labor, on the other hand, the contractions are usually felt in the lower back and extend in girdlelike fashion from the back to the front of the abdomen. They have a definite rhythm and gradually increase in frequency, intensity, and duration. In the course of a few hours, progressive effacement and dilatation of the cervix becomes apparent.

In general, primigravidas are advised to go to the hospital when their contractions are regular and five minutes apart. Multiparas should go when their contractions are regular and about ten minutes apart. The nurse can assure the prospective parents that it is no disgrace to come to the hospital in false labor and be sent home. It is better to be safe in coming to the hospital to be checked, because it could be the real thing!

Another sign of labor is a pink discharge. After the mucous plug is dislodged from the cervix, the pressure of the descending presenting part of the fetus (usually the head) causes the minute capillaries in the mucous membrane of the cervix to rupture. Thus, it is only a small amount of blood-tinged mucus which appears. However, any substantial discharge should be reported to the doctor. Some authorities feel that this is one of the least reliable signs of impending labor because the mucous plug can be dislodged when the woman is being examined vaginally or rectally during one of her antepartal visits.

Occasionally rupture of the membranes is the first indication of approaching labor. It used to be thought that this was a grave sign, heralding a long and difficult labor, possibly ending in a "dry" birth. However, present statistics show that this is not true. Because amniotic fluid is being produced continuously there is no such thing as a "dry" birth. And rupture of the membranes is often followed by a shorter than average labor.

If the membranes rupture, the mother-to-be should go to the hospital immediately or notify her doctor. After rupture of the membranes there is always the possibility

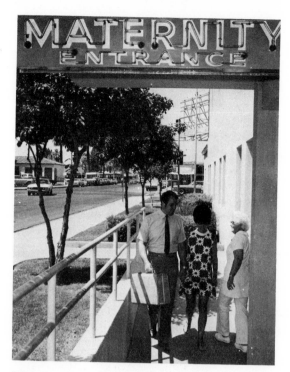

Figure 10-8. The expectant parents go to the hospital when signs of delivery are evident.

of a prolapsed cord if the presenting part does not fill the pelvis.

When labor is established, the pregnant woman and her husband usually leave for the hospital (Fig. 10-8). Generally there is someone on the hospital staff, such as the admissions clerk, to meet them when they enter the hospital. If the maternity department is any distance from the hospital entrance, the expectant mother is taken by wheel chair to that area. If she is in very active labor and delivery seems imminent, she may be transported by stretcher.

NURSING CARE DURING LABOR

The whole tone for the hospital stay is set by the way the nursing personnel greet the prospective parents when they arrive in the maternity department. A sincerely enthusiastic greeting by the nurse makes the couple feel welcome and assures them that this strange hospital environment is indeed friendly.

After introductions all around, the nurse

asks the woman pertinent questions about how many times she has been pregnant, how many children she has, are her membranes (bag of waters) ruptured or intact, how frequent are her contractions. Often the mother must sign permission slips before being admitted to the labor room, authorizing the doctor and staff to administer an anesthetic, do an episiotomy if necessary, take photographs, release information, and circumcise the baby if it is a boy. Because circumcision is often done in the delivery room soon after the birth of the baby, parents are asked to sign a circumcision permit on admission.

The nurse continues to go about admitting the expectant mother to the hospital. Many hospitals have specific admitting procedures for preparing the patient for the hospital routine. Emphasis in this chapter will be placed on nursing actions and their rationale in admitting and caring for a patient in labor.

Nursing History and Nursing Care Plan

As soon as possible after the patient has been admitted to the hospital, a nursing history should be taken. If one was taken during her pregnancy and is available at the hospital when she is admitted, this, of course, will suffice.

Otherwise, plan to sit down with the patient (and her husband or other family member) and informally interview her for the information needed. This will also help you to establish rapport with the patient and her family. With the information obtained on the nursing history, a written nursing care plan can be started. To formulate the nursing care plan it is helpful to have the suggestions and contributions of other nursing team members who have observed and taken care of the patient. A sample of a nursing history for a maternity patient can be found on pages 140 and 141.

Recording and Reporting

As the nurse continues to care for the patient in labor she frequently charts observations of the patient's progress. Lack of progress is significant also. It is suggested that the nurse record on the patient's chart (labor record or nurse's notes, or progress notes) at least once every hour or more frequently as indicated. Changes in the patient can occur suddenly, and they should be recorded and reported promptly. Sometimes immediate actions and decisions must be made for the safety and well-being of the mother and baby.

Pertinent observations about the following should be included:

1. The mother's general condition: is she restless or fatigued? Confident? Nervous? Fearful?

2. Does she have a full bladder?

3. Character of vaginal discharge: is it bleeding or "show"?

4. Rupture of membranes: color and odor of fluid? Is it meconium-stained? How long have the membranes been ruptured? What are the FHT's immediately following their rupture?

5. What is the mother's response to her progress? Is she relaxing well between contractions? Using breathing techniques during contractions?

Social Factors

Social factors can have a tremendous impact on the patient's reactions to childbearing. It is fascinating to observe how each mother responds uniquely to labor and delivery. Although all women go through basically the same physiological changes their attitudes toward childbearing and their behavior during labor varies considerably?

Was this a planned or unplanned pregnancy? What was the motivation for the pregnancy? The point is that it is often revealing to look at the social factors affecting the woman to gain an understanding of her in order to give her better nursing care.

If a woman is happily married, has her husband at her side, and is looking forward to having a baby, her attitude toward childbearing will most likely be positive. As a result her labor and delivery will probably be smoother and easier.

On the other hand, if a woman is divorced or separated from her husband, or unwed, this will naturally influence her attitude toward having a baby. If her husband is away, out of town, or overseas when she is in labor she is deprived of his support. Under these circumstances she might be angry, upset, or even resigned to the situation in which she finds herself.

There are several different resources available to the nurse to give her information about the social factors influencing the patient: the nursing history, doctor, prenatal record, family, and, of course, the patient herself.

Evaluating Labor

One of the first priorities for nursing care is to *observe* and *evaluate* the patient's progress in labor. Actually as soon as the patient enters the maternity department, the nurse begins to observe her. Experienced nurses can pick up clues as to how far the woman's labor has progressed by noting the expression of the patient's face, how she moves from the wheelchair to the bed, and how she gets undressed. Table 10-2 outlines the nursing care appropriate for the various phases of the three stages of labor. During the first stage of labor, nursing care will differ for each of the phases—the first phase, the mid-phase, and the transition phase.

Urine Specimen

In many hospitals the nurse routinely asks the patient for a voided urine specimen when she is being admitted to the labor room. The nurse checks the specimen for the presence of albumin as an indication of toxemia and then sends the specimen to the hospital laboratory for further urinalysis. (See Chap. 6 for a method of testing for albumin in the urine.)

If the patient has ruptured membranes there is no purpose in collecting a urine specimen at this time because the voided specimen would be contaminated with amniotic fluid. In this event, a urinalysis may be obtained at a later time—in the delivery room if the patient is catheterized, or sometime during the postpartum stay. It is routine to get a urinalysis on all obstetrical patients at some time during their hospitalization.

Vital Signs

The nurse will want to take the patient's temperature, pulse, and respirations. If her temperature is elevated over 100°F. (in some hospitals 99.2°F. is considered an elevation) this may signify that there is an infection present or that the woman is dehydrated. The nurse should remove the thermometer from the patient's mouth during a contraction and reinsert it when the contraction is over. Some women clench their teeth during a contraction and may break the thermometer.

Normal pulse range should be between 70 and 100 with the average being about 80. A pulse in excess of 100 might mean that an infection is present, especially if the temperature is also elevated, or it might indicate that the woman is dehydrated or simply excited. If it is below 60 then this is significant also and should be reported to the physician or nurse in charge.

The respirations should be between 18 and 24 per minute. Abnormally slow respirations (below 12) could mean respiratory depression perhaps due to a drug. Too rapid breathing (over 30) could signify that the patient is hyperventilating and should be advised to slow down her rate of breathing. Hyperpnea and dyspnea can, of course, signify lung pathology and should be reported.

Next, the patient's blood pressure should be checked. Blood pressure readings over 130/90 (or 140/90) may indicate toxemia of pregnancy or hypertension. A blood pressure below 90/60 may indicate shock. An initial blood pressure reading may be elevated because of the patient's excitement at coming to the hospital and being in labor. Therefore, if it is elevated on admission the blood

Obstetrical Nursing Care History*

NAME_____ Age_____ M. S. D. Keeping: Yes_____ No_____

G_____ P_____ Ab_____ Ages of children_____ EDC _____

Episiotomy: Yes_____No_____

Breast_____or Bottle_____

Previous hospital experience in this hospital? Yes_____ No_____

   Date_____ Service_____

When first saw Dr. while pregnant? _____Frequency? _____

Did you receive any teaching regarding AP care_____, labor and delivery_____,

   postpartum_____, or newborn care_____?

   Where?_____By whom?_____

   Do any reading? _____

Any complications during pregnancy? _____

Medications taken during pregnancy?_____, _____

Medication allergies? _____

Appetite while pregnant?_____ Weight gain?_____

Diet while pregnant? _____

	Breakfast	Lunch	Dinner	Snack
Time				
Usual Foods:				

Food dislikes? _____

Fluid preferences? _____

Sleep Habits:

   Usual bedtime?_____   Hours of sleep? _____

   Nap habits? _____

   No. of pillows desired? _____   Blankets? _____

   Windows open? _____   Curtains drawn? _____

   If unable to sleep at home, what things do you do that help you to fall asleep?

Elimination:

   Constipation? Yes_____ No_____

   What usually helps regularity? _____

Bladder irregularities? _____

Where stayed during pregnancy? _____

Will you have help when you go home? _____

What preparations have you made for your baby concerning:

Clothing_____

Feeding_____

Bed_____

Bathing facilities_____

Laundry_____

Desire for Rooming-In? Yes_____ No_____

Is there something special you would like to learn or do while you are in the hospital?

Desire to restrict visitors? Yes_____ No_____

Teaching "Check-off" List

_____Peri-Care	_____Baby bath
_____Lochia, fundus	_____Cord care
_____Stitch care	_____Formula prep., feeding
_____Bathing	_____Crying patterns
_____Breast care	_____Stool changes
_____Lactation	_____Circumcision care
_____Manual expression	_____Diapering and care
_____Diet	_____Positioning
_____Constipation	_____Rectal temp.
_____Rest, activity	_____2-week check-up
_____6-week check-up	_____Plans for pediatrician
_____Exercises	
_____Movie: "After You Go Home"	

Other Needs:

*Adapted from: Little, D., and Carnevali, D.: Nursing Care Planning. p. 124 Philadelphia, J. B. Lippincott, 1969.

Table 10-2. LABOR ROOM GUIDE FOR THE THREE STAGES OF LABOR*

Dilation	Physical Characteristics	Orientation of Patient	B.P. & P	FHT	TEMP.	BLADDER	Other	Appropriate Patient Activity
			NURSING CARE					
First Stage								
1-4 cm.	Contractions irregular or 4-5 minutes apart, lasting 30-40 seconds May be accompanied by: Backache, Abdominal cramps, and Slight bloody show	Excited; happy; some apprehension	every 4 hrs.	every hr.	every 4 hrs.	every 2-4 hrs.		Normal activity (if membranes not ruptured) Pelvic rocking Abdominal breathing
4-8 cm.	Contractions: 2-4 minutes apart lasting 45-90 seconds	Apprehensive; Does not want to be alone; Uncertain if she can cope with contractions;	every 2 hrs.	every 3 hrs.	every 4 hrs.	every 2 hrs.	Medications Back rub Environment: quiet dark Cool cloth Moisten lips Keep dry and clean	Abdominal breathing Assume most comfortable position Pelvic rocking
8-10 cm. (Transition)	Contractions: 2-4 minutes apart, lasting 45-60 seconds. Increased bloody show Ruptured membranes; Rectal pressure Leg cramps Marked restlessness Nausea Shaking of legs Perspiration on upper lip and forehead	Increasing apprehension Irritable and unwilling to be touched Frustrated and unable to cope with contractions if left alone Eager to be "put to sleep" Bewildered by intensity of contractions	every hr.	every 5-10 min.	every 4 hrs.	every 2 hrs.	Ice chips	
Second Stage								
Complete	Contractions 1-2 minutes, lasting 60-90 seconds; expulsive in nature Heavy bloody show Bulging of rectum and perineum	Relief Urge to push Desire to move bowels Rectal pressure Sometimes panics when head reaches perineum Splitting sensation due to extreme vaginal stretching Vague in communication Amnesia between contractions Tremendous satisfaction or great pain with each push.	aft. each contraction			Check for distention.		Respond to urge to pu Take *deep* breath, br knees toward shoulde with mouth closed, p back on knees while bearing down. Push duration of contracti Rest completely betw contraction.
Third Stage								
Placental stage	Rise of fundus Uterus assumes globular shape Visible descent of cord Trickle or gush of blood.	Alert, often euphoric Proud, happy Anxious to see baby Relief						
First 2 hrs. after delivery	Chilling	Euphoria to exhaustion Maternal feelings may or may not be in bloom. Hungry, thirsty	every 15 min.		once	Check for distention.	Offer fluid and diet as tolerated Check fundus, flow, perineum every 15 minutes	Sleep

*Courtesy of Arizona State University—College of Nursing.

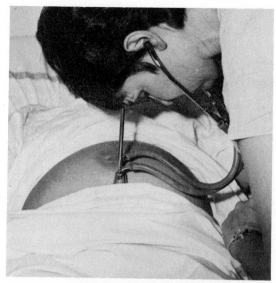

Figure 10-9. The nurse listens to the fetal heart tones. Note the position of the fetuscope.

pressure should be checked within 15 minutes to a half hour later to see if it has returned to normal limits. If it has there is no cause for alarm. The normal blood pressure of a woman in labor is usually between 100/70 to 120/80. Blood pressure during pregnancy is usually somewhat lower than it is when the individual is not pregnant. It is a good idea to check the patient's prenatal record so that her blood-pressure during her pregnancy can be used as a baseline to determine what is normal for *her*.

Fetal Heart Tones

The nurse will want to listen for the fetal heart tones with a special stethoscope called a fetuscope (Fig. 10-9). Some hospitals use a doptone, which is a special electronic device for amplifying the sounds of the fetal heart beat. In order to locate the fetal heart tones the nurse palpates the woman's abdomen to determine what position the baby is in. Usually, the fetal heart tones are best heard through the baby's back.

Palpating the abdomen to determine the position of the baby is called *Leopold's maneuvers*. For the first three maneuvers the nurse stands facing the patient.

First Maneuver. The nurse palpates the fundus with both hands to see if she can determine what part of the baby lies in the upper part of the uterus. As she palpates she asks herself these questions. What is the shape, consistency, and mobility of the object? If it is hard, round, and moveable, it is likely to be the head (indicating a breech presentation). If it is softer, more triangular, and not moveable it is probably the buttocks of the baby (which is a cephalic or vertex presentation).

Second Maneuver. The nurse moves her hands down to the sides of the abdomen. In this manner she stabilizes the uterus on one side with one hand and palpates the opposite side with the other hand. The purpose is to determine on which side of the uterus the baby's back (or spinal column) is located.

Then she alternates hands so that the opposite hand (from the one she used previously) stabilizes the uterus while the other palpates. If she feels a smooth, curved resistant plane on one side she has located the back. If on the opposite side of the uterus she feels smaller lumps, bumps, or irregular parts which sometimes move and kick as she is palpating, those are the knees and elbows of the fetus.

Third Maneuver. Still facing the patient with one hand she presses into the patient's abdomen just over the symphysis pubis. Exerting gentle pressure she can feel the presenting part between her thumb and fingers. If it is the head of the baby which is the presenting part, and if it is not engaged into the inlet, it will feel like a hard, round, moveable object.

Fourth Maneuver. For this final maneuver the nurse faces toward the patient's feet. With the first three fingers of both hands she presses on both sides of the medline about 2 inches above the symphysis pubis. She exerts gentle pressure downward toward the birth canal. If one hand meets an obstruction, it is probably the brow of the baby. This should confirm the findings of the second maneuver because the

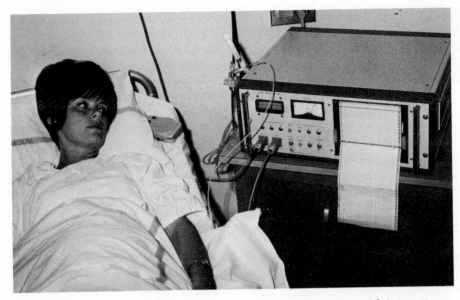

Figure 10-10.   The mother observes the fetal heart monitor with interest.

brow of the baby should be on the side opposite from where the back was located.

After determining the position of the baby she listens for the heartbeat in the appropriate spot. If the baby seems to be in an LOA position for example, the heartbeat should be heard best in the left lower quadrant. If the baby's heartbeat is best heard in either of the upper quadrants it would indicate a breech presentation. The fetal heartbeat is a rapid muffled sound, like a clock ticking under a pillow. The normal range is between 120 and 160 beats per minute. If the rate exceeds 160 or drops below 100 it should be reported immediately. Either of these extremes indicates fetal distress.

The uterine souffle may be heard as a swishing sound when the fetal heart tones are being checked. The difference between the two is that the uterine souffle will be the same rate as the mother's pulse rate. Some nurses like to keep their fingers on the patient's pulse at the same time that they are listening to the fetal heart tones to distinguish between the fetal heart tone and the uterine souffle.

Check the regularity of the fetal heartbeat by counting it for a full minute. During this minute, check the regularity by counting it for two consecutive 15-second periods. If there is a discrepancy in the number of beats in each 15-second interval, the fetal heart is said to be irregular. Sometimes as you listen you can pick up a definite slowing of the heartbeat. Irregularity of the fetal heartbeat should be reported promptly and charted.

Ordinarily, the fetal heart rate slows down at the height of a contraction but returns to normal within 10 seconds of the end of a contraction. You should check the fetal heart tones occasionally during a contraction, especially if an abnormality is suspected. However, in the interest of patient comfort, fetal heart tones are usually taken between contractions. (See Table 10-2, Labor Room Guide for the Three Stages of Labor, for suggestions as to the frequency of taking vital signs and fetal heart tones throughout labor.)

Fetal Heart Monitoring

Another way of checking the fetal heartbeat is to use an electronic monitoring device (Fig. 10-10). Although more hospitals are using this method, at present there are so few of these devices (except possibly in research centers) that they are being used on selected patients such as those who are having their labor induced or those who are considered high-risk maternity patients.

When the patient's cervix is dilated 2 cm. or more, her membranes are ruptured and a small metal electrode is attached to the presenting part of the baby. Of course, it is usually attached to the scalp, but it may be attached to the buttock or thigh in the case of a breech presentation. In this way the fetal heart is monitored throughout labor. A serial EKG (electrocardiogram) as well as the beeping of the monitor keeps tabs on the fetal heart rate.

What is the nurse's role in caring for a patient during this type of electronic monitoring? The nurse can reassure the patient and her husband about the safety of the equipment. Because it is electrical equipment they may be concerned that it can shock or even electrocute the mother or baby. The nurse can explain that the equipment will be attached throughout labor and will be removed right before delivery.

If the fetal heart rate drops, the nurse should immediately turn the patient on her side. This is, of course, true whether the fetal heart is being monitored or being checked with a doptone or fetuscope. When the patient lies on her back for long periods of time the weight of the baby presses on the large abdominal blood vessels, particularly the inferior vena cava. This interferes with the return of blood from the lower extremities and produces a drop in the fetal heart rate. Turning the patient on her side gets the weight off the vena cava and reverses the process. Often the FHT's quickly return to normal.

Timing Contractions

Valuable information about the patient's progress in labor can be obtained by timing the uterine contractions. When the patient first enters the labor room the nurse may ask her how frequently her contractions are occurring. Subsequently, the nurse or other team members will probably time them. Or if the husband knows how, he can time the contractions; it will help him feel more involved.

The patient herself should not be given the responsibility for timing her own contractions, the reason being that she may feel pains, twinges, or other sensations without being sure if they are contractions or not. Then too, the patient may not feel the contraction until after it has started or she may still feel the pressure and discomfort after the contraction is over. Therefore, she might not be very accurate or reliable in timing her own contractions.

Because the fundus is the active contracting portion of the uterus, the nurse palpates with the flat parts of her fingers in this region. She may want to explain to the patient why she is doing this because the patient feels the contraction down lower in her abdomen. Beneath her finger the nurse will feel the uterus becoming more firm as the contraction starts. It reaches a peak of hardness and then gradually becomes softer again. There is a period of relaxation between contractions when the uterus feels soft (less firm).

Contractions occur at about 15 to 30 minutes apart at the beginning of labor and may be 1½ to 2 minutes apart by the end of labor. If there is no definite pattern to the frequency of contractions, they are said to be irregular. The relaxation periods between contractions provide rest for the mother and the uterine muscle. They are also essential to the fetus, allowing it to receive enough oxygen.

In timing the frequency of contractions the nurse leaves her hand on the fundus, gently palpating the area. She times several consecutive contractions from the beginning of one to the beginning of the next. It may be helpful for an inexperienced person to record on a piece of paper the time when each contraction *starts*. Thus, one can see at a glance the frequency of contractions.

By the duration of the contraction is meant how long it lasts. Each contraction has three phases: (1) increment, the period during which the intensity of the contraction increases; (2) acme, the peak of intensity; and (3) decrement, diminishing intensity. The duration of a contraction in early labor can vary from 15 to 30 seconds; near the time of delivery the contraction may last 60 to 90 seconds. Remember, the frequency of contractions is recorded in minutes; the duration is recorded in seconds.

A contraction which lasts two minutes or longer is called a *tetanic* contraction and should be reported immediately. It could cause serious consequences to the mother and the baby—rupture of the uterus in the former and asphyxia in the latter.

Labor contractions are evaluated as to their *intensity*. They are termed mild if the uterine wall can be easily indented by the observer's fingers. If the uterine wall can only be indented slightly, they are moderate. And if the uterus cannot be indented at all the contractions are charted as hard or strong.

Even when contractions are regular and the patient is in good active labor, each contraction does not have the same intensity. A normal pattern may be for the patient to have a long hard contraction, followed by a milder contraction. Then she has another hard contraction, then a milder one, and so on.

Vaginal or Rectal Examination

Another valuable aid in determining the patient's progress in labor is to check the dilatation and effacement of the cervix. This may be done by the nurse or doctor as part of the admitting procedure. Depending on what part of the country you live in, a vaginal examination may be preferred over a rectal examination.

The nurse will help the patient get into as comfortable a position as possible, lying on her back with her knees flexed and feet either flat on the mattress or with the soles of her feet together. The patient should let her knees "fall apart." She will be more

comfortable if she has just emptied her bladder prior to the examination. Draped with the top sheet so that her abdomen and legs are covered, the patient should be instructed to relax as much as possible, breathe easily, and let her legs and pelvic muscles relax.

For a vaginal examination, the examiner dons a pair of sterile gloves and puts a small amount of sterile lubricant on the first two fingers of the examining hand. The labia are separated with the other hand, the fingers are inserted into the vagina until they reach the cervix. The cervix is felt to estimate effacement and dilatation. The fontanels may be palpated to determine the position of the baby. The depth to which the fingers can be inserted before they come in contact with the presenting part can serve as a measure of station.

A vaginal examination is more accurate than a rectal examination because the examiner is feeling the cervix directly, not through the rectovaginal septum. However, unless the examiner uses careful technique (wearing sterile gloves and avoids touching the rectum or surrounding contaminated area when inserting the fingers into the vagina), there is a possibility that infection will be introduced into the vagina. For this reason, as well as for the comfort of the patient, the number of examinations should be kept to a minimum.

A rectal examination is performed by putting on a clean rectal glove, using lubricant on the index finger, and then gently inserting the finger into the rectum. This may be uncomfortable for the patient, and she may have a tendency to tense up. Having her bear down as if to have a bowel movement for a second or two as the index finger is inserted may promote some relaxation of the anal sphincter.

The cervix is palpated through the rectovaginal septum to determine effacement, dilatation, position and presentation, and station. Those who prefer rectal examinations say that they can determine the station more accurately; they can locate the ischial spines more easily and then estimate where the presenting part is in relation to them.

Nurses should learn to do rectal and vaginal examinations on patients in labor. As with other skills it takes practice to maintain accuracy and proficiency. Student nurses should not be discouraged if they cannot tell what they are feeling at first.

A good opportunity for a student nurse to do a vaginal examination is immediately after a doctor has done a paracervical block on the patient. The student can check with the doctor and see if she obtained the same information as he did. Although the patient will not be able to feel, the student should be gentle so as not to rupture the membranes.

Another opportunity presents itself when the student nurse is prepping the patient prior to delivery. This is a wonderful opportunity to feel the fontanels and suture lines of the baby in addition to the fully dilated cervix. The nurse has already put on sterile gloves so that she can check the patient's vagina before cleansing the external genitalia.

Membranes

Whether or not the membranes are ruptured is an important factor in the progress of labor. The bag of waters can rupture at any time during the first stage of labor and, of course, may even rupture spontaneously before labor begins.

In order to speed labor along, the doctor will sometimes rupture the membranes with a hook or sharp instrument such as an Iowa forcep. It is believed (but has not been proven scientifically) that labor proceeds more rapidly if the hard head of the fetus acts as a dilating force rather than the softer action of the bag of waters.

When a women is in active labor and her contractions are close together and strong, if the membranes rupture spontaneously, she will frequently feel the urge to bear

down shortly after that. She should be watched closely for signs that delivery is imminent.

After the membranes are ruptured the fetal heart tones should be checked immediately. If the presenting part is not engaged, there is some danger that the cord may be washed down into the vagina and be compressed between the presenting part of fetus and the pelvis of the mother. Listening to the fetal heart tones would pick up any fetal distress. For this reason, the expectant mother is usually not permitted to get up and walk around or go to the bathroom after the membranes have ruptured.

The color and amount of amniotic fluid should be noted and described on the patient's record. There may be only a small or scanty amount or a moderate to a large amount. If the patient and bed are soaked with fluid this would be significant. *Polyhydramnios* is a condition (rare) in which an excessive amount of amniotic fluid fills the uterus (about 3000 cc.). It is often associated with a fetus having an abnormality of the gastrointestinal tract.

The color of the fluid is also important. It should be clear and colorless with perhaps some white particles (vernix caseosa) in it. A yellowish foul-smelling fluid may indicate that an infection (amnionitis) is present. If the fluid is thick and greenish it indicates that the fetus has passed some meconium and may be in distress *if in a vertex presentation.* When the fetus has a lack of oxygen (hypoxia), he struggles for breath, and the anal sphincter dilates resulting in passage of meconium into the amniotic fluid. Meconium-stained fluid in a breech presentation is normal because pressure from the contracting uterus on the baby's buttock forces meconium from his intestinal tract.

A record of the date and time that the membranes ruptured should be included in the patient's chart. Studies have shown that if the membranes have been ruptured longer than 12 to 24 hours there is a likelihood of amnionitis (infection of the amniotic sac). The nurse may want to call this to the doctor's attention.

Shave Preparation

If it has been ascertained that the woman is in true labor the nurse will usually shave her. As explained before, some doctors do not feel that this is necessary, but it is still a widespread practice throughout the United States.

The purpose of shaving the genitalia is to promote cleanliness and prevent infection. It is preferable to shave the patient earlier in labor instead of waiting until she becomes more uncomfortable and restless with contractions. In general the following equipment is needed: basin with several cotton balls, soap solution, a razor, paper towels, a wash cloth, and a hip pad or Chux.

A disposable "prep" tray containing all of the necessary items may be available. Proceed in this manner to shave the patient: wash your hands, assemble the equipment, and pour warm soap solution into the basin. Explain the procedure to the patient and instruct her to lie on her back with her knees bent. Place a hip pad (or Chux) and two paper towels under the patient's hips. The paper towels are used to catch the hair as it is being removed. Drape the patient as for a vaginal or rectal examination and instruct her to let her knees "fall apart." Soap the area with a cotton ball working crosswise from the mons veneris to the rectum. Since the rectum is a dirty area, terminate the washing here. Never return toward the vagina with the same cotton ball. Gentle traction in the opposite direction from which the razor is going will tighten the skin and make shaving easier. A paper towel in one hand will increase traction, since soap makes the skin slippery.

Begin at the mons veneris and, using short strokes, work downward on the labium to the vagina. Never lift the razor from the skin. Turn the razor over and repeat on the other labium. If hair is growing between the labia majora and minora, tilt the razor slightly and exert more countertraction to make the skin taut. Have the patient turn on her side so that you can shave around the rectum. Lift the upper cheek of the buttocks and shave *away* from the vagina *toward* the rectum. Turn the razor over and repeat on the other side.

When finished, remove the paper towels and equipment, and wash and replace the equipment. With a warm washcloth, rinse the genitalia, stroking from the mons veneris to the rectum. Dry the patient and remove the underpad. The main principles in shaving the genitalia are to avoid trauma to the skin and to prevent contaminants from entering the vagina.

If delivery is imminent and you only have a few seconds in which to shave the patient, a few strokes of the razor to remove hair from the perineum (area between the vagina and rectum) will suffice, since this is the area for "stitches."

Enema

It is assumed that the reader has learned the basic skills of giving an enema. Only the modifications necessary for a maternity patient will be presented here. As previously stated, enemas are not ordered routinely for patients in labor, and there are definite reasons for not giving them. If a patient is very nearly ready to have her baby she should not be given an enema. Nor should she be given an enema if she is having any vaginal bleeding, since an enema could increase it and thus be dangerous. However, an enema may be given in early labor to cleanse the lower bowel, provide more room for the baby's descent, and prevent contamination at the time of delivery.

The enema should be given in bed with the woman lying on her side. It is often convenient to give an enema just after the patient has been shaved. A small disposable enema may be used (such as a Fleets or Travad), or a standard soap solution cleansing enema may be ordered.

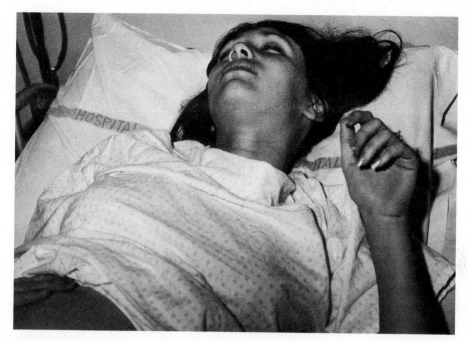

Figure 10-11. The patient is completely absorbed in concentration during a contraction.

Before administering the enema ask the woman to let you know when she is getting a contraction so that you can clamp off the flow of solution during the contraction. Pressure from the contraction plus the pressure from the solution entering the rectum is uncomfortable for the patient.

If it is a small disposable enema, it will only take a minute or two to give it. Instruct the patient to hold the solution for a couple of minutes or until she has the urge to evacuate. She is usually able to go to the bathroom to expel the enema if the membranes have not ruptured. It is well to check on her frequently while she is in the bathroom expelling the enema because she might feel weak or faint or may require assistance in getting to and from the bathroom. Record the procedure on the patient's chart in the usual manner.

Emotional State

Observing the patient's emotional state gives valuable information about the progress of labor, since there are definite emo-

tional changes that accompany labor. Typically the woman is excited, talkative, and apprehensive in early labor. Then, as her contractions become stronger she becomes quieter. Near the end of labor she is completely self-centered and absorbed in having the baby (Fig. 10-11).

Labor is a lonely experience for a woman. When she is first admitted to the hospital she is separated from her family and feels lonely and frightened. Also, she may feel trapped, because she knows that there is no way out for her. She is in labor and she must proceed and give birth to this baby. She should not be left alone; someone, it often doesn't matter to her who it is, should be with her. Of course, it is best if that person is someone in her own family, especially her husband.

It is sometimes very difficult for the nurse (or anyone) to stay with a patient in labor, particularly when she cries out or loses control of herself and pleads with you to help her. This is especially hard if the nurse has done everything she can think of to make the patient more comfortable. Some nurses escape these uncomfortable situations by leaving the patient alone. Hopefully, with the knowledge and understanding of labor and what is causing the behavior of the patient, the nurse can cope with her own feelings. Then she will be able to stay with the patient and husband and give them both the support they need. If the nurse must leave the room, the patient appreciates knowing when she will be back and how to use the call bell if she needs assistance.

Some nurses feel "in the way" when the husband is there in the labor room with his wife. They feel uncomfortable and intrusive when indeed the prospective parents have no such thoughts. If the couple wants to be alone they will usually say so. Actually, the husband and wife feel more secure and confident when the nurse is with them.

It has been traditional to ask the husband to leave the room every time a doctor or nurse does a rectal or vaginal examination on his wife. In fact he must leave for any procedure which involves exposing her genitalia. The rationalization often used is that they (the nurse or doctor) do not want to cause the couple any embarrassment. The truth is that they are the ones who feel uncomfortable and are protecting their own feelings. Instead of following this puritanical practice let us consult with the husband and wife on *their* preference. By all means let the husband stay!

Emotional Support

There are three team members, so to speak, who give important emotional support to the woman in labor: the husband, the nurse, and the doctor. It is the cooperative efforts of all of these people that help to minimize the mother's fears and build up her confidence.

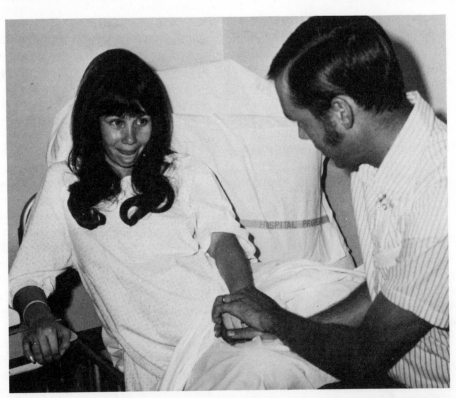

Figure 10-12.   The husband can give emotional support to his wife during labor.

Emotional support can help the mother make the best use of her own strength. Telling her that she is "doing a good job," and that she is breathing "beautifully" with contractions will encourage her to continue in her efforts.

What are some other specific ways that a nurse can give emotional support to the prospective parents? She can give the patient the best possible care from the time she enters the labor room. Through her actions she shows the parents that she realizes that this is a significant experience for them. She realizes that the parents came to the hospital because they need and want help. And it may be their first hospital experience.

She can also introduce others as they enter the room, include the prospective parents in the conversation when there are others in the room, and consult the mother about her care when possible.

It is the nurse who keeps the parents informed about the progress of labor. This includes going out to the father's waiting room to find the husband to tell him about his wife's progress. She can provide for the parents' privacy by keeping the door closed, if desired.

Talk in tones that are audible to the parents. Talking in hushed tones makes the parents anxious that you are discussing something about the wife that you don't want them to hear. Loud laughing and joking are also inappropriate because having a baby is a serious matter to the parents. However, this doesn't mean that the nurse cannot smile and be pleasant and cheerful. Explain special procedures to them and orient them to the hospital routine if this has not been done previously. Let the prospective parents listen to the fetal heart tones if they want to. Encourage the father to participate in his wife's care if he feels comfortable doing this (Fig. 10-12). Make it easy for him to leave if he becomes upset or tired. Use touch to provide emotional support. Physical contact, such as rubbing her back, holding her hand, timing contractions, etc., provides reassurance.

Comfort Measures

What can the nurse do to make the patient more comfortable in labor?

Positioning. A patient should not be flat in bed when in labor. The head of the bed should be elevated so that the forces of gravity can assist the labor process. Extra pillows should be used to provide support in positioning her, such as a small pillow placed in the curvature of her spine, or a pillow under her knees to take the tension off the abdominal wall.

The nurse can encourage the patient to change her position frequently and help her to get into positions that are more comfortable. The nurse can help the patient turn on her side and get into a position comfortable for late pregnancy and labor as described in Chapter 7. This is also an excellent position for back rubs and the application of sacral pressure.

Sacral Pressure. A patient's back often gets tired and may ache during labor. This is due to contractions starting in the back, to lying in one position for a long time, and to the weight of the uterus pressing on the spinal column. Some fetal positions, such as when the baby is lying in a posterior (rather than an anterior) position, produce more backache.

Most women really appreciate having their backs rubbed, and some women especially like sacral pressure applied during contractions. With the patient lying on her side, the nurse or the husband exerts firm even pressure with the heel of the hand in a circular motion in the sacral area throughout the contraction. Lotion or powder may be used to reduce friction. Sacral pressure is believed to provide comfort because it lifts the weight of the baby off the spinal column, particularly the lumbar and sacral regions, which are most vulnerable.

Muscle Spasms. If the patient gets leg cramps the nurse can relieve them by putting pressure on the knee and hyper-extending the foot.

Other Comfort Measures. Ice chips may be given to the mother to chew or suck on. This relieves the dryness of the mouth caused by medications or breathing through the mouth.

Another comfort measure for dry lips is to moisten them with vaseline or other lubricants, to prevent the patient from having sore, cracked lips after delivery.

A cool, damp cloth on the forehead, neck, and face feels very refreshing to the patient. Labor is hot work, and the uterus itself generates a lot of heat causing the mother to perspire profusely as labor advances. This can be continued as a comfort measure in the delivery room.

Changing hip pads (or Chux) frequently as they become soiled adds to the comfort of the patient. If the patient is having a lot of bloody "show" or the membranes are ruptured, she feels uncomfortably wet or sticky. Cleansing the patient's perineum may occasionally be necessary if there is a heavy amount of vaginal discharge. See the procedure for perineal care in Chapter 14.

Keeping the bladder and rectum empty will increase the patient's comfort during labor. There will be less pressure and more room for the baby to descend. A full bladder or bowel can actually retard the progress of labor. The patient should be encouraged to empty her bladder frequently. (See Labor Room Guide for the Three Stages of Labor.) If the bladder becomes full or distended the nurse should first try to get her to void by running water or pouring warm water over the perineum. Some patients cannot use the bed pan, so that assisting them to the bathroom often works. If these measures are unsuccessful then the nurse should get an order for catheterization from the physician.

The patient should not have any food or liquids after she is in active labor. The reason is that there is hypomotility of the stomach during labor and food or water ingested is likely to be vomited. An addi-tional reason is that if the patient receives a general anesthetic, it is best if she has had nothing by mouth for several hours before. If she vomits, the vomitus may be aspirated, producing serious lung complications and even death.

Helping the Patient to Use Breathing and Relaxation Techniques in the First Stage of Labor

The nurse should concentrate her efforts on helping the patient use the breathing and relaxing techniques as given in Chapter 7. Even though the patient has been well schooled in these techniques and has practiced them faithfully during her pregnancy, she will need reminders and encouragement from the nurse to keep them up.

A patient who does not know these techniques can be taught how to do abdominal breathing during contractions. Even though she doesn't do it perfectly it gives her something to concentrate on, and she feels that she can do something to help herself. Thus, it has psychological value.

When the labor progresses to the point that the patient says she can no longer do abdominal breathing, switching to costal breathing is in order.

Helping the Patient to Push in the Second Stage of Labor

When it has been determined that the cervix is fully dilated, the nurse will coach the woman on how to push with contractions. A primigravida may be fully dilated and pushing for a time in the labor room. Usually she is not taken to the delivery room until a small part of the scalp of the baby is visible at the vaginal introitus and does not recede back into the vagina at the end of the contraction. A multipara is often taken into the delivery room at 8 to 9 cm. of dilatation so that she pushes when she is on the delivery table.

With the head of the bed elevated or

with the nurse holding the woman around the shoulders so that her chin touches her chest, the nurse instructs her to "Push, push, push, just like you are going to move your bowels" or "Take a deep breath, hold it, and then push down hard."

If she can hold on to something around or under her knees or to the hand grips on the delivery table this will help to give her leverage. Her elbows should be bent in pushing. If she draws her knees up, so that her thighs act as splints to her abdomen, this helps too. In the delivery room she can brace her feet against the stirrups.

The nurse helps the mother to coordinate her pushing efforts with contractions by telling her when one is starting and by keeping her pushing throughout the contraction. Then when it is over, she can tell the mother to relax and rest as much as possible.

Some women tend to tense up the muscles of the perineal floor when pushing. The nurse can remind the mother to keep these muscles relaxed to facilitate the egress of the baby from the birth canal.

If there are too many people instructing the patient in what to do, this can lead to confusion. When one person has taken over the coaching and emotional support, others should not interfere.

Providing for Privacy and Modesty

The nurse will add greatly to the patient's comfort if she takes steps to provide for the patient's privacy and modesty. Sometimes two or more patients are in labor in the same room. Curtains between the beds should be drawn or screens put up when one of the patients is being examined or having a procedure done which requires exposure of the body.

Unfortunately, nursing personnel as well as doctors become lax in pulling the curtain or draping the patient for an examination or other procedure. Some patients are very sensitive about being exposed and are justifiably offended when hospital personnel show a lack of concern for their feelings.

Dependent Nursing Actions—Assisting the Physician

The nurse and physician must work closely together and cooperatively in the maternity department. This is especially true of the labor and delivery area, and it is certainly to the advantage of the patient. The physician often expects the nurse to keep him informed about the patient's progress in labor. Interns and residents also should be kept informed. The nurse (or resident) calls the doctor when the patient is admitted and then at periodic intervals throughout labor. Often she calls him to inform him that delivery is imminent. When the patient is first admitted in labor she may have a history and physical examination done, if there is no record of one during her prenatal visits (or if she did not have prenatal care).

For artificial rupture of the membranes (artificial amniotomy) the nurse assists by getting the patient ready and obtaining the necessary equipment. The patient is prepared and draped as if she were to have a vaginal examination. In addition, several hip pads or a bed pan is placed under her buttocks to catch the amniotic fluid.

A sterile instrument such as an Allis or Iowa forcep, or a disposable Amnihook is used. A sharp instrument or hook is necessary to puncture a hole in the membranes so that the amniotic fluid is released.

When the doctor has completed the vaginal examination and is ready for the instrument, the nurse removes the wrapper, using sterile technique. She hands him the handle of the instrument. After the membranes are ruptured, the nurse checks the fetal heart tones, observes the amniotic fluid for amount, color, and odor, and cleans and dries the patient. Then she charts the procedure in an appropriate manner.

ANALGESICS AND ANESTHETICS IN LABOR

Analgesics

An analgesic is any drug used to relieve pain. It is sometimes administered during labor to relieve the discomfort of labor con-

tractions. Usually, an analgesic is a narcotic such as Demerol. However, since it is
only given once or twice during labor there
is no danger of addiction. It is often administered intravenously and intramuscularly in combination with other drugs
such as tranquilizers and will act in about
20 minutes after it is given, taking the edge
off the pain. The mother will still feel the
contractions but will doze off to sleep between them.

The mother-to-be should know that she
can always ask for an analgesic if she becomes too uncomfortable. However, if given
too early it may stop or retard the progress
of her labor. If given too late it may make
the baby sleepy at birth. Therefore, the
woman cannot always have the medications
just when she thinks she needs them.

Sedatives

A sedative is a drug to promote rest and
sleep. It can be given early in labor, soon
after the expectant mother is admitted to
the hospital, to promote relaxation and
lessen fear. Drugs such as Seconal and Nembutal are classified as barbiturates and hypnotics and are given by mouth.

Tranquilizers

A tranquilizer is a drug that reduces
anxiety. It inhibits nausea and vomiting
and reduces the amount of narcotic drug
that a mother-to-be might require. This is an
advantage to the baby, since large doses of
narcotics given to the mother may slow the
baby's respirations. Therefore, tranquilizers
such as Phenergan, Vistaril, and Atarax
are usually given in combination with Demerol to produce the desired degree of pain
relief in labor. They are administered intravenously or intramuscularly, or half IV
and half IM. They are sometimes administered alone if the woman seems tense
when it is too soon to give her an analgesic.
Some women want to be "knocked-out"; to
have no recollections of labor and delivery.
A drug which produces this effect is Scopolamine. It seems to be used less frequently

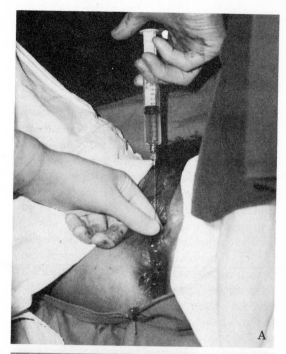
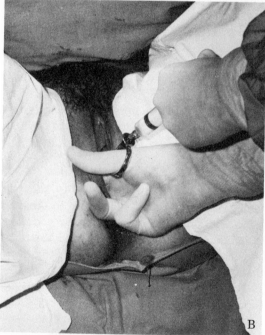

Figure 10-13. (A) Medication is injected into
the perineum to deaden the nerves for delivery
and repair of the episiotomy. Even though the
needle is about 3 inches long, the patient feels
only the initial prick as with any other injection.
(B) The physician uses his fingers inside the vagina to locate the ischial spines so that he can
tell where to inject the medication.

at present because of the number of women who want to be in conscious control during childbirth.

Anesthesia

Anesthesia is the loss of sensation brought on by the administration of certain drugs to *obliterate* pain and sensations. It may be used during delivery of the infant and the placenta and during perineal repair. It may be general or regional.

General Anesthesia. Inhalation anesthesia is an example of general anesthesia. The mother inhales gases through a mask held over her nose and mouth by an anesthetist or anesthesiologist. Nitrous oxide and cyclopropane are the agents most frequently used. Either one of them is used in combination with pure oxygen. The mother breathes the mixture in during contractions and is awake enough to be able to push with the contractions. She may be put to sleep following delivery of the baby when the placenta is delivered and the perineum repaired.

One advantage of inhalation anesthetics is that they do not impair uterine contractions. A disadvantage is that they should not be administered to a woman who has just eaten a meal because they cause nausea and vomiting.

Regional Anesthesia

Local Anesthesia. Local infiltration involves injecting an anesthetic drug such as Xylocaine or Procaine into the perineal area where nerves, including the important pain-producing pudendal nerve, are located (Figs. 10-13 and 10-14). This is a very safe method of anesthesia. It does not require an anesthetist, is safe for the baby, and does not impair contractions. A local or pudendal block, as it is called, is administered at the time of delivery or for repair of the perineum.

Other examples of regional anesthesia for childbirth are paracervical blocks, saddle blocks, and caudal anesthesia.

Paracervical block is one of the newer types of analgesia and anesthesia to come into wide use in obstetrics. Its main advantage is that the agent can be given to the mother in labor (this is why it is considered an analgesic) when the cervix is only partially dilated. It is administered by needle

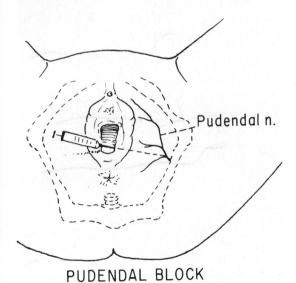

PUDENDAL BLOCK

Figure 10-14. Pudendal block.

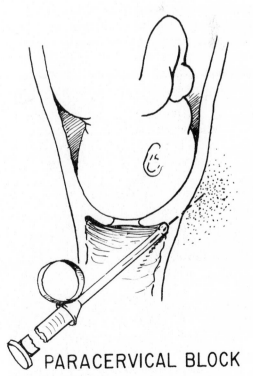

PARACERVICAL BLOCK

Figure 10-15. Peracervical block.

and syringe through the vagina, with the anesthetic drug being injected into the area around the cervix (Fig. 10-15). Thus, it relieves the pain caused by the cervix dilating. A medication such as Carbocaine is used for a paracervical block.

Spinal anesthesia, especially the saddle block is a popular form of regional anesthesia used for vaginal deliveries in the United States. In this form of anesthesia a suitable drug is injected into the spinal canal, while the mother is sitting up on the delivery table. Then after half a minute she lies down on the table with her head and shoulders elevated on pillows for the delivery.

Saddle blocks are of short duration and are therefore administered when delivery is anticipated within an hour.

The reason that it is called a saddle block is that the position of the anatomy anesthetized corresponds to the part of a rider's body that is in contact with the saddle. An advantage is that it is safe for the baby.

Some women fear spinal injections of any type because they have heard stories of people who became paralyzed as a result. This, however, is an extremely rare occurrence. They are also afraid of getting an unpleasant "spinal headache" following delivery. This is attributed to leakage of spinal fluid and can generally be prevented by the use of a small gauge needle.

Continuous caudal anesthesia and *analgesia* involves introducing a suitable drug into the caudal space, a space at the lowest tip of the bony spinal canal through which a large network of nerves passes. Blocking the pathways of the nerves anesthetizes the abdominal and pelvic areas. A chief advantage is that the mother may receive a caudal in early labor and throughout labor and delivery as needed. A small catheter is left in the caudal space so that analgesia can be continuous. It is truly painless childbirth.

It is also safe for the baby. However, the disadvantage is that in many areas only a few doctors know how to administer a caudal

(it requires skill). The doctor must also stay with the patient throughout labor—something many doctors are unwilling or unable to do.

Administering Sedatives and Analgesics

It is often the nurse's responsibility to decide when to give the patient sedatives and analgesic drugs. The doctor usually ordered that they be given as needed. If the patient seems tense and apprehensive she may be given a sedative, such as Seconal, or a tranquilizer, such as Vistaril, very soon after being admitted and prepared for delivery.

Analgesics are administered after the patient has demonstrated that she is in active labor (that her cervix is dilating and effacing). A primigravida should be having painful contractions every three to five minutes, and her cervix should be dilated at least 3 to 4 cm. The cervix of a multipara should be dilated at least 4 cm. before she receives an analgesic. The danger of giving analgesics too soon is that they may retard or even stop the progress of labor.

It is the nurse's responsibility to see that the fetus is in good condition before administering a narcotic such as Demerol. She checks the FHT's prior to giving it and then again 10 to 15 minutes later when the drug is taking effect (sooner, if the drug is given intravenously).

She makes sure that the room is darkened and the environment subdued so that the medication can take effect. To provide for the patient's safety, she raises the side rails of the bed after administering sedatives, tranquilizers, or narcotics.

If the nurse believes that delivery is imminent (within a half hour) she does not administer Demerol, because it will be too late to help the mother and it will have a maximum depressing effect on the respirations of the baby. If the baby is blue, makes little or no effort to breathe, and is sleepy this may be a result of administering an analgesic too late in labor. Thus, it is evident that proper timing is a critical factor in administering drugs to a patient in labor.

Assisting with Anesthesia

The nurse can render valuable assistance to the physician in helping him administer anesthetics to patients in labor. However, she should never allow herself to be put into the position where she is actually administering anesthetics. This is the responsibility of a trained anesthetist, anesthesiologist, or the doctor. Since obstetrical anesthesia differs from surgical anesthesia in several ways, certain considerations should be taken into account when it is being administered:

1. There are two persons to consider.
2. It is not absolutely necessary in normal labor.
3. Drugs which have little effect on uterine contractions should be used.
4. Drugs should not depress the respirations of the fetus.
5. The duration differs. The duration of surgical anesthesia can be predicted more accurately.
6. When the patient is prepared for surgical anesthesia food and fluids are withheld for 12 hours or more. This is not usually true for a maternity patient.

Certain general principles should be followed in administering anesthetics to maternity patients. They should not be started too soon—there must be proof of progressive dilatation and effacement of the cervix. Another principle is that safety precautions are necessary, such as not leaving the patient alone, taking precautions against possible explosions, having emergency equipment available such as oxygen, suction equipment, pressor drugs, and cardiac arrest equipment. The third principle is that the anesthetic should meet the three criteria for obstetric pain relief; it should (1) maintain fetal homeostasis, (2) be simple to administer, and (3) provide the patient with pain relief.

Needless to say, there is no perfect anesthetic as yet. However, there have been definite improvements made in techniques of using analgesia and anesthesia in obstetrics in recent years.

Hypnosis

Anesthetic hypnosis is always talked about but seldom seen. It has been used successfully in childbirth, dentistry, and surgery, and physicians and patients who have used it for childbearing have been enthusiastic about it. It provides pain relief for the mother without affecting the baby. The main disadvantages are that it is time-consuming (the patient must undergo hypnosis training on her prenatal visits and the doctor must stay with her throughout labor), and very few physicians have learned to use it.

Paracervical Block

The nurse may suggest to the physician when she thinks the patient is ready for a paracervical block. That is when the parturient is in good, active labor, is uncomfortable with contractions, and the cervix is dilated 4 to 5 cm. or more. A sterile paracervical tray is obtained which usually contains most of the equipment needed for the paracervical block. In addition, a pair of sterile gloves for the doctor, a sterile Iowa trumpet, and a 30-cc. vial of 1 per cent or 2 per cent Carbocaine or Metycaine (depending on the doctor's preference) may be needed. The patient is prepared for a vaginal examination. The procedure is explained and she is told that she should be relieved of the pain that is being caused by the cervix dilating.

Since a paracervical block sometimes causes a transient bradycardia in the fetus, the nurse should check FHT's before anesthesia is begun and every 5 to 15 minutes following. If the FHT's drop, the patient should be turned on her side immediately.

Unfortunately, not all paracervical blocks are successful. Some may take effect on only one side of the cervix. However, most of them produce the intended results. The patient may doze off to sleep within minutes after having a paracervical block, which demonstrates her freedom from pain. The paracervical block lasts for about an hour and a half and may be repeated during labor. The patient usually has a pudendal block for the actual delivery. The nurse is responsible for charting the following information: when the paracervical block was given, what medication was used, the strength of the solution, the amount given, the physician's name, and the patient's response.

Caudal

The nurse assists the physcian by obtaining the caudal tray, medication, and gloves as with a paracervical block. She also obtains equipment and solutions for skin preparation and draping of the sacral area if this is not included in the caudal tray. Tincture of Merthiolate or a suitable substitute may be used to cleanse the skin. Wide tape will be needed to tape the caudal catheter in place.

FHT's and the patient's blood pressure are checked before the caudal anesthesia is started. The patient is turned on her side in the Sims's position and prepped and draped. Explanations of the procedure are made before starting. (One doctor who does caudals on many of his patients has had a videotape of the procedure to use for patient teaching. It seems to be very effective.)

If the caudal is successful the patient should not feel any pain but may feel pressure. Her legs and feet will feel warm, but she will be able to move them. After the doctor has inserted the catheter into the caudal canal and taped it into place, the doctor and nurse help the patient to lie down on her back. Care is taken not to dislodge the catheter and other equipment (such as the vial of Carbocaine and syringe) which are left on the bed.

Because caudal anesthesia may cause the patient's blood pressure to drop, it must be monitored closely. A vasopressor, such as ephedrine or epinephrine, should be close at hand to be given immediately if the blood

pressure drops. Another way to relieve the hypotension is to elevate both of the patient's legs simultaneously. The continuous caudal will be used throughout labor and delivery. Because the patient does not have the urge to bear down, the baby will usually be delivered with forceps. It is an ideal anesthesia for delivering a premature infant because it has no effect on the baby, and the delivery is slow and controlled. Some patients cannot have a caudal because of a pilonidal cyst or infection in the area.

Charting will include: the time the anesthesia was started, by whom, medication, strength of solution, amount given, etc. In addition, an anesthesia record on which the patient's blood pressure and other pertinent information may be required by the hospital.

When an additional amount of medication is given to the patient (since it is a continuous caudal anesthesia), the quantity, time, and other pertinent information are recorded. Assisting with other kinds of anesthesia, such as a saddle block will be included in the chapter on delivery.

SIGNS THAT DELIVERY IS IMMINENT

The transition phase is the name given to the latter part of the first stage of labor. It is usually the most difficult time for the mother (and is hard on the father too). In most instances there are fewer than 20 contractions in the transition phase, so if the nurse can remind the patient of that, it might help. Also, reminding the patient that with each contraction that is one less that she will have before the baby is born, may be encouraging.

When the patient exhibits the signs of transition, this indicates that delivery is imminent. The doctor should be called (if he is not already there), and the delivery room should be prepared. At this time a multipara is often moved into the delivery room.

A major concern of student nurses (or anyone who is new to the maternity department) is how to determine when the patient is ready to deliver.

The signs and symptoms of transition are:

1. Contractions are close together, 2 to 4 minutes apart, lasting about 45 to 60 seconds, and strong in intensity. With each contraction the nurse should observe the mother's perineum for (1) bulging of the vulva, (2) a slit of the baby's scalp visible at the vaginal introitus, and (3) dilation of the anal sphincter.

2. An increase in bloody show because of the pressure of the presenting part of the fetus as it comes through the cervix causing tiny blood vessels to rupture and the mucous plug to be dislodged.

3. Membranes rupture spontaneously.

4. Shaking of the legs due to pressure of the presenting part on the perineal nerves.

5. Marked restlessness because of the intensity of the contractions.

6. Rectal pressure. The patient says she feels like she has to move her bowels. Explain to her that she feels this pressure because of the presenting part of the baby, but don't give her a bedpan at this time.

7. Perspiration on her upper lip and forehead due to the heat generated by her body, especially the uterus.

8. Nausea, or sudden emesis caused by hypomotility of the stomach. Be ready with an emesis basin.

9. How the patient feels. She may be increasingly irritable and apprehensive, unwilling to be touched but afraid of being left alone, frustrated and unable to cope with contractions, eager to be "put to sleep," bewildered by the intensity of contractions. She may cry out, "Oh God, help me!" or "I can't take it any more."

She responds best to short positive directions from the medical and nursing personnel. With the confirmation by rectal or vaginal examination that the cervix is 8 to 10 cm. dilated the nurse knows that the patient is in transition and will soon be ready to have the baby.

BIBLIOGRAPHY

Bradley, R.: Husband-coached Childbirth. New York, Harper and Row, 1965.

Eastman, N. J., and Hellman, L. M.: William's Obstetrics. ed. 13. New York, Appleton-Century-Crofts, 1966.

Estey, G. P.: "Word From a Mother." American Journal of Nursing, *69*:1453-1454, July, 1969.

Goodrich, F.: "The Problem of Anxiety in Obstetrics." Child and Family, Winter, 1965, 4(1), 1962.

Hoff, F. E.: "Natural Childbirth—How Any Nurse Can Help." American Journal of Nursing, *69*:1451, July, 1969.

Kendall, B., and Farell, D. M.: "Use of Fetal Electrocardiography." American Journal of Nursing, *64*:75-79, July, 1964.

Langhorne, F.: "Supine Hypotension Syndrome." American Journal of Nursing, *70*:1260, June, 1970.

Matousek, I.: "Fetal Nursing During Labor." Nursing Clinics of North America, June, 1968, 2.

Newton, N.: "Childbirth and Culture." Psychology Today, *4*:74, Nov., 1970.

Poppers, P. J.: "Overventilation During Labor." Bulletin of the American College of Nurse-Midwifery, *13*(2): 4-7, May 1968.

Weidenbach, E.: Family-Centered Maternity Nursing. New York, G. P. Putnam, 1967.

Suggested Reading for Further Study

Barnard, J.: "Peer Group Instruction for Primigravid Adolescents." Nursing Outlook, *18*:42, Aug., 1970.

Bradley, R.: "Fathers As Labor Coaches." Bulletin of the American College of Nurse-Midwifery, 7(2), 34, Summer, 1962.

Ulin, P. R.: "The Exhilarating Moment of Birth." American Journal of Nursing, *63*:60-67, June, 1963.

Delivery and Immediate Care of the Newborn 11

Once it has been determined that the patient is ready to go to the delivery room, a team — usually the doctor, nurse, and anesthetist — swing into action. Hopefully, the nurse who has been supporting and coaching the patient throughout labor will be able to go with her to the delivery room.

In addition to caring for the needs of the patient, the delivery-room nurse finds herself involved in many technical tasks. As a circulating nurse, she is responsible for setting up the room, transporting the patient to the delivery room, keeping an accurate record of the events of the delivery, and assisting the physician and anesthetist. It is a challenging, but satisfying experience. After all, how many people are privileged to witness the beginning of a new life?

The nurse must be able to react quickly and respond well in stressful situations. You may notice that in a delivery room tension usually builds up until the baby is born; after the delivery when all is going well with the mother and baby, the tension quickly disappears.

In many ways a delivery room is similar to an operating room. The same principles of surgical asepsis and safety are carried out. The nurse wears a clean scrub dress and a cap that covers all of her hair. She wears conductive shoes or boots to prevent static sparks of electricity because she is working around explosive anesthetic gases. When she is circulating in the delivery room or has opened a sterile pack, she must have on a mask to prevent contamination of the sterile field.

Preparation of the Delivery Room

There are probably no two hospitals in which the setup of the delivery room is the same (Fig. 11-1). The nurse learns how to set one up by observing and participating in the procedure followed by her own institution. In setting up the room, the nurse must know where equipment is located, the principles of surgical asepsis, the needs of the patient, and the preferences of the physician. A file of index cards stating the individual preferences of each staff physician is usually kept in the maternity department.

Setting up the delivery table is usually the first task. In large maternity departments, the table may be set up in advance and only a few items must be added at the time of delivery. If the table is not used within 24 hours, everything is removed and resterilized. However, in a busy maternity department this rarely happens. In a small maternity department, the delivery table is not set up until the nurse is reasonably sure that delivery will occur soon.

Procedure for Setting Up a Delivery Room Table

Wash your hands well. A surgical scrub is not necessary because you will be using sterile transfer (pick-up) forceps or sterile gloves to set up the table. Put on a cap and mask. Pull the physician's file card if you know which doctor will be using the delivery room. Assemble the equipment: basic delivery pack, instrument set, gloves, and suction bulb for the infant. Pull the de-

161

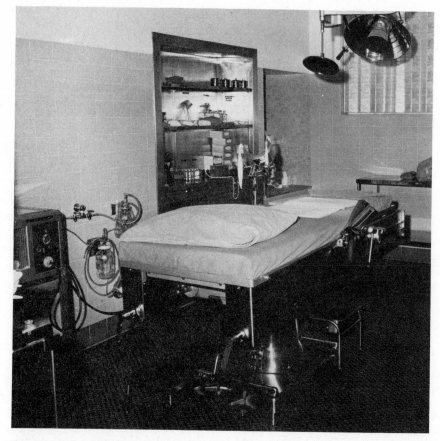

Figure 11-1. The nurse learns to set up the delivery room properly. Note the mirror attached to the overhead light so that parents may watch the birth of their baby. The table is divided into a top half and lower half. One of the metal stirrups is in place.

livery table away from the wall. Center the pack so that the drape will open properly and check the tapes on the outside of the pack to see if they have dark lines on them (if this method is used to indicate the sterility of the pack). Also, check the expiration date on the pack to make certain that the contents are still sterile. (Or check the indicator inside the pack for changes that indicate it is sterile.) Open the basic delivery pack which contains drapes and equipment used during a delivery. The following sterile equipment is usually included:

1 set of drapes for the patient: 1 for under the buttocks, 2 leggings, and 1 abdominal drape
4 extra sterile towels
2 gowns and towels—one each for the doctor and his assistant

1 drape for the interior of the incubator
1 baby blanket
2 perineal pads
1 T-binder, for fastening the patient's perineal pads
1 vaginal pack (or tail sponge)
1 medicine cup for local anesthetic (if used)
1 cord clamp
1 small basin for suture material
1 basin or cup for sterile soap solution (if used)
1 Luer-lock syringe (50-cc. size) with 3-inch spinal needle

Add to these supplies from the room: Two pairs of gloves, one bulb syringe, appropriate suture materials and needles (if needed), and cord blood tube if the patient is Rh negative.

Using transfer forceps or sterile gloves,

arrange the contents of the pack for convenient and orderly use. When using the transfer forceps, remember to keep the tips down. The instrument pack is opened and added to the table. Instruments are autoclaved separately since it takes less time to sterilize them, and the sharp instruments become dull through prolonged sterilization. An instrument set will probably include:

1 pair curved scissors to cut the cord
1 pair straight scissors for the episiotomy
2 curved hemostats for clamping the cord
1 straight hemostat
4 towel clips
Instruments for repairing the episiotomy
   1 needle holder
   1 tissue forceps with teeth
   2 straight Kelley hemostats
   2 sponge forceps (Ring forceps, sponge sticks) to sponge away the blood when inspecting the cervix and vagina for lacerations.
   2 or 3 Allis forceps to rupture membranes or aid in repairing the episiotomy.

Add the bulb syringe and gloves for the doctor. Since these require less sterilization time than instruments, they must be added separately. If the table is not to be used right away, cover it with a double cover and mark the date and time that you set up the table. If there is going to be a delivery soon, proceed with setting up the rest of the room.

Check the incubator to see that it is plugged in and warm for the baby. Set up the basin set which is usually in a double ring stand. If two basins are provided, one is for the placenta. The other is the splash basin into which sterile water or saline is poured. The doctor uses it for lubricating instruments, rinsing his gloves, or cleansing the patient. Set up the perineal preparation tray. This tray usually includes:

Basin for the cleansing solution
Sterile gauze sponges or cotton balls
Sterile gloves or sponge sticks
Flask of sterile water or saline for rinsing
Antiseptic to be used on the skin following the cleansing of the area.

While opening sterile packs and circulating in the delivery room, make sure you

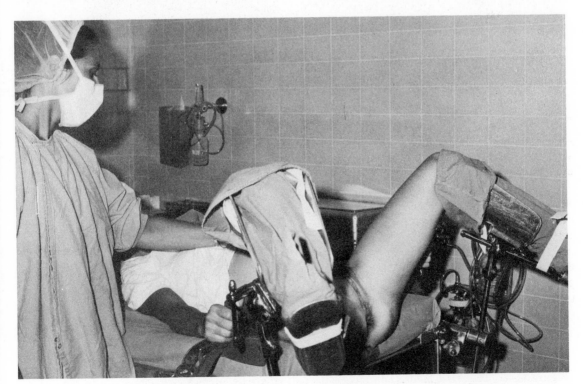

Figure 11-2. The patient is positioned on the delivery table ready for delivery.

apply the following principles of surgical asepsis:

Never turn your back on a sterile field.

Do not reach across a sterile field.

In pouring solutions, do not allow the unsterile outside rim of the container to touch the sterile receiving basin and do not hold the container so high that the solution splashes when poured.

Keep the tips of the transfer forceps down.

Hold your hands and elbows high, above the waist, when setting up a pack or table.

Be careful not to brush up against anything sterile with your scrub dress.

After the patient has been draped for delivery, slide your hands carefully under the drapes to time contractions (Fig. 11-2).

After you have set up the delivery room two or three times, you will discover how quickly and easily you can do it.

Transporting the Mother to the Delivery Room

In some hospitals the patient remains in the labor bed which is equipped with wheels and is narrow enough to fit through doorways. Before moving the bed, make sure all of the electrical attachments have been removed or unplugged. If the labor bed cannot be used, the patient will have to be moved by stretcher.

If it is a hospital that does not allow the husband in the delivery room, or if he does not plan to be there, the husband and wife should have a few moments to embrace and say good-bye. If the husband is going to be in the delivery room, now is the time for him to change into his "attire." He may wear essentially the same delivery room attire as the doctor.

If the patient is pushing very actively,

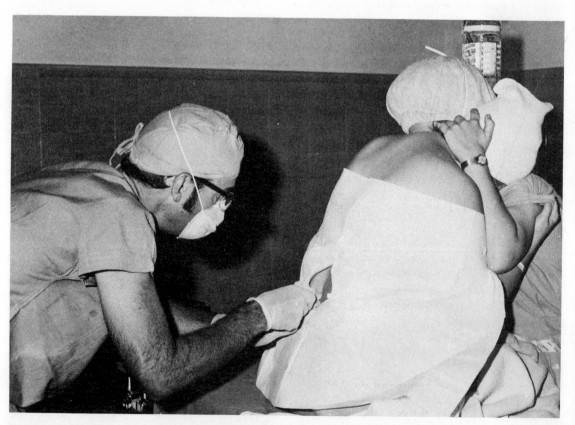

Figure 11-3. The nurse holds and supports the patient while the physician administers a saddle block for delivery.

and you would like her to slow down at this point, have her pant with the contractions. Remember to give her short commands rather than lengthy instructions. Positive statements such as "pant" are preferable to negative ones such as "don't push." Demonstrating by panting along with her may be helpful.

The patient can usually move herself fairly well from labor bed to stretcher and from stretcher to the delivery table if you help her and wait until she is not having a contraction. If she has an intravenous infusion running, someone should hold her arm and the IV bottle as she is moving from one place to another to prevent the IV from infiltrating.

Safety should be uppermost in your thoughts as you transfer the patient. The bed and the stretcher should be firmly aligned while the patient is moving. If time permits, fasten the safety straps around her knees. And instruct her to keep her arms close to her body as you move the stretcher through narrow doorways.

Assisting with Anesthesia

Spinal (Saddle Block)

When the nurse knows that the patient is to receive a "saddle block," she has the patient sit up on the side of the delivery table with her feet supported on a stool. The spinal tray, sterile gloves, and an anesthetic agent such as Carbocaine, procaine, or Xylocaine have been placed in readiness for the anesthesiologist or obstetrician. At least two pillows are needed to support the patient's head and shoulders following the administration of the anesthetic.

The nurse supports the patient physically by standing in front of her and holding her; she supports her emotionally by being with her and explaining what is going to happen. The physician prepares the skin in the lumbar region, at about the level of the iliac crests, with a suitable antiseptic. Before the spinal needle is inserted, the patient is instructed to bend forward to widen the space between the vertebrae. The nurse continues to hold and support her and cautions her not to move when the needle is being inserted (Fig. 11-3). It may be difficult for the patient to hold still, because of frequent and hard contractions. The needle is in the proper position when the spinal fluid drips from its hub. Then the anesthetic agent is injected between contractions. After 30 seconds have elapsed, the patient is assisted to a recumbent position with her head and shoulders elevated on pillows.

Because the anesthetic agent used for a "saddle block" is hyperbaric, that is heavier than the spinal fluid, it settles into the lower part of the spine and anesthetizes the abdomen, the inner aspects of the thighs, the vulva, and the perineum. In addition, the patient is usually unable to move her legs. Pillows are used to prevent the level of anesthesia from rising which could cause paralysis of the diaphragm resulting in respiratory arrest.

Advantages of this type of anesthetic are that the patient is awake and can see the baby being born, and there is no effect on the baby. Low, outlet forceps may be used to deliver the baby because the mother frequently loses her urge to push. Disadvantages are that it must be given by a skilled person, and a small percentage of patients develop a spinal headache in the postpartum period.

Trilene

This is a self-administered anesthetic which is commonly found in hospital delivery rooms. The patient can use it in a Duke inhaler. A capful of Trilene is poured into the metal cylinder, and the vapors are inhaled through a rubber mask. The Duke inhaler may be fastened to the patient by means of a wrist strap.

The nurse instructs the patient to breathe in the Trilene during a contraction. When the patient begins to fall asleep, her hand and the mask fall away, so that there is no danger of her receiving too much anesthetic. Since it is a potent anesthetic, there is danger if the nurse holds the mask for the patient. The nurse helps the patient use the Trilene mask chiefly by telling her when to use it (by feeling when she has a contraction) and encouraging her to use it with contractions.

An advantage of Trilene is that it can be used in smaller maternity departments where anesthetists or anesthesiologists are not available. A disadvantage is that the patient cannot be given an anesthetic following the use of Trilene, which is administered by the closed circuit method, because this has been known to produce cardiac irregularities.

Positioning

It is ideal to have two people assist the patient onto the delivery room table, one on each side. However, if this is not possible, one person can manage alone. After the patient is situated on the delivery table, have her move down so that her buttocks are at the separation between the upper half and lower half of the table. Usually the bottom half is rolled away during prepping and delivery so that the nurse and doctor are in close proximity to the perineum. This is called "breaking the table."

Then the stirrups are put into place and are adjusted in height and length so as to fit the patient and be as comfortable as possible. Cloth leggings are put on, and the patient's legs are lifted together to help prevent undue strain on the inner thigh muscles and pelvic ligaments. The nurse may put the patient up in stirrups when she knows the doctor has almost finished scrubbing and will soon be in the room or when the anesthetist gives her a signal to do so. The lights have been turned on, the sterile covers removed from the delivery table, sterile packs and basins opened, solutions poured, and the patient's chart brought into the room.

Sterile Perineal Prep

The next step in preparing the patient for delivery is to do a sterile perineal prep. The purpose is to cleanse the skin and remove secretions that have accumulated on the external genitalia and surrounding parts during labor.

Although the procedure and equipment vary among hospitals, the principles are the same: (1) Cleanse away from the vagina to prevent infection. Cleanse the rectum last. (2) Rub briskly enough to remove the secretions. (3) Work rapidly—if delivery is imminent, there may not be enough time to do a complete prep.

Suggested Procedure

As soon as the table is broken, the circulating nurse moves the sterile prep tray in close proximity to the patient's perineum. She uncovers the tray and puts on a pair of sterile gloves. Then she proceeds to cleanse the abdomen, thighs, and entire perineal area with soap or an antiseptic solution. For the comfort of the patient the solutions used should be warm.

Picking up a sponge (or cotton balls) that has been immersed in the soap solution, she starts at the mons pubis and washes from side to side on the abdomen until she reaches the umbilicus. The sponge is then discarded. With the second and third sponges she washes the thighs, starting at the outer aspect of the labia majora and continuing outward using an up-and-down motion to the knee. Each sponge is discarded after use. The fourth and fifth sponges are used to cleanse the labia on the right and left sides of the vagina. A single stroke from the mons pubis to the rectum is made on each side. However, care is taken to avoid touching the rectum. The last cleansing sponge is brought down the midline, from the clitoris over the urinary meatus, vagina, and down over the rectum.

Using the same technique, the nurse rinses the patient with sterile water or saline and an antiseptic such as aqueous Zepharin 1:1000, or she sprays or paints on Tincture of Merthiolate. Having completed the prep, the nurse removes the pad from under the patient's buttocks and stands by to "guard" the perineum until the doctor is ready to take over. With the patient's legs up in stirrups and with the patient pushing, the baby could be born at any minute.

The Delivery

While the doctor is draping the patient, the circulating nurse moves the delivery table and basin set into position. She adjusts the overhead light so that it focuses on the patient's perineum and she adds any additional supplies or instruments, such as forceps, to the delivery room table.

If there is no anesthetist, the nurse can stay with the patient at the head of the table, talking to her, coaching her, and giving her support. She should continue to monitor her blood pressure and the fetal heart tones. If the husband is there, he should also be at the head of the table, perhaps seated on a stool where the anesthetist usually is. Often a mirror is attached to an overhead light which can be adjusted so that the couple can watch the birth of the baby, if they so desire.

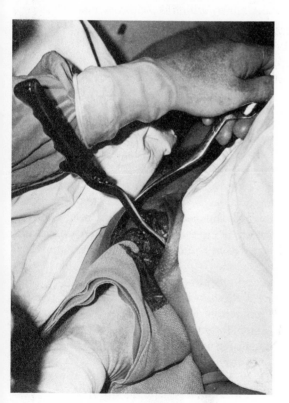

Figure 11-4. A forceps delivery.

If the mother is a primigravida, the doctor will frequently do an episiotomy and apply forceps to shorten the second stage of labor. He may also deliver a multipara in this manner if he feels that it is warranted.

Forceps Deliveries

The main use of forceps is for traction, that is, drawing the baby's head through the birth canal (Fig. 11-4). They may also be used for rotation. If the baby is in an undesirable position for delivery, the doctor may turn him so that he can be delivered more easily. Forceps deliveries are classified according to whether they are elective or indicated. Elective forceps deliveries are by far the most frequent, ranging between 15 and 50 per cent of all deliveries.

Indicated forceps deliveries occur in only 1.6 to 10 per cent of all deliveries. Some of the maternal indications are toxemia, heart disease, and exhaustion. Examples of fetal indications are irregular heartbeat, fetal heart tones below 100, and prolapsed cord. One reason for the large number of forceps deliveries in the United States is that mothers receive medications in labor which dull their urge to push.

Many obstetricians deliver almost all of their primigravidas with low elective forceps. It saves many minutes of exhaustive bearing down for the mother and prevents excessive pounding of the baby's head on the perineum. In some primigravidas there is a great deal of resistance by the perineum and vaginal outlet; they are said to have "tough" perineums.

Forceps deliveries are classified according to the station of the presenting part when they are applied. The most frequent are low or outlet forceps deliveries; the head must be well down on the perineal floor and the scalp partly visible at the time the blades are applied. Mid-forceps delivery is used when the head is higher in the pelvis but has already become engaged. High forceps delivery means that blades are applied before engagement has taken place. It is rarely used and is a very dangerous practice.

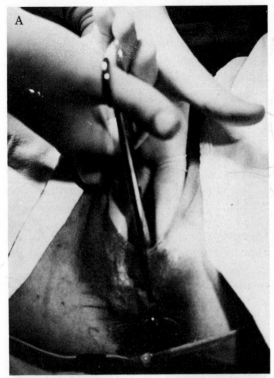

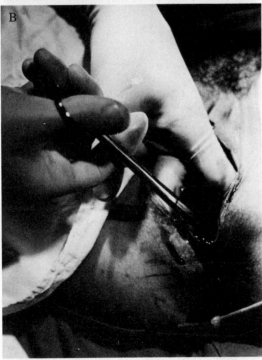

Figure 11-5. (A) In making a midline (median) episiotomy the scissors are pointed down toward the rectum. (B) The incision is completed.

There are many different kinds of forceps in use, including Simpson's, Kielland's, Elliott's, Luikart's and Tucker McLean forceps. All of them are used for cephalic presentation, but some are used for special maneuvers, such as a forceps rotation. If the baby is in a breech position, Piper forceps are often used. However, a baby in a breech presentation can deliver spontaneously. Piper forceps are unusually long forceps used to extract the head, which comes last. The nurse may anticipate the doctor's needs by having Piper forceps on hand if she knows it will be a breech birth.

Before applying forceps, the doctor checks to make sure that the cervix is completely dilated, the membranes are ruptured, and the bladder is empty.

Episiotomy

An episiotomy, which is an incision into the perineum to facilitate delivery, is the most common operation in obstetrics. An episiotomy which is properly repaired leaves the pelvic muscles and perineal tissues in almost the same condition as before the baby was delivered.

Episiotomies are done almost routinely on primigravidas, although they are frequently done on multiparas as well. They prevent undue stretching of the vaginal vault and perineal muscles, which can lead to prolapse of the uterus, cystocele, and rectocele in later life.

There are two kinds of episiotomies: the median, which is directed straight down toward the rectum, and the mediolateral, which is directed laterally and downward away from the rectum. Thus, there may be a right mediolateral episiotomy or a left mediolateral episiotomy.

A median episiotomy (Fig. 11-5) is more comfortable for the patient, heals better, is easier to repair, and presents fewer problems with dyspareunia (painful intercourse). The chief disadvantage is that it is more likely to extend down through the rectum than a mediolateral episiotomy.

In addition to shortening the second

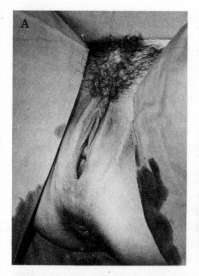 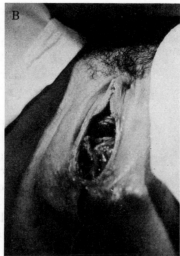 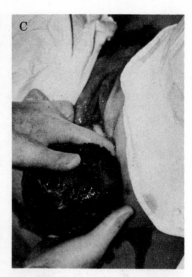

Figure 11-6. (A) In a spontaneous delivery the head appears at the vaginal introitus and distends the perineum. Note that the anus is dilated. (B) Crowning takes place. (C) The head rotates to one side (external rotation) and is again in the same position as it was when the baby was within the uterus.

stage of labor, an episiotomy prevents a ragged contused laceration, is easier to repair and heals better, and spares the baby's head from battering on the perineum (prolonged pounding may cause brain injury).

When the nurse observes that the physician has performed an episiotomy, she can bring suturing material (usually 00 or 000 chromic catgut) to the delivery table. Since chromic catgut is absorbable, the stitches do not have to be removed.

Lacerations

During delivery, lacerations of the perineum and vagina may occur because the head delivers too suddenly or "pops" out. In these instances the doctor probably has not had time to do an episiotomy. Even in the most carefully controlled deliveries, lacerations are often unavoidable because the tissues are so friable.

Perineal lacerations are classified according to the extent of the tear as first degree, second degree, and third degree. First degree lacerations involve tearing of the skin and mucous membrane only. They are fairly common and may require only a

few stitches or maybe none at all. Second degree lacerations involve skin, mucous membrane, and the muscles of the perineum (including the perineal body). They require repair similar to that of the usual episiotomy. Third degree lacerations include tearing of the rectal sphincter. They require extensive repair and could cause permanent damage. A third degree laceration can result from the extension of a midline episiotomy.

Spontaneous Delivery

When the mother is awake for delivery, she is able to bear down with her contractions and push the baby out. As she bears down, the baby's head gradually distends the perineum to a diameter of from 6 to 8 cm. To prevent lacerations the physician supports the perineum with one hand covered with a sterile towel. With the fingers of the other hand he gently controls the egress of the head from the birth canal (Fig. 11-6).

If the skin of the perineum appears tight and blanched, he performs an episiotomy at this time. There should be no hurry in delivering the baby, and the head should pref-

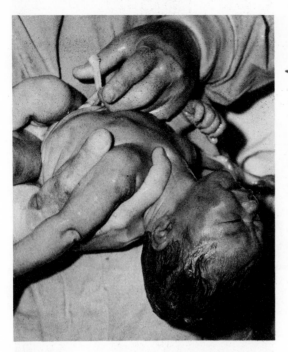

Figure 11-7. The physician must have a secure grip on the baby when clamping the cord.

the birth certificate and other legal documents.

The infant usually cries immediately, and the doctor holds him up for the mother to see. The cord is then clamped and cut (Fig. 11-7). If the patient is Rh negative, the nurse may remind the doctor. A sample of cord blood from the placenta is taken to be sent to the laboratory for a stat Coombs test.

After making sure that the baby is breathing satisfactorily and after inspecting it, the doctor hands the baby over to the nurse. She is ready to receive him into a sterile blanket or drape which covers the front of her scrub dress. Thus, when the doctor hands her the baby, he will not contaminate his gloves. Along with the baby,

erably be delivered between contractions. The mother may complain of a splitting sensation at this moment, due to the extreme stretching of the vagina as the head is born.

Often the doctor begins to suction the baby's mouth and nose as soon as the head has rotated to the side (external rotation). Then he feels around the baby's neck to see if the cord is wrapped around it. If so, and it is loose, he slips it over the baby's head. If the cord is tight, he must clamp and cut it immediately before delivering the rest of the baby.

In delivering the anterior shoulder, the physician exerts traction downward until it slips under the symphysis pubis. Then he lifts upward to deliver the posterior shoulder. The rest of the baby slips out easily accompanied by a rush of waters and blood. The nurse notes the exact time when the baby was born by looking at the delivery room clock when *all* of the baby (not just the head) has been delivered. This is the official time of birth which is recorded on

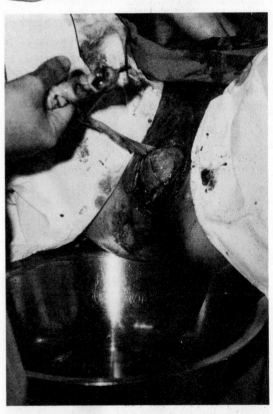

Figure 11-8. The doctor exerts mild pressure on the fundus and pulls gently on the cord to deliver the placenta. After the placenta is delivered, the intact placenta, membranes and cord are placed in a sterile placenta basin.

he gives the nurse the bulb syringe he has been using to suction the infant. Returning to the mother, he sees if she is bleeding too heavily, then turns his attention to the delivery of the placenta or repair of the perineum.

Delivery of the Placenta

If the mother is awake, she will also be able to cooperate in pushing out the placenta. During most deliveries an oxytocin such as Pitocin, Methergine, or ergonovine is given either intravenously or intramuscularly to the mother at the time that the anterior shoulder is being born. Contractions of the uterus start up again shortly thereafter due to the action of the oxytocic medication.

Frequently the physician delivers the placenta by manual expression; that is, he exerts pressure on the fundus (Fig. 11-8).

However, he must be sure that the placenta has *separated* from the uterine wall. Too firm pressure on the uterus, particularly if it is relaxed, accompanied by pulling on the cord may cause inversion of the uterus, a very serious complication.

Signs which indicate that the placenta has separated are: (1) the uterus rises up in the abdomen to or above the umbilicus (evidence of a retroplacental hemorrhage). (See normal physiology of the third stage of labor.) (2) The cord lengthens a few inches through the vulva. (3) There is an increased amount of bleeding from the vagina, ranging in amount from a trickle to a gush of blood.

After the placenta is delivered, it should be inspected to make sure it is intact. Then the doctor inspects the cervix and vagina for lacerations and repairs the episiotomy or any perineal lacerations.

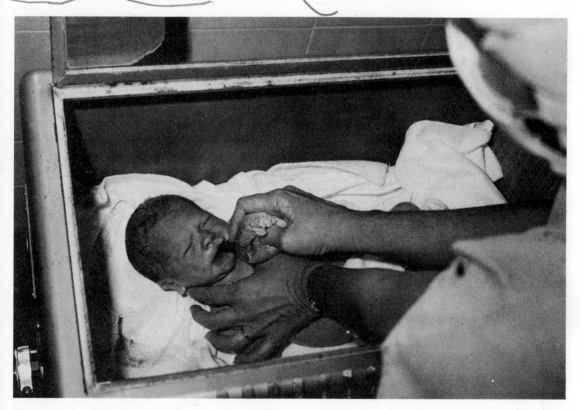

Figure 11-9. Immediately following delivery the baby is placed in a heated incubator where the nurse suctions the newborn with a rubber bulb syringe.

IMMEDIATE CARE OF THE NEWBORN

Establishing Respirations

The first principle in the immediate care of the newborn is to clear his airway in order to establish respirations. The lungs immediately take over the respiratory function of the placenta; this is why the newborn needs prompt attention to see that he begins breathing almost at once. Most normal babies begin breathing within one minute after birth. A strong cry is evidence that his respiratory system has begun to function well.

Some babies have a delay in the onset of respirations, or respiratory movements are made shortly after birth but are not sustained. With these infants, resuscitation must be carried out to prevent asphyxia. Asphyxia progresses rapidly if not treated and will result in damage to brain cells or in the death of the infant.

Clearing the Air Passages

Fluid, mucus, and sometimes blood and meconium are present in the baby's mouth, nose, and pharynx at birth. To prevent the baby from aspirating this material with his first breath, postural drainage is instituted immediately after birth. The baby is held by his feet with his head down and neck extended. Various equipment is used to suction the baby, but a bulb syringe and a mucous trap with a soft rubber catheter on the end are most common (Fig. 11-9). The catheter may be more effective than the bulb syringe because it reaches farther into the throat. The baby is placed in a supine position with his head lowered. Suctioning must be gentle to prevent injury to the mucous membrane, and brief—less than one minute is recommended. If the baby seems sleepy, gentle rubbing of his back along the spine or flicking the soles of his feet may stimulate him to cry.

Another high priority is to keep him warm. He should be wiped dry with the blanket and wrapped in a clean warm blanket. Modern delivery rooms are equipped with incubators and/or radiant warmers to maintain the temperature of the baby. In an air-conditioned delivery room, the baby's temperature will drop suddenly if he isn't kept warm. The infant is placed on his right side when placed in the incubator because this causes increased pressure in the left side of the heart to close the foramen ovale.

Observation of the Newborn

The Apgar Scoring System was developed in 1952 by Dr. Virginia Apgar, an anesthesiologist. It serves as a basis for comparing newborns collectively to better evaluate obstetric practices, obstetric analgesics, and the effects of resuscitation.

Five signs are evaluated within 60 seconds of birth, and again 5 minutes after the birth of the infant. Each sign is given a score of 0, 1, or 2 (Table 11-1); a combined score of 10 is considered perfect. The eval-

Table 11-1.   APGAR SCORING CHART

Sign	0	1	2
Heart rate	absent	below 100	above 100
Respiratory rate	absent	slow, irregular	good, crying
Muscle tone	limp	some flexion of extremities	active motion
Reflex irritability	no response	grimace	cough or sneeze
Color	blue, pale	body pink; extremities blue	completely pink

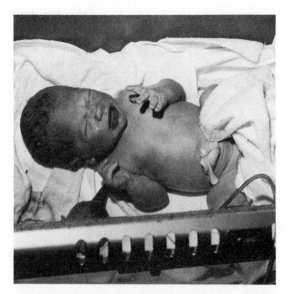

Figure 11-10. This infant probably rates a good Apgar score. Note the crying and the good muscle tone.

uation can be done by the doctor, nurse, anesthetist, or student nurse.

The heart rate is the first and most important sign to assess. If it is below 100, usually some other signs will be lacking. The reflex irritability sign is elicited by a brief tangential slap on the sole of the foot. The color is the least important sign in scoring. Almost all infants have cyanosis of their hands and feet at birth. According to the scoring system, a baby receiving an Apgar score of from 7 to 10 is considered vigorous (Fig. 11-10); a score of 4, 5, 6 indicates that the baby is mildly to moderately depressed and may require resuscitation; an 0 to 4 score indicates the baby is depressed and definitely requires resuscitation.

Resuscitation of the Newborn

Prevention of Asphyxia

The old saying "An ounce of prevention is worth a pound of cure," is applicable here. Since asphyxia of the newborn can result in permanent brain damage and even death, there are several principles of prevention that deserve our consideration as nurses.

Thoughtful prenatal care. Proper pre-

natal care reduces the probability of complications in the mother and infant which may result in asphyxia.

Cautious and individualized selection and use of drugs. Because individuals vary greatly in their response to medications, analgesics and anesthetics should not be routinely administered to women in labor.

Diligent observation throughout labor for causes and signs of fetal distress. For example, making an early detection of irregular or too rapid or too slow fetal heart tones, and reporting them promptly to the physician may prevent asphyxia of the newborn.

Judicious use of oxytocics to induce labor. If it is an elective induction, the patient should be at full term; her pelvis, large enough; and her cervix, ripe.

Use of appropriate operative procedures. Rather than allowing the patient to remain in labor for a prolonged period of time which could cause fetal distress, a decision to do a forceps delivery or cesarean section may prevent asphyxia.

Careful selection of techniques for pain relief. In the absence of experienced anesthetists, a local or pudendal block is the safest procedure for pain relief.

Free discussion of problems through consultation. When a physician encounters an abnormality or problem, he should consult with one or more experts, such as a board-certified obstetrician and gynecologist, before deciding on treatment and management of the patient.

Causes of Asphyxia

The most common cause is the use of drugs and anesthesia. The combination of depressant drugs such as Demerol with inhalation anesthesia will result in asphyxia in the infant. The main sign is slowed fetal heart tones. Treatment is aimed at delivering the baby as soon as possible, since mental retardation is caused by an anoxic condition in labor or during birth.

There are many other causes of asphyxia, such as infections in the mother or fetus (amnionitis); partial separation of the placenta, which reduces the blood supply to the fetus; a knot in the cord; a cord wrapped around the neck; compression of the cord; and aspiration of meconium.

Treatment and Nursing Care
What You Should Do:
1. Monitor the baby's heart rate; if oxygen is getting through, it will increase. *Do not* use drastic measures such as jack-knifing the baby, hot and cold tubbing, etc.
2. Place the baby in a warm crib; the baby will have no desire to breathe if it is cold. *Do not* let the baby get cold.
3. Place the baby in Trendelenburg position. *Do not* squeeze the baby. You could rupture the liver.
4. Hold the baby's chin forward.
5. Start giving oxygen immediately.
6. Resuscitate at 14 mm. of pressure.
7. Give oxygen 3 seconds on and 3 seconds off. Pressure must be intermittent. The pressure does not expand the alveoli, but delivers oxygen to the respiratory bronchioles. First effort of the baby to breathe is convulsive; then apply the oxygen according to the baby's respiratory rhythm.

If no other method is available, mouth-to-mouth breathing may be used. The principles of resuscitation are: get the baby's airway open; get oxygen into the lungs; keep the baby warm; handle the baby gently.

Use of Drugs. The use of respiratory stimulant drugs, such as α-lobeline and nikethamide, should be avoided. The reason is that they have a narcotic effect after the initial stimulating effect. Circulatory stimulants, such as caffeine sodium benzoate, may be occasionally used as supportive therapy. Opiate antagonists such as Nalline, are indicated only in cases of specific opiate depression.

Resuscitation Measures
Sensory Stimulation. Often a mildly to moderately depressed baby can be stimulated to take deep breaths and cry by slapping the soles of his feet or flicking a finger against his heels a few times.

Oxygen. A funnel or mask attached to freely flowing oxygen and held close to the baby's face increases the oxygen he inspires during his first breaths.

Mask and Bag Inflation. An Ambu bag or the Kreiselman resuscitator may be used. The mask is held snugly over the baby's face, and his chin is held up and forward. Oxygen is administered for a few seconds by intermittent pressure on the bag.

Mouth-to-Mouth Resuscitation. The baby is placed on his back, and the operator places his mouth over 2 to 3 layers of clean gauze if available or directly over the baby's mouth and nose. If the nose is not covered, it must be held closed so air will not escape through it. Breaths should be gentle so as not to injure the baby's lungs, and should be at the rate of about 20 per minute.

Direct Laryngoscopy and Tracheal Intubation. This method may be used first on a severely depressed baby but requires a skilled and experienced person, such as a pediatrician, or anesthetist. However, the nurse should know where the equipment is kept, should keep it in good repair, and should see that all parts are there.

Resuscitation of the newborn is a highly specialized skill which requires teamwork of the nurse, anesthetist, obstetrician, and pediatrician. When a resuscitation problem is anticipated, the nurse should notify the pediatrician or pediatric resident to be there for the delivery.

Care of the Umbilical Cord

The cord may be clamped immediately after birth or postponed for a few minutes until pulsation of the cord ceases. If there is a delay in clamping the cord or if the cord blood is stripped toward the baby before the cord is clamped, the baby will receive an added 50 to 100 cc. of blood from the placenta.

However, there are some instances when it is desirable to clamp the cord immediately. It may be necessary if the mother is deeply anesthetized to avoid further anesthesia to the baby. If there is an Rh problem, it may help to keep the serum bilirubin lower.

Various clamps are used, some of which are removed in 12 to 24 hours. Others are left on and drop off when the cord stump separates and falls off. Since there is danger of hemorrhage from faulty application of the cord clamp or tie, the nurse should observe for bleeding from the cord.

The cord is usually thick, white, and glistening in appearance. The white jelly-like material in the cord is called Wharton's jelly, and its function is to prevent compression of the blood vessels. It is important to observe and record the number of blood vessels in the cord. There should be three vessels: two arteries and a vein. If there are only two, this may be a clue that the baby has other congenital anomalies.

Care of the Eyes

The baby's eyes may be infected during birth if gonococcal organisms are present in the birth canal. Since the incidence of gonorrhea has increased in recent years, this is a real danger.

The Credé method of prophylactic eye treatment was introduced in 1881. Two

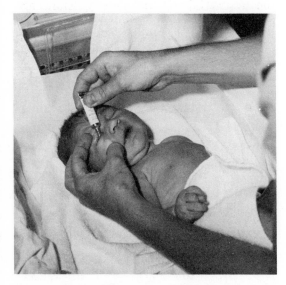

Figure 11-11. The nurse applies prophylactic antibiotic ointment to the newborn's eyes.

drops of a 1 per cent solution of silver nitrate are instilled into the conjunctival sac. The infant's eyes are then irrigated with distilled water or sterile saline solution, from the inner canthus outward. If the eyes are not irrigated, some infants develop a chemical conjunctivitis with marked edema of the eyelids and a thick yellow discharge. Treatment is required by law in all states in the United States to prevent blindness (ophthalmia neonatorum) caused by the gonococcus organism.

Antibiotic ointments may be used in some states instead of silver nitrate (Fig. 11-11.) They have the advantage of not being as caustic and irritating to the infant's eyes. Penicillin or Terramycin Ophthalmic Ointment, 1 per cent solution, is applied to the lower eyelid. A thin line of ointment is spread from the inner to the outer canthus and diffused over the infant's eye. Any excess ointment may be gently wiped away 15 minutes or so after the ointment has been applied. Prophylactic eye treatment may not be carried out in the delivery room, but will be done soon after the baby arrives in the newborn nursery.

Temperature

Because it is so vital to keep the newborn warm, the nurse takes the baby's temperature in the delivery room. If the baby has been placed under a radiant warmer, the temperature monitor is attached to his skin with paper tape.

Identification

The baby must be identified before the infant and mother are transferred from the delivery room. Plastic bands are attached to the wrist and ankle of the infant, and a matching band is attached to the mother's wrist. These three bands have the same serial number on them.

The minimum of identifying information includes the baby's sex, surname, mother's given name, and date and time of birth. Once the bands are applied, they should not be

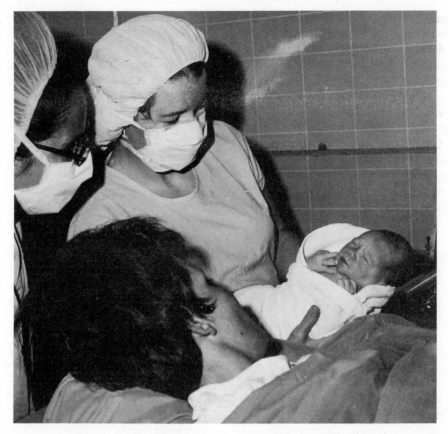

Figure 11-12.   The mother gets a good look at her baby.

removed until after the baby is discharged from the hospital.

Some hospitals footprint the baby and add the mother's fingerprint on the same sheet of paper as a supplemental means of identifying the baby in case doubt arises. However, unless footprinting or finger-printing is done by an expert, it is doubtful if it has any real value in establishing proof of identity.

Observe for Abnormalities

Careful inspection of the baby for gross abnormalities such as supernumerary dig-its, clubfoot, hypospadias, imperforate anus, birthmarks, should be carried out by the delivery-room nurse. The nurse should also check the general appearance of the baby to see if it needs to be placed in an incubator or isolette or requires any other special care such as oxygen.

Before the mother and infant leave the delivery room, the mother may wish to hold her infant (Fig. 11-12). In case the mother is still sleepy, the nurse should remain at her side while she is holding the infant. Then the infant is placed back in the in-cubator and wrapped warmly, to be taken to the newborn nursery. The bulb syringe or mucous trap should be left in the incubator with the infant in case he needs suctioning along the way.

IMMEDIATE CARE OF THE MOTHER

Following delivery, the mother's legs are lifted simultaneously from the stirrups and placed close together in order to prevent ex-cessive bleeding. Perineal pads are applied, and a T-binder may be used to hold them in place while the patient is being transported from the delivery room to the obstetrical recovery room.

The mother may be very happy, exhilarated, and relieved that it's all over. The mother is very tired, but she usually wants to see and hold her baby and be reunited with her husband, if only briefly. Some mothers, especially those who have had their babies by natural childbirth methods, may want to nurse the baby right away on the delivery table.

The new mother may have a shaking chill which is due to sudden release of intraabdominal pressure and emotional tension. A woman who has a rapid labor and delivery is more prone to this reaction following delivery because she has not had enough time to adjust physically or emotionally to the rapid sequence of events. The nurse can reassure the mother that this is normal and can help her change into a clean dry hospital gown and apply warm cotton blankets until the chill passes.

The patient's blood pressure and pulse, the condition of the fundus, and the amount of lochia (vaginal bleeding) are checked before she leaves the delivery room. The fundus should be firm and at the level of the umbilicus, or slightly below. If there is no excessive bleeding and the fundus is firm, and the pulse and blood pressure are within normal limits, the mother and baby are transported to the recovery room and nurs-

ery respectively. If the husband, grandparents, or other family members are there, the family is reunited, and they all have a chance to see the baby. This is often an exciting and joyous moment for the new parents, the relatives, and the members of the labor and delivery room team.

BIBLIOGRAPHY

Bonica, J.: Principles and Practices of Obstetric Analgesia and Anesthesia. Philadelphia, F. A. Davis, 1967.

Eastman, N. J., and Hellman, L. M.: Williams Obstetrics, ed. 13. New York, Appleton-Century-Crofts, 1966.

Fitzpatrick, E. et al.: Maternity Nursing, ed. 12. Philadelphia, J. B. Lippincott, 1971.

Hazlett, W.: The male factor in obstetrics. Child and Family, *6(4)*: 3, 1967.

Iorio, J.: Effective support during labor and delivery. R.N. *25*: 70-74, 88, 1962.

Juziviak, M.: A common sense approach to labor and delivery. R.N., *27:*53-58, 1964.

Leifer, G.: Principles and Techniques in Pediatric Nursing. Philadelphia, W. B. Saunders, 1965.

Marlow, D.: Textbook of Pediatric Nursing, ed. 3. Philadelphia, W. B. Saunders, 1969.

Montgomery, T.: Immediate care of the newborn. Clin. Obstet. Gynec., *5:*30-43, 1962.

Newton, N., and Newton, M.: Mothers' reactions to their newborn babies. J.A.M.A. *181:*206-210, 1962.

Suggested Reading for Further Study

LaFever, J.: View from the side of the table. Amer. J. Nurs., *63:*67, 1963.

Maternity Center Association: A Baby Is Born, ed. 3. New York, 1960.

Deliveries by the Nurse and Emergency Deliveries *12*

There are numerous circumstances in which a nurse may be called upon to assist with or conduct a delivery. Sometimes she helps to deliver a baby in the emergency room or the labor room, on a stretcher, or in an elevator or car. In any such situation the nurse will need her ingenuity to use whatever materials and equipment she has on hand.

PRECIPITATE DELIVERY

When a nurse spends any length of time in a labor and delivery department, sooner or later she will probably have the experience of "catching" a baby. This situation arises when a woman has a rapid labor or when the doctor has not been called in time or is delayed in arriving at the hospital. These are often called precipitate deliveries, which usually means that the delivery was unsterile and/or the doctor was not there. (A precipitate labor is something else. It is by definition a labor which lasts 3 hours or less.)

An unsterile delivery occurs when there has not been time to do the sterile skin preparation and apply the sterile drapes prior to delivery. It is important to note on the delivery room record if a delivery is unsterile. There is a greater probability of infection in the mother and infant as a result. However, an unsterile delivery is no disgrace. It can happen to anyone. If a labor and delivery department has a high percentage of unsterile deliveries, it may indicate that patients in labor are not being closely observed. It is well to remember that in other countries of the world cleanliness for deliveries rather than sterility is emphasized.

It is important to remember that when a woman is about to deliver it is dangerous to do anything to hold the baby back, such as holding the mother's legs together or giving the mother general anesthesia to prevent her from delivering. It is much safer to allow the baby to be born. Holding the baby back could cause possible brain damage to the baby and could tear or even rupture the mother's uterus.

Most labor and delivery departments of any size have a compact set of equipment called an Emergency Delivery Pack. The nurse should know where this pack is located so that she can get it at a moment's notice. If delivery may be close at hand it is wise for the nurse to take this pack along, if the woman is going to another department, such as x-ray, which is outside the labor and delivery department. This sterile pack should contain a bulb syringe or mucous trap, a baby blanket, placenta basin, instruments and scissors for cutting the cord, a cord clamp or tie, and so forth.

EMERGENCY DELIVERY*

In any emergency situation the nurse should know the basic principles of conducting a normal delivery. A nurse may also be

---

*Source: This section is adapted from Assisting at the Birth of a Baby after Enemy Attack if No Doctor is Available. Maternal and Child Health of the New York State Department of Health.

called upon to teach lay people, such as policemen and firemen, how to deliver babies. Since most deliveries are uncomplicated, anyone can be taught how to help.

The nurse or any other person who is called upon to assist in delivering babies should remember first and foremost the importance of staying calm. It is a tall order to stay calm if you do not feel calm. However, nothing will be gained by being panicky. In fact, all it will do is increase the anxiety of the mother. Secondly, stay with the expectant mother. It may not be possible to stay during the entire first stage of labor, but as delivery becomes imminent, during the transition phase, there should be someone with the mother constantly. If it is not possible for the nurse to be with her, then her husband or any other responsible person will reassure her by being at her side.

If the emergency delivery occurs at the side of a road or in a bomb shelter, the nurse will have very little equipment with which to work. She may use her finger to stroke the infant's throat to remove mucus, wrap the baby and placenta together in a coat for warmth, and leave the cord uncut until such time as sterile scissors and cord tapes are available.

The following procedure can be followed by the nurse or lay person in conducting a delivery.

During Labor

Try to select as clean a place as possible for the birth to occur. When the contractions come close together (every two minutes in a primigravida and every four minutes in a multipara) have the expectant mother lie down. Prior to this time the woman can walk, sit, squat, or get into whatever position is most comfortable for her. If the membranes rupture, have her lie down; the cord might prolapse if she is walking about. Have her lie down if it appears that the baby is about to be born.

Keep your hands clean by washing them frequently. Keep your hands away from the mother's vagina and instruct her to do the same. The hands-off policy is to prevent infection from entering the vagina and spreading into her reproductive organs.

Reassure the expectant mother. Tell her frequently that she is doing a good job. If you can tell her that everything is progressing normally, without false reassurance, this information will boost her confidence. Allow her to sleep and rest as much as possible. There is a natural relaxation and resting phase during the first stage of labor in which the woman can relax and even doze off to sleep between contractions.

You can take some of the following comfort measures which may help her. Tell her that deep slow breathing with each contraction will ease her discomfort. Rub the lower part of her back (sacral region) if she is experiencing the back pain that frequently accompanies labor. Suggest that she urinate every two hours. A full bladder may retard the progress of the baby as it descends. An empty bladder is also more comfortable for the expectant mother.

If her labor is long, offer her easily digestible foods and fluids. Offer drinking water if you are sure it is safe. A woman in labor needs the energy that food provides. Fluids prevent dehydration. Do not let the mother push down or strain during early labor. It does no good and only makes her tired. Pushing before the cervix is completely dilated may cause the cervix to become edematous and may retard its dilatation. Look at her perineum frequently to see if there is bulging or if the scalp of the baby appears at the vaginal opening.

If possible, prepare the following items in order to tie the baby's cord:

1. At least two pieces of strong white cotton tape, strips of strong cloth, or strong ribbon one half inch wide and 12 inches long. It would be desirable to have extra pieces of tape in case one is dropped. Flat-type shoelaces would be acceptable also. Never use string or thread because it may cut through the baby's cord.

2. A pair of scissors

3. Boil the tapes and scissors for at least

five minutes in a covered pan of water to sterilize them. The tapes and blades of the scissors should be covered by the water. Remove from the flame and drain off the water without touching the materials in the pan. Leave them in the covered pan until needed.

During Delivery

When the contractions are coming about every two minutes, scrub your hands and under your fingernails carefully for five minutes. Keep close watch on the mother and her perineum while you are scrubbing to observe for signs that delivery is imminent. Have the mother lie on her back with her knees bent up toward her abdomen. It may help her to push if she grasps under her thighs or over her knees during contractions. Place a clean piece of cloth, towel, sheet, or newspapers under the mother's hips. Have the mother push during contractions only when she has an urge to do so. You can explain that pushing may give her the feeling that she has to move her bowels. However, this feeling is due to pressure from the baby's head. Do not let her get up to go to the bathroom at this time as she may have the baby in the toilet.

Just before delivery, the contractions will be longer, stronger, and closer together. The membranes may rupture, if they have not already broken. When they break, there will be a sudden gush of water-like fluid. This is normal. The top of the baby's head will then be seen at the vaginal opening. The head will not recede between contractions as it may have previously.

As the baby's head begins to emerge, apply gentle pressure on the scalp to prevent the baby from popping out and tearing the vagina. With the other hand give support to the perineum using a towel or a part of the mother's clothing, such as her slip or dress. This is to prevent tearing of the perineum. Make sure that the mother stops pushing as the baby's head emerges so as not to tear the vagina and perineum. It will be easier for her to stop pushing if she opens her mouth and takes quick, short breaths, like panting.

As the baby's head is born, before the shoulders are delivered, check to see if the cord is around the baby's neck. If it is, gently slide it over the baby's head or shoulders. Next, you should gently but firmly direct the baby's head downward in order to deliver the top (anterior) shoulder. After the anterior shoulder is expelled lift the baby up toward the pubic bone to release the bottom (posterior) shoulder. Do not act in a hurry doing these maneuvers. Slow and easy does it. As the baby is born, support its head and body and let the baby slide into your arms. Providing support for the baby is especially important if the baby is small. Keeping the baby out of the amniotic fluid and blood which is between the mother's legs is also important, since the baby may aspirate the fluid as it takes its first breath.

Sometimes a baby is born surrounded by the membranes. As soon as the whole head appears, break the membranes immediately with your fingernails. This is so that the baby will not aspirate the amniotic fluid. It is usually easier to break the membranes just below the baby's nose because it is less tight there. Another suggested spot is at the back of the baby's head in the occipital region.

As the baby's feet are born, grasp his ankles firmly with one hand. Lift the baby by his ankles using your other hand to support his head. You will need to grasp him firmly since he will be very slippery. Holding him like this will keep him out of the fluid before he breathes and will let mucus drain from his mouth and respiratory passages. After the baby emerges, try not to touch the cord because of the danger of infection. Do not pull on the cord because of the danger of tearing it or turning the uterus inside out (inversion). A torn cord will bleed, and it is difficult to stop the bleeding.

Usually the baby will cry and breathe within a few seconds after birth. Since the mother has probably not had analgesics or anesthetics the baby is not sleepy and should have a good respiratory effort.

If the baby does not start breathing, you may institute the following procedures:

Try to clear the baby's throat of fluid and mucus by placing him on his side with his head lower than his feet. With the side of an index finger gently stroke the baby's throat in the center starting at the bottom of his neck and continuing to his chin. Massage the trachea in this way five or six times. It is important to get as much mucus out as possible before the baby takes a breath.

Gently rub his back to help stimulate his breathing.

Try to make the baby take a breath and cry by gently snapping the bottoms of his feet two or three times.

If these methods fail, start mouth-to-mouth resuscitation. With the baby's head back (hyperextended), cover his mouth and nose with your mouth and gently puff air into his lungs at the rate of one breath every five seconds.

Once the baby has started to breathe continue to observe him to make sure he does not stop. Place him on his mother's abdomen without pulling on the cord. Wrap him in a warm blanket or whatever is available. Have somebody keep a hand on the baby to prevent him from falling. The mother may be able to do this if you are alone.

Wait for the placenta to emerge by itself. It may take 15 to 30 minutes or more for the placenta to be delivered. You can tell if it has separated from the wall of the uterus when the cord lengthens three or four more inches. There may be a sudden gush or trickle of about a pint of blood. Ask the mother to push down with her next contraction in order to expel the placenta. Support the placenta with your hands as it comes out to prevent it from pulling on the cord.

After the placenta is delivered, wrap the baby and the placenta together in the blanket, towel, or coat with which you covered the baby. Then place them in the mother's arms. Every 15 minutes for an hour or two after delivery, feel the uterus to make sure that it is firm. It should have the consistency of a grapefruit and be at the level of the umbilicus or slightly below. The firmness of the uterus indicates that it is contracted and that blood vessels are closed off. This prevents excessive bleeding. Putting the baby to breast will help the uterus to remain contracted and thus control excessive bleeding.

If the uterus becomes soft (you can no longer feel it), bleeding may start. When this happens, use the flat parts of your fingers to gently but firmly massage the mother's lower abdomen. Use a circular motion while massaging until you feel that the uterus has become firm again.

Sometimes there is a great deal of bleeding, no matter what you do. If this should happen, get help to take the mother immediately to a doctor. Massage the uterus as necessary to keep it firm. Lower the mother's head as you would do for a patient who is in shock. Keep her warm by using blankets, coats, or anything available. Many women, after having a baby, have a chill and shaking of the extremities, especially the legs. The mother should be reassured that this is normal.

Care of the Baby

The same basic concepts apply to taking care of a baby in an emergency delivery situation as in a hospital or home situation where a doctor or midwife is in charge. First, respirations must be established, then warmth provided and the baby protected from injury and infection. Finally the baby should be observed for abnormalities and then identified.

There is no hurry about cutting the baby's cord. However, if other priorities in the care of the mother and baby have been or are being taken care of, and if you have scissors and tapes which have been boiled, you may want to tie and cut the cord. It is better to wait for boiled equipment because of the danger of infection. One of the organisms to be feared is the tetanus bacillus.

To tie and cut the cord scrub your hands again for five minutes. With one tape, tie a square knot around the cord about four to five inches from the baby's umbilicus. Be sure to tie it tightly enough so that there will not be any bleeding from the cord when it is cut. Use a second tape to tie a square knot around the cord about an inch or two nearer to the placenta. Cut the cord between the two ties.

After the cord is cut and you are ready to dispose of the placenta, wrap it in several thicknesses of newspaper, tie the package with cord, and dispose of it as you would refuse. If you are concerned that the placenta and membranes are not intact take it with you to the hospital or first-aid station for inspection.

If you do not cut the cord, and the placenta is left attached to the baby, be sure it is tucked snugly into the blanket or robe with him so that it does not fall and tear the cord if he is moved.

It is possible in the confusion which will exist in a disaster or other emergency situation that the mother and baby may be separated. For this reason some identifying information must be placed on both the baby and the mother. On a piece of smooth cloth write the full names of the mother and father, the date, the sex of the baby, and the time and place of the baby's birth. Then tie the cloth to the baby's ankle or wrist. Tie it tight enough so that it will not slip off, but not so tight as to stop circulation. Write the same information on another piece of cloth and tie it to the mother.

Do not wash the baby. The material which covers the baby at birth is a protection for its skin.

Later Care of the Baby

Keep the infant wrapped and warm and handle him gently. If the baby has trouble breathing because of mucus, lay him on a firm surface with his head to the side and with his head lower than his feet to facilitate the drainage of mucus. If he has a great deal of difficulty in breathing because of mucus or if he chokes on mucus, hold the baby up by his ankles with his head down for a short time.

The baby and mother will probably sleep for several hours after the birth. After about eight hours, the baby may be put to breast for feeding. Thereafter, have the baby nurse every three to four hours unless he is small. Low-birth weight babies (under five pounds) should not be fed for 24 hours. If the baby is under five pounds, try to get a doctor's advice about orders for his care, including when and what to start feeding him.

Later Care of the Mother

Make the mother as comfortable as possible. After washing your hands, place a clean pad, such as a folded sheet or towel about two feet square, under the mother's hips to receive the lochia. Change this pad as often as necessary. Sanitary pads may be used if they are clean.

Have the mother lie quietly on her back for two hours after delivery. Have her rest a few more hours if possible. After six to eight hours, have her get up for a short period of five to ten minutes. Try to have the mother void, if she has not done so before. Give her water to drink if safe water is available. Or offer her other fluids and foods. After the first eight hours, the mother may be able to do things for herself if she feels able. However, she should rest as much as possible for a few days.

When a Doctor is Required

If one or more of the following signs are present, it is necessary that the mother be taken to the nearest aid station or hospital and the condition reported to the doctor or nurse in charge:

1. If the mother has been told by her doctor that she has a serious condition which will require medical care during delivery, such as severe heart disease, diabetes, or a pelvis which is too small or narrow for the baby to be born.

2. If the mother has convulsions.

3. Excessive bleeding before delivery, or

a sudden gush, flow, or continuous trickle of blood or clotted blood.

4. Severe, continuous abdominal pain in addition to labor contractions.

5. Contractions which continue for more than 20 hours.

6. Excessive continuous bleeding after delivery. If the mother is saturating (soaking) a sanitary pad every half hour or is passing large blood clots, this is considered to be excessive bleeding.

7. Symptoms of shock: a rapid weak pulse, pale color, cold, clammy skin.

8. Unconsciousness.

9. "Shaking" chills and fever, other than the chills and shaking which occur immediately after delivery.

10. If the placenta has not been delivered one hour after the delivery of the baby.

11. If any part of the baby, other than the head, appears first at the vaginal opening.

BIBLIOGRAPHY

Fitzpatrick, E. et al.: Maternity Nursing, ed. 12. Philadelphia, J. B. Lippincott, 1971.

Melber, R.: The nurse's role in obstetrical emergencies in the hospital setting. Nurs. Clin. N. Am. 2:261-269, 1967.

Intrapartal Complications 13

TWINS

The birth of twins is a time of excitement for both the parents and the maternity department staff. Frequently, the parents have been told that they should expect two babies instead of one, but sometimes it comes as a shock and a surprise.

In general, there has been an increase in multiple births of all kinds in recent years. One of the reasons is the use of antisterility drugs, such as Clomid, which can cause multiple ovulation. There is a rising number of quintuplets and sextuplets being born throughout the world, but they do not receive quite as much publicity as they once did when such an event was extremely rare. The much publicized Dionne quintuplets born in Canada in the 1930's are said to have developed from a single ovum! Not too long ago, a woman who had been taking fertility drugs gave birth to nine infants, all weighing around one or two pounds each. All of them succumbed within about ten days of birth.

Incidence and Diagnosis

Twins occur approximately once in every 52 white births, but are more frequent among nonwhite races. There is definitely a genetic factor involved, because if there are twins on either side of the family, the father and mother are more likely to produce twins themselves. Another interesting fact is that if the woman is of higher parity and is older, her chances of having twins are greater.

A twin pregnancy may result from the fertilization of two separate ova or a single ovum. If two separate ova are fertilized, the twins are called dizygotic (two zygotes) or fraternal twins. When a single ovum is fertilized, monozygotic (one zygote) or identical twins develop. Fraternal twins may or may not be of the same sex and do not necessarily resemble one another more than other children of the same parents.

During pregnancy twins are suspected if the woman has an unusually large uterus for her period of gestation. Generally she has more of the discomforts and pressure symptoms than if she were carrying one baby. Complications such as toxemia and nausea and vomiting throughout pregnancy are more frequent. Dyspnea, edema, and varicosities are also more common and severe. The mother has greater difficulty in locomotion and is more tired because there are two active, kicking fetuses instead of one. The doctor makes the diagnosis by palpation, (two fetuses can be felt) auscultation (two heartbeats are heard), and x-rays. Listening to fetal heart tones is a very good way to make a diagnosis of twins. If two people, listening simultaneously, count the fetal heart rates for a full minute, and there is a difference of at least 10 beats between the two rates, twins are highly probable.

Ordinarily when a woman is carrying twins, each fetus occupies about one half of the uterus, with both lying longitudinally. Generally speaking, twins are smaller and

185

weigh less than single infants. However, their combined weight is usually greater than a single child's. Then too, one of them may die in utero while the other goes on to full development.

Labor and Delivery

It is not unusual that the onset of labor occurs two weeks or more prior to the expected date of delivery. This can be a blessing, but the parents may still be worried about the size of the babies. There is a difference in opinion about the length of labor; some authorities say that the majority of twin births are shorter than an ordinary single labor. The reason is that the cervix is completely effaced before labor actually begins, and the babies are usually smaller. Other experts disagree, because women carrying twins have a higher incidence of false labors and uterine inertia (dystocia).

The main difference in preparing for the delivery of twins is to get ready for two babies: have two heated incubators, two cord clamps, two bulb syringes, two identification bands, and so forth.

After the first twin is born, commonly designated as baby A, the doctor may have to rupture the membranes and deliver the second twin, baby B. Sometimes, he does a version, turning the baby from a cephalic to a breech presentation, and delivers the baby in that manner. Although it is a routine practice to give an oxytocin with the birth of the head or anterior shoulder of the baby, the mother should *not* be given an oxytocin with the birth of the first baby because this would cause the uterus to contract and make the delivery of the second baby difficult.

A frequent question is how does one know if the twins are identical or fraternal. Just because the babies are of the same sex, or size, or because they look alike, does not necessarily mean that they are identical. Examination of the placenta and membranes may offer some important clues. In identical twins there is one placenta with two umbilical cords. There is a single chorion with two amnions. (The amnion is the

membrane that lies closest to the baby.) For fraternal twins there are two placentas (but they may be fused giving the appearance of a single, large placenta), and there are two chorions and two amnions. Another definitive test is to compare all blood factors; there must be complete agreement for identical twins. Chromosomal studies may also establish whether the twins are identical or fraternal.

Postdelivery

The mother who has given birth to twins is more prone to postpartum hemorrhage as a result of the sudden release in intra-abdominal pressure and the abnormal over-distension of the uterus, with a resultant loss of tone (atony). Another cause of hemorrhage is that the doctor may have to remove the placenta manually due to the increased length of time between the birth of the two infants. Manual removal of the placenta is twice as frequent in twin births as in single deliveries.

Once the mother has passed the critical period following delivery, she begins to think about how she is going to feed and take care of two infants. It is perfectly possible for her to breast feed both infants if she so desires. Since breast milk is produced according to the law of supply and demand, she will be able to produce a sufficient quantity of milk.

In most instances, however, the mother decides to bottle feed, especially if the babies are small or if her husband or another person will be able to help her at feeding times. In the hospital the nurse usually feeds one of the babies while the mother feeds the other twin. Then they alternate the babies at the next feeding so that the mother becomes acquainted with both before discharge.

She should definitely be encouraged to have help at home for the first few weeks. Referrals to homemaker's service, a visiting nurse (in some communities), or the public health nurse may be appropriate. Diaper service should be advised if at all possible;

some diaper services offer special rates for twins. Parents can also be referred to child care books specifically about twins* and Parents-of-Twins clubs, which are found in some communities. Other parents who have had the experience of raising two children are good resource people and can provide a great deal of emotional support to the new parents. The nurse can steer the parents to these resources if they are not familiar with them.

INDUCTION OF LABOR

Having a baby "by appointment" is a fairly common practice throughout the United States. Although it is often done for the sake of convenience for both the mother and the doctor, there are definite medical indications for inducing labor. Induction of labor is defined as the bringing on of labor artificially after the period of viability.

When labor is to be induced, the patient arrives at the hospital at the appointed time and is admitted to the labor room in the usual manner. However, preparation of the patient may be more leisurely since she is not having contractions. Usually an enema is ordered to clean out the lower intestinal tract and possibly to stimulate uterine contractions. The mechanism by which this stimulation occurs is not fully understood.

The nurse may be responsible for setting up the intravenous infusion of Pitocin or may assist with rupturing the membranes. These are the two methods employed to stimulate the onset of contractions. In determining if the patient is a suitable candidate for induction, the physician checks the patient vaginally. The cervix should be ripe — soft and partially effaced and dilated. In addition, the fetus should be at term with the presenting part engaged in a vertex presentation.

An advantage of an elective induction of labor is that the attitude of the patient is

good. She also has an opportunity to arrange for care of her children at home, and her anxiety about reaching the hospital in time is obviated. Then too, she receives additional attention by having a physician sit with her throughout labor. There is some question as to whether the contractions of induced labor are more painful; however, there are fewer contractions.

In setting up an intravenous for induction, usually 5 units of Pitocin is added to 500 cc. of 5 per cent glucose in water, or 10 units in 1000 cc. The number of drops per minute can be regulated so that the IV is running very slowly; 14 to 20 drops per minute is average. The advantage of giving Pitocin by this method is that it can be better controlled because it can be stopped quickly. Pitocin acts directly on the muscles of the uterus, causing them to contract. Rhythmic contractions occur with intermittent periods of relaxation. However, because it is a powerful drug, it can cause a tetanic contraction. If a contraction is prolonged, lasting over 90 seconds, or if there is a change in the rate or regularity of the FHT's or signs of fetal distress, the IV should be stopped. This is one reason that the physician sits with the patient with his hand on the uterus. Severe lacerations of the cervix, rupture of the uterus, and anoxia of the baby are the dangers of tetanic contractions.

One way to set up IV's for induction is called the piggy back method. Two IV bottles are set up, one with the Pitocin added, and the other with plain glucose water. If it is necessary for the doctor to leave the patient's room, he can switch off the IV containing Pitocin and turn on the plain solution so that access to the vein is kept open.

Assisting the doctor with the rupturing of membranes is described in Chapter 10. Some physicians are somewhat reluctant to rupture the membranes because if the patient does not deliver, she is more susceptible to infection. Once the membranes are ruptured, the physician is committed to delivering the patient.

---

*Gebman, B.: Twins, Twice the Trouble, Twice the Fun. Philadelphia, Lippincott, 1965.
*Graham, P. The Care and Feeding of Twins. New York, Harper and Row, 1955.

Nursing Care

Even when a doctor is sitting at the bedside of the patient timing contractions, the patient still needs nursing care. Some doctors may make the nurse feel as if she is interfering, but the nurse is still responsible for providing nursing care. Checking the fetal heart tones, blood pressure, and pulse should be done more frequently than usual — every 20 minutes. If the nurse notices a prolonged contraction, in the event that the doctor has left the labor room, her first action is to shut off the IV immediately and then tell him about it.

The patient needs the same kind of physical care, emotional support, and comfort measures used throughout labor and delivery. The nurse and physician can cooperate to provide the best care for the patient.

Reasons for Induction

What are the medical and obstetrical indications for induction of labor? Patients with the following complications may have their labor induced:

Pre-eclampsia — because delivery of the baby may bring about remission of the disease

Diabetes mellitus — labor may be induced at 37 weeks because of the rapid aging of the placenta after this time if the pregnancy is allowed to continue

Premature rupture of the membranes with a viable fetus at term — to prevent amnionitis

Mild cases of premature separation of the placenta — to get the baby delivered as quickly as possible and prevent blood loss

Hypertensive cardiovascular and renal disease — to relieve the strain that pregnancy superimposes on these disease conditions

In summary, inductions have become commonplace and accepted practice in obstetrical management, and they are valuable in a wide variety of obstetrical difficulties. However, an induction in the hands of an untrained person is potentially dangerous to the mother and infant. Therefore, the physician, not the nurse, should take responsibility for administering Pitocin. This is not meant to scare the nurse, but to warn her against accepting responsibilities for which she is not prepared.

CESAREAN SECTION

Cesarean sections have become more common in recent years because refinements and advancements in surgical techniques have made them safer. A cesarean section is the delivery of the infant through an incision made in the abdominal and uterine walls (Fig. 13-1 A-D).

Indications

There are many reasons for performing a cesarean. The two most common reasons are: if the woman is known to have cephalopelvic disproportion (i.e., if the head of the baby is too large to pass through the maternal pelvis), or if she has had a previous cesarean section. The operation is usually scheduled about a week prior to the woman's expected date of delivery in hopes of allowing the fetus to reach full-term size before the mother goes into labor.

Other indications for cesarean section are toxemia, hemorrhage due to placenta previa or abruptio placentae, malpresentation of the fetus such as a shoulder presentation (transverse lie), and fetal distress. Since some of these difficulties obviously cannot be predicted ahead of time, emergency cesareans must be done in those cases. In an emergency situation, the patient is understandably frightened, and the nurse should be calm and yet carry out preparatory procedures with dispatch.

Types

There are four main types of cesarean sections.

Low Cervical. This type of cesarean section is considered the most desirable, because the incision is made in the lower uterine segment which is the area of least activity; hence the possibility of rupture of the scar is less likely with the next preg-

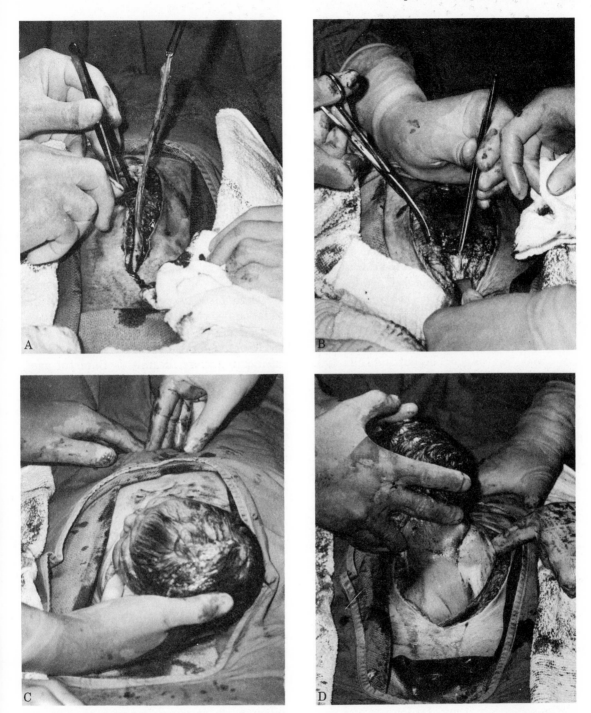

Figure 13-1. (*A*) In this cesarean section the incision is widened and an old scar from a previous section is removed. The scar tissue is the long, thin tissue being held up with a tenaculum. (*B*) The uterine wall is cut through with a pair of scissors and tissue forceps. The assistant is holding a small retractor with one hand and a gauze sponge with the other. (*C*) The head is delivered through the incision. (*D*) The surgeon exerts traction on the head to deliver the shoulders. The rest of the body will then slip out easily.

nancy. Also there is less danger of infection postoperatively than if the incision is made in the fundus.

A brief description of the surgical procedure follows: the abdomen is opened through a midline incision, and the peritoneum is dissected at its lowest portion. Either a transverse or longitudinal incision is made in the lower uterine segment, and the baby is delivered manually or with forceps. It is the method of choice, because it is as easy to perform and as quick as the classic operation.

Classic. The main advantage of a classic cesarean is that it is quick and easy to perform. One incision is made in the midline of the abdomen, and another in the fundus longitudinally. After the membranes are ruptured, the baby is grasped by the feet and delivered that way. It is sometimes done when there is an anterior placenta previa to avoid the danger of cutting into the placenta.

Extraperitoneal. This means that the peritoneal cavity is not entered. A transverse incision is made in the abdomen above the symphysis pubis. The lower uterine segment is exposed by peeling the peritoneum from the posterior portion of the bladder and the anterior portion of the uterus. A transverse incision is then made into the lower uterine segment, and the baby is delivered. The main disadvantage of this procedure is that it is difficult and time-consuming to perform. The advantage is that there is less danger of infection if spill of infectious material such as amniotic fluid occurs. However, since the advent of antibiotics, extraperitoneal cesareans have been rarely done.

Cesarean hysterectomy. This type of cesarean (also called a Porro's operation) is just what the name implies; after the baby is removed, a hysterectomy is done. Although a rare operation, it may be done on an older woman who has fibroid tumors or on a patient who has a Couvelaire uterus (a complication of a premature separation of the placenta). If the ovaries are healthy, they are not removed, so that the patient will

still have the benefits of hormone production.

Nursing Care

Nursing care differs in some ways from that given a patient who will deliver vaginally.

Preoperative Care. A more extensive shave is done. The entire abdomen is shaved from side to side starting from the xyphoid process and extending down over the perineal region. Care is taken to cleanse the umbilicus adequately.

A foley catheter is inserted; this is to keep the bladder empty so that it won't be in the way or accidently cut during the operative procedure. The patient is observed for signs of labor, and the doctor is notified if labor begins. He may want to do the cesarean section right away.

Atropine may be the only preoperative medication given. Rarely is Demerol used, because it may depress the baby. The patient is usually more apprehensive; thus she needs a lot of emotional support from her family and various members of the health team. For example, the anesthetist could come and talk to her before surgery.

She may be admitted to the hospital the day before surgery so that the necessary preoperative blood work, lab tests, preoperative teaching, etc. can be taken care of. The charting differs, since the forms used for a surgical patient are used.

Intrapartum. A registered nurse may be responsible for the immediate care of the newborn delivered by cesarean. In some hospitals a pediatrician is called to be present at the delivery. These babies frequently need to be resuscitated for the following reasons: (1) Excess secretions will need to be removed since the mother will not have been in labor (Fig. 13-2). The process of normal labor with uterine contractions helps to force out the mucus and fluid from the baby's respiratory passages.) (2) If the cesarean section is done for fetal distress, obviously the baby will need to be resuscitated. (3) If the mother has had a general

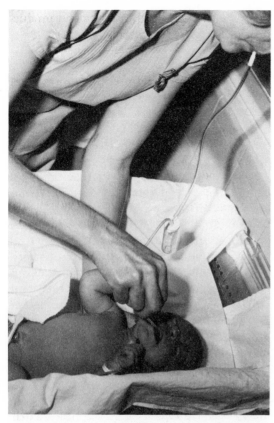

Figure 13-2. The nurse is suctioning mucus from the infant's stomach with a plastic disposable gastric tube. The mucus is drawn up into the container and does not go into the nurse's mouth. Note the infant's gag reflex.

inhalation anesthetic (spinals are more usual and are preferred for a cesarean section) the baby might require resuscitation.

The nurse or anesthetist prepares an oxytocin to be given as soon as the baby is born. She should have forceps for the doctor to use in delivery and other equipment available for resuscitation and the immediate care of the infant.

Postoperative Care. Most patients are taken to a recovery room for several hours. Vital signs are taken frequently, the amount of lochia is noted, and the fundus is checked by palpating it gently from the sides. If the patient has had spinal anesthesia, she won't be able to feel her uterus being palpated until the anesthetic wears off. Usually the patient is receiving an IV or

a blood transfusion; it should be checked for rate of flow, infiltration, and side effects. The foley catheter should be checked for the patency of the tubing, and the drainage bag should be emptied as necessary. Remember to inspect the abdominal dressings for bleeding.

In order to prevent hypostatic pneumonia, the patient should start as soon as possible, to turn, cough, and deep breathe, supporting her abdominal incision. It is hoped that she was taught how to do this as a part of her preoperative preparation.

The baby is placed in an isolette for approximately 24 hours and is treated as a premature infant. This is a routine practice for babies delivered by cesarean section, as they are more prone to respiratory distress and need to be observed more closely at first. The parents should have been prepared for this previously, and they can be reminded that this procedure is not unusual and doesn't mean that there is anything wrong with the baby. The husband and other family members can go to the nursery and look at the baby as much as they like; this may be reassuring to them.

As mentioned earlier, spinal anesthesia is frequently given for a cesarean section, after which the patient must lie flat in bed for 8 to 12 hours in hopes of preventing postspinal headaches in the postpartum period.

After the effects of the anesthetic wears off, the patient may begin to have pain in her abdominal incision. She will require sedation in the form of Demerol, or a substitute, for the first 24 to 48 hours following delivery. Since the physician has usually indicated that the medication should be given when needed, (a P.R.N. order) it is up to the nurse to decide when to give it. The patient should be kept as comfortable as possible, but should not be overly sedated, lest she develop postoperative complications from inactivity. If the patient is nauseated or is not permitted to eat or drink, other medications such as Ergotrate can be given intramuscularly to keep the uterus contracted and to control bleeding.

Later Care. Usually, within 24 hours after delivery, the IV's are discontinued and the patient begins to eat. She progresses from a liquid to a soft diet and then to a regular diet as tolerated. Her foley catheter is removed about the same time, and it is the nurse's responsibility to make sure that the patient is emptying her bladder.

The patient should be ambulated gradually. First the head of her bed is elevated, then she is allowed to dangle her legs over the side of the bed, before actually walking around the room. She may be apprehensive at first and afraid that her incision will open up. She needs to be prepared for the increased lochial drainage when she gets up for the first time. Each day she should walk about more to prevent complications and to promote return of normal bodily functions.

Depending on the size and location of her abdominal dressing, the nurse may or may not be able to check the descent of the uterus. Usually, the mother begins to feed the baby in about 24 hours following delivery. Because of her abdominal incision, she needs more assistance in handling and burping the baby. The nurse should stay with her at first to render all possible assistance. If the mother becomes tired or is in a great deal of discomfort, the nurse may decide to finish the feeding.

Because of the lochial discharge, the patient needs frequent perineal care, at least every four hours during the day, until she is able to provide her own care.

She has the same emotional changes as any postpartum patient and may have the postpartum blues. Since a vaginal delivery is a psychologically fulfilling experience for a woman, some patients may feel cheated because they were unable to have a normal vaginal delivery. In addition their concept of their own femininity may be shattered. Allowing the patient to vent her feelings to an understanding person such as the nurse, can be therapeutic.

The third day postpartum is often uncomfortable for the mother because of flatus. A cathartic or enema may be given to relieve it. Avoiding large quantities of iced drinks or ice water, and walking around as much as possible, will help relieve gas. A special enema such as a Harris flush or a Mayo enema may be given. An injection of Prostigmine, followed by insertion of a rectal tube is another way to relieve this distress.

Preparation for Discharge. The mother should definitely be encouraged to have help at first when she returns home because she has had major abdominal surgery in addition to having a baby. An appointment is made for her to return to the doctor or clinic in two weeks instead of six weeks, to see if her incision is healing and to check for possible complications. Family planning methods should be discussed, since it is advisable that the mother not become pregnant for at least a year following her cesarean section. Pregnancies too close together may put a strain on the uterine scar.

Instructions regarding bathing and douching are similar to those given to a mother who has delivered vaginally. However, the patient who has had a cesarean section will have to take sponge baths until her dressing is removed.

STERILIZATION PROCEDURES

At the time of a normal vaginal delivery, or when a cesarean section is done, the woman may have her fallopian tubes tied, because she and her husband have decided that they have as many children as they want and can provide for. They may feel that this is the best form of contraception for them, especially if the wife cannot take oral contraceptives and if other methods have not been entirely satisfactory for them. The increasing emphasis on population control has also prompted many couples to limit the size of their families.

Medical reasons may also dictate that a woman have her tubes tied, especially if she has heart disease, diabetes, severe varicosities, or any other condition which would rule out pregnancy. Although medical opinion varies concerning the number of cesarean sections a woman may have, often sterilization is done after the third one. Thus, the woman may be advised by the doctor to have a tubal ligation at that time.

There are several different methods of tubal ligation; the one which has the lowest number of failures is the *Irving procedure*. A brief description follows. The tubes are ligated and cut near their attachment to the uterus. Then the proximal ends of the tubes are buried in a stab wound in the myometrium and anchored by suture materials. The other methods of tubal ligation involve clamping, crushing, and cutting a portion of each of the fallopian tubes. In the Irving technique, burying one end of the tube into the uterine wall, appears to be a more reliable method.

If a woman is going to have a sterilization procedure, a written consent form is provided. It is preferable to obtain signatures of both the husband and the wife, but the consent of the woman alone is all that is required by law. In the case of an unmarried woman, if she is of age and mentally competent, she can sign for permission for sterilization. When the couple are contemplating sterilization, it is important to emphasize to both partners that the operation will prevent pregnancy but will not interfere with sexual functions or with menstruation.

When is a tubal ligation done? It is most commonly done at the time of cesarean section or within 12 to 24 hours of a vaginal delivery. However, it may be postponed for a few days. The operation is simple, and recovery usually takes place rapidly with no complications.

The couple may want to consider vasectomy, a sterilization procedure that is done on the man. This is gaining increasing acceptance throughout the world. The operation is even more simple than the female sterilization technique, and it can be done in the doctor's office. The man can also be assured that a vasectomy will not interfere with sexual desire or performance.

RUPTURED UTERUS

Fortunately a ruptured uterus is a rare complication. It is usually fatal to the infant and about one third of the mothers die. The uterus simply bursts because the strain put on it is more than its musculature can withstand.

The most common cause is rupture of a scar from a previous cesarean section. For this reason many physicians feel that once a woman has had a cesarean section, regardless of the reason for the original section, she should always be delivered by the abdominal route. Further it is safer to do a repeat section before the woman goes into labor, and the number of cesarean sections should be limited. Other causes of a ruptured uterus are a prolonged and obstructed labor, a traumatic delivery (such as a version and extraction), and injudicious use of oxytocin in labor.

Signs and Symptoms

Rupture of the uterus should be suspected if the patient is restless and anxious and seems to be aware of impending danger. Despite having strong contractions, she is making no progress even though she is pushing with contractions, she begs for relief incessantly, and she has panting respirations and a rapid pulse.

When rupture occurs, the patient may say that she felt something burst. She becomes quiet, and the pain usually ceases. If the uterus has ruptured completely, contractions cease because a torn muscle cannot contract. She may have referred shoulder pain due to the irritation of the diaphragm by the intra-abdominal hemorrhage. Often, the fetus can be felt in the abdomen (the outline is more distinct than when it is within the uterus) and there are no fetal heart tones. The patient exhibits signs of shock, her skin is pale, cold and clammy, her pulse is rapid and weak, and she is apprehensive.

Medical Treatment

Unless immediate action is taken, the

patient will die of hemorrhage. The treatment is to do an immediate hysterectomy. Replacing the blood loss via whole blood transfusions and combating infection by the use of antibiotics are essential to the recovery of the patient.

Nursing Care

The patient must be rapidly prepared for surgery. If time permits, the bed is put into Trendelenburg position and warm blankets are applied because the patient is in shock. Vital signs are checked almost continuously. Emergency equipment for cardiac arrest and oxygen and intravenous cut-down sets should be readily available. Whenever possible, the nurse who has been taking care of the patient during labor should stay with her and go with her to surgery. This will provide the best continuity of care and emotional support for both the patient and her family.

DYSTOCIA

When labor is prolonged and the parturient senses that she isn't getting anywhere, she may become very disheartened. For this reason, the nurse is often the key person to keep up the patient's morale, alert the physician to changes in the quality of the uterine contractions, and carry out measures to prevent further complications such as exhaustion and dehydration.

Dystocia simply means a difficult labor; there is a cessation of progress as a result of abnormalities in the mechanics involved. There are three separate and distinct forces involved in labor: the uterine contractions, the fetus, and the pelvis and surrounding structures. If an abnormality occurs in any one of them, dystocia results.

Causes

The most common cause of dystocia is called uterine dysfunction or uterine inertia. The uterine forces are not strong enough to overcome the natural resistance to the birth of the baby offered by the maternal soft parts and the bony birth canal. The fetus may cause dystocia if the presentation is faulty or if the fetus is large or abnormally developed. Abnormalities in the size of the pelvis and birth canal which form an obstacle in the descent of the fetus is another causative factor in difficult labors.

Evaluating Contractions

How can the nurse tell about the uterine forces? The best clinical evidence of the quality and intensity of the uterine contractions is obtained by palpating the fundus at the height of a contraction. If the uterine wall can be indented with the fingers, then the contraction is not of good quality. Remember that the complaints of the patient about her contractions are not always indicative of the actual intensity of contractions. Because there are differences in pain thresholds among patients, and because a patient who is having inefficient contractions is especially bitter in her complaints, the nurse should rely on her own evaluation of the quality of the contraction.

Uterine Dysfunction

In normal labor there is a latent phase which lasts several hours; the cervix effaces but dilates only slightly. This phase is followed by an acceleration and active phase when the cervix dilates rapidly and progressively. A declaration or slowing occurs just before full dilation.

If the patient has hypertonic uterine dysfunction (or primary inertia), this refers to a prolonged latent phase of labor. Hypotonic uterine dysfunction (or secondary inertia) indicates an abnormality in the active phase. Table 13-1 compares the symptoms of hypertonic and hypotonic uterine dysfunction.

Causes. The main cause of uterine dysfunction is the ill-timed and excessive administration of the analgesic. Other factors are minor degrees of pelvic contractions, slight extension of the fetal head as occurs with occiput posterior positions, and overdistension of the uterus. In some women, particularly in an elderly primigravida (a

Table 13-1. COMPARISON OF SIGNS AND SYMPTOMS

Hypertonic	Hypotonic
Contractions are very painful	Contractions become infrequent and of poor quality
Fetal distress appears early	Fetal distress does not appear until infection has developed
Does not respond favorably to oxytocin	Responds favorably to oxytocin
Sedation helps a great deal	Sedation has little value

woman over 35 who is having her first baby), the cervix is too rigid to dilate. However, in many patients the cause is unknown.

Treatment and Nursing Care. For a patient who has hypertonic dysfunction, the treatment is to stop the abnormal contraction by giving morphine (usually 1/4 gr.). In addition, a short-acting barbiturate may be given to promote relaxation and rest. If the patient is dehydrated, fluids are given intravenously. In the vast majority of patients normal labor will start when the patient wakes up.

A patient who has hypotonic dysfunction is examined vaginally to reevaluate cervical effacement and dilatation and the position and presentation of the fetus. X-ray pelvimetry is done to determine accurately the measurements of the pelvis and minor abnormalities of fetal position. Giving the patient an enema may stimulate the normal progress of labor. Rupturing the membranes or giving Pitocin intravenously, using all the precautions as with an induction of labor, is often carried out.

Supportive nursing care at its finest is required for a patient who has uterine dysfunction. Both parents will wonder why there has been no progress and why the doctors or nurses don't do something. Explanations should indicate the plan of action to be taken, what methods of treatments are being used now, and assurance that this is not an absolutely unique situation. It is essential that the parents know that the various diagnostic procedures take time, and they must be patient and wait. Repeated explanations, along with positive statements concerning any progress being made will be helpful. The nurse should avoid being trapped into making any predictions as to how long labor will last or what the outcome of any procedure will be. She can get feedback from the parents on their understanding of the situation and thus may be able to clarify any misunderstandings.

Physical care and comfort measures are basically the same as for any patient in labor, but probably more extensive: relaxation and breathing techniques, back rubs and sacral pressure, cool cloth to the forehead, and so forth. A close check of the fetal heart tones should be done, since fetal distress is more likely to occur in this instance. Observation for signs of dehydration, exhaustion, and infection should be made. Thus, an elevated temperature, rapid pulse, or any other similar sign, should be reported immediately. Dehydration may be prevented by seeing to it that the patient has lots of fluids to drink—between 2000 to 3000 cc. in 24 hours. However, IV's may be given instead. Urine output should also be observed.

If the patient has been given sedation, she shouldn't be left alone in a darkened room unless it is certain she is sleeping. Even when she is sleeping, she should be observed frequently. The quality and frequency of contractions and the reactions of the patient are very important for the physician to know in evaluating whether the patient is making any progress or if her labor is at a standstill.

Disproportion

A disproportion between the size of the infant and the birth canal is called cephalopelvic disproportion, commonly abbreviated C.P.D. The most frequent cause is a contracted pelvis. A narrowing can occur in any of the three parts of the bony pelvis, the inlet, midpelvis, or outlet. (See Chap. 5.)

In an inlet contraction the *diagonal conjugate* is 11.5 cm. or less. The most common cause for this occurrence is rickets, which is found in a higher percentage of Negroes than white women. Improved diets which contain a sufficient amount of vitamin D have greatly reduced the incidence of rickets and, therefore, of contracted pelvis. Another cause of inlet contraction is general poor development. It is usually found in small women in whom all pelvic measurements are shortened. Fortunately, women with inlet contraction tend to have smaller infants. Ninety per cent of these women deliver vaginally, but there is much molding of the infant's head, so that the infant may have extensive caput succedaneum (edema of the scalp).

A midpelvic contraction occurs when the distance between the ischial spines is below 9.5 cm. There is no satisfactory method of measuring this manually; the patient must have an x-ray. This abnormality frequently causes a transverse arrest; that is, the occiput is stopped in the transverse part of the pelvis, rather than being able to rotate anteriorly. It may cause a difficult midforceps delivery. However, the best plan is to wait and allow nature to take its course.

In an outlet contraction, the woman has a narrow pubic arch with the distance between the ischial tuberosities measuring 8.0 cm. or less. Even if it doesn't cause serious dystocia, it often produces perineal tears because the head of the baby goes backward, and the perineum becomes more distended. The incidence of forceps deliveries is greater, and a deep episiotomy is usually necessary.

Large or Excessive Size of the Baby

A child at birth rarely weighs over ten pounds; if it does, dystocia may result. The difficulty is generally due to the fact that the head is not only larger but also harder. The shoulders may also be large and difficult to deliver, a condition referred to as shoulder dystocia. The three usual causes for a large baby are the size of one or both parents, diabetes in the mother, and multiparity. A major problem is that the diagnosis of a large baby is often not established until after fruitless attempts to deliver the baby have been made. If the child is large, the mother should always be investigated for diabetes.

Hydrocephalus

Hydrocephalus is an excessive accumulation of cerebrospinal fluid in the ventricles of the brain. It accounts for 12 per cent of all malformations at birth. Breech presentations in these instances are common because the head is too large to fit into the pelvic inlet. Diagnosis is made by x-ray: the face is small in relation to the large head, and the skull is paper-thin. The treatment is to reduce the size of the head. The excess cerebrospinal fluid is drained by puncturing the skull with a spinal needle. In and of itself, this does not harm the baby. However, there is an infant mortality of around 70 per cent with this abnormality.

Summary

In summary, dystocia due to cephalopelvic disproportion again points up the importance of prenatal care. If pelvic contractures are found early by taking pelvic measurements, or if abnormalities of the fetus are discovered, plans can be made ahead of time for a cesarean section if need be. When the mother's pelvis is borderline, she may be given a trial labor of from 6 to 12 hours. Then if progress is not satisfactory within that time, the infant is delivered by cesarean section.

ABNORMAL FETAL POSITIONS

Persistent Occiput Posterior

In most women occiput posterior positions undergo spontaneous anterior rotation and are delivered either spontaneously or with low forceps. The second stage of labor is prolonged because more contractions and expulsive efforts of the mother are needed to rotate the head through a larger arc. The mother complains of backache more when the baby is in the occiput posterior position. In a small percentage of women, about 5 per cent, rotation does not occur; this is called a persistent occiput posterior. Delivery may be accomplished by rotating the infant gently by hand or with forceps. The Scanzoni maneuver is the double application of forceps to first rotate and then extract the head. Or Kielland forceps may be used to do the rotation. If the mother's pelvis is large enough, it is perfectly possible to deliver the baby in the occiput posterior position.

Breech Presentation

The incidence of breech presentations is about 3 per cent. There are three types of breech presentations: frank, complete, and incomplete. The most common is a frank breech in which the legs are extended along the child's body. In a complete breech, the child is sitting tailor fashion; in an incomplete breech, either a double or a single foot is presented.

Breech deliveries are more common in premature than full-term labors and among multiparas than primigravidas. The diagnosis is made by palpation (Leopold's maneuvers), x-ray, and the location of the fetal heart tones.

The mother may be frightened when she learns that she is going to have a breech birth. She may have heard that labor is longer and more painful. In truth, labor is not longer; a median duration is 9.2 hours in primigravidas and 1.6 hours in multiparas. So she and her husband can be reassured on that point. Remember, that meconium-stained amniotic fluid is *normal* in a breech presentation.

There is a higher risk to the infant, however. The risk to the full-term breech infant is nearly three times that associated with a vertex presentation. This is because the cord is more likely to be compressed during delivery. Prolapse of the cord is a common complication. Another factor that increases the risk to the infant is that there is more likely to be tentorial tears (the tentorium covers the brain) with subsequent intracranial hemorrhage. This can happen if the cervix is not completely dilated and the head is trapped.

The use of Piper forceps to deliver the after-coming head is considered good treatment. The buttocks of the baby may be bruised or the labia or scrotum quite swollen for a few days after delivery. The parents can be reassured that this will disappear in due time.

Prolapsed Cord

What should the nurse do if the cord prolapses? This is a very serious complication because if the cord is compressed, it will cut off the oxygen supply to the fetus. The nurse will observe the white glistening cord protruding from the vulva. Her first action is to change the patient's position to try to get pressure off of the cord. This may be accomplished by putting the patient into the knee-chest position or the Trendelenburg position. Another alternative would be to have the patient turn on her side in the Sims' position and elevate her hips on pillows so that her hips are higher than her thorax. Stay with the patient; she will be very frightened, not because this is painful, but because she knows that the baby is in danger. Listen to the baby's heartbeat frequently, if possible.

If the cord is left exposed for more than 15 minutes, it may start to dry. Warm, moist, sterile, saline compresses may be wrapped around it, but it should be handled gently, and no attempts should be made to replace it in the vagina. If a doctor is immediately available, the patient is usually taken directly to the delivery room to be delivered as soon as possible.

Transverse Lie or Shoulder Presentation

In a shoulder presentation, the fetus lies crosswise in the uterus rather than longitudinally. When labor begins, this type of presentation usually converts to a longitudinal lie. Abnormal relaxation of the uterine walls due to grand multiparity, pelvic contraction, and placenta previa are the causes. The diagnosis may be made by inspection, because the abdomen is unusually wide from side to side, and the fundus scarcely extends above the umbilicus. X-ray, palpation, and vaginal examination can all be used to confirm the diagnosis. This complication is an indication for elective cesarean section several days before term in a primigravida. It is very important to maintain intact membranes because of the danger of infection.

BIBLIOGRAPHY

Barter, R.: Induction of labor: helpful or harmful. Postgraduate Med., *43:*141-144,1968.

Eastman, N., and Hellman, L.: Williams Obstetrics, ed. 13. New York, Appleton Century Crofts, 1966.

Fitzpatrick, E., et al.: Maternity Nursing, ed. 12. Philadelphia, J. B. Lippincott, 1971.

Gonzales, B.: Voluntary sterilization. Amer. J. Nurs., *70:*2581, 1970.

Suggested Reading for Further Study

Bruce, S.: Reactions of nurses and mothers to stillbirths. Nurs. Outlook, *10:*88–91, 1962.

Melber, R.: The nurse's role in obstetrical emergencies in the hospital setting. Nurs. Clin. N. Amer., *2:*261–269, 1967.

UNIT STUDY QUESTIONS

1. One of the distinctive features of the first stage of labor is that
   a. it is involuntary in character
   b. the contractions are influenced by the mother's will
   c. its progress is aided by walking about
   d. the membranes rupture

2. Station plus two means
   a. the presenting part is 2 centimeters above the level of the ischial spines
   b. the biparietal diameter is at the level of the ischial spines
   c. the presenting part is 2 centimeters below the level of the ischial spines
   d. the biparietal diameter is 2 centimeters above the ischial spines

3. The forceps used exclusively for the delivery of the after-coming head in a breech presentation are called:
   a. Keilland's
   b. Piper's
   c. Simpson's
   d. Elliott's

4. Position of the fetus refers to
   a. the relationship of the long axis of the fetus to the long axis of the mother
   b. the relationship of the presenting part to the mother's pelvis
   c. the relationship of the fetal parts to each other
   d. the portion of the fetus which engages at the superior strait

5. A midline episiotomy has all of the following advantages over a mediolateral episiotomy *except*:
   a. it heals faster.
   b. it is more comfortable for the patient.
   c. it is easier to repair.
   d. there is less danger of extension of the incision.
   e. there is less bleeding.

6. A second degree laceration of the perineum involves:
   a. mucous membrane of the vagina, skin and muscles of the perineal body.
   b. mucous membrane of vagina and the skin of the perineum.
   c. the sphincter ani only.
   d. the mucous membrane of the vagina, perineal skin and muscles and the sphincter ani.

7. When the cervix is described as being effaced, this means
   a. the cervical canal is elongated
   b. the cervix is obliterated
   c. the cervix is thickened
   d. the cervix is dilated

8. During a contraction fetal heart tones usually:
   a. stop
   b. become slower and return to normal about the time the contraction ends
   c. become slower and irregular
   d. remain the same

9. Precipitate labor is defined as:
   a. a labor in which no medication is needed.
   b. a labor that is painless.
   c. a labor that is unattended by medical personnel.
   d. a labor lasting three hours or less.

10. The range of the fetal heart rate per minute is normally between
    a. 90 - 120
    b. 100 - 150
    c. 120 - 160
    d. 120 - 170

11. The *principal* danger in administering analgesic medication before the establishment of good labor is:
    a. respiratory depression of the newborn.
    b. lowering of maternal blood pressure.
    c. postpartal hemorrhage resulting from suppressed uterine contractions.

d. retardation of the progress of labor.

12. During the first stage of labor, the patient should not be given any solid foods because:
    a. when a patient is in labor she is not able to digest any solid food
    b. she may have a general anesthetic when it is time for delivery and might vomit and aspirate solid food
    c. her stomach will be upset and she would probably vomit solid food
    d. she will not be able to have an enema for two days after delivery

13. Separation of the placenta is *primarily* the result of:
    a. the sloughing off of the weakest layer of the decidua.
    b. inversion of the placental membranes.
    c. a disproportion between the unchanged size of the placenta and decrease in size of the placental site.
    d. peripheral detachment according to the mechanism of Schultz or Duncan.

14. A foley catheter is inserted *prior* to performing a cesarean section primarily to:
    a. prevent injury to the bladder during the operation.
    b. empty the bladder if the patient has been unable to void.
    c. instill a urinary antiseptic to prevent bladder infection.
    d. keep an accurate record of intake and output.

15. The two most common indications for a cesarean section are:
    a. cephalopelvic disproportion and fetal distress.
    b. fetal distress and repeat section.
    c. repeat section and cephalopelvic disproportion.
    d. toxemia and hemorrhage.

16. The first few days after a cesarean section is performed, the patient often has signs or symptoms of:
    a. respiratory distress.
    b. abdominal distension.
    c. hypertension.
    d. pelvic thrombophlebitis.

17. The term currently in use which describes cessation of progress in labor as a result of abnormalities in the mechanics involved is:
    a. dystocia
    b. dyspareunia
    c. decrement
    d. dysfunction

18. In a vertex presentation the head is born across the perineum by
    a. expulsion
    b. restitution
    c. flexion
    d. extension

19. If the fetal heart tones are below 120 or over 160, the patient should lie on her side to:
    a. close the foramen ovale.
    b. relieve pressure on the aorta.
    c. relieve pressure on the vena cava.
    d. prevent congestion in the heart.

20. Prior to an amniotomy the nurse should:
    1. have the patient void.
    2. check the fetal heart tones.
    3. check the pulse.
    4. check the blood pressure.
        a. 1 and 2
        b. 1, 2, 4
        c. 2, 3, 4
        d. All of the above.

21. Prior to delivering a baby in an emergency along a street the nurse should:
    a. perform a vaginal examination to be sure the cord has not prolapsed.
    b. help the mother lie down in the cleanest area possible.

    c. wash her hands.
    d. ask someone to boil a pair of scissors to cut the cord.

22. As the baby's head begins to emerge in an emergency delivery the nurse should:
    a. exert gentle pressure against the head to prevent maternal laceration
    b. encourage the mother to bear down so that the baby will be able to breathe as soon as possible.
    c. encourage the mother to pant to get more oxygen to the baby.
    d. hold the mother's legs together to allow time to get to the hospital to deliver the baby.

23. As soon as the baby is born in an emergency delivery he should:
    a. be put to breast to encourage uterine involution.
    b. be wrapped in a clean cloth and given to a bystander to hold.
    c. be handled as little as possible to prevent infection.
    d. be taken by someone to the hospital.

24. In an emergency delivery, if the placenta has not been expelled within 15 minutes after the birth of the baby, the nurse should:
    a. pull gently on the umbilical cord.
    b. massage the fundus.
    c. ask the mother to bear down.
    d. wait patiently.

25. Cutting of the umbilical cord in an emergency delivery:
    a. should be accomplished within five minutes of the baby's birth.
    b. should be accomplished within 30 minutes of the baby's birth.
    c. may be done with a clean pair of scissors if nothing else is available.
    d. should not be done without a sterile pair of scissors no matter what period of time elapses.

Nursing Care During the Puerperium 14

The puerperium is the period immediately postpartum. It begins as soon as delivery is complete and lasts approximately six weeks.

There are three major physiological changes that occur in the mother during this period: regressive as well as progressive changes take place; the reproductive system gradually reverts to the nonpregnant state; and if the mother is going to breast feed, changes occur to prepare for nourishing the baby.

PHYSIOLOGICAL CHANGES

Uterus

Each day the uterus, which is at the level of the umbilicus immediately after delivery, gradually becomes smaller and descends toward the pelvic cavity. By the end of the tenth day postpartum, it can no longer be felt above the symphysis pubis. This is believed to be caused by the breakdown, absorption, and excretion in the urine of protein material within the uterine wall. The rapid shrinking of the uterus until it returns to the nonpregnant state is called *involution.*

Endometrium

While the uterus is decreasing in size, the lining regenerates. The decidua vera differentiates into two layers. The top layer becomes necrotic, sloughs off, and is discharged as *lochia.* The second layer, next to the myometrium, is well-preserved and provides the foundation for the new endometrium.

Within a week to ten days the inner surface of the uterus, except for the placental site, is covered with a new epithelium. The placental site requires about six weeks to disappear.

It is believed that a process of exfoliation brings about the disappearance of the obliterated arteries and organized thrombi and undermines the site where the placenta was formerly attached. Thus, there is no scar tissue formed in the uterus. This is a significant fact for subsequent pregnancies, because scar tissue has a poor blood supply. If the uterus were filled with scar tissue, where would the placenta attach?

Cervix and Vagina

Right after delivery, the cervix is soft and flabby. There may be some lacerations present, but they usually heal rapidly. The external os usually remains slightly open even after involution of the uterus is complete. It never completely reverts to its prepregnant state.

The vagina recovers slowly from its great distension. The vaginal opening may remain somewhat gaping. The labia also becomes somewhat flabby and atrophic. About the third week the rugae reappear in the vaginal walls.

Lochia

Lochia is the name given to the normal vaginal discharge which diminishes in amount in the early postpartum period. It may persist approximately two weeks. In women who breast feed it is said to be less. Lochia consists of red and white blood cells, fatty epithelial cells, shreds of decidual tissue, and bacteria. It has a characteristic fleshy, stale odor.

Lochia progresses through three stages. From the first day to the third or fourth day postpartum, it is called lochia rubra and is primarily a reddish or pinkish-red discharge. From the fourth day to the tenth day, it is called lochia serosa because the lochia takes on a brownish appearance. The third stage is from the tenth day on and is called lochia alba, which is whitish or yellowish in appearance.

The total quantity of lochia discharged is approximately 200 grams. If the reddish color persists, it suggests that involution is not taking place as it should or that fragments of the placenta have been retained.

Bladder

In the early postpartum period the bladder has an increased capacity and is less sensitive to fullness than normal. In addition, if the mother has received analgesics or an anesthesic during labor, the sensation of a full bladder may be further diminished. Therefore, overdistension of the bladder occurs frequently in the postpartum period.

Another common problem is incomplete emptying of the bladder, which results in residual urine. Urine which remains in the bladder becomes stagnant and is a good medium for the growth of bacteria. This is one reason for the increased incidence of urinary and bladder infections among postpartum patients. Some mothers have difficulty in voiding at first. This is a result of labor itself which causes the tone of the bladder to be temporarily impaired and the tissues at the base of the bladder and urethra to be edematous.

Another important consideration is the fact that marked diuresis occurs during the first 24 to 48 hours following delivery as the body tries to get rid of the large amount of fluid retained during pregnancy. Some diuresis continues up to the sixth day postpartum. The mother may void 3000 cc. daily as compared with 1000 to 1800 cc. normally.

In addition, the parturient may perspire profusely (diaphoresis) during this period.

Abdominal Wall

The abdominal wall tends to be soft and flabby after delivery because it was stretched during pregnancy. Women, especially multiparas, tend to look pregnant after delivery. This can be discouraging! Because of the diastasis recti, the mother will tend to look this way until the muscles regain their tone. If the mother is helped with simple exercises, this will help her to regain her figure. If not, the muscles may remain permanently flabby.

Breasts

The breasts are usually very soft during the first two postpartum days. On the third to the fifth day they may become engorged (firm and full). Engorgement is brought about by the hormone prolactin (see Chap. 5), which is stimulated by the baby sucking at the breasts and by adequate function of the adrenal and thyroid glands.

When the milk comes in, the breasts often become painful and firm. In primigravidas, especially, the breasts are almost boardlike and hot to the touch, and the skin is stretched and shiny. Engorgement is due to the pressure from the increased amount of milk in the ducts and lobes as well as from the increased blood and lymph circulation in the breasts.

EMOTIONAL CHANGES AND NURSING CARE

During the puerperium there is a reversal of the changes that took place during labor. Labor is characterized by a gradual turning inward (introversion), a narrowing of interests, and a progressive withdrawal of social energy. Conversely, during the postpartum period, the mother is slowly able to extend the scope of her physical and mental energy, first to her baby and husband,

and later to people and events outside of her immediate environment.

Taking-in Phase*

This phase usually lasts for two or three days postpartum. The mother is passive and dependent and has difficulty in making decisions for herself. She tries to do as she is told and initiates little or no action. Her needs are expressed more in relation to herself than in relation to the baby. She needs to take in food and sleep a great deal to restore her energy. Some mothers show a preoccupation with food by storing it in their bedside stands or ordering double portions to be served on their trays. If the mother does not get sufficient sleep and rest, she may suffer from sleep hunger, which results in irritability and fatigue.

She needs to relive the experience of her delivery and go over all the details in order to integrate it with reality. She frequently talks on the telephone to her friends and relatives for hours telling them about her experience. An understanding nurse will provide her with an opportunity to talk by sitting down with her and asking her about it. Asking her "How did it go?" or "Was it like you expected it to be?" may get her started.

Taking-Hold Phase*

During this phase the mother becomes more independent and autonomous. Her interests gradually turn from herself to others in her immediate environment. She begins to make her own decisions and to take the initiative for her own actions.

She becomes interested in the mothering tasks, such as holding and feeding the baby. At first she seems awkward and unsure of herself. Her feelings of inadequacy are intensified because the nurses seem so confident. However, when she succeeds at a task, her delight and pleasure are wonderful to behold. No one but a new mother can

---

*Rubin, R.: Puerperal change. Nurs. Outlook, 9:753–755, 1961.

be so thrilled at being able to get her infant to burp!

She becomes concerned about the return of her bodily functions to normal, especially her bladder and bowels. If they don't behave as she expects them to, she is anxious and upset. If she is breast feeding her baby, she wants to be reassured about the quality and quantity of her milk, and the nurse or doctor is frequently asked, "Do you think I have enough?" The point is that the mother needs to be reassured continually that she is performing well and that her bodily functions will return to normal.

The taking-hold phase lasts about ten days, so that most of it will take place after she goes home. Because this phase requires a great deal of energy, the parturient should be cautioned about overdoing and becoming overtired when she goes home.

Postpartum "Blues". Another emotional reaction that is frequently seen following childbirth is the postpartum "blues." It often occurs on the third day postpartum, but it may not appear until after the mother goes home. Typically, after the baby is born, the mother is very excited, happy, and euphoric. Suddenly, she feels depressed and blue, and has a let-down feeling that she can't explain. She cries more easily for no apparent reason, is more irritable, loses her appetite, and has difficulty in sleeping. Seeming to be more vulnerable to stress at this time, she faces the responsibility of returning to her family and home with a new baby.

To help the mother get through this difficult period, the nurse can recognize and interpret the mother's behavior and be kind and understanding. Both the mother and father should know that the blues are not unusual. The woman benefits from increased affection and attention. She may feel that all of the attention and love has been shifted from her to the baby. In fact, she may be experiencing some jealousy for which she, in turn, feels guilty.

There may also be physical reasons that contribute to postpartum depression. Some authorities believe that unmet needs for sleep cause the blues, while others think that the tremendous hormonal, physiological, and glandular changes which take place following birth might be responsible.

It is interesting to note that this phenomenon occurs more frequently among women in the middle and upper socioeconomic groups in the United States. Women of other countries and cultures throughout the world and of the lower socioeconomic group in the United States are less likely to have postpartum depression. Perhaps it is because they accept child-bearing and child-raising with more equanimity. Women of other cultures, countries, and socioeconomic conditions are said to accept motherhood as an integral part of their lives and as part of their feminine role, whereas the middle or upper class American woman is more emancipated. These are only speculations; the cause of postpartum depression is not definitely known.

CARE OF THE MOTHER IN THE IMMEDIATE POSTPARTUM PERIOD

The first hour after delivery is a very critical period and is sometimes referred to as the fourth stage of labor. The reason is that the uterus may continue to contract and relax rather than remain firmly contracted. When the uterus is firmly contracted, the open blood vessels and sinuses at the placental site are compressed. Therefore, the uterus has to remain firm and contracted continuously to control bleeding. To make sure this happens, oxytocics, such as ergonovine, Pitocin, and Methergine, which act by contracting the smooth muscle of the uterus, are given.

When these medications are not available, such as in a home or emergency delivery, the contraction of the uterus is brought about by the action of the sympathetic nervous system. The mother's joy in hearing the newborn cry, in seeing it, or in holding it, brings about this response.

Whether the patient goes to a post-partum recovery room or is taken to the postpartum bed where she will be for the remainder of her hospital stay, she should be observed carefully for the first 12 to 24 hours following delivery. This is the most likely time for a postpartum hemorrhage to occur. For the first two hours her fundus, flow, blood pressure and pulse are routinely checked every 15 minutes for the first hour, and then every half hour subsequently.

The nurse observes where the top of the fundus is in relation to the umbilicus (Fig. 14-1). If it is above the umbilicus, the uterus may be filled with blood clots, or the bladder may be full and pushing it up. The nurse would either express the clots or get the patient to void. If the patient has a full bladder and is unable to void, check to see if a catheterization order is included among the postpartum orders written by the physician. There is usually such an order included.

The fundus should be in the midline of the abdomen. However, the uterus moves easily from side to side immediately after delivery. The nurse may observe that it is deviated to the right or left. This may be caused by the pressure of a full bladder or bowel. Aside from encouraging the patient to void, there is no other nursing intervention.

The consistency of the fundus is either firm or boggy. If it is firm, it will be the size and consistency of a small grapefruit. If the uterus is soft or boggy, the nurse will be unable to feel it at all. The first nursing action taken following the discovery of a boggy uterus is to massage in the general area where the uterus should be, using the flat part of the fingertips in a circular fashion. Usually within a short time the uterus becomes firm again.

If bleeding is heavy, and the fundus is boggy, and the uterus does not respond to massage, the nurse should inform the doctor right away. He may order additional oxytocics to be given either intravenously or intramuscularly, or he may order an intravenous infusion of 1000 cc. of fluids with one ampul of an oxytocin added, to be started

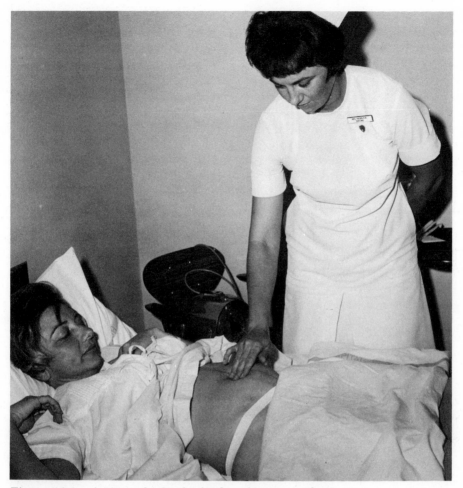

Figure 14-1.   A nurse checks the fundus of a new mother.

immediately. Overmassage of the uterus should be avoided because it is painful and may actually cause fatigue of the uterine muscle which leads to relaxation.

Blood clots should be expressed with firm pressure in the direction of the vaginal canal. It is important to make sure that the uterus is well contracted first because excessive pressure on the fundus could cause inversion of the uterus. When first learning to express clots, student nurses tend to be too gentle because they are afraid of hurting the patient. However, in order to prevent excessive bleeding it is necessary to exert enough pressure so that any or all blood clots are expelled. The patient can be taught to massage the fundus if she is awake enough. However, she should not have to assume the responsibility for doing it.

The patient's pulse should be taken. If it is over 100, it is too rapid and may be a danger sign indicating shock or hemorrhage. A rapid pulse is an earlier indication of shock than a drop in blood pressure.

Blood pressure determinations may be significant. If the patient's blood pressure is elevated, it may be a transient reaction from an oxytocic she received in the delivery room, or it may be due to toxemia. Low blood pressure indicates that the patient is in shock. It is wise for the nurse to compare the patient's blood pressure and pulse with the rates recorded during labor. If the rates deviate considerably, she should report her findings immediately to a physician for prompt treatment.

The amount of lochia is an important observation in the immediate postpartum period. A moderate amount of lochia is usual; the perineal pad is fairly well covered in about one hour. The patient usually wears two perineal pads because of the normally heavier flow during the first 24 hours. Not only should the pads be inspected, but the hip pad under the patient's buttocks should be checked, since the lochia may tend to flow to such a dependent area.

If the bleeding is heavy or excessive, the patient will be saturating a pad every half hour or will be expelling blood clots. The size of blood clots can vary from about the size of a dime to about the size of a lemon. They look very much like raw liver and should be saved for inspection by the doctor. If a part of the placenta was retained inside the uterus and then expelled, it will have a rougher fleshy appearance. It should also be saved to be shown to the doctor.

Depending on how long the patient is in the recovery room, she may be given a bath and perineal care. She is encouraged to void; if she is able to do so, her first voiding is measured. The reason for measuring the amount of urine is to determine if she is emptying her bladder. If the patient voids 150 cc. or more, this usually indicates that she is.

It is very interesting to observe the different reactions of patients following delivery. Some of them are excited and talkative; others are quiet and seem only to want to sleep or to rest; still others are thirsty and hungry and want something to drink and eat right away. Unless the mother was put to sleep with an inhalation type of anesthetic, she can have ice water right away. The nurse can call the diet kitchen for a tray for the patient or fix her a snack from the foods that are available on the postpartum unit. Often a beverage and light, easily digested foods such as broth or soup, jello and custard are all that the pa-

tient requires at this time. In fact, she may think she is ravenously hungry, and then can eat but a small amount of the food served to her. If the patient had an inhalation anesthetic or is nauseated, eating is contraindicated for several hours.

It is more difficult for the nurse to meet the patient's need for sleep and rest because it is necessary to check the blood pressure, and the fundus and lochia frequently. However, if the checks can be done with a minimum of time and as unobtrusively as possible, the patient may still be able to get some naps between checks.

The husband is welcome to visit his wife in the recovery room. If space is limited, usually only one visitor is permitted. Another important visitor is the baby! Frequently the baby is brought from the nursery for the mother to hold and inspect. The identification bands and the sex of the baby are checked with her at this time. The physical care of the mother includes keeping her clean and dry, i.e., changing her perineal and hip pads frequently. Giving her an opportunity to brush her teeth or rinse her mouth with mouthwash is often appreciated.

Perineal Care by the Nurse

After delivery of the baby, the perineal area of the mother needs special attention. Washing with warm water reduces the possibility of infection, contributes to the general comfort of the parturient and reduces odor. It is a clean rather than a sterile procedure.

Perineal care, commonly referred to as "peri-care," is done by the nurse until the mother can go to the bathroom by herself. While the mother is confined to bed, she receives perineal care after each voiding or defecation. If she is not voiding, the perineal area should still be cleansed every four hours. Mothers who have been delivered by cesarean section should have more frequent perineal care at least every three hours, because the presence of the indwelling catheter and the dark moist environment created by the combination of lochia, perspiration, bed covers, and inactivity encourages the growth of bacteria.

Many hospitals supply each new mother with a maternity kit which contains the necessary supplies. Although the equipment varies in different hospitals, the following is considered basic.

1 plastic irrigating bottle
A package of cleansing tissues
Sterile perineal pads
Newspaper or a paper bag
Bed pan and cover
A measuring pitcher

The nurse begins by explaining what she is going to do. Since the patient will most likely be doing her own perineal care after this first time, she needs instructions while the nurse is doing the procedure. The nurse can modify her teaching if the patient remembers the procedure from a previous childbirth.

After washing her hands, the nurse removes the patient's perineal pads from front to back and disposes of them by placing them in a paper bag. The patient is given a warmed bed pan and encouraged to void if she can. A measured amount of warm tap water from the irrigating bottle is poured over the patient's vulva and perineum.

Removing one tissue at a time from the container, the nurse wipes from the mons veneris to the rectum on one side of the labia. She repeats this step on the other side of the labia. With the third tissue, she wipes straight down the midline from the mons to the rectum, wiping very gently over the stitches. Using each tissue once only, she discards the tissue after each front-to-back stroke. Removing the bedpan, she has the patient turn on her side into the Sims's position.

Lifting the upper cheek of the buttock, she dries the area between the vagina and rectum using as many fresh tissues as necessary. She wipes *away* from the vagina. (This is an excellent opportunity to observe the patient's perineum.)

Finally, she applies the sterile perineal pads from front to back, handling them only on the outside. The inside of the pad which goes next to the vulva and stitches is kept sterile. The nurse then removes the equipment. She measures the amount of liquid in the bed pan and subtracts the amount poured over the patient's perineum from the irrigating bottle. The amount remaining is the patient's urinary output. She charts the amount that the patient voided, the amount of lochia, and the condition of her perineum.

Instructing the Patient in Perineal Care

The patient should know the "why" of perineal care as well as the "how." The procedure and equipment should be simple enough that the patient can continue to use it after she goes home. She should be instructed to wash her hands before and after the procedure, and to remove and replace her pads always from front to back to prevent bringing organisms around the rectal area forward to the birth canal. She should use a separate tissue for each stroke, wiping from front to back, and discarding the tissues after each use to prevent infection. As a further guard against infection she should handle the pads only on the outside and avoid touching the inside. She should not borrow or loan equipment. And she should give herself perineal care each time after she urinates or defecates.

Many maternity departments have printed instructions for perineal care on the wall in the patient's bathrooms. They also provide separate shelves in a convenient location near the toilet so that the equipment can be kept readily at hand.

LATER POSTPARTUM CARE

Physical Care

Although the postpartum patient quickly becomes independent and self-sufficient, she still requires a certain amount of physical care. Soon after delivery, when the mother's condition has stabilized, the nurse may offer her a bath. If she is still confined to bed, she usually prefers to bathe herself as much as she is able, with the nurse bathing those areas that she cannot reach, such as her back and legs.

The postdelivery bath is aimed at preventing infection, especially in the breasts and the perineum. The mother is instructed to bathe her breasts first, since this is the area to keep the cleanest. If the mother is breast feeding, she should use plain water to wash her breasts because soap tends to remove the protective oils from the nipple and areola. She should wash her breasts with circular strokes, from the nipple outward (Fig. 14-2).

Then she should proceed with her bath in the usual manner, with the exception of washing the perineum. A clean bra or breast binder should be applied. Many patients have their own bras which can be most satisfactory if they are clean, large enough, and give adequate breast support. If the patient does not have a bra, or is waiting to have them brought in from home, the nurse should apply a supporting breast binder whether the mother is nursing or not.

A breast binder should be fitted to the patient by taking tucks in the sides if nec-

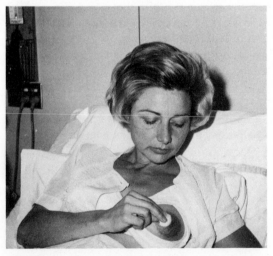

Figure 14-2. A mother cleanses her nipple with a moistened cotton ball, using a circular motion, prior to breast feeding.

essary and fastening them with safety pins. The breasts should be elevated on the chest wall and lifted toward the opposite shoulder while the binder is being pinned. The patient can support her breasts in the proper position while the nurse does the pinning. It should be pinned down the front so it can easily be undone for nursing the baby.

Vital Signs

On a postpartum unit, the patient's temperature, pulse, and respirations are taken once in the morning and again in the afternoon or evening unless otherwise indicated. Elevations in temperature over 100°F. (some hospitals use 99.2°F.) should be taken every four hours until the temperature has returned to normal for 24 hours. The pulse and respirations should be within normal limits. A pulse rate over 100 may indicate pathology or a complication.

Some postpartum patients have a slow pulse, usually in the 60's. If it has a good quality and is not associated with any other abnormalities, it is not significant.

Even if not ordered by the physician, the patient's blood pressure should be checked at least once a day during her hospital stay. The reason is that toxemia can develop in the postpartum period. A blood pressure of 130/90 or above may be significant.

Early Ambulation

Most postpartum patients may be up to the bathroom between six and eight hours after delivery. This, of course, depends on the amount and type of anesthesia used during delivery. If the mother had a saddle block, she may lie flat in bed for about 12 hours. (This time varies among hospitals and doctors.) Or, if she had a blood loss of 400 to 500 cc. at the time of delivery or in the recovery room, the nurse might decide that the patient should not get out of bed this soon.

Early ambulation has several advantages for the postpartum patient. She gets her strength back more quickly and feels better and stronger; her circulation is improved; she has fewer complications with thrombophlebitis, bowel and bladder complications and is less likely to need catheterizations; she has less abdominal distension and constipation.

Just because the mother is able to get up early does not mean she should feel that she is on her own. She may be afraid to ask the nurse to do things for her. The nurse should encourage the mother not to hesitate to ask for help. The nurse should watch for clues to the patient's emotional status regarding independence and should consider this in the nursing care plan. Some parturients resent being forced to independence too quickly; others resent an enforced dependency.

When the mother gets up for the first time or showers or takes a sitz bath, the nurse should be with her for safety reasons. In a shower, faintness may occur because of lack of oxygen, or the mother may suddenly feel weak, dizzy, and faint during any of these "first time" activities. This is a frightening experience for both the mother and the nurse. If the patient suddenly feels "woozy," ease her into a chair or to the floor, protecting her as much as possible from injury, and call for help to get the mother back to bed as quickly as possible. If the mother is conscious, have her lower her head between her knees to hasten the flow of blood to the brain. It is a good idea to carry a glass ampul of aromatic spirits of ammonia (smelling salts) in your uniform pocket just in case such an emergency arises. Upon returning the patient to bed, raise the side rails and check her vital signs as well as the amount of lochial discharge. Stay with the patient to reassure her and make sure that she recovers satisfactorily before leaving her.

Frequently, a postpartum patient is concerned that she is bleeding too heavily the first few times when she gets out of bed. While she is lying in bed in a supine or reclining position, lochia collects in the vaginal vault. Then when she stands or changes her position abruptly, gravity causes the sudden increase in vaginal drainage. Assure her that this is normal.

Sleep and Rest

The mother needs an abundance of sleep and rest during the puerperium. The hospital routine is such that there are many activities going on which make it difficult to meet this need. However, if the mother is comfortable and relaxed, she can be encouraged to sleep whenever possible. Some maternity departments make it a practice to have a rest hour after lunch. Visitors are restricted, and the patient's environment is subdued so that she can get some uninterrupted rest. The need for rest is even more important if the mother is breast feeding. Fatigue and tension are known to inhibit the milk supply. Also, inadequate rest can contribute to emotional problems and the mother's ability to cope with her new responsibilities.

It is the nurse's responsibility to adjust the hospital routine whenever possible to provide for periods of sleep and rest. A bottle-fed baby may be fed by the nurse occasionally if the mother is sleeping and does not want to be awakened. If the patient is having difficulty in getting to sleep at night, the nurse should refer to the nursing history and nursing care plan to modify factors in the environment to conform to the patient's usual sleep habits.

Nutrition

Because most women have good appetites following delivery, the nurse is mainly concerned that the meals provide for the general nutrition of the patient and meet the needs of a lactating mother. Good nutrition promotes a rapid recovery, helps the mother resist infections, and improves the quality and quantity of breast milk.

The daily diet of a lactating mother should be similar to her diet during pregnancy. In addition, she needs an extra pint of milk (a quart and a half a day), an extra serving of meat, citrus fruit, one egg, and a vegetable. A daily addition of about 1000 calories is required for milk production. She should avoid consumption of foods which might disagree with her. The old belief that certain food eaten by the mother causes gas and intestinal disturbances in the baby has been disproved. An addition of about 20 grams of protein to the diet (making a total of 98 grams of protein daily) is advised by the National Research Council. This is to ensure that the protein content of the milk is adequate.

Ample fluids are advised for the lactating woman. She should increase her intake to between 2500 to 3000 cc. daily. This favors milk production. Because nursing mothers are especially hungry in the hospital, the nurse should offer between-meal snacks three times a day. Offering her milk, ice cream, custards, and fruit juices helps her meet her additional nutritional and fluid requirements. Other new mothers may want these between-meal nourishments too.

Postpartum Observations

The nurse makes daily observations in a systematic way when she is giving nursing care to the parturient. These observations are to ascertain if the expected involutional changes are occurring and to detect any deviations from normal.

The following areas are included in her daily observations:

The Breasts.   Are they soft, or firm and engorged? Are they lactating or nonlactating? If the mother is breast feeding, what is the condition of the nipples? Are they intact, or are they cracked and fissured? Are they sore or painful?

The Fundus.   Is it firm or boggy? Where is it in relation to the umbilicus? (If the fundus is one finger below the umbilicus, it is recorded as U/1; two fingers below, U/2, etc.) Usually the fundus descends about one or more finger breadths below the umbilicus each day. Be sure that the patient has voided recently before you check her fundus.

The Lochia.   Is it rubra or serosa? Is the amount excessive, heavy, moderate, or scanty? How often does she change her perineal pads? Is she passing any clots? Note the odor of the lochia; a foul odor may indicate infection.

The Perineum.   Have the patient turn on her side to inspect her perineum. Is the suture line well approximated? Is there any redness, edema, purulent drainage, or bruises? Are there any hematomas? Hemorrhoids?

In addition to the specific areas of the mother's anatomy, the nurse should note the color of the mother's skin. Does she look pale and washed out? Checking the records to see how much blood the patient lost in the delivery room or recovery room or checking her hemoglobin and hematocrit (usually done routinely the morning of the second day postpartum) may explain the pale, washed-out look. In such instances, you should protect the patient from infection, have her ambulate more slowly, and provide for nutritional requirements.

Observe the mother's appearance and her affect. Does she take an interest in her appearance, or does she seem to not care? Does she appear worried or apprehensive? Or does she appear rested, happy, and relaxed? Inquiries by the nurse, when appropriate, into the mother's concerns may reveal a problem to be referred to the social service department or public health nurse.

Physical Discomforts and Their Nursing Care

Painful Sutures

Often the patient is too shy or embarrassed to complain or to tell the nurse that her perineum is causing her much pain. The nurse can often pick up clues by noting the way the patient sits, walks, or moves. She moves very slowly and painfully, or she sits down very gingerly and tries to sit on one buttock at a time. There are several comfort measures to relieve a sore episiotomy.

Perineal Lamp.   A perineal lamp may be used to provide comforting dry heat to the area. Heat from the lamp increases blood circulation to the stitches and reduces edema; hence the patient is more comfortable. In many maternity departments "peri-lights," as they are called, are used as a routine part of perineal care for any patient who has stitches. The patient is placed in the dorsal recumbent position with her legs flexed and knees comfortably spread. The lamp is placed about 12 inches from the perineum and left in place for approximately 20 minutes.

It is important that the patient lie flat in bed (the head of the bed is *not* elevated) for maximum exposure of the perineum to the lamp. Although lamps are equipped with low-wattage bulbs (usually 60 watts), care must be taken not to place the lamp too close to the patient or leave it on too long because it might burn the patient. If the perineal light is used for more than one patient, it should be wiped with a disinfectant solution after each use.

The patient is covered with the top bed sheet during the treatment; she may want to read or have some other form of diversion during the treatment. The perineal lamp treatment is usually given twice a day.

Sitz Baths. Sitz baths help to relieve the discomfort of a sore perineum. Unlike a perineal light, which the nurse gives as a routine part of perineal care, a sitz bath generally must be ordered by the physician. They are frequently given two or three times daily.

The sitz bath, like the perineal light, gives comfort by increasing circulation to the perineum, thus reducing edema and soreness through the use of moist heat. Because they stimulate circulation, perineal lights and sitz baths are usually not started until the day after delivery (or at least 12 hours after delivery).

The temperature of the water should not exceed 105°F because of the danger of burning the patient and because the perineal region is tender and more sensitive at this time. The patient stays in the tub approximately 20 minutes. However, the sitz bath

may need to be terminated sooner if the patient has any untoward effects.

Although a regular bathtub may be used, it is more difficult for the patient to get in and out of and it is more difficult to clean. Many of the hospital maternity departments have built-in sitz tubs which are small, low, square tubs usually made of porcelain. They are equipped with a temperature gauge which automatically controls the temperature of the water.

Whatever type of tub is used, the nurse fills it with a few inches of water, just enough for the patient to sit in. She provides the patient with something soft to sit on such as a turkish towel or cotton hip pad. If necessary, she helps the patient in and out of the tub and either checks on her frequently or places a call bell within her reach. The tub should always be cleaned with a disinfectant after use.

Recently a personal sitz bath kit has appeared in many hospital maternity departments. Its advantages are: it belongs to one patient only; there is no waiting to use communal equipment; and the patient can continue to use it at home. The kit consists of a lightweight plastic pan that fits on the toilet bowl, a large plastic irrigating bag, and tubing which attaches into the pan. Thus, the patient can take a sitz bath in her own bathroom.

Other Relief Measures. Topical sprays, such as Americaine or Dermoplast, which contain a local anesthetic agent, may also be used for temporary relief. After doing her own perineal care, the patient sprays the medication directly on the stitches and allows it to dry before replacing her perineal pad.

Applying ice bags or ice gloves to the perineum may also provide relief or may be used to reduce perineal or vulvar hematomas. To prepare an ice glove the nurse fills an ordinary surgical glove (or rectal glove) with ice chips, secures the end, and places a small sterile towel around it. The glove or bag is then applied directly to the perineum.

The perineal exercise of alternately contracting and relaxing the muscles of the anal sphincter and the vagina, may also relieve soreness if practiced several times a day. The practice of pinching the buttocks together tightly before the patient sits on a hard chair (which is preferable to a soft one) may help. Finally, an analgesic medication, such as codeine, will relieve pain.

Constipation

It is not uncommon for the parturient to experience some difficulty with intestinal functioning. Because the intestines were crowded into such a small space before the baby was born and are now, once again, occupying a relatively large space, they tend to lose their tone. Although doctors' orders vary, it is common for the patient to be given a stool softener each night after delivery or a laxative on the evening of the second day postpartum. By the third day, usually the day of discharge, the patient is given a suppository or an enema. Generally the suppository is effective, and the patient prefers it to an enema.

If the patient has had a third degree laceration or extension of her episiotomy, stool softeners are frequently given daily along with mild lubricating laxatives until the patient begins to have normal bowel movements.

Afterbirth Pains

Many women complain of discomfort from afterbirth pains in the immediate postpartum period. These pains are caused by the uterus contracting, indicating that it is returning to the nonpregnant state. The pains occur more frequently among multiparas than primigravidas because presumably the latter have better muscle tone. These pains, of course, are more severe when the mother is breast feeding or after she has received an oxytocic. There should not be any hesitation on the nurse's part to give the patient an analgesic medication promptly. There is little danger of a maternity patient becoming addicted to a drug during her short hospitalization. An explanation to the mother as to why she is having afterbirth pains is appropriate and may be reassuring.

If the mother would rather not take oral analgesics, the nurse could suggest abdominal breathing, the same type of breathing used during labor. It usually helps.

Hemorrhoids

Hemorrhoids are frequently exaggerated in the puerperium because of the pressure of the presenting part and the amount of pushing done by the mother during delivery. They may be very painful or so swollen that they cannot be replaced until their size is reduced.

Measures which provide relief for painful hemorrhoids include the application of witch-hazel compresses, sitz baths, soothing local anesthetic ointments such as Nupercainal, or analgesic-anesthetic sprays such as Dermoplast or Americaine.

Engorgement

Nursing care includes having the mother wear a good supportive brassiere 24 hours a day. If the mother does not have a bra which gives her good support, the nurse may apply a breast binder. If the mother is not breast feeding, ice bags are applied to reduce the heat, and analgesic medications such as aspirin or codeine may be given. The nurse can also suggest that she might restrict her fluid intake during this period.

HELPING THE MOTHER TO BREAST FEED

The nurse is in an excellent position to get the mother off to a good start in breast feeding. Although the hospital nurse only has a limited time to work with both the mother and baby, she can teach her the fundamental principles of breast and nipple care and feeding techniques.

The mother and baby must learn to work together. One reason that breast feeding is so psychologically satisfying is that it continues the symbiotic relationship that existed in utero. The baby derives pleasure from sucking, from the close warmth and body contact with his mother, and the relief of his hunger pains when his stomach is full. The mother receives pleasure because the baby relieves the tension and fullness in her breasts, and she too enjoys the closeness and warmth of the infant sucking at her breast. Thus it is a mutually satisfying dependent relationship.

Cleanliness is one of the most important principles in breast feeding. Before handling the breasts, the mother should always wash her hands. Indeed, the mother should have clean hands before handling the baby. If handwashing facilities are not readily available, the mother may wipe her hands with a towelette moistened with a bacteriostatic soap.

If the mother desires privacy while nursing, the curtain should be pulled around her bed. The nurse should stay with the patient, especially a mother who is breast feeding for the first time. She needs a great deal of emotional support and teaching, which is time-consuming and requires patience. When the baby begins to show signs that he is learning to grasp the nipple and suck well, the nurse should leave the mother and infant alone for short intervals. This will help to increase the mother's confidence in her own abilities.

Acquainting the mother with the various feeding reflexes of her infant and how she can elicit them is helpful. The most important one is the rooting reflex. The infant will turn his head automatically to hunt for the nipple in response to having his cheek touched. If you touch his left cheek, he will turn his head to the left, and vice versa. Thus, when the mother first receives her infant, she should give him time to root. As he nuzzles and feels the breast beside his cheek, he will turn his head and start to search for the nipple. Infants can often smell the milk which also elicits this response. If the infant is having difficulty in finding the nipple, the nurse shows the mother how to cup the infant's head in her hand and guide his mouth to it. Once the infant finds

the nipple in his mouth, he usually starts to suck right away.

When helping the mother to breast feed, the nurse does not take over the infant or interpose herself between the baby and the mother. No matter how awkward and inept the mother seems to be, it is she who will be feeding the baby. The mother must learn to evoke the responses she wants in the baby. It may be difficult for the nurse to patiently stand by while the mother learns.

The position of the mother during breast feeding should be comfortable and relaxing. The nurse encourages the mother to experiment to find any position that is most satisfactory. Because she may feel somewhat weak following delivery, the mother may start off breast feeding lying down. A side-lying position, with one arm raised and the head supported on a pillow, may be recommended. The baby also lies on his side, or he may lie on his back, whichever seems best.

Another position is sitting up in a comfortable chair. The mother may use a footstool for support, with a pillow under her arm on the side on which she is nursing. It may be desirable to have the baby lie on a pillow so that he is elevated enough to reach the breast easily without straining. Many mothers find this to be the position they use most after they are at home because they can use both hands to support the baby.

The nurse should emphasize that the sucking behavior of infants varies considerably and that there is no single "right way" to breast feed. One baby takes the nipple eagerly and hungrily; he is aggressive and vigorous in his sucking movements, and he may be satiated in 10 minutes. Another baby may be a procrastinator and tends to put off taking the breast; when he has the nipple in his mouth, he just lets it lie there. Still another baby seems to be a "rester." He gets the nipple in his mouth, takes a few sucks, and then rests for a time. All babies need some rest periods in between sucking. However, a baby who is a "rester" tends to rest longer and more frequently than others.

In the actual nursing process, the mother

should make sure that her nipple is on top of the baby's tongue. Otherwise, his sucking will be to no avail. She should try to get as much of the areolar tissue into the baby's mouth as possible so that the baby's sucking movements compress the milk ducts and sinuses. If the breast tissue compresses the infant's nose and interferes with his breathing, he won't be able to nurse. The mother should compress the breast tissue with her forefinger and hold it away from his nose.

If the baby seems disinterested in the nipple, show the mother how to moisten the nipple by expressing a few drops of colostrum. Once the infant tastes the colostrum, his interest frequently revives.

It takes patience and time for the mother and baby to learn breast feeding. Everyone will have to work at it, and it takes at least a couple of weeks for a routine to be established. Encourage the mother to persevere, and she will be rewarded. If the baby is upset and crying when he comes out to nurse, he should be held, soothed, and cuddled until he calms down. Or if the baby is sleepy and the mother or nurse can't wake him, there is no need for concern. It won't hurt him to miss the feeding, and he will probably be more hungry the next time. The mother may not get upset that the baby is missing a feeding if the nurse seems to take it as a normal happening.

Care of the Nipples. The nipples should be kept clean and dry. After nursing, the mother may apply a cream such as Masse or Vitamin A and D ointment. These creams contain oils to keep the nipple and areola soft and supple.

To keep the nipples dry and prevent excoriations of the skin, the nurse may use a heat lamp on them for approximately 20 minutes twice daily. Just exposing the nipples and breasts to the air is often satisfactory. If the nipple becomes cracked or eroded, time for healing should be allowed. A nipple shield which is a glass or plastic cover fitted with a rubber nipple may be used temporarily. If the nipple begins to

bleed, breast feeding should be discontinued, at least until healing has taken place. However, this is a decision that the patient should discuss with her doctor.

Length of Nursing. The mother should start out gradually until her nipples become toughened up. Prolonged nursing initially may cause the nipples to become sore and the tissues to break down. It is usually recommended that the mother start out nursing the baby for three to five minutes on one or both breasts. She gradually increases this to about 20 minutes, which is the average length of time for breast feeding. Actually, the baby gets most of the milk in the first five to ten minutes; the rest of the time is spent sucking to satisfy the baby's needs for sucking. If the baby is spending 30 to 45 minutes, this is too long a time and may indicate that the mother has an insufficient milk supply.

A breast-fed baby does not swallow as much air as a bottle-fed baby; hence he does not need to be burped as frequently. The best times to burp him is when the mother changes breasts, midway in the feeding, and at the end of a feeding.

Complemental Feedings. There is controversy over whether the baby should be given additional feedings from a bottle. Many proponents of breast feeding are against this practice, because they feel that it interferes with the baby's eagerness to nurse which results in the mother having a diminished milk supply. In any case, it is a good idea for the mother to know how to prepare a relief bottle which may be given to the infant occasionally. She will also want to give him plain water or glucose water at times.

Mechanical Aids for the Lactating Mother

Breast Shields. Breast shields are used to draw out the nipple when the nipple is flat or inverted or if the nipple is flattened out because of the engorgement of the breasts. It fits snugly over the patient's breast, with the nipple centered within it. However, it should only be used for a few minutes until the nipple is erect enough for the infant to grasp. The breasts cannot be emptied when a nipple shield is used because the lacteal sinuses are not compressed. After use, a breast shield should be washed, dried, and then autoclaved.

Hand Pump. The nurse may use a hand pump to express milk, if the mother is producing more milk than the baby is taking, if nursing has been temporarily interrupted, or to relieve engorgement. After cleansing her breasts and hands, the mother places the cup-shaped portion of the pump over her nipple and alternately compresses and releases the rubber bulb. This should be done for no longer than 15 to 20 minutes. A clean receptacle should be provided for collecting the milk, and the amount is frequently measured and recorded.

Electric Pump. This pump provides intermittent pressure in expressing milk from the breasts and is used for the same purposes as the hand pump. A glass funnel fits over the patient's breast. Low pressure should be used to avoid trauma to the nipples. The funnel and glass container which collects the milk should be sterilized between use.

Referrals. If after working with the nurse on breast feeding the mother still seems tense and apprehensive, the nurse can refer her to several different community resources. The public health nurse, visiting nurse (in some communities), and the La Leche League are all appropriate sources. The nurse should be prepared to interpret the services to the mother so that she knows what to expect.

BIBLIOGRAPHY

Cahill, I.: The Mother from the Slum Neighborhood: Current Concepts in Nursing Care. Ross Laboratories, 1964.

Fitzpatrick, E., et al.: Maternity Nursing, ed. 12. Philadelphia, J. B. Lippincott, 1971.

LaLeche League International: The Womanly Art of Breast Feeding, ed. 2. Franklin Park, Ill., Interstate Printers Publishers, Inc., 1963.

Riker, A.: New parent blues. Child and Family, 6:10–17, 1967.

Rubin, R.: Basic maternal behavior. Nurs. Outlook. 9:683–86, 1961.

———— Maternal touch. Nurs. Outlook, 11:828–31, 1963.

———— Puerperal change. Nurs. Outlook, 9:753–55, 1961.

Schmitt, M.: Superiority of breast feeding: Fact or fancy. Amer. J. Nurs., 70:1488, 1970.

Williams, B.: Sleep needs during the maternity cycle. Nurs. Outlook, 15:53-55, 1967.

Yunek, M.: Postpartum care is more than routine. Nurs. Outlook, 17:50, 1969.

Suggested Reading for Further Study

Clark, A.: The beginning family. Amer. J. Nurs., 66:802–805, 1966.

Pryor, K.: Nursing Your Baby. New York, Harper and Row, 1963.

Patient Teaching and Family Planning 15

One of the major jobs of the nurse in the postpartum unit is to teach the mother how to take care of herself and the baby after they leave the hospital. Opportunities for teaching the postpartum patient are unlimited; herein lies one of the challenges of maternity nursing. Since there is relatively little physical care needed by most postpartum patients because they quickly regain their independence, the nurse can spend a great deal of time teaching.

ANTICIPATORY GUIDANCE

One important aspect of teaching the mother is to tell her what she might expect once she goes home. Many women do not realize that the postpartum period lasts for six weeks and that it takes this length of time for the woman to restore herself. The nurse can impress upon her the necessity for taking it easy and getting enough rest. Otherwise, if the mother overworks and gets overtired as she might in the "taking-hold" phase, it may take her a much longer time to regain her former energy.

The nurse can ask her who is going to help her when she goes home and can encourage her strongly to get someone to help if she hasn't done so. (See Chap. 8 for further discussion.) Mothers who are unsure of themselves and feel inadequate in taking care of the baby or in breast feeding might be referred to the public health nurse.

For a mother who has other children at home a discussion of sibling rivalry is often appropriate. It is important that parents anticipate the reactions of their other children to the new baby—jealousy, envy, perhaps regressive behavior. Specific measures to deal with these problems can be suggested by the nurse. (See Chap. 30.)

The mother may also be interested in discussing with the nurse the differences in maternal feelings and in mothering patterns. Many women think that they should be overcome with maternal feelings the moment that the baby is put in their arms. Some mothers are. However, many mothers do not feel motherly at the start, and this may worry them a great deal. Pointing out to the mother that it may take some time for her and the baby to get acquainted may be very reassuring. Taking care of the baby physically, seeing his enjoyment, and cuddling and playing with him will all help in the development of mother love.

To some mothers the baby is a real person as soon as they feel quickening during pregnancy. Other mothers do not have maternal feelings for some time after the baby is born. No mother should be alarmed if she doesn't feel motherly at first. She will with time.

INDIVIDUALIZED TEACHING

A rooming-in unit provides an excellent opportunity for the nurse to teach both the mother and the father. However rooming-in is more a philosophy than a physical setup, and opportunities to teach the parents can be found on regular postpartum units as well as in rooming-in units.

A major objective is the development of the mother-infant relationship. If the husband is there, the nurse can do much to include him too (Fig. 15-1). When both parents are involved the nurse is really helping the development of the parent-child relationship. When the nurse has this objective in mind, her nursing actions reflect it. Instead of bathing the baby in the nursery, she takes the baby out and shows the mother how to bathe him; or perhaps the mother would like to bathe the baby herself. The mother is usually fascinated when the nurse points out to her the characteristics and reflexes that her baby has.

Helping the mother to breast feed or bottle feed the baby in the most comfortable and relaxed way also promotes a good mother-infant relationship. The mother can be told about self-demand feeding of the

infant, and how the healthy infant, in adjusting his appetite to his own rhythmic metabolic needs, will set up his own feeding schedule. It seems far better to satisfy an infant's normal desires than to force him to adopt a predetermined schedule.

Rooming-in seems to offer the most ideal physical arrangements to promote self-demand breast feeding, since the baby and mother are in close proximity.

The nurse can include the father in her teaching program by showing him how to hold the baby, how to diaper, bottle feed and burp the baby, and how to give him a bath (Figs. 15-2 and 15-3). Many husbands like to attend classes on formula preparation and family planning with their wives.

ASSESSING THE PATIENT'S TEACHING NEEDS

So far we have been making an assumption that the patient has a variety of teaching needs. Student nurses often feel that because a woman has had a baby previously she must know all about infant care, so that there is nothing more to teach her. Of course, it is true that in general, primiparas have the most obvious and greatest need for teaching. However, if it has been a long time since the woman has had a baby (even three or four years), or if the woman has a boy this time, and she has had all girls previously, she will probably need to learn some things.

The point is that the nurse will have to make an individual assessment of the patient's teaching needs. She can use the obstetrical nursing history form as one method of finding out what these are. (See p. 138.) Once the needs are identified, they can be incorporated into the patient's nursing care plan, and specific ways of meeting these needs can be spelled out on the Kardex. As the nurse is working with the mother she will also pick up clues as to what her teaching needs are.

Some principles of teaching are: (1) find out what the patient already knows, and begin at that point; (2) make sure that what

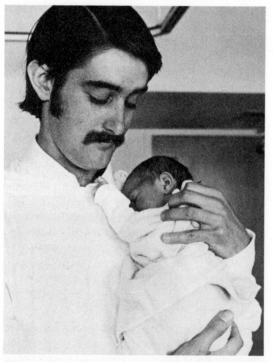

Figure 15-1.   Holding his newborn is a wonderful experience for father and baby. (Peter Whitney)

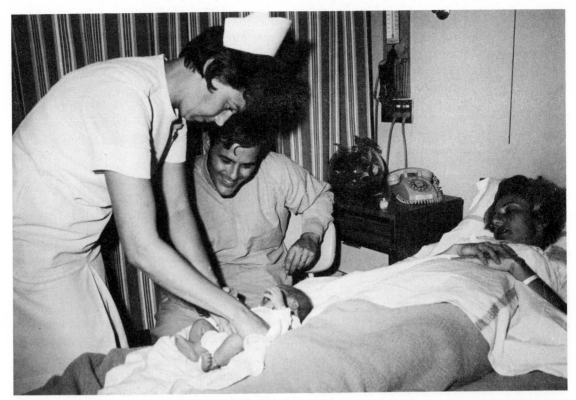

Figure 15-2. The nurse shows the parents their new baby.

you are teaching the mother is consistent with the teaching of the doctor and other members of the hospital staff; (3) make sure the patient is ready to learn; if she is uncomfortable or in need of other kinds of nursing care, these needs must be met first; and (4) try to teach her according to what she will be doing at home by finding out what equipment she will be using.

POSTPARTUM EXERCISES

Exercises are usually recommended during the postpartum period to restore tone to those muscles which were overstretched during pregnancy—mainly the abdominal muscles and the perineal muscles. It is also important to exercise the pectoral muscles which underlie the breast tissue (Fig. 15-4). Postpartum patients are frequently interested in knowing what they can do to help get their figures back. The nurse can tell them about simple exercises they can start right away while in the hospital.

Anything in the way of exercises should be mild and not tiring and designed to promote comfort as well as to lay a foundation for more vigorous exercises. The following exercises have been carefully tested to meet the above criteria. They should be done slowly, gently, correctly, and consistently to have the desired results. The purpose of these exercises is to enhance the mother's sense of well-being, promote rest, prevent the common discomfort of poor body position and alignment, and begin postpartum restoration. They have been specifically designed to be done progressively and in order, so that the first exercises prepare the muscles for the exercises that follow. In this way the muscles are protected and the most effective results are ensured. The exercise should be done with the head of the bed flat. The series should be done three times a day, with each exercise repeated four times. The nurse may explain the exercises to the mother in the following manner.

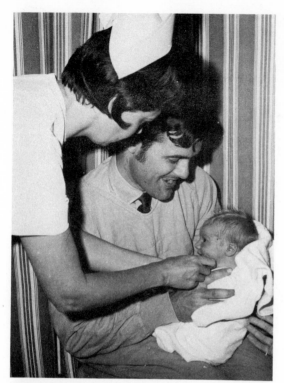

Figure 15-3. The nurse shows the father how to burp the baby.

Exercise Schedule

Delivery Day

Deep Breathing. (Designed to promote relaxation and prepare for the exercises.)

Take a deep breath. Let it out in a big sigh. Relax all muscles of the body as you exhale.

Abdominal Tightening

Take a deep breath. Let it out slowly through the mouth. *Gently* pull in and up on the abdominal muscles in a rippling motion (i.e., tighten first above the pubic bone, then progressively upward until all of the muscles from the pubis to the umbilicus have been tightened).

Hold the muscles tight to a count of three. Relax the muscles slowly from the top (umbilicus) downward to the pubic bone. Take a deep breath. Let it out in a big sigh. Relax all your body muscles as you exhale.

First Postpartum Day

Repeat deep breathing and abdominal tightening. (On each succeeding day all exercises learned so far will be done before the new one.)

Chin Lift

Do abdominal tightening as outlined. While holding the muscles to the count of three, lift head so chin is on chest. Relax your head back on the pillow. Relax the abdominal muscles slowly from the top downward as you exhale. (See Fig. 15-5.)

Pelvic Rock

Do abdominal tightening as outlined. While holding the muscles to the count of three, press your lower back into the mattress. Relax the muscles from the top downward, making a tunnel under the lower back as you exhale. Take a deep sighing breath and relax completely as you exhale.

Second Postpartum Day

Repeat all first-day exercises.

Pelvic Tilt

Do abdominal tightening while the abdominal muscles are held to a count of three. Slide the right leg down the mattress. As you exhale, relax the abdominal muscles from above downward and return the leg to its usual position. Take a deep sighing breath and as you exhale repeat, sliding right arm down the mattress. Repeat with left leg; left arm.

Third Postpartum Day

Repeat second-day exercises.

Leg-Raising (modified)

Do abdominal tightening. While muscles are held to a count of three, press your lower back into the bed, and raise the right leg so the right heel rests on the toe of the left foot (no higher!). As you exhale, relax the abdominal muscles from the top downward and return your right leg to the bed. Take a deep breath and relax all of your muscles as you exhale. Repeat with the left leg. Continue the series until the six-week postpartum examination.

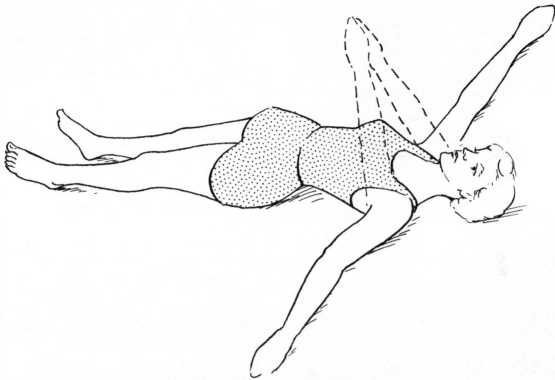

Figure 15-4. To help firm the pectoralis muscles which underlie the breast tissue, lie flat on the back with the arms outstretched. Raise the arms slowly and press the fingers together sharply and firmly. Relax and repeat 10 times. This exercise can also be done in a standing position or lying flat with a book in each hand.

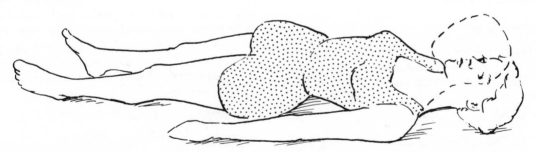

Figure 15-5.   Chin Lift.

Other Exercises

More strenuous abdominal exercises consist of leg raising and sitting up from a recumbent position. These are illustrated and described in Figures 15-6 (A and B) and 15-7 (A and B).

In the leg raising exercise it is recommended that only one leg be raised at one time since the diastasis recti (separation of the rectus muscles) will not permit the patient to raise both legs simultaneously. Similarly, sit-ups may be too strenuous at first and chin- and head-raises may be about as much exertion as is advisable.

As leg-raises and sit-ups require much effort, they should only be done once or twice at first and increased gradually. They

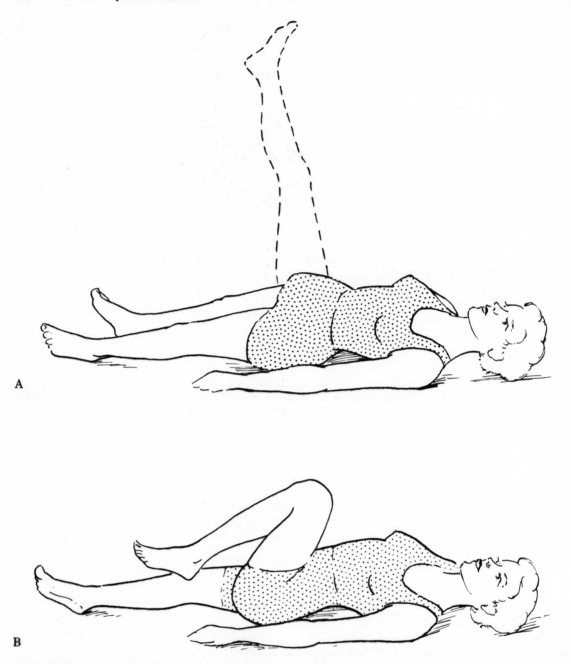

Figure 15-6. (A) To strengthen the abdominal muscles the mother lies on her back and raises her right leg as far as possible without bending the knee or raising the head and then lets it down slowly. Next the left leg is raised and lowered in the same way. Right and left legs are alternately raised and lowered. This may be started when the patient is five days postpartum.

(B) A variation of a leg exercise is to bend the right knee and draw the thigh up over the abdomen and then straighten the leg and lower it. Next the left leg is drawn up and lowered in the same way. Right and left legs are alternately raised and lowered. This exercise can be begun about the eighth day postpartum.

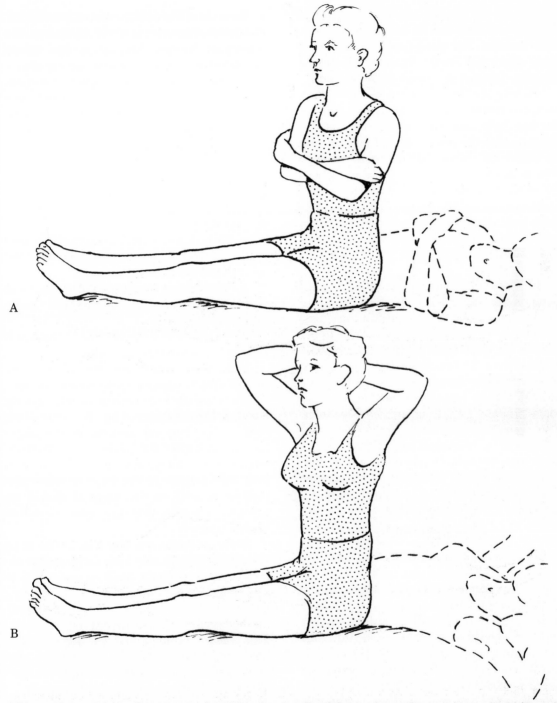

Figure 15-7. (A) Another exercise for strengthening the abdominal muscles is to lie on the back, without a pillow, and cross the arms on the chest. Raise the head and shoulders just enough to clear the floor at first and gradually raise a little farther. If the mother does not find it too strenuous, this exercise, which may be started on about the 10th day, may later be carried to the sitting position.

(B) For sitting up, the mother may clasp her hands behind her head and then bring them forward and reach for her toes. Crossing the legs at the ankles may facilitate sitting up from the recumbent position. This exercise may be started about the 12th day postpartum.

should not be carried out to the point of fatigue, and they can be continued for several months. The pelvic contraction exercises (described under Painful Sutures in Chapter 14) may be taught to the patient.

To help the uterus return to a good position, the mother may lie in a prone position for one half hour once or twice a day. A pillow under the abdomen and feet, as well as under the head, may promote comfort. The knee-chest position is sometimes used for several months after delivery to correct a retroversion of the uterus. *This should be done only when recommended by the physician* since a few cases of fatal air embolisms have been reported due to air entering the vagina.

In assuming this position the patient rests on her knees and chest for a few minutes, being sure that the thighs are perpendicular to the floor and that the upper part of the body rests on the chest instead of the elbows. The back must not be allowed to sag. Prior to assuming this position, the patient should empty her bladder and remove any tight clothing around her waist. The knee-chest position favors the return of the uterus by causing it to fall forward into its normal position. It also increases circulation to the pelvis. It should be done twice daily for one minute at first and gradually increased to five or ten minutes.

FAMILY PLANNING

An important aspect of patient teaching in a postpartum maternity unit is teaching the mother about family planning methods. The philosophy behind family planning or birth control is to make every child a wanted child. Responsible parenthood is inherent in the philosophy, meaning that the parents are able to provide for the physical and emotional needs of the child. Depending on the aspirations of the parents, they might also want to be able to give their children certain educational advantages or a certain standard of living which they would not be able to achieve if the size of their family becomes too large.

Because of the public concern over the implications of expanding world population, the American Nurses Association has issued the following pronouncement, noting that it is the responsibility of all registered nurses:

1. To recognize the right of individuals and families to select and use such methods for family planning as are consistent with their own creed, and mores.

2. To recognize the right of individuals and families to receive information about family planning if they wish.

3. To be responsive to the need for family planning.

4. To be knowledgeable about state laws regarding family planning and the resources available.

5. To assist in informing individuals and families of the existence of approved family planning resources.

6. To assist in directing individuals and families to sources of such aid.*

It is clear from these statements that nurses should assume an active role in family planning. It is unrealistic to delay giving the parents information on the assumption that patients do not resume sexual intercourse until after the six-weeks postpartum examination. Thus, the opportunity to present information to the parents while the mother is still in the hospital should be grasped. Usually they are most receptive at this time.

Some patients are shy and hesitant to ask about family planning information directly. Other patients have no hesitation at all; one such patient asked the doctor several questions about family planning methods while he was delivering her baby. This was the problem that was uppermost in her mind. Even patients who appear shy about asking questions display a great deal of interest when the subject is broached.

Teaching about family planning methods

---

*This is a quotation from the American Nurses Association statement on family planning approved Sept. 1966, Board of Directors, American Nursing Association.

varies according to the hospital. Some post-partum units have group discussions or more structured classes taught by a qualified nurse. It is usually very interesting to sit in on one of these classes and observe the patient's reactions and their questions. In the more formalized class a wide variety of films and flip charts are used. Samples of the various contraceptive methods can be passed around the room while the class is discussing the advantages and disadvantages of each method. In other hospitals the nurses do more individualized instruction.

Discussing family planning on an individual basis is best accomplished if the nurse has first established rapport with the patient. She must use the language that is appropriate to the patient's level of understanding because using the same words that the patient uses for male and female reproductive organs, as well as those that describe sexual activities will increase nurse-patient communications. During the discussion about family planning methods the patient may regard the nurse as a friend, a mother substitute, or a giver of information. As a friend, the nurse helps the mother confide in and trust her by being a sympathetic listener to the woman's problem. The young mother may confide her views on sexual matters to the older nurse as someone who will not judge her harshly for her opinions. This is a subject teenagers have difficulty discussing with their parents. As the information-giver, the nurse gives the woman correct information about contraception and sex, teaches anatomy, and explains how conception occurs.

How does a nurse introduce the subject of family planning if the patient does not bring it up? She can say, "Do you want help in planning your family?" or "Do you want birth control information?" Or less directly, "How soon would you like to have your next baby?" or "Do you know what family planning methods are available?"

The nurse should be able to discuss the various methods, explain the advantages and disadvantages of each kind, and teach the parents how to use them. The patient and her husband are the ones to decide which method they prefer to use. Their choice will depend on such practical considerations as frequency of intercourse, the expense involved, and the bathroom facilities available. Other factors to be considered are their moral and religious convictions and the aspirations of the family.

If the nurse feels that in her conscience she cannot give contraceptive advice, she should tell her patients so. This will give them an opportunity to get the information from another source.

Oral Contraceptive

It is generally accepted that the synthetic hormones (estrogen and progesterone) act by inhibiting ovulation. There are two ways in which these hormones are used in oral contraceptive pills. In the most commonly used method, each pill contains a combination of both synthetic estrogen and progestin to assure that ovulation is inhibited. It is considered to be slightly more effective in preventing pregnancy.

The other method is called the sequential method; it involves taking two different pills each month. For the first 15 or 16 days of the menstrual cycle a pill containing synthetic estrogen is taken to inhibit ovulation. Then a combination of estrogen and progesterone is taken for the rest of the cycle to produce the onset of menstruation within three to five days after the last pill is taken.

The pills are usually taken for 20 or 21 consecutive days each cycle. A variation of the 21-day pill schedule includes taking seven additional inactive pills so that the woman is taking a pill every day. This simplifies the schedule.

The combination pill is the most reliable method of contraception known at the present time. The sequential pill is only slightly less effective. The disadvantages are that about one third of women experience some unpleasant side effects during the first cycle or two of use. Some of the side effects are similar to the discomfort of early pregnancy:

nausea, breast enlargement and tenderness, weight gain, and fluid retention. Also, spotting or unexpected breakthrough bleeding may occur. Usually, these symptoms disappear after the woman adjusts to taking the pill. Switching to another kind or brand may also help.

Blood clotting disorders, although rare, have been associated with use of the pills. Women who have endocrine disorders or any suspicion or evidence of cancer should not take them. A woman should be under a doctor's care and should have regular Pap smears done while taking the pill.

The high degree of effectiveness and acceptability makes it the most widely used form of contraception. Most women have little difficulty in following the pill schedule correctly. Since taking a pill is dissociated from the sexual act itself, it has a high degree of acceptability. However, the woman must be motivated to take a pill each day.

Points in Patient Teaching

The 20 or 21-day Combination or Sequential Pills. A pill must be taken every day during the number of days that pills are to be taken (20 or 21 days). A missed pill means there is a chance of becoming pregnant. After the 21 pills have been taken, no pill is taken for one week.

The next sequence of pills is begun on the same day one week from the day the last series was finished. A woman must continue taking pills in this manner even if there is spotting or bleeding between periods or if the woman is still menstruating when her new package is to be started.

A woman must take her pills at approximately the same time every day. She should put them in a safe place out of reach of children, but also where she will be reminded to take them. With some pills a woman will have a reduction in the amount of menstrual flow.

The 28-day Pill. A pill must be taken every day. There is never a day in which the pill is not taken. When a woman takes the last pill in her package, she takes the first

pill of her new package the very next day. All other instructions are the same as for any other oral contraceptive pills.

Intrauterine Devices

IUD's are small objects (loops, spirals, rings) made of plastic or stainless steel, which are inserted into the uterus by the physician. They may be left in place indefinitely.

It is not clearly understood how they prevent pregnancy. Evidence suggests that they may speed the descent of the egg so that the sperm cannot fertilize it. Since these devices do not require much attention on the part of the user, they are good for women who lack the motivation to use other contraceptive methods regularly. The level of protection is about the same as for other traditional methods such as the diaphragm. Some women cannot use them because of expulsion, bleeding, or discomfort.

Points in Patient Teaching

The woman may feel some cramping when the device is inserted. She will have some spotting or bleeding for a day or two after insertion. There is about a three-month adjustment period during which time she will have more bleeding than usual and cramping. The woman must check herself periodically to see if the device is in place. It is most likely to come out during a menstrual period. Since some devices have strings, she should feel for the strings once a week. Another device is called the Majalin spring. After a menstrual period she should feel at the cervical os for metal. If she does not feel metal, she can assume that the spring is in place.

Diaphragm

This is a round rubber cap which fits over the cervix. It is used in combination with a spermicidal jelly or cream. It serves as a barrier to prevent the sperm from gaining entrance into the cervix. After having intercourse the woman should leave it in place from six to eight hours. It must be fitted by a physician because the sizes vary and may change after a woman has a baby or gains or loses a great deal of weight.

It is a safe method offering a high level of protection if used properly. Some failures result from improper placement or a hole in the diaphragm. A rate of two to three pregnancies per 100 women per year is an estimate for consistent users. If motivation is weak, the pregnancy rate is much higher. Some women dislike using a diaphragm because they dislike the procedure involved in inserting it.

Points in Patient Teaching

The woman should be instructed as follows. Insertion of the diaphragm must be a part of your daily routine prior to the usual time of sexual intercourse. Empty bladder and wash hands. Thoroughly spread spermicidal preparation over the inside of the dome of the diaphragm and around the rim. Compress the sides of the diaphragm and insert, pressing downward and inward with the inside of the dome facing up. After insertion, check and make sure the cervix is covered and that the rim is snug behind the symphysis pubis.

The diaphragm must be left in six to eight hours after the last intercourse in order to protect against pregnancy. If a woman douches she may douche at the time she removes the diaphragm, six to eight hours after the last intercourse and no earlier. If a woman douches at the time of removing the diaphragm she must take half of the douche before and half after removing the diaphragm.

A diaphragm is removed by catching hold of the rim behind the symphysis pubis, pulling it down, and then pulling it out compressing the side as it comes. If sexual intercourse is repeated within six to eight hours, the diaphragm is left in and an applicatorful of spermicidal preparation is inserted.

To care for the diaphragm, wash with mild soap, rinse well, and dry thoroughly. Check for holes by holding it up to the light

and gently stretching the rubber. Dust with cornstarch, *never* talcum powder or perfumed powder, as this will cause the rubber to decompose. Store in a dry container away from the heat.

A diaphragm will not get lost in the body or fall out. The woman can walk around and do her usual activities. However, the position should be rechecked after a bowel movement to make sure it is still covering the cervix.

Rhythm

The rhythm method of contraception depends on abstinence from sexual intercourse during the period of the month when the woman is fertile. This is the method that has the approval of the Roman Catholic church. Due to menstrual irregularities and inability to determine accurately when the ovum is released, the method may require abstinence for as long as half of the month.

One way for the woman to determine when ovulation takes place is to take her basal body temperature daily. She takes her temperature either rectally (more accurate) or orally every morning and plots it on a temperature graph. During the secretory (estrogen) phase of the menstrual cycle the temperature is at its lowest. When ovulation occurs, the temperature rises suddenly and sharply, about .5 to 1 degree. Progesterone is responsible for the increase in temperature. If pregnancy occurs, the woman's temperature remains at a higher level. But if she is not pregnant, the temperature drops a few days before the onset of menstruation.

When the woman takes her basal temperature daily for a couple of months, a pattern emerges as to what days are likely to be her fertile period, and she should abstain from having intercourse for a couple of days before and after ovulation. While some couples have worked this out successfully for themselves, most require assistance from a doctor or rhythm clinic.

If the rhythm method is correctly taught, understood, and practiced, its effectiveness in women with regular menstrual cycles is similar to that of mechanical and chemical contraceptives. Self-taught rhythm, haphazardly practiced, is one of the most ineffective methods of family planning.

Other Contraceptive Methods

Condom

A condom is a thin, strong sheath or cover made of rubber or similar material and worn by the man. It covers the penis and prevents sperm from entering the vagina. The woman may use a spermicidal cream, jelly, or foam for added protection.

A condom offers a high degree of effectiveness if used correctly and consistently. Some couples find the use of condoms objectionable because it cuts down on sensation and pleasure. Failures are due to the condom tearing or slipping off after a climax. It rates in effectiveness with the diaphragm.

The condom must be on the male penis before it approaches the female external genitalia or is inserted into the vagina. If the condom is plain-ended an overlap allowance of one fourth to one half inch must be made for collection of the seman. The man must withdraw his penis immediately following ejaculation before the penis becomes flaccid. As the man withdraws his penis he must hold on to the condom near the base of the penis to prevent its falling off or leaking semen while withdrawing. Condoms are used once and thrown away.

Spermicidal Preparations

Creams, jellies, and foams capable of killing sperm are inserted into the vagina. The purpose is to coat the cervical os and vagina with a substance which will destroy sperm and act as a mechanical barrier as well. They provide protection for about an hour. The effectiveness of chemical contraceptives alone is believed to be less than when used with a mechanical barrier, such as a diaphragm or condom. Nevertheless, the likelihood of pregnancy is significantly reduced with these simple methods.

Some couples feel that the drainage of material from the vagina is objectionable or that stopping to use one of the spermicidal preparations spoils the spontaneity of the sex act.

Points in Patient Teaching

Fill applicator and lie down. Insert applicator into the vagina as far as it will go pressing downward and inward. Withdraw applicator one half inch and then push plunger thereby depositing spermicidal preparation at cervical os.

If sexual intercourse does not take place within one hour of insertion of the spermicidal preparation, a second applicatorful must be inserted before intercourse. If sexual intercourse is repeated, another applicatorful must be inserted prior to each act of coitus. If a woman douches, she must *not* douche for at least six to eight hours after the last sexual intercourse in order to be protected.

Coitus Interruptus or Withdrawal

The man withdraws his penis from the woman's vagina prior to ejaculation. This requires great self control. This method has been responsible for many failures in family planning, probably because it is possible for a few sperm to escape into the vagina before the climax and semen may be deposited without the man being aware of it. While statistical studies show it to be moderately effective, coitus interruptus is unacceptable to many couples because it may limit sexual gratification.

Douche

This is flushing of the vagina immediately after intercourse to destroy or remove the sperm. Douching is considered a poor method of contraception because the sperm enter the cervical canal within 90 seconds after ejaculation.

Lactation

The patient should know that breast feeding is not a reliable contraceptive measure. Because the menstrual flow may cease during the time the mother is breast feeding, she may think that she cannot become pregnant. However, the absence of menstrual periods during lactation should not be taken as evidence that ovulation has not occurred. The nursing mother should use some method of contraception if she does not wish to become pregnant.

In summary, teaching the patient about family planning methods helps the couple to space children and limit the size of their family to the number that they desire.

GOING HOME

Before the mother leaves the hospital the physician gives her instructions on how to take care of herself, when to resume certain activities, and the importance of rest and good nutrition. Frequently, printed instructions are given to the mother so that she has something to refer to in the weeks ahead. She is usually advised to get plenty of sleep and rest and to take a nap once in the morning and again in the afternoon. She should avoid climbing stairs as much as possible for two weeks. The mother is usually advised not to have sexual intercourse until the six-weeks examination because of the danger of infection and possible injury to her episiotomy. Douching may be permitted somewhat earlier, around the third or fourth week postpartum. A douche which helps to restore the normal acidity of the vagina is often recommended.

For the care of a sore episiotomy the mother may be advised to take sitz baths. Shampooing the hair can be done at any time, and tub baths or showers are permissible. If the mother is not breast feeding and if she does not continue taking a medication to dry up her breasts, she may experience some fullness of her breasts and leakage from the nipples. The mother who is breast feeding is instructed as to her diet, what supplemental vitamins to take, and what to do if her nipples become tender or cracked.

The mother may be wondering when her menstrual cycle will return. She is usually advised by the doctor that the menstrual cycle in a non-nursing mother usually starts within six to eight weeks following delivery. In a nursing mother it begins a few months later. There is tremendous variation in whether the first few menstrual periods are scanty or unusually heavy. In general, the mother can be told not to be concerned about any pattern of bleeding or menstruation for the first three months postpartum unless she is concerned that the amount of bleeding is too heavy.

After a week or two of being at home, the mother is encouraged to get out at least one afternoon or evening a week, without children. This helps to relieve tension.

The doctor who is taking care of the baby, either a general practitioner or pediatrician, may give the mother going-home instructions about feeding, bathing, cord

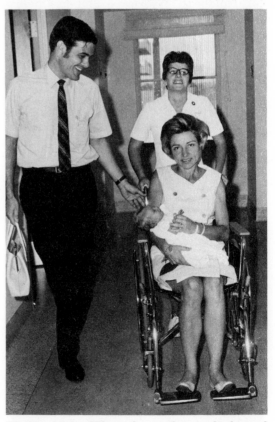

Figure 15-8. When the mother is discharged from the hospital she may be taken to the door in a wheelchair and holding the baby. This is done for reasons of safety.

care, bowel habits, behavior of the newborn, and early growth and development. The nurse should emphasize to the mother how important follow-up care is for both herself and her baby. The baby is usually checked in four weeks, and the mother usually returns in six weeks for her postpartum examination.

The typical postpartum patient is very excited and anxious to go home, and she may leave the hospital in such a flurry of excitement, that she forgets part of her belongings. However, considering all that she has accomplished and experienced in the last few days, it is amazing that she is as well organized as she is. It is a gratifying experience for the nurse to be able to discharge the new family from the hospital and to feel that she has helped them to have a rewarding childbirth experience and has helped them off to a good start.

BIBLIOGRAPHY

American Nurses Association Statement on Family Planning, approved Sept., 1966, Board of Directors of the A.N.A.

Calderone, M.: Manual of Family Planning and Contraceptive Practice, ed. 2. Baltimore, Williams and Wilkins, 1970.

Cameron, J.: Postpartum Restoration. Unpublished paper, Oct., 1967.

Cantor, N.: The Teaching-Learning Process. Buffalo, New York, Dryden Press, 1953.

Cassidy, J.: Teenagers in a family planning clinic. Nurs. Outlook, *18:*30, Nov., 1970.

Day, G.: Early discharge of maternity patients. Nurs. Outlook, *11:*825–827, Nov., 1963.

Maternity Center Association: Psychophysical preparation for childbearing: Guidelines for teaching, ed. 2. New York, The Association, 1965.

Mitchell, H.: How do I talk?–Family planning. Amer. J. Pub. Health, *56:*738–741, May, 1966.

Rossi, A.: Transition to parenthood, Journal Marriage and the Family, *30:*26–39, Feb., 1968.

A summary of contraceptive methods (pamphlet). Chicago, Ill., G. D. Searle Co., April, 1969.

Suggested Readings for Further Study

Guttmacher, A.: Family planning, the needs and the methods. Amer. J. Nurs., *69:*1229, June, 1969.

Postpartum Complications *16*

HEMORRHAGE

The most dangerous time for hemorrhage to occur is after the doctor has gone home, the family has left, and the patient has drifted off to sleep. As you may recall, the first hour after delivery is the *most* crucial period, sometimes referred to as the fourth stage of labor. However, the first 12 hours postpartum are when the majority of hemorrhages occur; 12 to 24 hours after delivery is the period when the second highest number of hemorrhages occur. Therefore, the nurse cannot relax her guard for the first 24 hours after delivery, and since she is frequently left alone with the patient during this time she has a great deal of responsibility for her safety. Knowing what to do and being able to carry out the necessary measures promptly may be life saving.

The usual blood loss during delivery amounts to about 150 to 200 cc. A postpartum hemorrhage is 500 cc. or more.

UTERINE ATONY

The most important cause of postpartum hemorrhage is uterine atony. Due to prolonged labor the muscles are fatigued and fail to contract. This is likely to occur in women who have had many children (grand multiparas) because the uterine muscles have been stretched many times and have lost their tone. Another reason is uterine overdistention from a multiple pregnancy, a large baby, or hydramnios (excessive amniotic fluid). Premature separation of the placenta also predisposes to uterine atony because blood may have been forced into the muscle fibers of the uterus rendering them incapable of contracting. If the nurse notices any of these predisposing factors on the patient's delivery room record, she should be particularly alert for signs of postpartum hemorrhage.

Hemorrhage from uterine atony may be external, internal, or both. The most significant characteristic is that the uterus is large and boggy. As bleeding continues the patient may develop symptoms of shock, such as a pallor, weak rapid pulse, cold perspiration, air hunger, restlessness and anxiety, and drop in blood pressure.

Treatment and Nursing Care. The most important aspect of care is to stay with the patient and massage the uterus. It usually responds well to massage and becomes firmer and contracted in a few minutes. When you are certain that the uterus is contracted, press down on the fundus in the direction of the birth canal to express any clots. There may be some large ones.

If the patient continues to bleed excessively despite massage, have someone call the doctor to come and check the patient. Continue to take the patient's vital signs and massage the fundus. Usually, the doctor will order additional oxytocin or start an intravenous infusion with Pitocin added. If the patient has a distended bladder and is unable to void, a catheterization may be done. A full bladder pushes the uterus up and may contribute to increased bleeding. If

231

the patient is in shock, warm blankets are applied and the foot of the bed is elevated. Usually the patient responds well to these measures and quickly passes through the crisis. By keeping calm and staying with the patient, the nurse can provide reassurance.

LACERATIONS AND TEARS OF THE REPRODUCTIVE TRACT

Sometimes there are tears or lacerations of the cervix, vagina, or perineum that continue to bleed. Or if a suture has slipped off a "bleeder," a large hematoma can occur near or at the site of the episiotomy. Sometimes these hematomas can contain 500 cc. of blood! One of the most significant characteristics of this kind of bleeding is that the uterus is firm and contracted, but bright red blood continues to trickle steadily from the vagina. This may be a more insidious type of bleeding than hemorrhage due to uterine atony, but the amount of blood lost may be just as great. The patient may go into shock and have the same signs and symptoms as previously described.

Treatment and Nursing Care. In the case of a hematoma, an ice glove or ice bag is covered with a sterile towel and applied directly to the perineum. The patient may have to be returned to the delivery room for examination to locate where the bleeding is coming from. Repair of the laceration or debridement of the hematoma follows. Intravenous fluids or blood transfusions and antibiotics to prevent infection may be administered. If the patient is to be returned to the delivery room or operating room, oral fluids should be withheld, since a general anesthesia may be given.

RETAINED PLACENTAL TISSUE

The most common cause of late postpartum bleeding is retained fragments of the placenta. This is why careful examination of the placenta after delivery is so important, to make sure that no part of the placenta or membranes has been left inside the uterus. As long as *any* tissue remains inside the uterus the muscle fibers cannot contract

properly to occlude the blood vessels. Then too, as the placental fragments separate from the uterine wall, bleeding accompanies the process.

Although the bleeding may take place while the woman is in the hospital, occasionally she may hemorrhage sometime later. She should be instructed to notify the doctor at once if she starts to bleed excessively at home or passes any tissue.

Treatment and Nursing Care. The treatment for retained placental fragments consists of giving Ergotrate by mouth to help expel them. If bleeding is more severe, intravenous fluids with Pitocin added may be given for basically the same reason. Any tissue or parts of the membranes which are passed should be saved for inspection by the doctor. If bleeding continues despite the administration of oxytocins, a dilatation and curettage (D and C) may be necessary.

PUERPERAL INFECTION

A puerperal infection is a postpartum infection of the birth canal. When the oral temperature taken four times daily reaches a level of at least 100.4°F on any two of the first ten postpartum days (except the day of delivery), then puerperal infection is suspect. Of course temperature elevation in the postpartum period may be due to the excitement of going home, upper respiratory infections, kidney infections, cystitis, or engorgement.

Puerperal infection is one of the most important causes of maternal mortality, along with hemorrhage and toxemia. The morbidity associated with it is also very significant, because the disease processes may require a long recovery period or they may be irreversible. If the mother needs to be hospitalized, this means that she has to be separated from her family and her new baby with whom she is just beginning to establish a relationship. Understandably, she is upset and depressed and needs a great deal of emotional support.

Causes. How does a puerperal infection get started and what causes it? Puerperal infection almost always is the result of pathogenic organisms being introduced into the genital tract from the outside. There are a variety of ways by which infection may be introduced, such as the use of improperly sterilized gloves or instruments or careless vaginal or rectal examinations. If the patient involuntarily touches her genitals during labor in an attempt to control pain she may introduce pathogenic organisms. Attendants who are harboring streptococci or staphylococci organisms in the nasopharynx, or those with upper respiratory infections may also infect the highly susceptible parturient. Then too, there is always the possibility that the mother may pick up an infection from another patient.

Another cause of puerperal infection is an alteration in the virulence of the normal bacterial inhabitants of the vagina. These pathogenic organisms can easily ascend into the uterine cavity during labor and delivery after the mucous plug is dislodged from the cervix and the membranes are ruptured.

What bacteria are most commonly responsible for puerperal infection? The streptococcus is the organism most often responsible. Since streptococci are commonly found in the nasopharynx of most individuals, there is an ample source for infection. Another organism, the staphylococcus is often responsible for the local or superficial infections in perineal or vaginal lacerations or incisions. There is a low incidence of puerperal infections due to other organisms such as the gonococci, *E. coli*, or *C. welchii*.

Predisposing Factors. A patient who develops anemia following an acute hemorrhage is less able to combat infection. Also, a patient who is anemic during her pregnancy is more susceptible to a postpartum infection. For this reason it is important to prevent or treat anemia during pregnancy before the woman goes into labor.

Exhaustion, dehydration, and prolonged labor are all factors which lead to infection. After being in labor for 24 hours, many patients are apt to become infected, particularly if the membranes have been ruptured for a long time. Another factor is retained placental tissue because the fragments may become necrotic. The uterus which is warm and dark and contains a good blood supply is a favorable environment for infection due to anaerobic organisms.

Frequent examinations during labor may lead to infection, since the greater the number of examinations, the greater is the chance for infection. These examinations should be kept to a minimum, and the patient's progress in labor can be judged by other methods.

Types of Puerperal Infection. Postpartum infections may involve the lining of the uterus (endometritis) or the pelvic area surrounding the uterus (parametritis). It may extend via the blood vessels or lymphatics to other areas in the body far removed from the original site of infection. If the extension of infection is along the vein it is known as thrombophlebitis. It is most often localized, but it can become a generalized peritonitis or septicemia.

Signs and Symptoms. Along with fever, the uterus may be unusually large and tender and afterbirth pains may be severe and prolonged. The patient may complain of headache, insomnia, and anorexia. If she is breast feeding, her milk supply may be suppressed. Her lochia may be increased in amount, may appear brownish, and may have a foul odor which pervades the room. However, very severe infections may be associated with scanty, odorless lochia.

Treatment. Treatment would include isolating the patient. She will most likely be placed in a Fowler's position to promote the drainage of lochia. Ergotrate is given to promote the tone of the uterus, and antimicrobial drugs are used to combat the infection.

Extension of Infection. The nurse should observe for signs of extension of the infection or generalized peritonitis. Severe abdominal pain and tenderness, nausea and vomiting, and distension, in addition to the previously listed symptoms, are indications of peritonitis. If the patient has chills accompanying a sudden rise in temperature, this usually means extension of the process.

Thrombophlebitis

The extension of infection may involve the veins of the legs (the femoral, popliteal, or saphenous) and is referred to as *femoral thrombophlebitis*. If the veins of the uterine wall and broad ligaments such as the ovarian, uterine, and hypogastric arteries are involved, it is called *pelvic* thrombophlebitis.

During the postpartum period, clots or thrombi may form in the pelvis or lower extremities due to a slowdown in the circulation. A common site of thrombophlebitis is the thigh or calf.

Symptoms. In addition to chills and fever, the patient may complain of pain in her leg, and one leg may feel hot. Sometimes circulation is impeded so that the leg, usually the left one, swells considerably, and there may be red streaks or locally inflamed areas. If a great deal of swelling occurs, the skin may be so tense that it appears white and shiny. Because of the white swollen extremity the old-fashioned term for this condition was milk leg. It often occurred about the same time that the milk came in, so it was falsely attributed to this cause.

Treatment. The treatment consists of giving the patient anticoagulants such as Coumadin or heparin to thin the blood. The nurse should recognize that the use of anticoagulants significantly increases the possibility of postpartum hemorrhage. Her observations of abnormal bleeding should be reported immediately. Prothrombin or clotting times are done to safely control the amount of anticoagulants given. The affected leg is elevated on pillows to prevent pooling of blood, and a bed cradle may be used to relieve the pressure of bed clothing. Some doctors believe in applying ice bags intermittently to the leg, whereas others

believe in using a heat lamp under the cradle. Massage of the leg is contraindicated owing to the danger of a pulmonary embolus.

Bed rest is recommended at first, and the patient is ambulated cautiously because of the danger of emboli. Elastic stockings or ace bandages are commonly ordered. If they are applied correctly, they help speed the venous circulation back to the heart and discourage the formation of clots.

Peritonitis

Peritonitis occurs when the infection extends through the pelvic lymph nodes to the peritoneal cavity. It is similar to surgical peritonitis except that the patient's abdomen does not become rigid due to flaccid abdominal muscles postpartum. The patient is very ill with constant and excrutiating pain, vomiting and diarrhea, and a high fever (103°F to 104°F). She may be restive and unable to sleep.

The treatment is to relieve the abdominal distension by suctioning the gastrointestinal tract via a Levine tube. Large doses of antibiotics may be given intramuscularly or in the intravenous fluids. Since the patient is not to have anything by mouth, intravenous fluids are given. Blood transfusions may also be beneficial. Analgesics are given to relieve pain.

Nursing Care
Prevention. The following is a list of ways to prevent postpartum infection.

Aseptic technique is carried out in the maternity department. If the nurse notices anyone not following this technique she should remind them gently and tactfully.

Equipment and supplies must be properly sterilized.

Masks should be worn at all times and changed frequently in the delivery room because the upper respiratory tract is a reservoir for streptococci.

Anyone who has an upper respiratory infection or skin infection should not take care of maternity patients.

The maternity department should be kept as a clean area, segregated from other patients who have infections.

The baby should not be brought to the mother if her temperature is elevated over 100.4°F, until the source of the fever is determined or until the mother's temperature has returned to normal for 24 hours.

Solutions should not be allowed to run into the vagina during perineal preps, perineal care, or catheterizations.

The patient should be instructed to wash her hands before giving herself perineal care to avoid the possibility of introducing infection.

The patient's resistance should be kept up during prolonged labor with rest and fluids.

Vaginal and rectal examinations should be kept to a minimum. The patient's progress in labor may be accurately evaluated by observing her reactions and contractions.

Cure. The nurse has the first opportunity for detecting the signs of infection and alerting the physician to them. The patient should be well hydrated so that her fever is reduced. Around 3,000 cc. in 24 hours may be given. Her diet should consist of easily digested foods which are high in calories and vitamins. Another goal of the nurse may be to promote adequate sleep and rest to facilitate recovery. She should administer analgesics to alleviate pain and keep the uterus contracted by giving ergonovine. The latter drug prevents extension of infection and absorption of toxins. Keeping the patient in Fowler's position helps to prevent upward extension of infection. Isolation technique should be used to prevent the spread of infection to other patients.

MASTITIS

Mastitis is another form of infection that may develop postpartally. Symptoms of inflammation of the breast do not usually develop until the third or fourth week after delivery. The breast becomes hard, red, and painful and the patient has chills, fever, and a rise in pulse rate. If the infection localizes in one area of the breast with a collection of purulent material, it is called a breast abscess.

The organism which most commonly causes mastitis is the staphylococcus. It most frequently gains entry through cracks or fissures in the nipple. Another mode of transmission is from the infant himself who may harbor the organism in his nose and throat. While the baby is nursing, the staphylococcus gains entrance even though the mother's nipples are intact.

Prevention. Preparing the breasts for breast feeding is an excellent way to prevent mastitis. If the nipples and areola are toughened for nursing ahead of time, they are less likely to be traumatized. Other means of prevention are to avoid nursing the baby too long, cleansing and drying the breasts well, and using nipple creams.

Treatment. When mastitis develops it is often treated with broad spectrum antibiotics or penicillin. The mother must stop breast feeding, and supportive measures, such as restricting fluids, wearing a good supporting bra, applying ice packs, and administering analgesics, may be helpful while the breasts are drying up. If a breast abscess is present, heat may help to localize it. The physician may prefer to aspirate the pus rather than resort to incision and drainage. When incision and drainage is done, the patient is prepared for surgery and general anesthesia in the usual manner. Packing is left in the incision until purulent material is completely evacuated. Complete recovery is usually prompt.

POSTPARTUM PSYCHOSIS

Occasionally, a patient may experience a postpartum psychosis. Actually, this is not a separate mental disease; it is referred to as postpartum because it occurs after the birth of a baby. Childbirth is the factor that triggered the psychosis. One third of these patients have had a mental illness prior to pregnancy.

Symptoms. The symptoms run a wide gamut. The patient may be withdrawn, depressed, hostile, or suspicious. She may reject the infant and express fear that she is going to kill or otherwise harm him. She may have unreasonable fears, hallucinations, or feelings of inadequacy. The earlier symptoms of postpartum psychosis are similar to those of the postpartum "blues": the patient may have insomnia and be depressed or irritable.

Nursing Care. The nurse can recognize and report early symptoms, such as any unusual or bizarre behavior. She should be concerned about safety measures, so that the patient doesn't harm herself or her baby. If the mother is disturbing other patients or may do harm to them, she should be segregated. The patient should receive psychiatric help promptly; some patients may make a fairly rapid recovery with psychotherapy and the use of tranquilizers.

Because it is possible to present only the briefest outline of this complication, the reader is encouraged to consult a psychiatric nursing text for a more comprehensive discussion. See suggested readings at the end of this chapter.

BIBLIOGRAPHY

Eastman, N. J., and Hellman, L. M.: Williams Obstetrics, ed. 13. New York, Appleton-Century-Crofts, 1966.

Goodrich, F.: Obstetric hemorrhage. Amer. J. Nurs., *62*:96-98, Nov., 1962.

Jewett, J. et al.: Childbed fever—a continuing entity. J.A.M.A., *206*:344-350, Oct. 7, 1968.

Tucker, J.: Nursing care in obstetric hemorrhage. Amer. J. Nurs., *62*:98-98, Nov., 1962.

Suggested Readings for Further Study

Leifer, G.: Rooming-in despite postpartal complications. Amer. J. Nurs., *67*:2114, Oct., 1967.

Normand, W.: Postpartum disorders, *In* Freedman, A. et al. (eds.): Comprehensive Textbook of Psychiatry. Baltimore, Williams and Wilkins, 1967.

The Unwanted Pregnancy 17

An unwanted pregnancy is any pregnancy unwanted by the people involved or by society. In our present era where there is more knowledge available about contraceptive methods and more liberal abortion laws, it is true that more means are available to prevent an unwanted pregnancy. However, there is a large gap between knowledge and practice. There is still a substantial number of women who have unwanted pregnancies and carry them through to term. The concept of an unwanted pregnancy encompasses a broader scope than just the unwed mother, although a major portion of unwanted pregnancies falls into this category. It also includes the mother who is separated or divorced from her husband, or a mother who has too many children and feels that she is unable to take care of another baby. It may also include the girl or woman who becomes pregnant as a result of rape or incest.

THE UNWED MOTHER

Much has been written and said about unwed mothers because they account for the largest number of unwanted pregnancies. Therefore, in order to dispel some common misconceptions about unmarried mothers, it seems appropriate to discuss some reasons why a girl or woman becomes pregnant outside of marriage.

"Unwed mother" is not a medical, psychiatric, or psychological term; it is a socio-legal designation. In our culture, the emphasis is on the importance of the family and the belief that a child should be raised in a home with both a father and a mother. The unwed parent is often seen by society as having violated the culture's social and ethical standards.

The unwed mother can be found in any age group from 12 to 44 (see Table 17-1). Statistics show that the number of adolescents who become pregnant out of wedlock is higher than in other age groups. One of the reasons for this is the increase in sexual permissiveness in our society. Earlier dating has led to earlier sexual experiences including intercourse.

The conflict in today's culture about the acceptance of sex as a basic drive and the disapproval of pregnancy out of wedlock, is as confusing to teenagers as it is to the older

Table 17-1. ILLEGITIMATE LIVE BIRTHS FOR THE UNITED STATES FOR 1968*

Total number of illegitimate births	339,100
White	155,200
Nonwhite	183,900
Percent of all births	9.7%
By age of mother	
Under 15 years	7,700
15–19 years	158,000
20–24 years	107,900
25–29 years	35,200
30–34 years	17,200
35–39 years	9,700
40 years and over	3,300

*U. S. Bureau of the Census Statistical Abstract of the United States: 1972 (93rd Ed.) Washington, D.C. 1972.

members of our society who attempt to meet their responsibilities to these younger people. As one writer put it: "There seems to be widespread tolerance of extramarital sexual intercourse—as long as there is no baby."*

The young unmarried mother runs the whole gamut of psychological problems and conflicts. Her unmarried state may be incidental; the real problem may be that she has attempted to solve identity problems through her sexual behavior. Each unwed mother must be considered as an individual to see what problems she is attempting to solve and to see what kind of nursing care she should receive.

What are some of the broad psychological problems among unmarried mothers, irrespective of their ages? Dr. Irene Josselyn, noted psychiatrist and author, believes that we have abandoned a concept commonly held in the early part of the century, namely, that unmarried mothers are promiscuous. In fact she says that they are usually not mature sexually, and their sexual drive has played a very minor part in their sexual behavior. They are using their sexuality simply as a tool for solving their problems.

A frequent characteristic of unmarried mothers is the wish to be loved, not in a sexual sense, but in a much broader sense. Thus the sexual act itself may give them a transient experience of feeling loved. Common in the history of these girls is a feeling of being unloved. They feel that nobody likes them and that their parents, particularly the mother, does not like them. In addition, these girls may not be physically attractive and may be approached by boys who are rather unattractive and immature. The boy often feels the same way as the girl and is incapable of loving just as the girl is; they both want to *be* loved.

The majority of girls who become pregnant outside of marriage have no conscious

wish for pregnancy, according to Dr. Josselyn. At the time of ovulation there is, in most women, an increased desire not only for intercourse but for pregnancy. Often the wish for pregnancy is unconscious. Thus the girl or woman may be led into having intercourse at that phase of the menstrual cycle when she has the strongest sexual desire without having any conscious thought of pregnancy.

Another group of unmarried mothers has a strong wish for a child as an object toward which to direct their love. Once they find they are pregnant, they lose all interest in the father. Because a child is dependent upon a parent and therefore must love the parent, they see the child as their security against ever feeling unloved.

An unmarried girl may have become pregnant because she is acting out her hostility toward men, or because she feels insecure about her own femininity and has intercourse as a means of holding the man's interest.

In some cases the young parents are involved in a meaningful relationship. They love each other and are loyal to each other, so that the sexual act is an expression of love. However, when faced with the problems of pregnancy, they decide that they do not wish the permanency of marriage. This is particularly true for the adolescent boy. An unmarried adolescent father needs counseling and guidance. Those who have worked with teenage fathers have found that these boys feel more responsibility and concern than had previously been thought. They need someone to help them work out their confused, troubled feelings.

Prenatal Care for the Teenager

An adolescent girl does not have the motivation to seek antepartal medical care as an older, married woman might. She thinks of herself as a young girl, not an expectant mother. She may even deny her pregnancy. Pregnancy may mean being excluded from school, being rejected by her family, and facing a strange, frightening immediate

---

*Garland, P.: The community's part in preventing illegitimacy. *Children, 10*:71, 1963.

future. Small wonder then that she lacks enthusiasm for traveling across the city to a prenatal clinic to join a group of patients with whom she feels no bond whatever.

Yet these girls require close medical supervision during their pregnancy, because there is a higher incidence of complications of pregnancy among unmarried mothers. There is a higher incidence of anemia, toxemia, and pelvic contractures resulting in prolonged labor. A higher proportion of premature and low-birth-weight babies are born to unmarried mothers, and there is a higher infant mortality rate.

A greater effort must be made to reach the young people and provide them with the necessary medical care as well as with counseling and guidance. If a school nurse has established a good relationship with the students, a troubled girl is very likely to take this problem to her. The nurse, the teacher, or the social worker can help the girl arrange for physical care and continuing education, and work toward an emotional adjustment.

The Attitude of the Nurse

The unwed mother or the mother who is giving her baby up for adoption because she can't take care of another one represents problems which arouse strong feelings. The nurse is not insulated from such feelings. She may find that she can be nonjudgmental in taking care of an unmarried girl who is pregnant for the first time because she feels that anyone is entitled to one mistake. But how does she feel toward the patient who has several illegitimate pregnancies? The point is that the nurse must first examine how she feels about illegitimacy and the practice of giving a baby up for adoption before she can be of any assistance to the mother. The mother will not be helped by a nurse, or any other person, who is judging her actions, imposing her values and standards of conduct, or displaying a punitive or cold and aloof attitude. The patient does need the help of a nurse who understands, cares, and has empathy for her situation.

Nursing Care

Antepartal Care

To meet the needs of an expectant mother who has an unwanted pregnancy it is necessary to find out from her what she thinks she might need, how she sees her situation, and what she might like to have done for her. The patient should be involved in her own plans; ready-made plans should not be imposed upon her.

In addition, she will probably need information and reassurance about the ordinary progress of pregnancy. Because of the guilt which the mother may feel concerning the circumstances surrounding her pregnancy, she may be especially concerned as to whether or not the baby will be normal. Some women may have attempted abortion in the early months and may wonder if this has harmed the baby. Thus, reassuring the mother about the normal condition of the fetus (insofar as it is possible to tell) and listening to her in a nonjudgmental way when she talks about her guilt feelings are ways that the nurse can help. Since many of these women have misconceptions about their own bodies and the process of pregnancy, the nurse can provide more accurate information through appropriate explanations.

Support During Labor and Delivery

Are the needs of a mother who has an unwanted pregnancy any different than those of any other mother? If she is an adolescent she may not be as physiologically or emotionally mature to meet this experience as the older mother. In the young primipara there are increased hazards from toxemia, prolonged labor, and cephalopelvic disproportion. This leads to higher numbers of cesarean sections and a higher perinatal loss. Thus, the medical problems are greater among this younger group of mothers.

The emotional needs may be greater for the girl or woman with an unwanted pregnancy. The anxiety which is present in some degree in all patients is increased, especially if she does not have the support of her family or friends to sustain her during childbirth. In some cases where the patient's mother or the father of the baby or another significant person is available, his or her presence in the labor room can provide support during labor. However, sometimes these people can be very upsetting to the patient, and the nurse may be able to see that they are doing more harm than good. Perhaps she can suggest that they "go and get a cup of coffee" if she sees that they are upsetting the patient.

Another factor which may make childbirth more emotionally upsetting is that as the symbiotic relationship of the mother and infant draws to an end, the mother may be concerned about the fate of her child. She may regress into a childish state or become more withdrawn during labor than the mother who wants her baby. The patient's loneliness may provoke her to act out her feelings of anger and frustration. The nurse must meet these outbursts with firmness and kindness. Setting limits on behavior may be necessary in some instances.

In general, the physical and emotional needs of the mother with an unwanted pregnancy are met through warm, considerate comfort measures and good physical care. Nonverbal communication by means of the nurse's facial expression, the warmth of her smile, and her touch are very important. However, the nurse should not be oversolicitous either, because this can be degrading to the patient.

Postpartum

At first, as with other mothers, the patient is pleased with the flatness of her abdomen. If she is an unwed mother she may wonder if the signs of pregnancy will disappear. Other questions she frequently asks are, "Will anyone be able to tell about the pregnancy?" "When will I be back to my old self?" The nurse can be helpful in telling her about the normal involutional processes and what to expect in relation to them.

The woman who relinquishes her baby

goes through a separation crisis. She may react with depression, irritability, hostility, anxiety, and grief. In the case of an unwed adolescent mother who gives up her baby for adoption, the one who has a healthy relationship with her parents usually weathers the separation crisis best. On the other hand, the adolescent whose pregnancy was an act of open rebellion against her parents may suffer considerable anxiety and guilt. This may lead to feelings of failure and further self-destructive behavior. Or, on the other hand, there may be a positive result, with the girl determining to do better.

Nursing care is aimed at providing opportunities for the mother to discuss her feelings without fear of criticism. The nurse can do this best by being an understanding and sympathetic listener. She can encourage the mother to use professional services on a preventive basis rather than only during a crisis. She can help the patient to focus on the future by asking about her plans for school or a job.

A wide variety of resources are available in many communities and the nurse should be familiar with the services. For example, she might refer an unmarried mother who wishes to conceal her pregnancy to a maternity home. For a patient who is not keeping her baby, a social service agency which handles adoptions would be appropriate. The family planning clinic, the public health nurse, and child care facilities are a few of the other possible resources that could help this woman. (See Chap. 3 for information about the various services available.)

One additional comment in regard to the hospital care of a patient who has an unwanted pregnancy. Many maternity departments make an effort to provide for the patient's wishes for anonymity by designating the patient as "confidential" or "no information." This means that the hospital does not give out any information concerning the patient's presence in the hospital. This helps the patient maintain secrecy if she so desires. In some hospitals the patient who is designated "confidential" or "no information" may be cared for after delivery in a separate unit or wing off the maternity departments. It may be that the medical and nursing staff believes that this may be less emotionally upsetting for the mother who is giving up her baby for adoption. There are others who believe it is better for the mother to remain in the maternity department with the other mothers and babies. Their reasoning is that it will help the mother accept reality and go through the grieving process where she will receive support. They believe that sending the mother to another area may only reinforce her denial of the situation and postpone her grieving to a time when she may not have someone to talk to and support her. Since each side of the question seems to have merit, the patient should be consulted about her wishes.

In summary, the nursing care of these mothers provides a challenging task for the nurse. The main key lies in how well the nurse can relate to the patient, support the patient in her own decision-making, and encourage the strengths of the patient. Better sex education, more acceptable contraceptives, more liberal abortion laws, and the changing attitudes of society may reduce the problem of unwanted pregnancies in the future.

EDUCATIONAL PROGRAMS FOR PREGNANT GIRLS OF SCHOOL AGE

Traditionally, if a schoolgirl became pregnant she was obliged to drop out of school as soon as her pregnancy became known. This applied to married as well as unmarried girls. In many school systems, married students, pregnant or not, have also been discharged from school or have been allowed to continue their school work but denied participation in extracurricular activities. Eventually it became evident that this was essentially a throw-away policy. It was seen as contributing to a girl's lack of belief in her own worth to society. As long as her baby was taken from her and she herself

became an outcast, society took little interest in what became of her.

The maternity homes set up to salvage these girls unwanted by society attempt to meet their emotional and educational needs. Regular scholastic classes are held in many of these homes, so that the girls can receive credit on their school record. These girls are usually prepared to resume their regular classes after delivery. Unfortunately, only a minority of pregnant girls are reached through these maternity homes.

Public school boards began experimenting with means for providing continuing education for "girls with the temporary problem of being pregnant"*, as one school system puts it. Various programs were created to meet the needs of girls who had to leave school because of pregnancy. These programs vary from strict rules concerning school attendance to rules permissive enough to allow a pregnant girl to remain in her own class if she so desires.

Traditional rules are still maintained in many school districts. A pregnant girl, married or unmarried, must leave school immediately. If the girl wishes to return to school after delivery, she must attend a different school. An unmarried student who has had more than one child cannot return to regular school. Unmarried fathers may not be welcomed in school or may be counseled to attend evening school. Other policies stipulate that a pregnant schoolgirl continue her education at home through correspondence courses.

A program with more insight is one which provides for special schools, usually within the public school program. One such program was created in a rural area with the help of a federal grant.† This is a program for middle class, average girls, whose ages range from 14 to 18 years. Most of the

*McMurray, G. A.: Community action on behalf of pregnant school-age girls, educational policies and beyond. Child Welfare, 49(6):342, 1970.
†Zober, E.: The pregnant schoolgirl. Child Welfare, 48(6):362, 1969.

girls are 16 or 17 years of age, in the 11th or 12th grade. A house in a residential section serves as the schoolroom. A full range of high school subjects is offered, including vocational as well as academic subjects.

A number of city school boards have adopted similar plans. In most of these, the student may attend on a regular school basis as long as she feels able to do so before delivery. She is allowed to resume classes at the special school after delivery until her doctor allows her to return to her regular class. Grades and credits earned are sent to her regular school. Some of these schools provide nurseries for the babies while their mothers attend classes.

The question remains, however, whether even this is the best way of helping the pregnant schoolgirl. Some schools are now allowing pregnant girls to stay in their regular classes. Convincing arguments are given for both solutions. It is not necessarily easier for a girl to leave the school environment with which she is familiar. Too often she may view this as a form of punishment or of nonacceptance. Advocates of the special schools point to their warm, friendly atmosphere as more favorable to the girl's adjustment. Perhaps there is need for both.

BIBLIOGRAPHY

Auerbach, A., and Rabinow, M.: Parent Education groups for unmarried mothers. Nurs. Outlook, *14*:38, March, 1966.

Cassidy, J.: Teenagers in a family planning clinic. Nurs. Outlook, *18*:30, Nov., 1970

Cyesis Center-Homebound Program of the Phoenix Union High School System. Phoenix, Arizona.

Daniels, A.: Reaching unwed adolescent mothers. Amer. J. Nurs., *69*:332, Feb., 1969.

Festinger, T.: Unwed mothers and their decisions to keep or surrender children. Child Welfare, *50*:(4):253, April, 1971.

Josselyn, I.: The Unwed Parent. Speech presented at Arizona State University, Tempe, Arizona, April 8, 1967.

Malo-Juvera, D.: What pregnant teenagers know about sex. Nurs. Outlook, *18*:32, Nov., 1970.

McMurray, G.: Community action on behalf of pregnant school-age girls: Educational policies and beyond. Child Welfare, *49*(6):342, June, 1970.

Pannor, R.: The forgotten man. Nurs. Outlook, *18*:36, Nov. 1970.

Ross Roundtable on Maternal and Child Nursing #2, The Adolescent Unwed Mother, 1965, Ross Laboratories, Columbus, Ohio.

The Double Jeopardy, The Triple Crisis—Illegitimacy Today. National Council on Illegitimacy, 1969.

Vincent, C.: Unmarried Mothers. New York, The Free Press of Glencoe Inc., 1961.

Zober, E.: The pregnant schoolgirl. Child Welfare, *48*(6):362, June, 1969.

Suggested Readings for Further Study

Daniels, A.: Medical, legal and social implications of contraceptives for teenagers. Child Welfare, *50*(3):150, March, 1971.

Polk, L.: Unwed mother or unwed mother. Nurs. Outlook, *12*:38, Feb., 1964.

Shanas, B.: Help for girls in trouble. Parents, June, 1971, pg. 42.

UNIT STUDY QUESTIONS

1. Which one of the following complications is responsible for the largest number of maternal deaths?
   a. cardiac disease.
   b. infection.
   c. toxemia.
   d. hemorrhage.

2. Mrs. Lee will not be breast feeding her baby. The measures that may be employed in the management of breast engorgement are:
   1. the use of a breast pump
   2. the application of ice packs
   3. the administration of analgesic medication
   4. the application of a breast binder
      a. 2, 3, 4
      b. 3, 4
      c. 1, 3, 4
      d. All of the above

3. Failure of the uterine musculature to contract sufficiently to control bleeding from the blood vessels of the placental site is called:
    a. uterine dysfunction
    b. uterine dystocia
    c. uterine hypoplasia
    d. uterine atony

4. A new mother is breast feeding her baby on a self-demand schedule. A self-demand schedule means:
    a. feeding the baby every four hours and then as often as the baby desires.
    b. a feeding schedule to fit the baby's individual needs.
    c. feeding the baby whenever he cries.
    d. feeding the baby more frequently to satisfy his sucking reflex.

5. An abnormal lochia would be indicated if one noted:
    a. a bloody discharge for the first three days postpartum
    b. a fleshy odor
    c. a foul odor
    d. a whitish-yellow discharge on the tenth postpartum day

6. Mrs. Miller told the nurse that each time she breast feeds, she experiences some pain similar to the discomfort she had during labor. This most likely is indicative of:
    a. uterine atony
    b. improper sucking of the baby
    c. suppression of lochia
    d. the uterus involuting

7. About five hours after delivery, Mrs. Smith began to bleed excessively. Factors influencing the increased incidence of excessive bleeding four to six hours after delivery are:
    1. the aftereffects of anesthesia.
    2. a full bladder.
    3. the oxytocic drug wearing off.
    4. postpartum pain medication.
        a. 1 and 2
        b. 1,2,3

c. 2 and 3
d. all of the above.

8. If a patient has a diagnosis of thrombophlebitis it is particularly dangerous to massage the affected area because massage predisposes to the development of:
    a. an embolism
    b. endocarditis
    c. a coronary infarct
    d. varicose veins

9. Which of the following drugs is *not* used in the treatment of puerperal infection:
    a. sulfa drugs
    b. antibiotics
    c. Ergotrate
    d. magnesium sulfate

10. Conditions which predispose to puerperal infection are:
    1. pre-existing anemia
    2. trauma at the time of delivery
    3. hemorrhage
    4. multiparity
    5. overweight
        a. 1, 2 and 5
        b. 2, 3 and 5
        c. 1, 2, and 3
        d. 1, 3 and 4

11. Which one of the following seems to predispose the patient to mastitis:
    a. fissures of the nipple
    b. inadequate breast support
    c. manual expression of milk
    d. incomplete emptying of the breasts.

12. The nurse places a patient with endometritis in Fowler's position. The purpose of this is:
    a. to eliminate tension on the uterus.
    b. to relieve pressure on the diaphragm.
    c. to facilitate lochial drainage.
    d. to decrease pulmonary congestion.

13. If a new mother asks you if breast feeding can be considered to be a reliable contraceptive measure which reply would be most appropriate?

a. "Yes, breast feeding is a reliable contraceptive measure."

b. "Breast feeding should not be considered a reliable contraceptive."

c. "Breast feeding is a reliable contraceptive measure during the first eight weeks following delivery."

d. None of the above.

14. Basal body temperature is used:

a. to indicate the presence of secretory epithelium.

b. to determine the estrogenic activity.

c. to determine the approximate time of ovulation.

d. to determine the regularity of the menstrual cycle.

15. When used according to instructions the most reliable contraceptive method we have today according to the lowest percentage of pregnancies is the:

a. rhythm method

b. diaphragm

c. condom

d. oral contraceptive

16. The "combined" pill uses

a. Estrogen and progesterone in each pill

b. Estrogen in some pills and progesterone in others

c. Estrogen in some pills, progesterone in some pills, and iron in the pills taken during menstruation.

d. Estrogen, progesterone, and iron combined together in each pill

17. A contraceptive method that can be obtained without seeing a doctor is:

a. a diaphragm

b. an oral contraceptive

c. a condom

d. an I.U.D. (intrauterine device)

Matching—Place the correct answer in the blank provided under Column I.

COLUMN I

_____ Endometritis

_____ Version

_____ Septicemia

_____ Frank breech

_____ Puerperal sepsis

_____ Thrombophlebitis

_____ Parametritis

_____ Mastitis

COLUMN II

1. Thrombosis combined with inflammation of a vein or veins.

2. The use of piper forceps.

3. Inflammation of the breast.

4. An infection during the puerperium arising in the pelvic organs.

5. Entry of the feet and buttocks into the pelvic brim.

6. Inflammation of a vein.

7. Inflammation of the cellular tissue around the uterus.

8. An operation in which the baby is turned to a more desirable position.

9. Inflammation of the lining of the uterus.

10. Presentation of the buttocks at the pelvic brim.

11. A morbid condition due to pathogenic bacteria in the blood stream.

12. A disease caused by monilia albicans.

Unit Five: The Neonatal Period

Characteristics and Care of the Newborn
18

CHARACTERISTICS OF THE NEWBORN

The newborn period of life is a highly vulnerable time, during which many adjustments to extrauterine life must be made. The successful transition from uterine life to independent physiological functioning is dependent on the smooth functioning of physical resources. In this chapter the normal development of the infant at birth is discussed.

The Respiratory System

The first and most important task of the newborn is to oxygenate his own red blood cells, which he starts to do with his first cry. Respiratory movements probably begin late in fetal life, although there is no functional respiration before birth.

Respirations of the newborn are mainly abdominal and diaphragmatic. Changes toward the adult type of thoracic breathing usually begin when the infant starts to sit up several months later. Breathing in the healthy newborn is quiet and shallow at a rate between 30 and 80 per minute. Character and rhythm vary with the state of the infant's activity. Grunting, labored respirations, with a rate over 50 to 80 per minute when resting may indicate respiratory difficulty and should be reported to the physician.

The Cardiovascular System

The heart beat is also variable, ranging from 120 to 180 beats per minute according to the infant's activity. Adjustments in blood circulations occurring at birth are

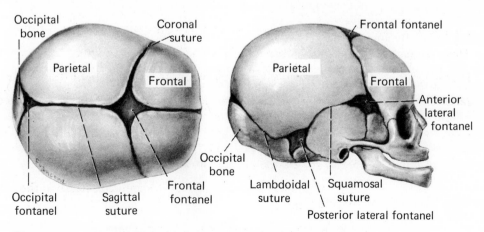

Figure 18-1. Infant skull showing fontanels and cranial sutures.

245

discussed in Chapter 38. In the newborn, blood does not circulate freely to the extremities, therefore the hands and feet may have a dusky hue and feel cool, while the rest of the body is red and warm.

Blood pressure is characteristically low in the newborn, and is difficult to measure. Normal pressure is about 80/46 at birth, rising to 100/50 by the tenth day.

Body Temperature

Temperature regulation is unstable at birth. The infant's relatively greater skin surface permits a relatively greater loss of heat, and his heat regulation system is immature.

Immediately after birth the infant's temperature drops to about 96° F., a normal reaction to the change from the warm uterus to the outside world of the delivery room. During the first 12 to 24 hours, the body temperature gradually rises to 98° to 99° F. where it stabilizes. Infants who are slow to adjust body temperature are placed in heated cribs or incubators in the nursery until they stabilize. A newborn at home can be protected from chilling by being wrapped in a light blanket and kept in a warm room. Care must be used not to overdo this protection. Hot water bottles and heating pads should be avoided, as a young infant can be easily burned.

Digestive Tract

The gastrointestinal tract is functional, with meconium passed between 8 to 24 hours after birth. The nurse should check to make sure an anus is present, and also watch carefully for the first stool to rule out any higher rectal atresia. Meconium is a sticky greenish-black substance composed of bile, mucus, cellular waste, intestinal secretions, fat, hair and vernix caseosa swallowed during fetal life with the amniotic fluid.*

The newborn infant is able to digest the

protein, fat and carbohydrate in breast milk, or modified formulas. Sucking and swallowing reflexes are present before birth.

The Genitourinary Tract

The kidneys secrete urine before birth, and some collects in the bladder. After birth, the kidneys are sufficiently mature to handle the load suddenly presented them. A record of the first urination is important in order to establish the fact that the kidneys are functioning adequately and that there are no severe constrictions of the urinary outlet system.

In the male infant the prepuce of the penis is normally tight and adherent. Circumcision may be done for cultural or religious reasons (see page 255). In the female the labia are prominent due to the effects of the mother's estrogens. The female infant may also have a slight bloody vaginal discharge, also due to hormonal stimulation from the mother.

The Head and Skull

In order to facilitate the passage of the large head of the newborn infant through the birth canal, the skull bones are not united but can mold and overlap. The seven bones of the skull are divided by narrow spaces called sutures. At the point of juncture of these bones, triangular spaces called fontanelles are present. The two palpable fontanels at birth are the anterior, at the juncture of the frontal and parietal bones, and the posterior, at the juncture of the parietal and occipital bones (Fig. 18-1).

The brain is covered with a tough membrane, making it difficult to injure the child at the fontanels, with ordinary handling. Mothers need to be assured that the baby's scalp can be washed over these points without harm, and ordinary cleansing can be helpful in preventing the frequent accumulation of crusts composed of oil, serum and dirt popularly known as *cradle-cap*.

The head of the newborn is large in proportion to the rest of his body. It

---

*Breckenridge, Marian E. and Murphy, Margaret Nesbitt: Growth and Development of the Young Child, p. 169. Philadelphia, W.B. Saunders, 1969.

measures about 12 to 14 inches (30.5 to 35 cm.) in circumference. During the first few months of life, the sections of bony skull calcify and join together; the posterior fontanel disappearing after four to six weeks, and the anterior fontanel closing between the end of the first year and the 18th month. During delivery the head has molded along the suture lines, so that it may have asymmetrical proportions after birth. Usually normal shape is assumed within a few days. (Fig. 18-2).

Caput Succedaneum is an edematous swelling of the soft tissues of the scalp involving the presenting part during labor and delivery. The edema usually disappears within a few days.

Cephalhematoma is a collection of blood between the periosteum and a skull bone. The swelling of the overlying scalp is usually not visible until several hours after birth. Most cephalhematomas are absorbed within a few weeks. Aspiration of the contents of the swelling is contraindicated because of the danger of infection.

The Chest

The chest in the newborn has a smaller circumference than the head. The breasts of both male and female may be enlarged as a result of maternal estrogens in the blood stream. A pale milky fluid can be expressed. The condition clears up in 4 to 6 weeks. In the meantime, the breasts should be handled gently and not manipulated in any way.

The Skin

Sluggish peripheral circulation and vasomotor instability are manifested in the deep red color the infant acquires when he cries, and in the pale hands and feet of many newborns. The infant in good condition shows a good skin turgor.

Fine downy hair, called *lanugo* covers the skin of the fetus, and may have virtually disappeared in the full term infant. A cheeselike, greasy substance, vernix, protects the skin of the infant in utero. Vernix is a water and oil mixture containing

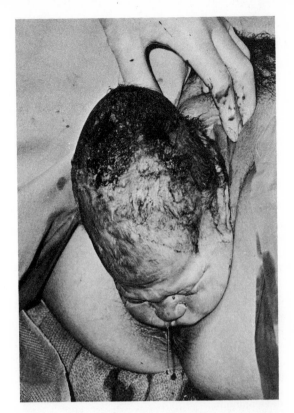

Figure 18-2. The head of this newborn is elongated owing to the pressure applied by forceps.

a mixture of cells flaked off from the skin and fatty substance secreted by the sebaceous glands. It is believed to protect the skin during uterine life. At birth the skin may still be covered with vernix, or it may be accumulated in the folds of the skin.

In some hospitals the vernix is believed to be protective and is not washed off. It eventually dries spontaneously. In other nurseries, the infant is bathed when its temperature stabilizes.

Skin blemishes are common. Many disappear in time. "Strawberry marks" (nevus vasculosus) are the most common of the vascular nevi. These are raised, bright red collections of blood vessels appearing at birth or shortly after. They usually break up and disappear spontaneously in later childhood.

Pigmented nevi (moles) in infants are benign areas of rough brown or black areas.

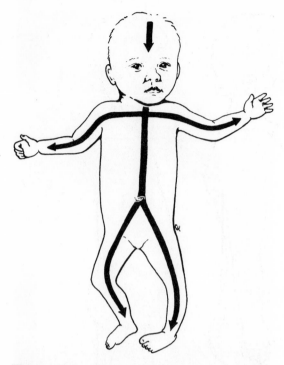

Figure 18-3. The arrows indicate the cephalo-caudal and proximal-distal progress of infant development.

They may be located at any site on the body. Large flat surfaces of brown pigment called cafe-au-lait are sometimes present. Although some of these nevi are unsightly, they are benign. Nevi in areas where they are subject to repeated irritation probably should be removed during later childhood.

Milia are pinhead-size papules which may occur on the face of the newborn. They are small collections of sebaceous gland secretions that have been trapped beneath the skin. They eventually disappear spontaneously.

Forcep marks are noticeable on the face but disappear in a day or two. (Fig. 18-2). Bruises may be present on the head or scalp after a difficult delivery. They are also common about the genitalia and buttocks in breech-delivered infants. These gradually clear up without treatment.

Physiological jaundice occurs in a large number of newborn infants and has no medical significance. The yellowing of the skin does not appear until after the second day of life. *Any jaundice appearing during the first 3 days of life should be promptly called to the physician's attention.* The nurse needs to be alert to the possibility of hemolytic disease of the newborn in such cases.

The skin or head blemishes or marks can be very distressing to the new mother who does not understand their relative lack of significance. A mother may worry excessively about such marks but may be afraid to ask for an explanation. The nurse can do much to relieve her worries by carefully explaining in simple terms about these minor marks or bruises. Any significant condition should be explained by the physician, with follow-up by the nurse.

The Bony Structure

The arms and legs of the newborn infant are short in comparison to his trunk. Prenatal development proceeds in a cephalocaudal — head-to-feet — progression, and in a proximal to distal sequence. This means that his head and trunk are well developed, but the distal areas develop later. Development also proceeds from the general to the specific, the gross muscles coming under control before the finer muscles.

Height and Weight

The newborn infant's birth weight is of great interest to all concerned. Average birth weight is 7-1/2 lbs. (see Table 26-2 and growth chart in Chapter 26.) Average length is 20 inches. These measurements are based on white children in the United States. Infants in other countries or of other races may differ slightly.

Neonatal Activity

The newborn infant makes uncoordinated, random movements. At this age his movements and responses to stimuli are built-in reflexes, or as we might say, instinctive reactions. The healthy newborn infant when placed on his abdomen face downward will lift his head or turn it to one

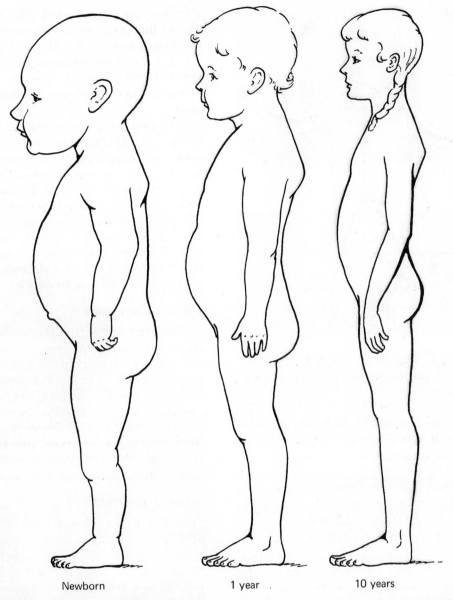

Newborn   1 year   10 years

Figure 18-4. There is a startling change in body proportions during infancy and childhood.

side to clear his airway. He can hiccup, sneeze, yawn, stretch, blink and cough. He also swallows and sucks his thumb, having practiced before birth.

Neonatal Reflexes

The newborn infant's behavior is governed by reflexes triggered by his immature nervous system. He startles easily when his equilibrium is disturbed. Put him down suddenly on a flat surface and he will tense, throw his arms out in an embracing motion and usually cry. This is the Moro reflex, also called the startle reflex (Fig. 18-7). This reflex disappears by 4 to 6 months of age.

The tonic neck reflex (TNR) is a position many infants assume particularly

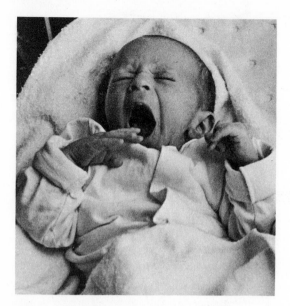

Figure 18-5. The newborn infant yawns frequently.

for sleeping. The infant turns his head to one side, extends his arm on the same side and flexes the opposite arm in a sort of fencing position (Fig. 18-8). Not all young babies assume this position, however, and it disappears in normal infants at about 6 or 7 months of age.

Other Reflexes in the Newborn

Rooting reflex. The infant turns his head toward any warm object touching his cheek, and actively seeks the nipple. Thus, when a nurse places her hand on the infant's cheek to turn his face to his mother's breast, he turns instead toward the nurse's hand.

Sucking reflex is elicited whenever a finger or nipple is placed in the infant's mouth.

The grasp reflex. Pressure on the palm of the newborn causes him to close his fist tightly around the examiner's finger. The grasp is so strong in a healthy infant that he can be lifted up off the examining table. This reflex grasp fades, to be replaced by a voluntary grasp in a few months.

The stepping reaction is seen in most normal newborns. When held in an upright position, the infant makes stepping movements. This reflex is not seen after 3 or 4 months of age.

Sensory Development

Sight. The infant sees at birth in a limited manner. His eyes are sensitive to bright light, and he appears to be aware of differences in light intensity. By the end of 2 weeks he looks at large objects, but he is not following them with his gaze. His eyes are gray or blue at birth, changing to their permanent color over the following months.

Hearing. The newborn responds to noise

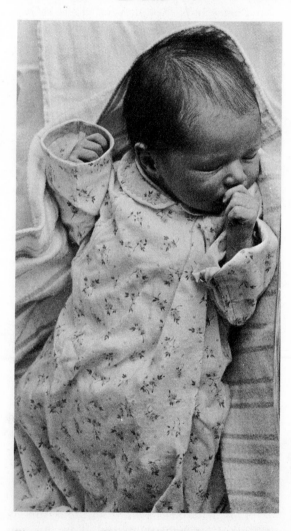

Figure 18-6. The newborn infant sucks his thumb.

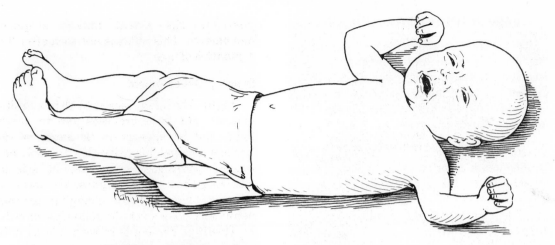

Figure 18-7. The Moro, or startle, reflex.

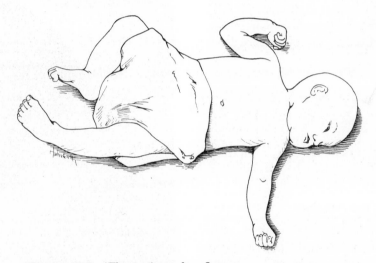

Figure 18-8. The tonic neck reflex.

as soon as the pressure in his ears has equalized. He startles at a loud noise and ceases his crying or postural activity momentarily when spoken to in a soft, soothing voice.

Touch. Sensitivity to touch is present from birth. The newborn uses his sense of touch in feeding; both tongue and lips are sensitive to touch at a very early age. Newborn infants do not appear to be very sensitive to external pain, although they do definitely respond to needle pricks. However they do respond strongly to hunger pains or internal discomfort.

Muscular Activity

The infant immediately commences, or rather, continues, his *developmental task* of exercising his muscles. His arms and legs are moving constantly when he is awake, and even in sleep he frequently moves to change a position or to stretch a muscle. His muscles are maintained in a tensed state as though for ready action, his legs are drawn up, and his fists are clenched. A newborn infant who habitually lies in a relaxed manner, with supple, soft musculature, needs to be watched closely for central nervous system inadequacy.

CARE IN THE HOSPITAL NURSERY

In the delivery room the newborn infant has been observed and identified and has received his prophylactic eye drops. If his mother is awake she has seen her child, and may have held him in her arms; perhaps his father has also.

The Newborn Nursery

The infant can now be transported to the nursery, either warmly wrapped and carried in the nurse's arms, or in a movable heated crib, depending on his condition and on hospital policy. In some maternity departments, the newly born are admitted to a receiving or admitting nursery where they are under constant supervision and care for a period after delivery. Premature or high risk infants are admitted to the infant intensive care unit.

On acceptance in the nursery, the infant is identified, weighed, and checked over carefully; he also has his temperature taken. The foot of his bassinet is elevated at an angle of 15° to 20° for the first 24 hours because of the possibility of respiratory distress. The infant should be turned from side to side every 2 or 3 hours.

Temperature of the Newborn

If a rectal temperature is taken, care must be used not to insert the thermometer for more than 2 cm. Instances of bowel perforations from rectal thermometers and infant rectal tubes or catheters are on record. Many nurseries make a practice of taking axillary temperatures. This is done by placing the bulb of the thermometer in the infant's axilla, holding his arm to his side, and keeping the thermometer in place for 1-1/2 to 2 minutes. Maintenance of a stable temperature in the newborn is important. An axillary temperature of 96° to 99° is considered within normal limits. Means employed for stabilization of the infant's temperature are warm clothing, a nursery temperature of approximately 75°, and, if necessary, a heated crib.

In many nurseries, an injection of 1 cc. of

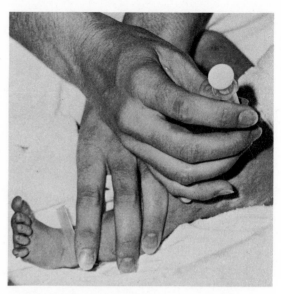

Figure 18-9.   Receiving vitamin K injection.

vitamin K intramuscularly is given shortly after birth. This is given in order to correct any coagulation defect related to vitamin K deficiency.

Bathing

Nurseries differ in the way the admission bath is given. In some nurseries newborn infants are cleansed with a sterile cotton ball soaked in liquid detergent containing 3% hexachlorophene as a precaution against infection.* In other nurseries, the blood and vernix are wiped from the infant's face for esthetic reasons, and no other admission cleansing is attempted. The major concern is to avoid chilling the newborn, whose temperature is not yet stabilized. The infant is then dressed in shirt and diaper, and wrapped loosely in a light blanket.

Observation of the Newborn in the Nursery

The newborn is kept in the admitting nursery until his temperature has stabilized, he has been examined by his physician, and his mother has rested. In some nurseries this is a routine period of 12 hours. If his con-

*The Academy of Pediatrics now recommends against the use of hexachlorophene for bathing newborn infants.

dition is satisfactory, he is then moved into the central nursery or to his mother's bedside if rooming-in is used. The first neonatal day is a hazardous period. The nurse caring for infants in the admitting nursery needs to know what to look for as well as how to respond to any emergencies. Her observations should be carefully recorded.

1. *Infant's cry and state of activity.* The healthy full term infant should have an excellent muscle tone. Muscle tone is defined as the resistance to passive movement when a limb is moved by the examiner.* During the first hours after delivery many infants are quite sleepy and inactive, but a healthy full term baby does not relax his muscle tone even in sleep. The infant's cry should be deep and vigorous, a lusty cry. A weak or high pitched shrill cry should be reported.

2. *Respirations* are noted, with particular attention to indications of respiratory distress. Mucus in the nasopharynx may cause considerable distress and gagging episodes during the first hours of life. Usually postural drainage will help remove the mucus. Treatment in periods of apnea or severe respiratory distress is discussed in Chapters 19 and 21.

3. *Condition of the cord.* The cord site is checked frequently, and any bleeding or oozing is reported promptly.

4. *The infant's skin* is checked for appearance of jaundice or pallor. Jaundice during the first 24 hours should be reported (See Chapter 21). If the infant has been circumcised in the delivery room, the site is also inspected for bleeding.

5. *Elimination.* First urination and defecation must be watched for and reported. The nursery nurse should be advised if the infant voided in the delivery room.

Care in the Central Newborn Nursery
The Infant's Emotional Needs

A newborn reacts to being held closely and lovingly. His distress subsides, he can

*Egan, D.F. et al: Developmental Screening: 0-5 years. p. 6

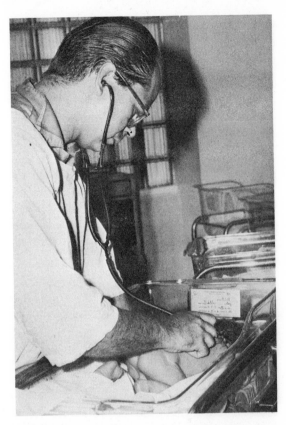

Figure 18-10.   Examination by physician.

even ignore his physical needs momentarily while he responds to the comfort of his mother's intimate presence. Not for long, of course, because during this period of his life his emotional needs are met principally through the complete physical care he receives. The optimal care combines cuddling, rocking and soft, soothing voices with the comfort of feeding in his mother's arms, of being warm and comfortable. The security the newborn feels helps him develop the sense of trust he needs to cope with his new environment. Emotional support is not as easily supplied in a central nursery as it is in a rooming-in setup. If a restless or distressed infant can be held and soothed in the nursery and taken to his mother promptly when he indicates hunger, he will receive much of this necessary emotional support. Rocking chairs are needed in the newborn nursery.

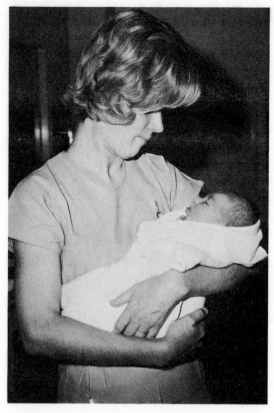

Figure 18-11. He needs to be held closely and lovingly.

Physical Care

In the United States the present length of stay for a healthy newborn in the hospital is 3 days. Infants delivered by cesarean section generally stay 5 days.

Daily care. The infant should be undressed and inspected daily. The *bath* may be similar to the admitting bath. However, if the mother is given a demonstration bath and returns the demonstration, a complete sponge bath should be given.

Care of the cord. No dressing is put over the umbilical cord stump. In some hospitals the stump is painted daily with a triple dye to guard against infection. Triple dye contains acriflavine, gentian violet, brilliant green and water. In nurseries where triple dye is not used, the base is wiped daily with alcohol.

The cord tie is left in place until the cord drops off, but the clamp is removed in 24 hours. Mothers should understand that sponge baths only are given until the umbilicus is healed.

Blood Test for Phenylketonuria (PKU) Babies are routinely tested for PKU before being discharged in hospitals in most states in this country. The Guthrie assay method is most commonly used. In this test, one or two drops of blood are obtained by heel prick and are placed immediately on filter paper. The specimen is sent to the laboratory where the phenylalanine level of the infant's blood is determined (See Chapter 31).

Regulations for Newborn Nurseries

Standards for newborn nurseries have been set up by the American Academy of Pediatrics. Nurses, parents, anyone handling a newborn infant should first wash his hands

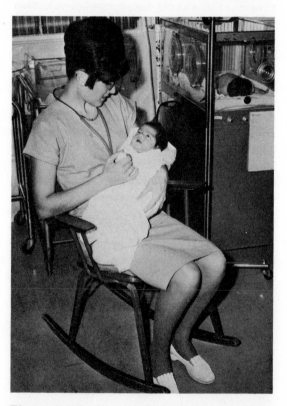

Figure 18-12. It's a good idea to have a rocking chair in the nursery. (Courtesy Good Samaritan Hospital, Phoenix.)

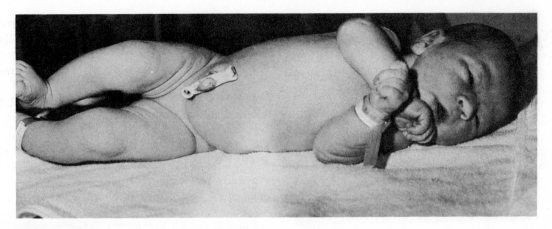

Figure 18-13. The cord stump is examined frequently.

thoroughly with an antiseptic or soap containing hexachlorophene.

Nursery personnel put on clean gowns when caring for newborn infants, preferably gowns with short sleeves. All members of the nursery staff should have a pre-employment physical. No staff member should enter the nursery or handle the babies if she has any infection, whether respiratory, skin lesion, or gastrointestinal.

Circumcision is a surgical procedure in which the foreskin or *prepuce* of the penis is removed. Traditionally it has been performed for religious or cultural reasons. In the United States it has been believed to be of medical significance as well, and circumcision of the newborn has become almost routine. However, circumcision is not practiced to any great extent in Europe, South America, or Japan.*

Physicians in this country are now beginning to question routine circumcision of newborn males. No surgery is entirely benign, and the arguments against routine mutilation of the bodies of newborn infants are potent. Many physicians now advise circumcision in selected cases only where in their judgment a reason exists for this procedure.

Circumcision is frequently performed in

the delivery room shortly after the child's birth, unless it is to be a religious ritual circumcision. The raw incision is covered with sterile, Vaseline-saturated gauze. The infant is checked frequently for bleeding. The incision heals rapidly. When the gauze falls off, it need not be replaced.

Rooming-in

The practice of rooming-in has much in it to be commended. In this plan, the infant's crib is placed beside the mother's bed in order to permit mother and child to be cared for together. It is interesting to note that many of the so-called "under-developed" countries have followed this practice throughout history, and that many more sophisticated countries use it without question.

The American Academy of Pediatrics, in setting standards for hospital care for newborn infants, presents the following special features of rooming-in: (1) provides the mother and infant with a natural mother-child experience beginning as soon after delivery as the mother is capable of assuming the care of her baby; (2) fosters infant feeding on a permissive plan; (3) facilitates instruction of mothers and fathers in infant care, and (4) reduces the incidence of cross-infection among infants.

Types of plans. Rooming-in plans have been worked out in various ways. Some

---

*Shepard, Kenneth S.: Care of the Well Baby. p. 294

nurseries permit the baby to stay at the mother's bedside throughout the day, returning him to the nursery at night. Others provide continuous rooming-in, but nearly all make some provision for the baby to be taken into the nursery when necessary for the mother's comfort.

Rooming-in has done much for mothers who are unhappy with the rigid schedule and enforced separation that a nursery fosters. There are many good mothers, however, who, for various reasons, do not wish to use the rooming-in plan. A mother with several small children may appreciate the short period of rest, quiet, and absence of responsibility that the hospital can provide.

Nutrition of the Newborn Infant

The timing of the newborn child's first feeding depends partly on his condition and partly on the philosophy of those responsible for him. Some physicians would prefer to allow the infant a period of rest immediately following birth, bringing the child to the breast after a period of 6 to 12 hours. Others advocate putting the child to breast when he shows a definite readiness and the mother has recovered sufficiently.

Breast Feeding

Breast feeding appears to be coming back into favor in the United States after a period during which many women rejected it in favor of artificial feeding. Even the woman who returns to employment outside the home after a month and a half or two may feel that there are advantages to breast feeding during this short period.

That there are advantages is true. Breast milk is easily digested, needs no preparation and is available as needed. It does not sour or become contaminated in a healthy mother.

There are few contraindications to breast feeding. Certain maternal illnesses such as tuberculosis or severe malnutrition are reasons against breast feeding. An infant's inability to nurse due to physical causes such as prematurity or cleft lip defect makes special feeding measures necessary. Another

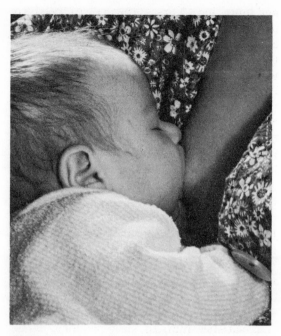

Figure 18-14. Breast feeding has emotional and physical benefits for both mother and baby.

pregnancy will make breast feeding too much of a drain on the mother.

The healthy mother must be entirely free to make her own decisions in this matter. If she does not desire to breast-feed her infant, she must not be made to feel guilty or inadequate as a mother. The advantages of breast-feeding may be enumerated if she is undecided: the absence of milk contamination, the ready supply of milk, and the absence of formula preparation (Fig. 18-14).

The infant who is loved, and held for his feedings, who experiences the same kind of closeness that the breast-fed infant receives, probably does not suffer emotionally because he is bottle-fed. A certain number of infants, however, do appear to have allergic reactions to cow's milk, which are not evident when these infants are breast-fed. This, of course, does not include those infants who, because of some metabolic defect, cannot tolerate any form of milk.

Probably the majority of women can successfully breast-feed their infants if they understand and follow principles of hygiene and nutrition. Nurses themselves need to understand the principles underlying successful breast feeding. A normal infant is born with a "rooting" reflex, so that he seeks with his mouth the source of nourishment. Anything that touches his cheek is interpreted as a source of food, and if he is hungry, he immediately turns his head in that direction. Therefore, a nurse who puts her hand on a baby's cheek and tries to turn his head toward the breast, is defeating her purpose. A better policy is to let the breast lightly brush the infant's cheek, and he will then turn in that direction to seek the nipple. He may need some help in learning to grasp the nipple properly.

We have learned much about the behavior of young infants. The baby who is allowed to eat when he is hungry, to determine for himself the amount of food that satisfies him, to sleep as long as he chooses without being disturbed, appears to have a much better chance to develop a sense of security as well as physical well-being.

Self-demand feeding is often considered impractical in the newborn nursery. Nurses are apt to react in a conservative manner to new ideas. Certainly there are practical difficulties, but it is actually poor nursing to reject an idea that is for the welfare of the patient without meaningful consideration. Almost always, the sole insurmountable obstacle to carrying out a new but desirable technique is a closed mind.

The healthy infant soon adjusts his appetite to his own rhythmic metabolic needs and sets up his own feeding schedule if allowed to do so. In the majority of vigorous, full-term infants, this schedule approximates a 4-hour interval. Smaller infants may need food every 3 hours, or, occasionally, at a 2-hour interval. The rate of stomach emptying also varies in individuals. It appears far better to satisfy an infant's normal desires than to force him to adopt a predetermined schedule. After a short period of adjustment, the household can learn to plan activities around the infant's schedule.

The nursing infant may be permitted to suck for the period of time it takes to satisfy him, provided of course that there is sufficient milk. Some babies seem to get right down to business and get all they want in 5 or 10 minutes. Others may be more leisurely and enjoy 15 or 20 minutes at the breast. An infant who is not satisfied in 20 to 30 minutes is signaling that things are not entirely right. Perhaps the mother has found it difficult to relax, or has not had enough rest or proper nourishment. This results in an interruption in the flow of milk, causing the baby to be irritable and unsatisfied. In turn, baby's unhappiness causes more worry and unrest for mother. Frequently, a third person—such as a nurse — understands the difficulty and helps to straighten things out.

Artificial Feeding

The mother who, for whatever reason, chooses to feed the baby a formula, can be assured that present day formulas approximate human milk and are entirely satisfactory.

Probably of greater importance to the average infant than the type of feeding is the feeling of acceptance and security he receives. The bottle-fed baby needs to be held closely and lovingly in the same manner as the breast-fed baby. Bottle propping has no place in either the newborn nursery or in the home. It is dangerous for the infant and deprives him of needed physical contact.

Babies are apt to swallow air when they nurse and need bubbling once or twice during feeding. This is true both of bottle-fed and breast-fed infants. The baby may be held up over his mother's shoulder and his back gently rubbed, or he may be sat upright on her lap with his head supported.

The formula is usually warmed, although recent studies have shown no ill effects from cold milk, and it appears to be well accepted this way. Mothers should be made aware that healthy babies regurgitate small amounts of formula at times. They should know that there is a difference between regurgitation and vomiting.

Regurgitation means the simple spitting

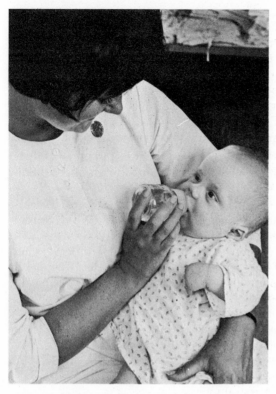

Figure 18-15. Positioning of an infant for bottle feeding.

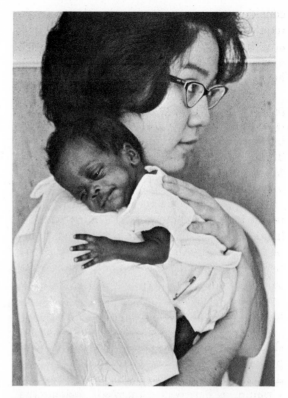

Figure 18-16. Bubbling a baby against the shoulder.

up of small amounts, actually an overflowing, perhaps from an air bubble, too rapid nursing, or just too much milk for the stomach to hold.

Vomiting is used to designate the expulsion of an appreciable amount of fluid. Although this also may be the result of rapid feeding or inadequate "burping," it may also indicate an abnormal condition, and requires careful watching.

Types of Formulas

Commercial formulas. Commercially prepared formulas come either completely ready for use, or may require dilution with sterile water. Some preparations are available to the consumer completely prepared in their own disposable containers, with nipple attached. These formulas have been prepared to approximate quite closely human milk and are easily digestible. They are a great help to mothers who have to

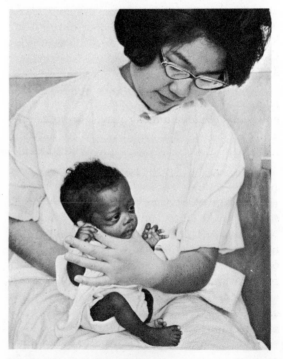

Figure 18-17. Bubbling a baby sitting upright.

consider the amount of time and work required in the preparation of formulas. They are, however, rather expensive, and the mother may prefer to do the preparation herself.

Evaporated milk is probably the most popular form of milk for home preparation. It is inexpensive, safe, and easy to use. It can be kept in the can until opened, is easily diluted and well tolerated by most infants. Most brands have been irradiated with vitamin D.

Whole milk is not so frequently used today for young infants. It requires careful handling, is easily contaminated, and must be fresh. Grade A pasteurized milk should be used, and it should be boiled before use, both to soften the curd and to destroy harmful bacteria. Whole milk may also have been irradiated with vitamin D.

Dried milk may be either whole milk or skim milk that has been processed into powdered form. When reconstituted, whole dried milk is similar to liquid milk, although vitamin A has been destroyed during the processing. It is useful while traveling or in areas where refrigeration is not available.

Any of these forms of milk must be kept refrigerated; whole fresh milk immediately following production, evaporated milk after the can is opened, and dried milk after being liquefied.

Special formulas are available for infants allergic to milk. These are usually made from soy beans or have a meat base. Formulas are also available for infants with certain metabolic defects, such as phenylketonuria.

Preparation of Formulas

The type of milk used needs dilution with sterile water and the addition of a carbohydrate in order to meet the infant's needs. The carbohydrate may be in the form of simple sugar, or a dextrin-maltose preparation. Formulas for full-term babies are calculated to provide 20 calories an ounce. The average infant takes 2 to 3 ounces at a feeding during the first weeks of life, with gradual increases in strength and amount.

There are two methods of preparing a formula at home. One, known as the *aseptic method*, requires that all utensils be sterilized before use, and that these utensils be used for no other purpose than formula preparation. This includes saucepan, mixing spoons, measuring cups and can opener. Bottles, bottle caps and nipples are boiled, the tops of cans washed with soap and water and rinsed in hot water. The person preparing the formula should scrub her hands and wear a clean apron or dress.

The method known as *terminal sterilization* is simpler and more commonly used. In this method, the formula is mixed in clean utensils and poured into clean bottles, nipples put in place and then covered with paper, metal or glass caps. The filled bottles are placed on a rack in a kettle, partially submerged in water, and covered and boiled for 25 minutes. They are then cooled at room temperature and placed in the refrigerator as soon as possible. Specially made utensils for sterilizing may be bought, but are not essential.

Additions to Feeding

Whether breast or bottle fed, the infant needs supplements of vitamins C and D. These can be fed directly with a dropper into the infant's mouth. Orange juice, of course, is an excellent source of vitamin C. If used, it should be diluted, and started in amounts of a teaspoonful. As some infants are allergic to orange juice, many prefer to start off with vitamin drops and switch to orange juice as the baby grows older.

Vitamin D may also be given in pediatric drops, or may not be necessary at all if the infant is getting enough irradiated milk to supply his requirements. This is seldom the case, however, and additional vitamin D must be supplied. An alternate source of vitamin D is cod liver oil. The chief objection to this is the possibility of the young infant aspirating the oily substance.

Milk is not a source of iron in the diet, but the normal, full-term infant has stored enough iron during the last month of fetal life to meet his needs for the first few months of his neonatal life, after which he needs iron-rich supplementary foods.

Fluorides. The role of fluoride in strengthening the calcification of dental tissues in formation has been documented in recent years. In areas where the fluoride content of drinking water is inadequate or absent, its administration in appropriate dosage to infants and children is recommended by the American Dental Association and by the majority of pediatricians.

Fluoride preparations come in tablet or liquid form. Drops may be started at approximately one month of age as prescribed by the pediatrician, the usual dosage at this age being approximately one drop daily, with dosage increases at intervals throughout childhood. Topical application of a fluoride preparation to erupted teeth is a recommended additive, rather than a substitute for the internal preparation.

CARE AT HOME

The mother may have many questions about the care of her infant, especially if this is her first child. The nurse needs to be able to answer intelligently.

Sleeping Arrangements

Many child psychologists advise that the infant should not sleep in his parents' room. The infant's room should be close enough so that his cry can be heard. However, most mothers are apprehensive about the newborn infant and prefer to have him within sight. For the comfort of both the parents and the child he should be moved out early. Dr. Spock advises moving the infant out of his parents' room by the age of 6 months. At a later period when he has become accustomed to sleeping in his parents' room, moving him out is apt to be emotionally traumatic to him.

Sleeping

The newborn may sleep as many as 20 out of the 24 hours during the first 2 weeks. He may waken only for feedings. Some infants seem to be constitutionally more active right from the start, and are awake more of the time. An infant who is healthy and well cared for can be relied on to set his own schedule.

There is no need to insist that the household be abnormally quiet while the baby sleeps. He quickly becomes accustomed to ordinary household noises. Older children should be allowed to play as usual.

Picking Up the Baby when He Cries

The idea used to be that children should be disciplined and trained to routine from birth. We now understand that an infant's greatest need is for security, love, and immediate attention to his needs. The new first-time mother may overdo this. She does not need to run to the baby whenever he moves about or makes a slight noise.

However, it is not spoiling an infant to pick him up when he cries, to comfort and cuddle him, to feed him if he is hungry, and to look for the cause if he is uncomfortable. These are all attentions that he needs for his emotional and physical well-being. A young infant acquires his knowledge of his environment mainly through tactile stimulation. He needs the feel of his parents' arms and their touch.

Feeding

This was discussed in the section on nutrition. The infant will soon set his own schedule if allowed to do so.

Elimination

Breast-fed infants usually have several soft, light yellow stools a day. Formula fed infants may have one to several stools daily. The stools are more solid and formed than those of the breast-fed baby. After the first weeks, some healthy infants may not have a daily stool.

Bathing the Newborn

Sponge baths are given until after the cord stump falls off and the umbilicus is healed. A demonstration for the new mother while she is still in the hospital will be helpful.

Routine for Sponge Bath

Gather together all equipment and supplies, place conveniently for use. Soap should be used sparingly if at all. If used, a mild infant soap with or without hexachlorophene is available.* Powders and lotions are unnecessary and may be irritating to the infant's skin. Cotton-tipped applicators may injure the delicate mucous membranes, and should not be used.

Equipment

1. Basin of warm water 98° to 100°F., or comfortable to mother's elbow.
2. Cotton balls.
3. Clean soft washcloth and a large soft towel.
4. Soap if used. Safety pins for diaper.
5. Clean diaper, shirt, light blanket.
6. Receptacle for soiled clothing, paper bag for used cotton balls.
   Note: Mineral oil or Vaseline may be used in diaper area for cleansing and protection against diaper rash.

Procedure

1. Wash infant's scalp, face, and neck, and dry. Cotton balls may be used if needed around eyes, behind ears, and in neck creases.
2. Remove infant's shirt and wash his trunk, arms, and legs. Turn him over and wash his back. No special cord care is necessary, except cleanliness. If the site is reddened, odorous, or if there is a discharge, the physician should be notified.
3. Remove diaper, wash the genital area from front to back. Circumcised area should need no special care. In uncircumcised males, it is now generally agreed that retracting the foreskin is not necessary.
4. Diaper the baby, and wrap loosely in a light blanket.

*Hexachlorophene is no longer desirable for bathing infants.

Dressing the Infant

In the heated homes of today, a shirt and diaper may be enough clothing, with a light blanket for cover. The mother should feel the infant's body with her hands occasionally. He should feel warm to her touch.

Putting a Shirt on a Newborn

If the shirt is one that opens out, with ties or snaps at the front opening, lay the infant down on the outspread shirt. Reach through the end of the sleeve, grasp the infant's arm, and pull it through the sleeve. Repeat with other arm, close front of shirt, and tie or snap.

If the pullover shirt is used, it should be one with an easily stretched neck opening. Gather the shirt in your hand and pull it rapidly down over the infant's head. Put his arms through the sleeves as previously described.

Diapering

Disposable diapers are used in many newborn nurseries. The mother may plan to continue their use at home. Some pediatricians believe infants are more prone to diaper rash if they are used all the time. They are useful for traveling and emergencies.

Diaper service is a great help to working mothers. If this service is used, containers for soiled diapers are furnished. If the mother plans to use cloth diapers, she may need a demonstration on folding the diaper. (See Figs. 26-23 and 26-24.)

Weighing

For the infant who sleeps well and appears satisfied with his feedings, weekly weighing is sufficient. If the mother has no scales, she does not need to go to the expense of scales if her infant is thriving, and if she takes him for his monthly checkup at the well baby clinic or the pediatrician's office. Such a monthly visit to the well baby clinic or the pediatrician is an excellent investment in health for an infant.

BIBLIOGRAPHY

Breckenridge, Marian E. and Murphy, Margaret Nesbitt: Growth and Development of the Young Child. Philadelphia, W. B. Saunders, 1969.

Duvall, Evelyn: Family Development. ed. 4. Philadelphia, J. B. Lippincott, 1971.

Egan, D. F., Illingworth, R. S. and MacKeith, R. C.: Developmental Screening 0-5 Years. London, Wm. Heinemann Medical Books Ltd., 1969.

Fitzpatrick, Elise, Reeder, Sharon, and Mastroianni, Luigi: Maternity Nursing. Philadelphia, J. B. Lippincott, 1971.

Hellmuth, Jerome (ed.): The Normal Infant. Seattle, Special Child Publications, 1967.

Ladas, Alice K.: How to help mothers breast-feed. Clinical Pediatrics, *9:*702, 1970.

Liley, H.M.I.: Modern Motherhood. New York, Random House, ed. 2, 1969.

O'Grady, Roberta S.: Feeding behavior in infants. AJN, *71:*736, 1971.

Shepard, Kenneth S.: Care of the Well Baby. ed. 2. Philadelphia, J. B. Lippincott, 1968.

Solomom, Laurence M. and Esterly, Nancy B.: The newborn skin, Journal of Pediatrics, *77:*888, 1970.

Suggested Readings for Further Study

Liley, H. M. I.: Modern Motherhood. New York, Random House, ed. 2. 1969.

Spock, Benjamin: Baby and Child Care. New York, Pocket Books, ed. 2, 1971.

Care of the Newborn in the Intensive Care Unit *19*

THE PREMATURE INFANT

The premature baby, or preemie as he is often called, is very special. Caring for him can be one of the most challenging, rewarding and exciting experiences a nurse can have. It can also be a frightening, threatening experience. Knowledge and skill make the difference. Knowledge and skill also make the difference to the baby, a big difference and for a whole lifetime.

The Concept and Definition of Prematurity

Simply stated the premature infant is one who was born earlier, smaller and physically less mature than the full term infant. A birth weight of 2,500 grams (5 1/2 lbs.) or less is one method of defining prematurity. Less than 36 weeks of gestation is also a criterion for identifying the preemie. The lack of development can also be measured by careful physical observation. Babies who lack

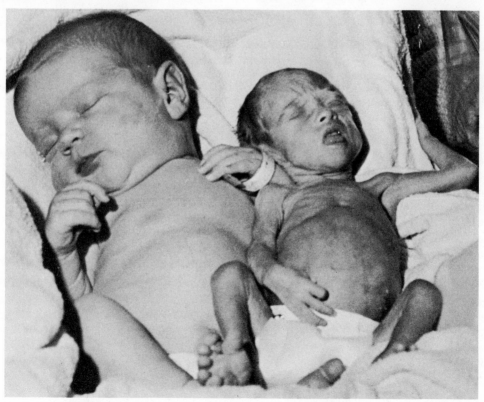

Figure 19-1. The difference between the full term and premature infants is striking. The "preemie" has a relatively large head and loose skin. Sometimes loops of intestine are visible through the thin abdominal wall.

263

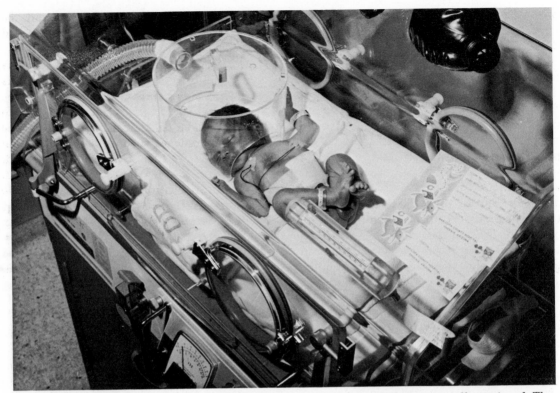

Figure 19-2.   In an intensive care nursery a twin is placed in an incubator specially equipped. The incubator is provided with the following: a plastic hood directly over the baby's head to increase oxygen concentration; air temperature thermometer (bottom right); temperature dial for servocontrol system (bottom center); lever for elevating mattress platform (left center); hinge which allows side to be opened down and out (above lever). On the baby's chest are two electrodes and leads to a vital signs monitor. (Courtesy of Maricopa County General Hospital.)

physical maturity are not always underweight. For example, the heavy babies of diabetic mothers are often immature. Careful physical examination should be used to establish a gestational age based on physical development rather than the calendar.*

Some babies do not grow in utero as well as expected. These babies are underweight for their gestational age. They may be more mature than one expects just from the birth weight. They are usually called small-for-date babies. Dysmaturity is also a term used in relation to these babies.

---

*For a more complete discussion of gestational age refer to: Battaglia, F. and L. O. Lubchenco, "A Practical Classification of Newborn Infant by Weight and Gestational Age," *Journal of Pediatrics*, 71:159, 1967.

The concepts of gestational age and immaturity are as important to the definition of prematurity as birth weight. In common practice, birth weight is often taken as the sole criterion. This has led many people to use and prefer the term low-birth-weight baby.

Characteristics of the Premature Infant

The physical appearance of the preemie is startling and dramatic. The baby is small. His extremities are thin with very little muscle and subcutaneous tissue. Toes and fingers are also very thin and relatively long. His head and abdomen are large for his body. The abdomen protrudes because of poor muscle tone. This poor muscle tone also gives the baby an exhausted, flaccid posture. The preemie's skin is thin, relatively translucent and wrinkled. However, the newborn preemie's skin may not be wrinkled because of edema, and he may temporarily have a deceptively plump appearance. The thin, translucent skin contributes to the baby's red color. The superficial veins of the abdomen and scalp are more visible than in the full term newborn. Typically, lanugo is plentiful and widely distributed over extremities, back and shoulders. It is important to note that the skeletal system is as immature as the muscular. The ears have soft, minimal cartilage in the auricles. They are very pliable and often fold over on themselves under the baby when he is placed on his side. The soft bones of the skull have a tendency to flatten on the sides, since the baby usually spends much time lying on one side or the other. The baby's flexible ribs give with each labored breath. Overall the preemie looks very much like an emaciated wizened little old man.

Physiologically, the premature has several important handicaps. His neurological system is immature. This can be demonstrated by eliciting reflexes which normally have disappeared by birth. Some important reflexes such as sucking, rooting and gagging are not yet well developed. Movement is obviously less coordinated. Temperature control is more difficult for the preemie than the full term infant. He cannot shiver nor is there the integrated reflex control of peripheral blood vessels. His body surface is great in relation to body mass, and sweat glands are not functioning well; this adds to the neurological deficit.

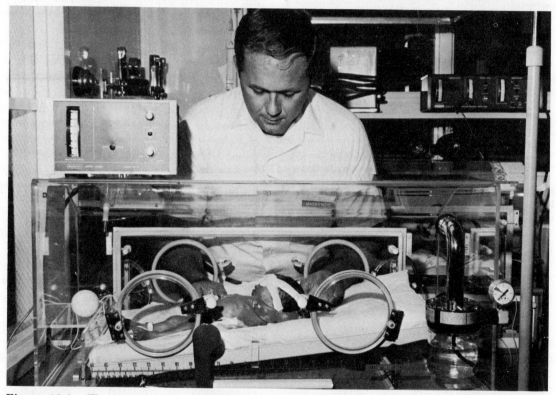

Figure 19-3. The second twin is placed in another incubator which shows the following: oxygen humidifier (bottom right); vital signs monitor (upper right); mask and bag for respiratory assistance (below vital signs monitor); bililamp (above monitor); flag indicating over 40% oxygen concentration possible (bottom center); bulb for aspirating nose or mouth (bottom left); air temperature thermometer (center left); apnea monitor (top left). The baby wears an eye mask for protection from fluorescent light of the bililamp and on his chest is a lead to the vital signs monitor. (Courtesy of the Maricopa County General Hospital.)

Respiratory difficulties are probably most critical for the premature. Typically his respirations are shallow and rapid but very irregular. Periods of apnea are common. Respirations may become so labored that the chest wall and perhaps even the sternum are retracted.

The digestive system of the premature is not as prepared for food and the responsibilities of digestion as the full term infant's system. The stomach is small with a capacity of 1 or 2 ounces. The sphincters at either end of the stomach are immature. This accounts for the baby's ability to regurgitate or vomit, particularly if fed quantities of formula which distend his stomach. The immature liver is unable to handle all the bilirubin produced by hemolysis and preemies are prone to jaundice and high blood bilirubin levels. The danger is that this will cause brain damage. The preemie is also immunologically immature. He did not receive the same quantities of antibodies from his mother as the full term infant, nor is he able to produce them.

Muscle weakness contributes to nutritional and respiratory problems. It also means that the preemie may not be able to position himself adequately or change his position. He is certain to be prone to fatigue and exhaustion, even from such simple things as eating and breathing. In summary, this little infant is simply physiologically premature, not yet as developed as the full term infant.

Nursing Care

The physical handicaps of preemies lead directly to nursing care. The aspects of nursing care to be discussed here are the incubator, cleanliness, monitoring vital signs, oxygen, hydration, feeding, bilirubin lights, medications, fatigue and stimulation, emotional support of the parents and preparation for discharge.

The Incubator

Placing the baby in an incubator is an essential part of his care. The incubator provides a means of maintaining the ideal temperature, humidity and O_2 con-

centrations to support the baby. It also provides a means of isolating the baby to protect him from infection. The baby should be cared for in the incubator. The nurse should organize her work so that even the portals are opened as seldom as possible.*

Cleanliness

Although the incubator provides a great deal of protection from infection, it cannot do the whole job. Careful handwashing is certainly very essential. It is obvious that if the baby is to be protected everyone must wash his hands and do it every time. Studies have shown that careful handwashing is more important in controlling nursery infections than caps and gowns and excluding important people such as parents or physicians from contact with baby. Some nurseries are asking parents and staff to wear gowns only if they are going to hold the baby or have other such contact.

In addition to handwashing and incubators, there is a third obvious line of protection: clean or sterile equipment. Modern incubators are designed to be as easy to clean as possible. Babies who are in incubators for long periods should be transferred to fresh incubators on a regular basis. Water in humidifiers should be changed frequently; every day is not too often, and every 8 hours may be preferable.

Monitoring Vital Signs

Close observation of the baby is a constant and primary responsibility of the nurse. Monitoring vital signs is one aspect of this responsibility. The vital signs monitored are temperature, pulse and respiration. Blood pressure measurements are not routinely made on premature infants. Axillary temperatures are taken frequently and recorded. How often temperatures are taken will be determined by how unstable the baby's temperature is. The incubator thermostat is adjusted to maintain an axillary temperature of 96° to 98°. Maintaining the humidity level in the in-

*Specific and detailed information about care of an infant in an incubator is available in Leifer, Gloria: Principles and Techniques in Pediatric Nursing, pp. 31-38. Philadelphia, W.B. Saunders, 1967.

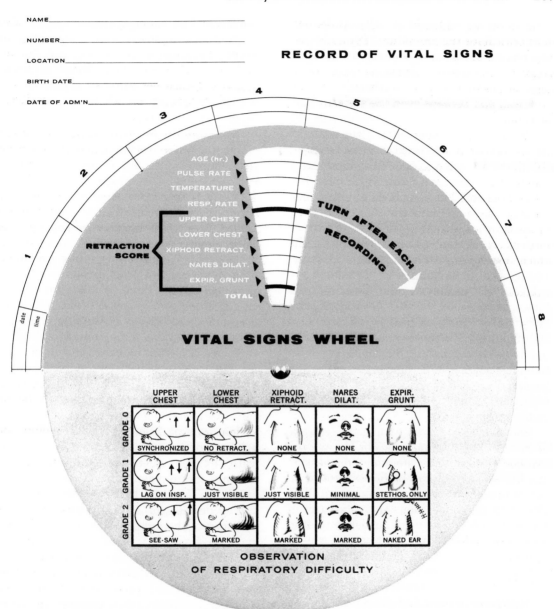

Figure 19-4. The vital signs wheel is used to follow up a baby's progress in the first hours of life. (Mead Johnson Laboratories)

cubator will help the baby to stabilize his temperature.* Most incubators are equipped with a servo control system for temperature regulation. A temperature-sensitive elec-

*For further study of temperature regulation read: Oliver, T.K., Jr.: Temperature regulation and heat production in the newborn, Ped. Clin. North Amer., *12:*765, 1965 and Lutz, L. and Perlstein, P.H.: Temperature control in newborn babies, *Nurs. Clin. North Amer.,* 6:15, 1971.

trode is attached to the baby's abdomen, and it connects with the incubator's thermostat. The incubator can then be set to turn the heater on and off according to the baby's skin temperature. It is still standard practice to take and record axillary temperatures when the baby is being monitored by servo control. In taking axillary temperatures be sure that the axillia is dry, that the arm is held closely to the body and that adequate time (5 to 10 minutes) is allowed for the temperature to register. Rectal temperatures are not regularly taken after admission in order to prevent damage and over-stimulation of the rectal sphincter.

Apical pulses are taken regularly as part of the care of the preemie, listening to the heart through the chest using a stethoscope. Observations should include rate, rhythm and strength. It is a good idea to listen for a full minute in order not to miss an irregularity in rhythm. It is also a good idea to take the pulse before rather than after such activities as taking the temperature or feeding which may stimulate the baby. The pulse rate is normally rapid (120 to 140/minute) and unstable. Preemies are subject to dangerous periods of brachycardia (down as low as 60 to 80/minute) and tachycardia (up as high as 160 to 200/minute). The nurse's observations of pulse rate, rhythm and strength are essential to understanding how the baby is tolerating treatments, activity, feedings and the temperature and O_2 concentration of the incubator.

Observation of the premature infant's respiration is obviously of utmost importance. Determining the rate of respiration and identifying retractions is essential to determining proper oxygen concentrations. One of the most hazardous characteristics of the premature infant is his tendency to stop breathing periodically. The hypoxia caused by this apnea and his general respiratory difficulty may cause mental retardation or other neurological problems.

It is so important and yet so difficult to observe respirations closely enough that frequently electronic apnea alarms are used. Electrodes are placed across the infant's chest with leads to the apnea monitor outside the incubator. The monitor gives a continuous reading of respiratory rate. It also has visual and audio alarms which can be set to alert the nurse when the rate goes too high or low or if the baby waits too long to take a breath.

In the fully equipped premature nursery, the apnea monitor is incorporated in a complete vital signs monitor. This vital signs monitor has temperature, pulse and respiration monitors. The pulse monitor gives a continuous rate reading and also has alarms to alert the nurse about extremes. The temperature monitor is similar. It is a nursing responsibility to place, check and replace the leads from the baby. The electrodes should be removed and relocated slightly at least every day. This will protect the baby's sensitive skin from being damaged by the electrode paste and adhesive. The skin should be cleansed carefully between applications of the electrodes. Many false alarms are the result of leads coming loose. Some of these can be prevented by using a very small amount of electrode paste and being careful to keep the paste inside the circle of adhesive on the electrode. Apical pulses, axillary temperatures and visual observations of the baby's respirations are still made at regular intervals by the nurse. The vital signs monitor serves as an extension of the nurse's eyes and ears, making her an even more constant, accurate and complete observer.

Oxygen

Not all premature infants need extra oxygen, but many do. Incubators are made with oxygen inlets and humidifiers for raising the oxygen concentration in the incubator from 20 to 21% (room air) to a higher percentage. This is the usual method of oxygen therapy. Observations that the baby is breathing rapidly, retracting and cyanotic indicate he needs more oxygen.

High blood concentrations of oxygen are dangerous. The immature retina is damaged, causing blindness. This condition is called retrolental fibroplasia. A baby with relatively healthy lungs is likely to have his eyes damaged by concentrations of over 40% oxygen. A baby whose lungs are unable to transmit oxygen to his blood readily may be safe at 80% or 90% oxygen. Blood gas tests to determine the arterial blood oxygen are the most precise way to determine the proper oxygen concentration to prescribe for a baby. In the absence of a laboratory to do blood gas determination, the doctor and nurse must rely on careful, recorded, continual observations of the baby. Observations should be made of the pulse rate, the respiratory rate, retractions, skin color, muscle tone, alertness and activity. In the absence of lung pathology it is safer to keep the incubator O_2 concentration below 40% unless hypoxia can be documented. For the baby's protection, incubators are constructed so that it is difficult to get over 40% concentrations without special maneuvers. It is part of the nurse's responsibility to measure the oxygen level in the baby's incubator at regular intervals. This is done by means of an instrument called an oxygen analyzer.*

Oxygen is also used in handling apnea. Usually a little gentle stimulation, such as wiggling a foot, is enough to remind the baby to breathe. There are times when respiration needs to be assisted by a bag and mask. Every nursery nurse should know how to "bag" a baby in order to be prepared for such times. The principles of this form of assisted respiration are very similar to those of mouth to mouth artificial respiration. The neck must be well extended to open the airway. The mask covers the baby's mouth and nose. A "tight seal" between the mask and the baby's face must be maintained. The bag, filled with oxygen or air, is squeezed quickly. The quantity of air needed is relatively small and the pressure very gentle.

Hydration

When he is born, a preemie may be too weak to suck or not yet have adequate sucking and swallowing reflexes. For several hours or even a day he may be able to manage without fluids, but soon he will need intravenous fluids. In many cases an I.V. "life line" will be established right after delivery. Fluids are given through a catheter passed into the umbilical vein in the stub of the umbilical cord if it is still fresh. I.V. fluids can also be given through other veins. Very small amounts of fluid are needed; perhaps as little as 5 to 10 cc. per hour or even less. When such very small amounts are needed they can be measured accurately and administered at a steady rate by using an

*Segal, S.: Oxygen: too much, too little, *Nurs. Clin. North Amer.* 6:39, 1971 contains more discussion about the use of oxygen.

infusion pump. Accurate and complete records of I.V. fluids are kept. The nurse should also observe and record such observation as the number of urinations, color of the urine and edema. Edema will change the loose wrinkled skin to tight, shiny skin. The open fontanels of the skull can also help in determining hydration. With a full-term child the fontanel will become soft and depressed in the case of dehydration.

Feeding

At first some preemies will get all their fluid, electrolyte, vitamin and caloric needs by I.V. routes. At the other extreme are the larger, older preemies who start with a nipple and bottle. Many "in-between" preemies will need gavage feedings. The frequency and quantity of the gavage feedings will be determined by the baby. Usually feedings are given every 2 hours. If the stomach is not being emptied by the next feeding more time needs to be allowed between feedings or smaller feedings need to be given. Usually the quantity given is just as much as the baby can tolerate and is increased cc. by cc. as fast as tolerated. Starting a baby on 5 to 10 cc. per feeding is not unusual. The feeding is not too large if the baby's stomach is not so distended that it causes respiratory difficulty, vomiting or regurgitation and if there is not much formula left in the stomach by the next feeding. The common preemie formula has 13 calories per ounce. A formula with 20 calories per ounce may also be used. If the formula is too rich the baby will have a tendency to vomiting and diarrhea. If he is not gaining weight, after the usual drop after birth, the calories may not be enough. Some preemies are fed breast milk contributed by their mother or a wet nurse.

When a baby who is being gavage fed begins to suck on the gavage tube, his fingers or hands, he may be ready for nipple feeding. He is ready if he can take the same quantity of formula by nipple that he was tolerating by gavage and not become too tired. Some babies need alternating gavage and nipple feedings to see them through the transition period. The nipple for a premature infant is of softer rubber than the regular nipple. It is also smaller, but no shorter, than the regular nipple.

There are other methods by which preemies may be fed if neither gavage or nipple feeding is tolerated and if I.V. fluids are not adequate. Some babies do better if fed with a rubber-tipped medicine dropper. For other babies it is necessary to provide gastrostomy feedings.

Prematures need to be "burped" after feedings. Sometimes simply changing the baby's position is enough assistance. At other times it may be helpful to rub or pat the baby's back gently.

The baby should be weighed daily at the same point in his feeding schedule. These daily weights will give an indication of the baby's overall health and whether he is getting enough calories. The baby's doctor and parents will probably want to know the baby's current weight each day. Weighing the baby on the same scales in the same clothing and at the same time will help insure accurate and comparable data.

Bilirubin Lights

Jaundice is a common occurrence in prematures. It is becoming quite common to expose the babies to "blue" fluorescent lights in order to prevent bilirubin levels from reaching dangerous levels.* The lights are placed over and outside the incubator. The baby is completely exposed to the light without diaper or shirt. The baby's eyes are shielded from the ultraviolet light. Nurses become creative in making miniature masks and eye patches to be taped over the baby's eyes with paper tape. The eye patches can promote infection if they are not clean, changed frequently and applied so that they stay in place. Nurses should be aware that the light can cause skin rashes, "sunburn" or tanning. Stools may be loose and green.†

Medications

The usual, healthy premature needs very little medication. The baby will probably be given an injection of Vitamin K at birth. Vitamins and/or iron may be added to his

*20 mgm./100 cc.
†For further study refer to: Williams, Sandra: Phototherapy in hyperbilirubinemia. *Amer. Journal of Nurs.*, 71:1397, 1971.

feedings to improve his nutrition. Some physicians will prescribe intramuscular antibiotics, such as penicillin, to prevent infections. Intramuscular phenobarbital may be used to prevent hyperbilirubinemia.‡ The dosage and quantities prescribed for a preemie are minute. Great care must be taken in figuring and measuring the dosage. Usually the best site for intramuscular injections is the anterior aspect of the thigh.

Fatigue and Stimulation

The small preemie has almost all he can do to breathe and pump blood. The nurse should plan the baby's day so that he does not become exhausted. Too much cannot be done with the baby at one time. Constant handling and moving about may be just as fatiguing. The baby's energy can be conserved by not bathing the baby regularly but giving only "face and fanny" care as needed. Preemies are not usually dressed in anything or perhaps only diapers. This conserves energy, provides more freedom of movement and allows better opportunity to observe the baby. Conserving the baby's energy should not mislead the nurse into ignoring or avoiding the baby. Nor should it mislead her into discouraging the mother-child contact essential to their establishing a normal relationship.

Older prematures have a special need for stimulation. Visual stimulation may be provided by mobiles hung over the incubator and toys placed in or on the incubator. Audio stimulation may be provided by a radio turned low, a music box or wind-up toy in the incubator. Some nurseries have radios playing in them. A very good form of audio stimulation is having the baby's parents, doctor and nurse talk to him. Tactile stimulation will be provided by the baby's bath and being held, cuddled and fondled. The contact between the baby and his mother and father can be very helpful to both the baby and his parents.

The nurse must position the premature carefully and change his position periodically. He can be positioned from side to side. If he is placed on his back or stomach

‡High levels of bilirubin in the blood.

special care must be taken to see that he does not aspirate emesis or bury his nose in sheets or diapers. Preemies have a knack of wiggling into corners and cracks from which they cannot extract themselves. After a feeding the best position is probably on the left side with the head of the mattress platform slightly elevated.

Emotional Support of the Parents

The premature baby creates a crisis for his parents.* The parents will need what is usually referred to as emotional support. Emotional support to the parents during labor and delivery may mean such things as keeping husband and wife together, providing as much information and explanation to them as is possible, recognizing that the fear and anxiety of the parents is natural, normal and acceptable and providing opportunities for them to express their feelings. Part of the parents' anxiety and fear may come from the excited, poorly organized or poorly prepared staff. Nurses can do much by being calm, well prepared and organized in their work. Probably the best emotional support the parents can have is excellent physical care for their child.

Emotional support after birth may be such things as reports on the baby's condition, perhaps even a talk with the nurse from the nursery. It will be helpful to give the parents a chance to talk about their feelings. The mother, particularly, may have feelings of failure and inadequacy. Either or both parents may have difficulty feeling the child is theirs and have difficulties developing typical parental feelings. As soon as appropriate the parents should see and then have physical contact with the baby and help to care for it.

When the mother goes home without the baby the nurse can help during this crisis by helping the mother make plans for continued

*For more complete discussion of this crisis read: Kaplan, D. M. and Mason, E. A.: Maternal reactions to premature birth viewed as an acute emotional disorder, *In*: Parad, E.J., ed.: Crisis Intervention: Selected Readings. New York, Family Service Association of America, 1965. p. 118.

contact with the baby and how she is going to handle the questions and reactions of friends and neighbors. Parents who cannot return to the nursery to see the baby, participate in care, and talk with the staff may receive support by telephone conversations with their baby's doctor and nurse.

Preparation for Discharge

Participating in the care of her baby in the nursery is a natural way for the mother to prepare for the discharge of the baby. The baby's nurse is her teacher. Sometimes informal classes are held but most of the instruction is individualized.

Before the baby goes home, the mother must know how to hold, feed, bathe, dress, diaper and protect the baby. She will need to become less fearful of his size, fragility and special needs. She needs to have learned what the real special needs of her baby are and how to meet them. Before the family takes the baby home the parents need to know that they can reach their doctor and nurse at any time. The parents should know their baby well enough that they can recognize changes to report to the doctor or nurse. A nurse, usually a public health nurse, is often asked to visit the home to which the baby will go. The nurse tries to determine if the home is adequately prepared for the baby and assists the family in making it adequate.

Premature babies are usually discharged when they weigh 5 to 5-1/2 lbs. and are gaining weight steadily. The baby needs to be able to eat with bottle and nipple. A preemie ready for discharge has demonstrated his ability to get along without an incubator by being in an open bassinet for several days or weeks. After the baby goes home a nurse, usually a public health nurse, visits the family. She checks the health of the baby, follows up on teaching the baby's care and helps incorporate the new member into the family.

The Intensive Care Nursery

There is a trend in many parts of the country to centralize the facilities for the care of the sick or very premature newborn. These intensive care nurseries are staffed by doctors, nurses and technicians with special education and experience. These people are provided with the equipment to provide care not often needed by the healthy bigger premature. They can provide respirators, exchange transfusions, umbilical catheters, gastrostomy feedings. They can do pulmonary function tests and determine blood gases.*

In most situations, an intensive care nursery is supported by a transportation program. The doctor and nurse attending the baby at delivery and immediately afterward identify the baby who needs especially sophisticated and intensive care. They refer him to the intensive care nursery. The baby is transported by air or surface ambulance in a portable incubator. Usually a nurse, and perhaps a doctor, from the intensive care nursery care for the baby during the trip. The nurses and doctors at the intensive care nursery keep in contact with the referring doctors and nurses. The family may not be able to visit at the intensive care nursery. If this is the case, contact can be maintained with the family by telephone conversations, visits from the public health nurse and contacts with the referring doctor and nurses who have contact with the family. A social worker may be an important member of the team caring for the intensive care patient and his family.

The Causes and Prevention of Prematurity

The causes of prematurity are many and obscure. In many cases a definite cause is not known. It must be made clear also that many conditions are associated with prematurity; but the fact that they cause prematurity has not been established.

Some of the conditions associated with early birth of small immature babies are multiple pregnancy, grand multiparity, poor maternal nutrition during pregnancy, trauma (such as falls), incompetent uteral os, placental insufficiency, placenta abruptio, placenta praevia, very young age of mother,

---

*For more information about intensive care nurseries the following articles are recommended: Lucy, I. F.: The newborn special care unit, *Hospital Practice*, 3:25, 1968, and DeMarco, J. P. and Reed, R.: Care of the high risk infant in the intensive care unit, *Nurs. Clin. North Amer.*, 5:375, 1970.

toxemia of pregnancy, no antenatal care and low socio-economic status of the family.

Prevention of many of the conditions mentioned above focuses on providing for good maternal health through improved socio-economic conditions, family planning and antenatal care. Some programs have provided for more antenatal clinics which are accessible and acceptable to women. Some programs make supplemental food commodities available to expanding families. Family planning clinics are being opened. Mobile trailer clinics and extended hours are being used. Some programs are providing services to unmarried mothers and to those under 18. These are indirect methods of preventing prematurity and they work as much to improve general health as to prevent prematurity. Direct preventative measures such as bed rest, hormone therapy and suturing the os of the uterus are of limited value. At this time progress in preventing prematurity is slow. More progress is being made in care of the infant so that he survives as a healthy individual. Nursing care is a key factor in this.

FURTHER READING

Several suggestions for specific further reading are identified in the footnotes. The following are some suggestions for general reading.

Babson, S. G., and Benson, R.: Primer on Prematurity and Pregnancy. St. Louis, C. V. Mosby, 1966.

Cross, M.: The Premature Baby. Boston, Little, Brown, 1957.

Ross Laboratories: The Premature Infant. Columbus, Ohio, Ross Laboratories, 1959.

Silverman, W.A.: Dunham's Premature Infants. ed. 3. New York, P. B. Hoeber, 1961.

Interesting Activities

1. Tour an intensive care nursery.
2. Visit a premature infant and his family in their home.
3. Take apart an incubator as if to clean its parts and reassemble it.
4. Participate in the care of a healthy premature in an incubator who needs gavage feedings and occasional respiratory assistance with bag and mask.

Nursing Care of the Newborn with Congenital Anomalies 20

THE INFANT WITH A CLEFT LIP

A young, prospective mother is naturally excited over the forthcoming birth and the prospect of bringing home her first baby. There have been charming new babies among her relatives and friends, and everyone is looking forward to the new arrival. There has usually been much preparation in anticipation of the homecoming.

Mary White was such a mother. She was told in the delivery room that she had a healthy son, but she became considerably puzzled when no one brought him to her for immediate inspection.

After she had rested, however, the nursery nurse appeared in her doorway, holding the newborn baby lovingly and tenderly in her arms. "Mrs. White," she said, "you have a husky son of whom you can be very proud. I am anxious for you to see him, but I must tell you first that he has a facial defect, a cleft in his upper lip. Fortunately, this defect can be repaired early. It is not pretty to look at now, but plastic surgery can give you a very good looking baby. He surely is a fine boy altogether."

Mary eagerly accepted her child, but could not help the feeling of shock that she experienced when she looked at his face. Perhaps one of the greatest dreads at the moment was the thought of the reaction of her family and friends when they saw her child's disfigurement.

Mary was not alone in her unhappiness, because this defect appears in about one out of 800 births. The cause is not entirely clear. There seems to be a genetic influence in some instances, for the incidence is higher in families in which there is a history of the defect, but it also occurs in isolated instances. It has been known to occur in infants whose mothers have had rubella during the first trimester of pregnancy, but, in this instance, this defect does not occur so frequently as do others.

The defect itself is the result of a failure of the maxillary and premaxillary processes to fuse during the fifth to eighth week of intra-uterine life. The cleft may be a simple notch in the vermilion line, or it may extend up into the floor of the nose. (Fig. 20-1)

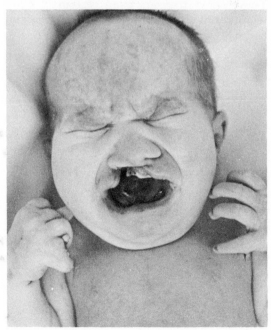

Figure 20-1. Unilateral cleft lip extending into the floor of the nose.

273

Plastic surgeons differ as to the best time for repair. Some are in favor of early repair, before the infant goes home. Another group prefers to wait until the infant is 1 or 2 months old.

There are certain obvious advantages to early repair. The mother's emotional comfort in being able to take home a normal-looking infant needs to be considered. Another advantage concerns feeding: because of the divided upper lip, he cannot suck, and has to be fed by dropper, spoon or Asepto syringe. This presents difficulties for both mother and child.

If early surgery is contemplated, the baby should be healthy, of average or above average weight, and must be placed where he can be—and is—watched constantly. A newborn child has greater difficulty dealing with excess mucus than does an older infant. Good results are obtained when these infants are in the hands of competent plastic surgeons and experienced nurses.

The surgeons who decide to wait can also cite advantages. They have more tissue to work with in an older child, of particular advantage when dealing with a wide defect. They believe they are more certain of good results, and also believe that the parents can be realistic enough to face facts as they are.

Nursing Care

There is little preoperative preparation for the infant who has surgery during the first few days of life. For the older infant, it would be well to accustom him to elbow restraints, for he has to wear them for several days following surgery. It is also helpful if the nurse becomes accustomed to feeding the infant with an Asepto syringe. This requires a special technique that is difficult to acquire without practice.

Immediate postoperative care. This demands continuous and intelligent observation. The swollen mouth tissues cause an excessive secretion of mucus that is poorly handled by a small infant. For the first few hours, he must never be left alone because he can quickly and easily aspirate the mucus.

A sore mouth calls for a comforting thumb, and this can quickly undo the difficult and costly repair. This is one occasion when the child's ultimate happiness and well-being must take precedence over his immediate satisfaction.

Elbow restraints. These must be properly applied and checked frequently. These are made with canvas and with tongue blades, which are tied firmly around the arm, and pinned to the infant's shirt or gown to prevent their sliding down below the elbow. (See Figs. 24-8 and 24-9) The child can move his arm around, but cannot bend his elbow to reach his face. The restraints must be applied snugly, but not allowed to hinder circulation.

Restraints need to be removed frequently to provide physical relief. This is done by removing them from one arm at a time and controlling movements of the child's arm. A sufficient supply should be kept on hand in order to change soiled restraints.

The baby suffers emotional frustration because of the restraints, so satisfaction must be provided in other ways. He needs rocking and cuddling as any baby does, but probably in larger measure. Mother is the best person to supply this loving care, and no doubt the most willing. Nurses come next.

Care of suture line. The suture line is left uncovered after surgery and must be kept clean and dry to prevent infection with subsequent scarring. In many hospitals, a wire bow—called a Logan Bar—is applied across the upper lip and attached to the cheeks with adhesive tape. This prevents tension on the sutures. (Fig. 20-2)

The sutures are carefully cleaned as often as necessary to prevent the collection of dried serum. Frequent cleaning is quite essential for the first two or three days, as well as after every feeding as long as the sutures are in.

A tray containing the articles needed for suture care is kept at the bedside and changed daily. It should contain a covered jar of sterile cotton-tipped applicators, a sterile container of solution for cleansing and a paper bag for waste. The solutions used are commonly hydrogen peroxide or sterile saline.

With clean hands, dip an applicator into the solution and gently clean each suture with a rolling motion. The sutures inside the lip also need cleaning. Application of an ointment following the cleansing may be ordered.

Technique for feeding. Have ready a sterile Asepto syringe with the tip protected by a piece of sterile rubber tubing about one inch long. Plastic tubing is unsatisfactory as it may slide off and lodge in the infant's throat.

Place the syringe and warmed formula on the bedside stand within easy reach. Hold the infant in your arms in an upright position. Pour the formula into syringe and place the rubber covered tip in the child's mouth, away from the suture line. The formula usually drips quickly enough without squeezing the bulb. The nurse must learn to regulate the drops to the infant's breathing and swallowing, but both she and the baby soon learn. The baby swallows considerable amounts of air and needs burping frequently. About 30 minutes should be allowed for a feeding.

The baby is much safer when placed in his crib after his feeding if he is positioned on his side, in order to prevent aspiration if he vomits or regurgitates. If he cannot be satisfactorily restrained in this position but must instead be placed on his back, his head should be kept elevated and the child watched carefully.

The sutures are removed 7 to 10 days after surgery. The infant will probably be allowed to suck on a soft nipple at this time. Following effective surgery and intelligent, careful nursing care, the appearance of baby's face should be very good.

The mother should be told that this baby can be fed and treated as any other. The scar fades as time goes on. She needs to know that he is probably going to need a slight adjustment of the vermilion line in later childhood. With today's surgery, she can expect that the child will not have the un-sightly, thickened tissue seen in early days. (Figs. 20-3 and 20-4)

Some infants who have a cleft lip also

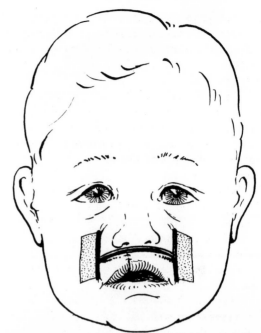

Figure 20-2. Logan bar for easing strain on sutures.

have a cleft palate. In such instances, the lip is repaired as described, but the palate repair is delayed until sometime during the second year. The baby is able to suck after the lip repair and should progress normally until ready for palate surgery. Some milk may seep through the cleft palate and out through the nose, but most of these babies learn to handle this without too much difficulty.

OBSTRUCTIONS IN THE DIGESTIVE SYSTEM

Esophageal Atresia with Fistula

A serious anomaly is esophageal atresia, with or without fistula into the trachea. There are several types of atresia, but 90% of them fall into one category. This most common type consists of the upper, or proximal end of the esophagus ending in a blind pouch, with the lower, or distal segment from the stomach connected to the trachea by a fistulous tract (Fig. 20-5*A*).

Incidence and diagnosis. Esophageal atresia and esophageal atresia with fistula into trachea are among the most common of anomalies causing respiratory distress. The incidence is about one in 2500 births.

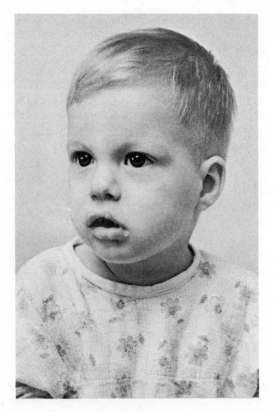

Figure 20-3. This child has returned for slight revision of cleft lip repair.

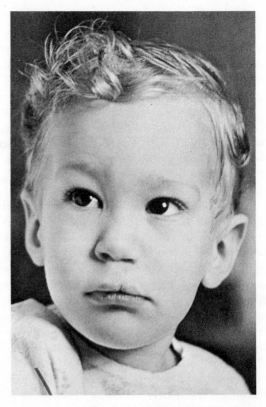

Figure 20-4. This child may need a revision of the vermilion line.

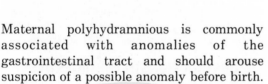

Maternal polyhydramnious is commonly associated with anomalies of the gastrointestinal tract and should arouse suspicion of a possible anomaly before birth.

Diagnosis. Diagnosis is not difficult to make if the possible presence of this condition is recognized. A rubber catheter passed through the infant's nose is blocked at the site of the atresia, and x-ray film shows the catheter coiled upon itself in the blind pouch. Usually the catheter alone is sufficient, but if contrast media is used, it should be a small amount of iodized oil. Barium is never used. The fistulous tract into the trachea may be demonstrated by the appearance of air in the gastrointestinal tract.

Clinical Manifestations. It is obvious that mucus, or any fluid that a newborn baby with this condition swallows, goes into the blind pouch of the esophagus. This pouch soon fills and overflows, with the usual result of aspiration into the trachea.

Probably few other conditions are as dependent on the watchful observation of the nurse for early diagnosis, which in turn, greatly improves the child's chances for survival. This newborn infant has frothing and excessive drooling. He has periods of respiratory distress with choking and cyanosis. It is true that many newborns have difficulty with mucus, but the nurse should be alerted to the possibility of an anomaly and report such difficulties to a responsible person. She may, and should, take the responsibility for delaying the first feeding until the infant has been checked.

If early signs are overlooked and the nurse tries to feed the child, she experiences a situation that she could very well do

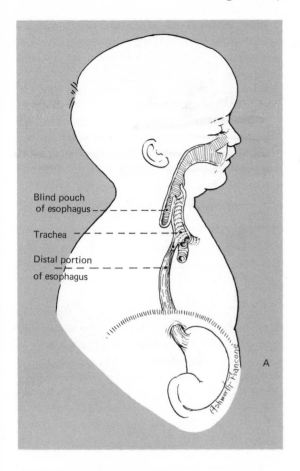

Blind pouch
of esophagus

Trachea

Distal portion
of esophagus

A

without. The baby chokes, coughs and regurgitates as the food enters the blind pouch. He becomes deeply cyanotic and appears to be in severe respiratory distress. During this process, he aspirates some of the formula with resultant pneumonitis. Naturally, this sequence does much to make surgery more of a hazard to the child. In a very real sense, the infant's life may depend upon the careful observation of the nurse.

Preoperative Care. The infant needs to be placed in an incubator where highly saturated air, constant temperature, and oxygen are available. He should be positioned with head and chest elevated 30° to prevent reflux of gastric juice into the lung. A nurse should be in constant attendance. Frequent intermittent nasopharyngeal suction—as often as every 10 to 15 minutes—is needed to remove secretions. Care must be used to avoid injury to the

Figure 20-5. (*A*) The most common form of esophageal atresia. (*B*) Both segments of the esophagus are blind pouches. (*C*) Esophagus is continuous, but with narrowed segment. (*D*) Upper segment of esophagus opens into trachea.

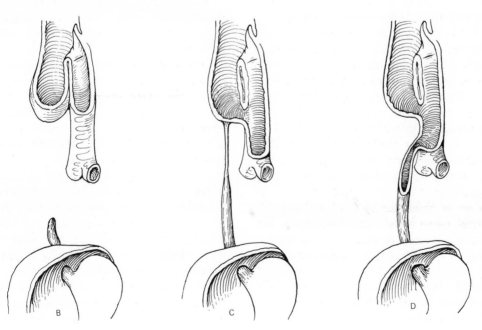

B   C   D

blind pouch. Intravenous fluids are given by slow drip. Broad spectrum antibiotics are used if pneumonitis or aspiration pneumonia is present.

Surgery may be delayed until the infant's condition is improved, and here again, the nurse must be constantly aware of his condition. She must watch for changes in color, temperature, pulse, and state of activity. She must keep in mind the ever present danger of pneumonia or pneumonitis. The child must be turned frequently.

Not the least of the nurse's duties is to give adequate attention to the infant's family. It must be remembered that this is a newborn infant who has never been home. Perhaps he is also premature; this increases the family's anxiety. Frequently, the infant has been removed from the place of his birth and taken to a center where more skilled care is available. This means that the mother does not get to see her child, and must rely on reports from her husband or from other members of the family.

Perhaps she is fortunate at that. It is certainly frightening to see the child enclosed in the incubator with so many tubes attached to his body. Families are often afraid to ask too many questions, and so bring back only gloomy reports to the anxious mother.

It does nothing for the family for the nurse to say, "The baby is doing as well as can be expected." They certainly hope he is doing a little *better* than the picture allows them to expect. However, the nurse must guard against giving a false impression of well-being and optimism. A brush-off of, "You will have to ask the doctor" is not well accepted either. If the nurse does not know what is going on, or is not interested, the child is indeed in a sorry plight!

Time must be taken to listen to the family, and to give honest answers. The nurse refers them to the doctor as necessary, but she can give much supporting care herself. She can explain the various types of equipment, thus removing their mystery. She can explain the defect and its repair in simple, nonmedical terms. She can show a

warm, human interest in the mother's progress and well-being. Above all, she does not show a feeling of irritation or hurriedness, but by her manner, she convinces the family that these interviews are an important part of nursing.

Postoperative Care. While the infant is still in surgery, his nurse prepares for his return. The incubator must be clean, warm, and functioning properly. Ample supplies must be readied so that she will have no difficulty obtaining them, because she must resume her careful, constant observation on the infant's return.

A waterseal chest tube may be put in place in the operating room (See Chapter 38). Ordinarily complete chest expansion occurs in a few hours. The gastrostomy tube is sutured to the skin following surgery. The dressing around the tube must be kept clean and changed as needed. An extra strip of adhesive around the tube at the site of insertion and attached to the skin will help prevent displacement of the tube. Following surgery treatment is resumed much as before. The child is placed in the warm, humidified incubator and kept free from excessive mucus by suctioning.

Feedings by gastrostomy tube are usually started on the second or third day. For this the nurse needs a sterile funnel or syringe barrel and a clamp. The funnel or syringe barrel is attached to the gastrostomy tube, and the solution placed in the funnel before the tube is unclamped. It is allowed to run in slowly, and the tube is again clamped when the feeding has reached the lower edge of the funnel or syringe barrel to avoid introduction of air. (Fig. 20-6)

For the first 2 or 3 days, glucose and water are used. In some hospitals, gastrostomy feedings are given by slow drip, using a special drip apparatus. After the physician is satisfied that the fluid is being well tolerated, warm formula is given according to the physician's directions.

Psychological Needs. The infant has psychological needs, one of which is the need to suck. Following an anastomosis, he can be given a sterile nipple stuffed with cotton or a pacifier to suck when he receives his gastrostomy feedings. After the feeding, he needs to be held and cuddled.

The infant who has not yet had an anastomosis cannot be permitted to suck, thus he has an even greater need for physical contact and warm acceptance. These infants continue to need gastrostomy feedings until further surgery.

Most of these infants, however, have had an anastomosis, and are ready for oral feedings after 8 to 10 days. A small-holed nipple should be used, and feedings given very slowly. Stenosis at the site of the anastomosis is not uncommon, so the nurse must be particularly watchful for choking or difficult swallowing.

When the mother is able to, she should be encouraged to spend some time observing and helping with the care of her baby. Remember that this child has never been home before, so the mother needs practice in the routine care of her newborn infant as well as in special procedures. She needs to develop confidence in bathing and weighing as well as in dressing a small infant.

Gastrostomy Feeding. The mother should also learn how to give gastrostomy feedings. Hopefully, she will not have to give them, but many babies develop strictures at the site of the anastomosis, requiring temporary use of the gastrostomy tube for feeding. The wound itself should be well healed at the time of baby's discharge and require no special care or any dressing, so that baby can be put in the tub for bathing.

The mother also needs to practice oral feeding, and to learn what symptoms indicate impending trouble, such as a stenosis at the site of anastomosis. She should be told to call her doctor or the hospital resident if baby chokes over feedings or regurgitates, and to stop feeding until baby has been checked. With all of this, she must not be made too apprehensive.

A fair proportion of these infants develop stenosis at the site of the anastomosis and require dilatation, which probably will be done at the hospital. Mother should also know of this possibility.

The gastrostomy tube may be left in place for several months until the surgeon is satisfied that all need for its use is past. Frequently, several dilatations of the esophagus are necessary during the months following surgery.

Prognosis is somewhat guarded, much depending on the infant's condition at time of surgery. Early diagnosis, especially before feedings are attempted, is an important factor in the infant's survival. For many infants, the condition is complicated by prematurity and by other congenital anomalies. However, through careful management, together with devoted nursing care, the mortality rate has been greatly reduced from the former prediction of

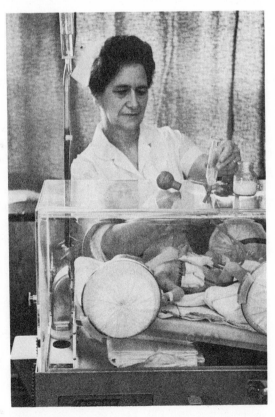

Figure 20-6. The infant is being given a gastrostomy feeding.

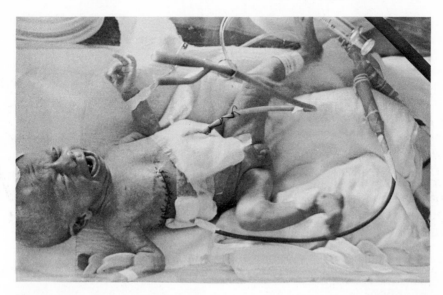

Figure 20-7.   Repair of tracheal esophageal atresia and fistula showing chest incision and drainage tube. Gastrostomy tube is also in place.

"hopeless," and a normal life is now possible for many.

Meconium Ileus

Meconium ileus is the presenting manifestation of fibrocystic disease in approximately 5 to 15% of the newborns who later develop additional manifestations. Depletion or absence of pancreatic enzymes before birth results in impaired digestive activity, and the meconium becomes viscid and mucilaginous. The inspissated meconium fills the small intestine, causing complete obstruction. Clinical manifestations are bile-stained emesis, a distended abdomen, and an absence of stool. Intestinal perforation with symptoms of shock may occur.

Treatment is surgical resection, employing one of several methods, but the mortality rate is high in spite of skillful surgery. The majority of infants who survive develop cystic fibrosis of varying degrees of severity.

Imperforate Anus

In this condition, the rectal pouch ends blindly at a distance above the anus, and there is no anal orifice. There may be a fistula between the rectum and the vagina in the female or between the rectum and the urinary tract in the male.

Etiology. Early in intrauterine life the membrane between the rectum and the anus should be absorbed, and a clear passage made from the rectum to the anus. If the membrane remains, blocking a union between the rectum and the anus, an imperforate anus results.

Diagnosis. In some newborn infants, only a dimple indicates the site of the anus. When a rectal temperature is attempted, it is perceived that there is no anal opening. However, there may be a shallow blind opening in the anus, with the rectum ending in a blind pouch some distance higher. For this reason it is imperative to understand that the ability to pass a rectal thermometer into the rectum is not a reliable indication of a normal rectal-anal canal. In fact, some newborn nursery personnel take axillary temperatures on infants from birth.

More reliable presumptive evidence is obtained by watching carefully for the first meconium stool. If the infant does not pass a stool within the first 24 hours, this should be reported to the physician. Abdominal dis-

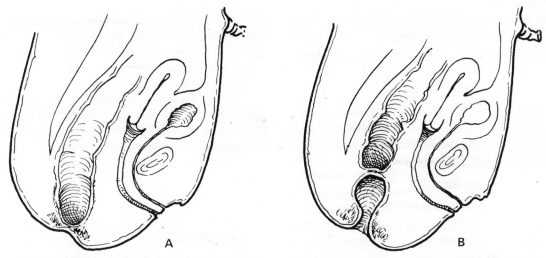

Figure 20-8. Imperforate anus (anal atresia). (*A*) Membrane between anus and rectum; (*B*) Rectum ending in a blind pouch at a distance above the perineum.

tention also occurs. Definitive diagnosis is made by x-ray studies.

Surgical Procedure. If the rectal pouch is separated from the anus by only a thin membrane, the surgeon can repair the defect from below. When a high defect is present, abdominal-perineal resection is indicated. In these infants a colostomy is performed, and the extensive abdominal-perineal resection is delayed until the age of 3 to 5 months, or later.

Home care. When the infant goes home with a colostomy, the parents will need to learn how to give colostomy care. The mother should be taught to keep the area around the colostomy clean with soap and water, and to diaper the baby in the usual way. Zinc oxide ointment is useful for protection of the skin around the colostomy.

Omphalocele

This is a rare anomaly existing at birth. Some of the abdominal contents protrude through into the root of the umbilical cord and form a sac lying on the abdomen. This sac may be large and contain much of the intestines and the liver. The sac is covered with peritoneal membrane instead of skin. Surgical replacement of the organs into the abdomen may be difficult with a large omphalocele, as there may not be enough

space in the abdominal cavity. Other congenital defects are present in many instances.

With large omphaloceles, surgery may be postponed and the surgeon will suture skin over the defect, creating a large hernia. The abdomen may enlarge enough as the child grows older so that replacement can be done.

Diaphragmatic Hernia

In this condition, some of the abdominal organs are displaced into the left chest through a diaphragmatic opening. The heart is pushed toward the right, and the left lung is compressed. Rapid, labored respirations and cyanosis are present on the first day of life, and breathing becomes increasingly more difficult.

Surgery is essential, and may be performed on an emergency basis. During surgery the abdominal viscera are withdrawn from the chest and the diaphragmatic defect is closed. A pleural tube is left in place, connected to a waterseal drainage bottle. Other anomalies may be present; the mortality rate is high.

This defect is not the same as the diaphragmatic hiatus hernia. In a hiatus hernia, a portion of the stomach protrudes into the chest through a normal opening in the diaphragm. This is a condition more common in adults.

ANOMALIES OF THE NERVOUS SYSTEM

Hydrocephalus

Hydrocephalus is a condition characterized by an excess of cerebrospinal fluid within the ventricular and subarachnoid spaces of the cranial cavity. Normally there is a delicate balance between the rate of formation and the absorption of cerebrospinal fluid. The entire volume is absorbed and replaced every 12 to 24 hours. In hydrocephalus this balance is disturbed.

Cerebrospinal fluid is formed by the choroid plexus, mainly in the lateral ventricles. It is absorbed into the venous system through the arachnoid villi. Cerebrospinal fluid circulates within the ventricles and the subarachnoid space. It is a colorless fluid, consisting of water with traces of protein, glucose and lymphocytes.

The *noncommunicating* type of congenital hydrocephalus occurs when there is an obstruction in the free circulation of cerebrospinal fluid. This blockage causes increased pressure on the brain or spinal cord. The site of obstruction may be at the foramen of Monro, the aqueduct of Silvius, the foramen of Lushka, or the foramen of Magendie. (Fig. 20-9)

In the *communicating* type of hydrocephalus, there is no obstruction of the free flow of cerebrospinal fluid between the ventricles and the spinal theca. The condition is caused by defective absorption of the cerebrospinal fluid, this causing pressure on the brain or spinal cord to build up. Congenital hydrocephalus is most frequently of the obstructive or noncommunicating type.

Hydrocephalus may be recognized at birth, or it may not be evident until after a few weeks or months of life. Occasionally, the condition may not be congenital, but may instead occur during later infancy or during childhood as the result of a head injury, or an infection such as meningitis.

When hydrocephalus occurs early in life before the skull sutures close, the soft pliable bones separate to allow head expansion. This is manifested by a rapid growth in head circumference. The fact that the soft bones are capable of yielding to pressure in this

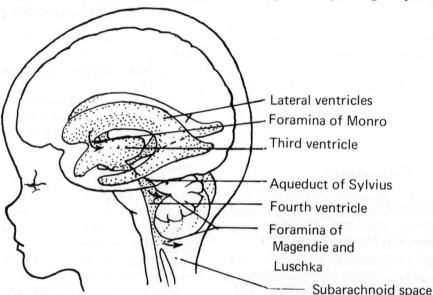

Lateral ventricles
Foramina of Monro
Third ventricle

Aqueduct of Sylvius
Fourth ventricle
Foramina of Magendie and Luschka
Subarachnoid space

Figure 20-9. Ventricles of the brain and the channels for the normal flow of cerebrospinal fluid. (Courtesy of Dr. A. J. Raimondi. From Raffensberger, J., and Primrose, R.(eds.): Pediatric Surgery for Nurses. Boston, Little, Brown and Co., 1968.)

manner may partially explain why many of these infants fail to show the usual symptoms of brain pressure, and may exhibit little or no damage to mental function until later in life. Other infants show severe brain damage, often occurring before birth.

Clinical Manifestations

A rapidly enlarging head may be the first manifestation of this condition. An apparently large head in itself is not necessarily significant. Normally, every infant's head is measured at birth, and the rate of growth is checked at subsequent examinations. Any infant's head that appears to be abnormally large at birth, or appears to be enlarging, should be measured frequently.

As the head enlarges, the suture lines separate, and the spaces can be felt through the scalp. The anterior fontanelle becomes tense and bulging; the skull enlarges in all diameters; the scalp becomes shiny, and its veins dilate. The eyes appear to be pushed downward slightly, with the sclera visible above the iris, giving the so-called "setting sun" sign. (Fig. 20-10)

As the condition progresses, the head becomes increasingly heavy, the neck muscles fail to develop sufficiently, and the infant has difficulty raising or turning his head. Unless the hydrocephalus is arrested, the infant becomes increasingly helpless, and symptoms of brain pressure eventually develop. These may include irritability, vomiting, failure to thrive, and arrested development.

Diagnosis

An excessively large head at birth is suggestive of hydrocephalus. Rapid head growth with widening cranial sutures is also strongly suggestive. Positive diagnosis is made through the use of pneumoencephalograms and ventriculograms.

Prognosis

Prognosis is guarded in all cases. Many affected infants show severe brain damage at birth. Surgical intervention is the only effective means for relieving brain pressure and preventing further damage. Some

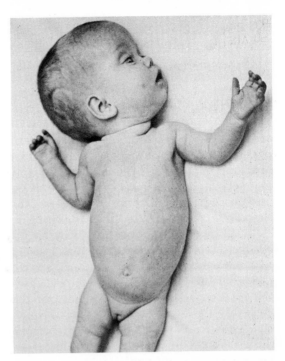

Figure 20-10. A child with hydrocephalus. Note the pull on the eyes giving the "setting sun" appearance. Note also the site of incision for a ventriculo-auricular shunt.

children who have suffered only minimal brain damage are able to function within a normal mental range. Motor function is usually retarded.

Surgical Treatment

For the majority of cases the only available procedure is a shunting device that bypasses the point of obstruction, draining the excess cerebrospinal fluid into a body cavity. This procedure arrests excessive head growth and prevents further brain damage. Installation of a shunting device is considered to be indicated for any hydrocephalic infant whose condition permits, most surgeons being unwilling to wait for a possible spontaneous arrest.

Shunting procedures. A number of types of surgery have been devised over the years for this condition with varying success. The most successful kind of surgery has consisted of a shunting procedure, using a rubber or polyethylene tubing to bypass the point of obstruction and to drain the excess cerebrospinal fluid into a body cavity. The pleural and peritoneal cavities have been used, but these procedures have short-term effectiveness. Use of a ureter has been more successful, and many children today lead normal lives after a ventriculoureterostomy. This, however, necessitates the removal of one kidney, and also requires the addition of measured amounts of salt to the diet, to be continued indefinitely. The amount of salt drained out of the body from the loss of cerebrospinal fluid seriously upsets the electrolyte balance unless it is replaced.

The procedure of choice, at present, is a bypass that uses the venous system, routing the excess cerebrospinal fluid into the right atrium of the heart. This procedure utilizes the jugular vein. A burr hole is made into the skull just above and behind the ear, through which the tip of a polyethylene or silicone rubber catheter is introduced into the ventricle of the brain. The catheter is then

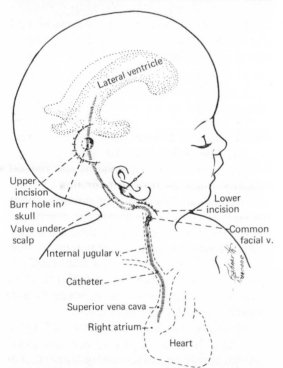

Figure 20-11. An operative procedure for hydrocephalus, in which a catheter drains the ventricular system into the right atrium. (Jacob, S.W., and Francone, C.A.: Structure and Function in Man. ed. 2. Philadelphia, W.B. Saunders, 1970)

threaded into the jugular vein, with the distal end draining into the right auricle of the heart. A one-way valve built into the tube prevents reflux. Valves commonly used are the Spitz-Holter and the Pudenz-Heyer (Fig. 20-11).

Difficulties are associated with the use of these valves. Complications include a need for revision in about 40% of the cases, and septicemia, usually staphylococcal. Treatment for the septicemia requires removal of the valve and tube and prolonged antibiotic therapy. Following clearing of the infection, the apparatus may be replaced, although reinfection may occur.

Postoperative Care

Following a ventriculoatrial shunting, the infant is kept with his head turned away from the operative site until the incision is well healed. If the child is able to turn his head, sandbags may be needed to keep it turned to one side. Vital signs are taken routinely as they would be after any surgical procedure. He should be watched carefully for change of color, excessive irritability or lethargy, and for abnormal vital signs. The fontanelle is frequently depressed after shunting; this is to be expected. A suction machine for removal of excessive mucus from the nose and the mouth should be readily available.

The side of the head on which the baby lies should be examined for pressure sores, particularly if the head is large and heavy. Sponge rubber under his head may be useful.

The child may receive intravenous fluids immediately following surgery, with oral feedings started when he is able to tolerate them.

Physical Care and Emotional Support of the Infant with Hydrocephalus

Every infant has the need, and the right, to be picked up, loved and held in a loving, comforting manner. When any child has suffered a painful or uncomfortable experience, his need for emotional support becomes much greater.

The chief way in which an infant can perceive such support is through physical contact, made in a soothing, loving manner. When a nurse has to be responsible for causing discomfort to a child, such as giving an intramuscular injection, she must realize that an integral part of the treatment is the immediate following of emotional support. Preferably, this support is given by the person who has caused the pain.

The nurse should *never* feel that she does not have time for this part of the treatment, any more than she would feel that she did not have time to wash her hands or put on sterile gloves when indicated. Occasionally, of course, it is not possible for physical reasons to pick up a child out of his crib. The nurse must convey her concern by her touch, her voice, her soothing manner. Convey it, however, she must.

Physical care is of course important. When the head is heavy and difficult for the child to turn, it must be turned for him to prevent skin breakdown. Tincture of benzoin applied to irritated places may prevent such breakdown. Any broken area should be reported at once.

Bathing. Sponge baths may be necessary if the infant has poor head control. Special care to the areas behind the ears and in the creases of the neck is important. As in everything done for these children, special attention can be a means of alleviating some of the inherent frustrations. There are many little comfort-promoting devices that nurses do not always consider important.

Comfortably warm bath water is soothing. Too often, one finds only a few inches of cool or lukewarm water in the bath basin, especially when the nurse has prepared the water before she has collected all of her equipment.

If back rubs are soothing for adults, might not a few minutes spent in giving a gentle rub be appreciated by an infant who must lie in his crib for long intervals? If a soft, gentle voice is pleasing to hear, this infant too may be soothed and pleased, perhaps even stimulated, if the nurse talks to him during the bathing process.

Feeding. Feeding technique also assumes importance for this child. These babies have a need to be held when they are fed even more than the healthy babies, but, in practice, this need is frequently not met. The nurse may need to select a chair with an arm on which to rest her elbow while supporting the heavy head. When these children have difficulty holding their heads erect, bubbling them becomes somewhat more difficult. Bottle feeding needs to be given carefully and slowly, with special attention to absence of air in the nipple.

When, for some reason, the baby cannot be held for feeding, there may be a temptation to prop the bottle; especially if the baby cannot move his head, and thus lose the nipple as easily as another child. There is no place for bottle propping in his care, however, or in the care of any hospitalized infant.

Head Measurement. The baby's head circumference should be measured daily, or at intervals ordered by the doctor. The tape measure is passed around the largest portion of the child's head, over the forehead and around the occipital region. In the interest of accuracy, it is better if the same person does the measurement each time, using the same tape measure.

Social Interaction. The infant in his crib needs social interaction. He needs to be talked to, played with, and provided with activity according to his ability. Toys commensurate with his physical and mental capacity must be provided for him.

If the child has difficulty moving about his crib, toys must be within his reach and within his ability to manipulate. A cradle gym tied close enough for him to reach may be good. If he cannot raise his head, or cannot turn in pursuit of an elusive toy, he receives additional frustration which he can well do without.

It is most important that the infant be allowed to become a part of the social environment, but this he cannot achieve if he is turned with his face toward a blank wall. Unless his nervous system is so impaired that all activity increases his irritability, he needs stimulation as much as any child. If turning an infant from side to side means turning him away from the sight of activity, turn the crib around so that he is not facing the wall or ward divider.

The effect of attention and stimulation on the average infant is amazing. One infant may lie in his crib day after day, receiving all necessary physical care, but no emotional stimulation. He is never played with, talked to, or picked up. Because of his limitations, he cannot provide self-stimulation. This child does not fit into our definition of a normal child, is not treated as one, and therefore does not act as one.

A second infant with the same handicap is given all the contact and support that any infant requires. His personality develops, growing by what it feeds on. His nurse uses the time she has for his physical care as a time for social interaction. She talks and laughs with him, plays with him, and visits him at times between the necessary occasions for giving physical care.

A person seeing the two infants might well remark about the personality development and mental alertness of the second child, finding the first child dull and

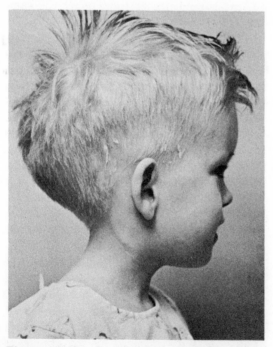

Figure 20-12. Arrested hydrocephalus after a ventriculo-auricular shunt.

apathetic. Yet both may have had the same capacity for development, but are products of differing environments. Once again, we become impressed with the concept that nursing is much more than the meeting of physical needs.

Help to Parents

A nurse does not find it difficult to understand the anxiety and apprehension parents feel if this condition is present in their child, but she may feel quite helpless in trying to give them support. Her own acceptance of the child with her tender care and concern for his welfare helps convey her warmth of feeling. Her matter-of-fact acceptance of his handicap, as well as her treatment of him as a baby with normal needs, helps put the situation on a more realistic basis.

Arrangements should be made to give much of the normal, daily care at times when parents are able to be present. They need to learn how to hold and handle the baby in as normal a manner as possible. Undoubtedly, they need much encouragement. Can they do him any harm by the way they care for him? Should he not be kept quietly by himself to prevent too much stimulation? Many other questions may be asked of the nurse, and many misapprehensions may be cleared away.

A mother should be encouraged to help with her child's care when there are others present to give her support. She can be encouraged to feel the valve in the ventriculo-auricular shunting device, and to develop an understanding of its function. Both parents need to understand the importance of careful observation for any abnormal developments, and, at the same time, attempt to create as normal a life as possible for their child. (Fig. 20-12)

Spina Bifida

Another congenital anomaly of the central nervous system is a spinal malformation called *spina bifida.* In this condition there is a defect in the neural arch, generally in the lumbosacral region; the posterior laminae of the vertebrae fail to close, presenting an opening through which the spinal meninges and spinal cord may protrude.

The bony defect occurring alone, without involvement of the tissues, is called spina bifida occulta. In most cases, it is asymptomatic and presents no problems. A dimple in the skin or a tuft of hair over the site may cause one to suspect its presence, or it may be entirely overlooked.

Clinical Features

When a portion of the spinal meninges protrudes through the bony defect and forms a cystic sac, the condition is termed spina bifida with meningocele. No nerve roots are involved; therefore, no paralysis or sensory loss below the lesion appears. The sac may, however, rupture or perforate, thus introducing infection into the spinal fluid and causing meningitis. For this reason, as well as for cosmetic purposes, surgical removal of the sac, with closure of the skin, is indicated.

Spina bifida with myelomeningocele signifies a protrusion of the spinal cord and the meninges, with nerve roots embedded in the wall of the cyst. The effects of this defect vary in severity from sensory loss or partial paralysis below the lesion, to complete flaccid paralysis of all muscles below the lesion. The complete paralysis involves the lower trunk and legs as well as bowel and bladder sphincters. It is not always possible however to make a clear-cut differentiation in diagnosis between a meningocele and a myelomeningocele on the basis of symptoms alone.

The condition myelomeningocele may also be termed meningomyelocele. The associated spina bifida is always implied, but not necessarily named. *Spina bifida cystica* is the term used to designate either of these protrusions.

In some hospitals the baby is placed on a Bradford frame to facilitate handling. The canvas frame must be covered with soft sheets to prevent skin irritation, and the edges of the open section below the perineal region protected with sheets of plastic that drape down into the receptacle placed on the bed below the frame.

The child is positioned on his abdomen with flannel restraints to hold him in place. A rolled towel under his ankles or a rolled blanket under his legs is needed to prevent pressure on his toes. It is possible to position a small infant on his side while on a Bradford frame, with the use of a rolled blanket against his back above the lesion, and restraints to hold him in place.

Nurses and parents are encouraged to hold the child at intervals, particularly for feedings. Of course he must be held in such a manner as to avoid pressure on the sac, but the child can be fitted comfortably into the nurse's arm. Parents may be frightened and need encouragement as well as help in correctly positioning the child.

Postoperative care. Following repair of a meningocele or myelomeningocele, the infant is placed in a prone or knee-chest position and not moved unnecessarily until the operative site is completely healed. This means that all procedures must be carried out with the infant in this position, including feeding and bathing.

Usual postoperative observations are followed. Perineal care must be continued, and special precautions for keeping the operative site clean and dry strictly observed. When feedings are begun, the nurse turns the baby's head to one side and holds the bottle, at the same time keeping the baby in the prone position. The surgeon decides when he can be moved or turned.

Continuing Care

It is difficult to predict the future for these infants. Many of those with hydrocephalus and myelomeningocele appear to have a hopeless prognosis at birth. Many who do survive in spite of severe handicaps, succumb to infection during early life. Some, however, live through the hazardous early years. These children, with skillful help and favorable circumstances, may be able to achieve useful, satisfactory lives.

The majority of neurosurgeons and orthopedists prefer to give the child every possible assistance, even if the prospect does not appear particularly favorable. Shunting devices and repair of spinal defects are made early in life. If satisfactory results have been attained, orthopedic procedures should be carried out in anticipation of the possibility of future ambulation. These may include casting for talipes equinovarus and hip dysplasia, as well as intensive physical therapy to prevent progression of deformities.

As the child grows older, he can progress from a stroller to a wheelchair, with the prospect for many of learning to walk with the help of braces and crutches. Increasingly, as medical knowledge advances, more such handicapped children are helped to a relatively normal way of life.

Urinary control. The most difficult problem is that of urinary incontinence. If voluntary sphincter control is absent, the infant cannot be toilet trained. Dribbling of urine does not keep the bladder emptied and reflux resulting in hydroureter and hydronephrosis is common, with resultant severe kidney damage.

The bladder can be emptied by mechanical expression, using the Credé method. Firm hand pressure is applied over the bladder region, with the hand moved slowly down below the symphysis pubis. This is done periodically to prevent the accumulation of urine in the bladder. The parents should be taught this procedure before they take the child home.

Associated conditions. Hydrocephalus of the obstructive type is frequently associated with these two defects. Bypass procedures may arrest the hydrocephaly, but cannot affect or restore the neural function involved in a myelomeningocele. It was formerly thought that surgical repair of the spinal defect would frequently cause hydrocephaly not previously present, and parents were so advised. This has not been proved, however.

The concept accepted by many neurosurgeons today is that hydrocephaly is already present, the surgical repair of the sac accelerating its development. Other defects are frequently present, the most common being talipes equinovarus. Hip displasia may also be present. (Fig. 20-13)

Surgical Treatment

Surgical repair of a myelomeningocele cannot be expected to decrease the neurological disability, although many surgeons believe that future function is improved to some extent in those carefully repaired. It has been observed that some newborn infants show a limited motor ability that rapidly decreases after birth. Many neurosurgeons advocate immediate repair.

A leaking sac calls for immediate repair to prevent meningitis. Some infants with a thin membrane over the sac, through which spinal fluid is leaking, show signs of meningitis at birth.

The primary objective of surgical repair is closure of the defect, with replacement of neural elements within the vertebral canal whenever possible. Nerve roots that can be freed are replaced in the canal, the sac amputated at its base or turned inward, and plastic surgery employed for covering the site of the defect.

Nursing Care of the Infant with Spina Bifida Cystica

Preoperative care. The infant needs the same kind of care outlined for the care of the child with hydrocephalus; in fact, he quite possibly has hydrocephalus. This infant's care, however, is complicated by the presence of the spinal lesion.

The infant with such a spinal lesion cannot be allowed to lie on his back, but must be positioned on his side or abdomen. His position must be frequently changed.

It is most important that the sac be kept clean and dry, with all pressure avoided. Any leakage of spinal fluid must be reported immediately. Avoidance of contamination from urine or fecal material is of particular importance. A sheet of plastic may be taped between the defect and the anus, and folded back on itself to form a barrier, and taped into place. If the sac covering is thin, a dressing may be ordered to be placed over it. This may be a dry, sterile dressing, or may be medicated. Adaptic, Vaseline gauze or Varidase may be used.

Perhaps the greatest nursing challenge is in keeping the perineum clean and in preventing excoriation when paralysis of the sphincter muscles is present, because the lack of sphincter control results in constant dribbling of urine and feces. Because the infant cannot be placed on his back, fecal material runs down over the perineum. The constant dribbling of urine and feces causes severe skin irritation. To help prevent excoriation, scrupulous cleanliness must be maintained. The perineum should be cleansed frequently with an unmedicated oil and left exposed to the air at all times.

A number of methods have been devised to achieve urinary continence for the child, none of which has proved to be entirely satisfactory. A very few children have achieved successful control after long-term, rigorous training. Control of fluid intake, with strict regularity of mechanical bladder emptying by the Credé method, combined with unlimited patience, has produced good results. Few parents or children are able to carry out these long-term programs. Even if control is achieved in this manner, the bladder may not be completely emptied.

Indwelling catheters may be useful for short periods, especially when an infection is being treated. Transplant of the ureters into the sigmoid is a procedure that has been widely used, but the ascending infection that usually results has been discouraging.

The most encouraging procedure employed at present is an ileal loop, or cutaneous ileoureterostomy. A small segment of the ileum is isolated, its distal end closed, and the proximal end brought to the skin surface of the abdomen. The remaining bowel is anastomosed for continuity of function. The ends of the ureters

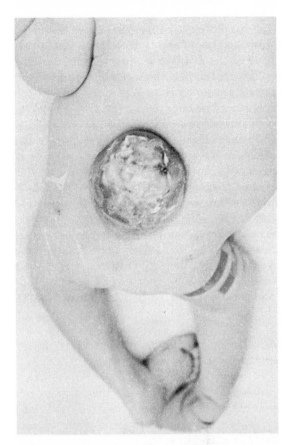

Figure 20-13. A myelomeningocele showing an additional defect of club feet.

are inserted into the sides of the ileal segment, which then acts as a conduit for the urine to the surface of the body. An ileostomy bag fitted over the stoma receives the urine. The parents and child need careful instruction and practice in learning to apply the bag correctly to prevent leakage.

Bowel control is not so difficult to achieve. A slightly constipating diet may be necessary at first. The parent places the child on the toilet at the time he usually has a bowel movement, perhaps using a suppository until habit is established. Accidents may happen at first, but intelligent regulation is usually effective.

The courage and persistence demanded from the parents of these children, as well as from the children themselves, is nearly more than the unaffected person can grasp. They deserve a great deal of emotional support and encouragement. Considerable physical and financial help is necessary for most families.

The child who does achieve ambulation through use of braces and crutches, and is able to take his place as a well adjusted member of society, rewards all those who gave so much time, effort and unending patience. The child in Figure 20-14 is such an example. A myelomeningocele was successfully repaired in infancy. He learned to walk with crutches and braces; at the age of five he re-entered the hospital for new braces, an Achilles tenotomy, and urinary tract evaluation. He was a friendly, outgoing child with a sunny disposition, a lively imagination and quick mental ability. The picture shows him ready to leave the hospital

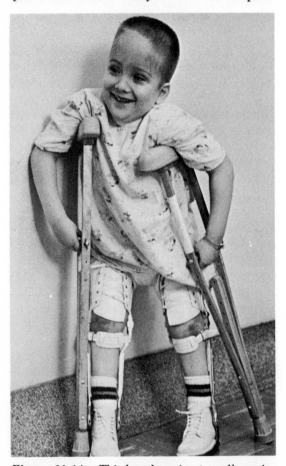

Figure 20-14. This boy, learning to walk again with new braces, underwent successful surgery for repair of a myelomeningocele during infancy.

with his new braces. Giving such a child hope for a relatively normal life seems well worth the effort put forth by so many—not the least of whom was the child himself.

Anomalies of the Genital System

Pseudohermaphroditism (Intersexuality)

Various abnormalities of the external genitalia may be found in the newborn. The most common is called the *adrenogenital syndrome*. Females with this congenital anomaly have an enlarged clitoris, resembling a penis. The labia are fused, resembling a biped scrotum. Internal sex organs are female and there is a female chromosomal pattern. The potentiality for fertility is normal.

Diagnosis should be confirmed as early as possible; the infant is raised as a girl. An exploratory laparotomy may be necessary to confirm the sex. Plastic surgery to the external genitalia to correct the structures is best performed between the ages of 18 months and 4 years.

In male pseudohermaphroditism, testes are present, but the external genitalia are ambiguous or completely feminine. In those who are completely feminine in appearance, breast development occurs at puberty, but menstruation is absent. Testes are usually in the abdomen; there are no ovaries. The testes should be removed at puberty; estrogens are given, and the child is raised as a girl. The child will, of course, be sterile.

True hermaphroditism, in which both ovarian and testicular tissue are present, is very rare. There is usually an ambiguity of external genitalia. Exploratory laparotomy is needed to determine sex. A child who has been raised as a male or female will adopt the role assigned to him. Decision should be made early before the sex of the newborn has been announced and before the birth announcement is made out. No changing of sex roles should be made in later childhood as this is extremely damaging psychologically. If internal organs are later discovered which do not correspond with the child's announced sex, these should be removed.

Hypospadias

Hypospadias is a congenital condition of a male child in which the urethra terminates on the underside (ventral) of the penis, instead of at the tip. A cordlike anomaly (called a *chordee*) extends from the scrotum to the penis, pulling the penis downward in an arc. Urination is not interfered with, but the boy is unable to void while standing in the normal male fashion. Surgical repair is recommended before the child starts to attend school to avoid the psychological damage he will suffer through ridicule from his male classmates.

Surgical repair is performed in two stages. The primary surgery is for the purpose of releasing the chordee. Later, during the preschool period, plastic surgery is used to extend the urethra to the tip of the penis and to close the ventral opening. These infants should not be circumcised, as the foreskin is used in the repair.

In *epispadias* the opening is on the dorsal (top) surface of the penis. This condition frequently occurs with exstrophy of the bladder. Surgical repair is indicated.

BIBLIOGRAPHY

Carrington, K. W.: Ventriculo-venous shunt: use of the holter valve as treatment of hydrocephalus, J. Mich. Med. Soc., *58:*373, 1959.

Gellis, Sydney and Kagan, Benjamin, eds.: Current Pediatric Therapy. Philadelphia, W. B. Saunders, 1970.

Hormoz, Azar, Chrispin, Alan R., and Waterman, David J.: Esophageal replacement with transverse colon in infants and children, Journal of Pediatric Surgery, *6:*3, 1971.

Nelson, Waldo E., Vaughn, Victor C., and McKay, R. James, eds.: Textbook of Pediatrics. ed. 9. Philadelphia, W. B. Saunders, 1969.

Raffensperger, John G. and Primrose, Rosellen Bohlen, eds.: Pediatric Surgery for Nurses. Boston, Little & Brown, 1968.

Wilson, C. B. and Raeburn, C. L.: The surgical management of meningocele and myelomeningocele, Journal of Pediatrics, *61:*595, 1962.

Suggested Readings for Further Study

Avery, Gordon B. et al.: Meningocele and Hydrocephalus, Clinical Proceedings of the Children's Hospital of Washington, D. C., *26:*135, 1970.

Bonine, Gladys N.: The myelodysplastic child—hospital and home care, AJN, *69:*541, 1969.

Leape, Lucian L. and Holder, Thomas M.: Temporary tubeless urinary diversion in children, Journal of Pediatric Surgery, *5:*288, 1970.

Wendel, Robert M. and King, Lowel R.: The treatment of urinary incontinence, Journal of Pediatric Surgery, *5:*543, 1970.

Medical Conditions of the Newborn *21*

CONGENITAL RUBELLA

Following a major rubella epidemic in Australia in 1941, the teratogenic* effect of the rubella virus on the fetus during the first trimester of pregnancy, as it passed the placental barrier, was noted and eventually well documented. A resulting combination of defects discovered in the newborn, consisting of congenital cataracts, heart disease, deafness and microcephaly, became known as the rubella syndrome.

In 1962, the rubella virus was successfully propagated in tissue culture. Techniques for isolation of the virus and detection of antibodies are now perfected.

The most extensive rubella epidemic in history occurred in the United States in 1964, resulting in a large number of babies with congenital malformations from maternal infection. It has been estimated that as many as 10,000 to 20,000 babies may have been so affected. One result of this epidemic with its unfortunate consequences has been an increase in our knowledge concerning congenital rubella.

It is now apparent that the rubella virus infection acquired by the fetus in utero generally persists throughout fetal life, is present at birth, and for an undetermined time after birth. Virus has been recovered from aborted fetuses and from infants throughout the first year of life. Persons coming into intimate contact with these babies may develop the disease, and such cases are on record.

---

*Teratogenic: producing serious malformations or deviations from the normal structure.

Congenital Defects

A large variety of defects have been reported in association with congenital rubella, in addition to those previously documented. Malformations constituting the rubella syndrome are now found to include the following: cataracts and other eye defects, occasionally glaucoma; deafness; cardiac anomalies, especially patent ductus arteriosus and septal defects; intrauterine growth retardation; subnormal head circumference and retarded functional development. Less commonly found, but seemingly associated with rubella, are meningocele, purpura, enlarged liver and spleen, defects of long bones, and many others.

An infant may be suspected of harboring rubella virus if there is a history of maternal infection during the first trimester of pregnancy and if the presence of one or more of the malformations described is observed. There does, however, appear to be evidence that some infants, infected in utero, excrete rubella virus even when no abnormalities are noted.

Cultures of rubella virus may be obtained from pharyngeal secretions, urine, cerebrospinal fluid, and other secretions or tissues. The infant with rubella may shed virus for a number of months after birth, some for as long as a year. As long as virus shedding continues, his secretions are capable of spreading the disease.

Indications for Isolation

All women of childbearing age who are not immune to rubella should avoid contact with an infected infant. This includes nurses in the newborn nursery, in clinics or physicians' offices, public health nurses and other personnel in nurseries and infant departments of the hospital. Reliance on immunization by presumed attacks of rubella during the individual's childhood is generally not enough because many rashes resemble that of rubella, and symptoms of childhood rubella are mild. Testing for the presence of rubella serum antibody is desirable in areas where adequate laboratory facilities are available.* A positive reaction shows the person to be immune either as a result of the disease itself, or from immunization. Parents of infected infants should understand the dangers presented to pregnant women.

Care of the infant is concerned with treating concomitant conditions and giving routine care accorded any newborn infant. Some infants are extremely ill from complications present at birth, and rates of permanent damage are high.

Prevention

A rubella vaccine is now available that produces long lasting immunity. This is a live virus vaccine administered in a single subcutaneous injection. In the United States, mass vaccination for children between the ages of 1 and 12 years is being attempted as vaccine becomes available. Priority is given to kindergarten and early school age children, as this is the age group most likely to disseminate the disease. History of rubella in a child is usually not reliable enough to omit vaccination.

Women of childbearing age in the United States are not given the vaccine unless there is no possibility of pregnancy within 2 months following vaccination. Each case is considered individually. Medically acceptable methods of contraception should be followed to insure against pregnancy. Vaccination with live rubella virus is contraindicated during pregnancy. At the

*Report of the Committee on Infectious Diseases 1970. P. 131. Evanston, Illinois, American Academy of Pediatrics, 1970.

present time it is not known to what extent infection of the fetus with potential damage may follow vaccination of the mother.

Pregnant women who have been exposed to rubella during the first trimester of pregnancy may be given immune serum globulin (human). Whether the fetus receives protection through this is controversial, as clinical signs of the disease in the mother may be suppressed, but the virus may still injure the fetus if she contracts the disease. There is some suggestion that the use of this gamma globulin may lessen the likelihood of fetal infection and damage, but infants with congenital rubella have been born to women who have received this protection. Rubella in a woman in the first trimester of pregnancy is now legally recognized as an indication for abortion in many states of the United States, and in many other countries.

IMPETIGO

This infection of the skin occasionally appears in newborn nurseries where strict aseptic technique is not carried out. Impetigo may be either a staphylococcal or streptococcal skin infection, but in the newborn period it is usually due to staphylococci. Lesions appear anywhere on the body.

Clinical manifestations. The lesion is vesicular, becoming rapidly seropurulent with an area of erythema surrounding each lesion. Rupture of the pustules causes spread to other areas.

Susceptibility among newborns seems to be general. The infecting organism may be carried by attending personnel with minor staphylococcal lesions. The condition can spread quickly through a nursery unless strict isolation of the infected infant is carried out.

Treatment. The lesions should be washed with a soap containing hexachlorophene. If crusts have formed they should be removed. Bacitracin or neomycin ointment may be employed locally. Systemic antibiotic therapy is usually not indicated except in severe infections with secondary complications.

Prognosis. The disease is generally mild with complete recovery if the infant is cared for properly. In the past, sepsis has occurred in sick and premature babies.

CONGENITAL SYPHILIS

Syphilis, whether congenital or acquired, is caused by the spirochete *Treponema pallidum.* Fetal infection does not occur much before the fourth month of fetal life after the fetal organs are formed, therefore, anomalies rarely occur. The infection is contracted through the mother by placental transfer. About one fourth of infected infants are stillborn. Infants born live may not show any clinical symptoms for months or years.

Diagnosis

A Wasserman test on cord blood at delivery is done when congenital syphilis is suspected. Passively acquired antibodies may give a false positive, therefore other seriological tests will be given later. If results are doubtful, treatment will usually be instituted to avoid a full blown infection.

In *early* congenital syphilis, symptoms may appear before the sixth week of life. Rhinitis, with a profuse, mucopurulent nasal discharge is usually the first symptom. A maculopapular skin rash next appears, heaviest over the back, buttocks and backs of the thighs. Bleeding ulcerations and mucous membrane lesions appear around the mouth, anus, and the genital areas. Anemia is present, psuedoparalysis and pathological fractures may occur. These symptoms usually subside without treatment while the infectious organism lies latent in the child's tissues.

Late symptoms, appearing after infancy, involve the skeletal framework, the eyes and the central nervous system. The child may acquire a flat bridge of the nose, known as "saddle nose." His permanent teeth are affected, the incisors are peg-shaped (Hutchinton's teeth). A condition of the eyes called *interstitial keratitis* frequently occurs later in the disease with lacrimation, photophobia, and opacity of the lens which may lead to blindness.

Treatment

Ideally, treatment is preventive, consisting of treatment of the affected mother early in pregnancy. Treatment for the affected infant consists of a course of penicillin. Aqueous procaine penicillin, 15,000 units per kilogram of body weight per day for 10 days, or benzathine penicillin (Bicillin) 50,000 units per kilogram of body weight once weekly for 3 doses is given intramuscularly to children under the age of 2 years. Over the age of 2 years, the dosage is increased. Conditions co-existing with the presence of syphilis such as anemia, malnutrition, and eyes lesions need to be treated symptomatically.

Prognosis

Early congenital syphilis usually responds to vigorous treatment, and growth and development will not be affected. Late congenital syphilis responds well to treatment, but pathological changes in the bones, eyes, and nervous system are permanent.

GONORRHEAL OPHTHALMIA NEONATORUM

Gonorrheal eye infection in the newborn is a serious condition usually resulting in blindness when prophylactic treatment at birth is omitted. The infectious agent is *Neisseria gonorrhoeae,* the gonococcus. The infant becomes infected as he passes through the birth canal of an infected mother.

Symptoms are acute redness and swelling of the conjunctiva with a purulent discharge from the eyes, occurring within 36 to 48 hours after birth. The condition is communicable for 24 hours after specific therapy is instituted, or when no therapy is used, until discharge from the eyes has ceased.

Prevention

In the United States, all states have mandatory laws requiring the use of specific preparations instilled into the eyes at birth. A number of states require instillation of 1% silver nitrate. In other states antibiotic drops such as penicillin, or 1% terramycin ophthalmic ointment are used. Silver nitrate itself causes a chemical irritation of the conjunctiva, with purulent discharge. Two minutes after instillation of silver nitrate, the eyes should be flushed with sterile water or normal saline.

Treatment

Penicillin is a specific for the treatment of gonorrheal infections, including gonorrheal ophthalmia.

HEMOLYTIC DISEASE OF THE NEWBORN

All that we presently know about hemolytic disease of the newborn has developed in the last thirty years. It is truly amazing that the cause, treatment, and method of prevention has been worked out in such a short span of time. Indeed, the development of Rhogam which is used to prevent the disease has been heralded as one of the remarkable achievements in obstetrics during this century.

Hemolytic disease is another name for *erythroblastosis fetalis*. In this disease the infant's red blood cells are broken down (hemolyzed) and destroyed producing severe anemia. As a result of the rapid destruction of red blood cells severe anemia, heart failure, and brain damage may result.

Incidence

The incidence of hemolytic disease is directly related to occurrence of certain blood groups in our population.* About 85% of the white population is Rh positive and 15% Rh negative. This percentage varies among different racial groups—for example, only 5% of the Negro population is Rh negative, so that they have a lower incidence of the disease. Thus only a small percentage of marriages, about 13% in the United States, provide the set-up for the development of this complication.

What is the Rh factor? The Rh factor is a protein substance called an *antigen* found on the surface of red blood cells.† It is called

---

*Fitzpatrick, Elise, et al.: Maternity Nursing, ed. 12. P. 522. Philadelphia, J. B. Lippincott, 1971.

†Rh hemolytic diseases of the newborn. Nursing Currents, *21*:2, 1972. (Publication of Ross Laboratories, Columbus, Ohio.)

Rh because it was first identified in the blood of Rhesus monkeys. Those people who possess the factor are called Rh positive (D), and those who are lacking it are Rh negative (d).

The blood type of an individual is inherited—the same hereditary rules are followed in regard to dominant and recessive traits with Rh positive being dominant. If a woman who is Rh negative marries a man who is also Rh negative, no problem will exist with their children. However, if the father is Rh positive and the child inherits Rh positive blood from his father, trouble may occur.

Another important point is whether the father is homozygous or heterozygous. If he is homozygous positive, that means that both of his genes carry the D (dominant) trait, but if he is heterzygous positive, one of the genes is a D and the other a d. Thus, if the husband is heterozygous positive and his wife is Rh negative, there is a 50—50 chance of their having a Rh negative baby (and no problem).

Because of the mechanism by which the mother is sensitized to the Rh factor, there is very little chance of the first baby being affected. Therefore, when all of the factors are taken into consideration, the chances of having a baby with hemolytic disease are rather slim, the incidence being about 1 in 200 births.

Pathophysiology

The pathology is based on the principles of the *antigen-antibody response*. Although the fetal and maternal circulations are completely separated, there may be a break in the placental barrier which allows some of the fetal red blood cells to escape into the maternal circulation. Often the break occurs at the time the placenta separates during delivery; or it may take place after an abortion. The Rh positive fetal cells entering the maternal circulation act as a "mini-transfusion" causing the mother to react by forming protective antibodies. It may take some time, however, for the antibodies to form so that the first baby is rarely affected.

With the next pregnancy, if any of the

baby's red blood cells enter the maternal circulation, there is a rapid formation of antibodies. Consequently, the maternal antibodies enter the fetal circulation and begin to hemolyze the baby's red blood cells (Fig. 21-1).

Due to the rapid destruction of red blood cells, there is a breakdown product called bilirubin which is excreted into the amniotic fluid. The baby's body makes a valiant attempt to replace the red blood cells being destroyed by sending out large amounts of immature red blood cells called "erythroblasts" into his blood stream. For this reason, the disease is called *erythroblastosis fetalis*. As the process of rapid destruction of the red blood cells continues the baby develops anemia which, if severe enough, can result in heart failure and death of the baby in utero.

Prenatal Care of the Rh-Negative Woman

An expectant mother should have her blood tested for blood group and Rh type at the time of her initial prenatal visit. If the woman is found to be Rh negative then she should be followed closely throughout her pregnancy.* At periodic intervals she should have blood titers done as a screening method to detect the presence of antibodies. This allows the attending physician to evaluate the health of the fetus and plan for the baby's delivery and care.

---

*Her husband's blood should also be typed and if he is Rh positive, a genotype may be done to determine if he is homozygous or heterozygous.

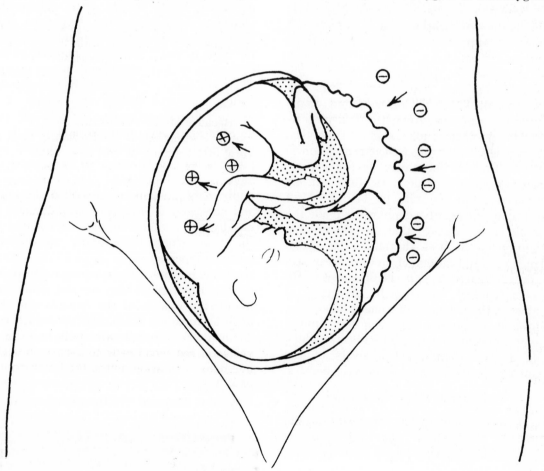

Figure 21-1. Antibodies from mother enter the child and begin destroying its blood cells.

Treatment

When titers show the presence of antibodies the doctor then tries to determine how much the fetus is affected. Since there is no direct way to sample the infant's blood to find out the degree of anemia, indirect means must be used. A recent advance in diagnosing fetal diseases has been through the use of a procedure called *amniocentesis*. By inserting a needle into the amniotic sac 10 to 15 cc. of amniotic fluid is removed. If done by a skilled person, it involves little risk to the mother or fetus. The fluid is sent to the laboratory for spectophotometric analysis which shows the amount of bile pigments (bilirubin) in the amniotic fluid. Thus it can be determined if the fetus is mildly, moderately, or severely affected.

Amniocentesis is a valuable diagnostic aid in Rh sensitization and is carried out when the expectant mother is in the third trimester of pregnancy. It is also being used to diagnose the presence of genetic abnormalities for such conditions as Mongolism, Tay-Sachs disease, and maple syrup urine disease. Amniotic fluid may be used for cytologic studies, chemical analysis, or enzyme assays.* When there is a reason to suspect that the fetus may have a genetic defect, a sample of amniotic fluid can be obtained about the 12th or 14th week of gestation. If a positive diagnosis is made the couple may decide that a therapeutic abortion is the best alternative for them. Thus, the implications of amniocentesis are far-reaching—not only in the diagnosis of Rh incompatibility but also in detection of babies with a variety of genetic disorders. However, at present there is a very limited number of centers in the United States which can do the complicated analysis of the amniotic fluid to diagnose genetic defects.

Intrauterine Fetal Transfusion

If spectrophotometric analysis of the amniotic fluid shows that the fetus is severely affected, then what? How far along

---

*Nitowsky, H.: Prenatal diagnosis of genetic abnormality, Am. J. Nurs., 71:1551, 1971.

the woman is in her pregnancy will determine the method of treatment. If she is past 32 weeks gestation, the attending physician will decide to deliver the baby, either by inducing labor or by cesarean section. The best treatment is to get the baby out of the uterus which is a hostile environment, as quickly as possible. Even though the baby is small, it is better to have it alive. After delivery, the baby is turned over to a pediatrician and will need to have exchange blood transfusions.

If the woman is under 32 weeks gestation a dramatic procedure called an intrauterine fetal transfusion may be her only hope of having a live baby. Developed in 1963 by Dr. William Liley, intrauterine transfusion is the injection of whole Rh negative blood into the peritoneal cavity of the fetus. There the blood is absorbed to combat the anemia. It is a very difficult procedure to perform because the fetus is small, and may jump out of the way when he feels the thrust of the needle. There is a danger of injecting the blood in the wrong spot and killing the infant. The mother should definitely be told all the hazards and risks involved and that it is likely to be an emotionally traumatic experience for her. However, if she desires to have a live baby (and has had several stillborn infants), and if the skilled physician and necessary facilities are available, she is usually quite willing to give her consent to the transfusions. Intrauterine transfusions must be repeated every 10 to 14 days until the fetus reaches a large enough size to be delivered. Although they are not done very frequently because of the hazards and difficulties in doing them, the procedure has about a 50% survival rate. It is truly marvelous to see even one woman carry home a live baby with her that she otherwise would have lost.

What is Rhogam? (Rh Immunoglobulin)

The most exciting recent development in the *prevention* of Rh isoimmunization is a specially prepared gamma globulin which contains a concentration of Rh antibodies. Unfortunately, prevention is only possible for mothers who do not have antibodies (have not been previously sensitized). These antibodies combine with the Rh antigen and neutralize it. Thus the mother's bloodstream is cleared of the Rh positive cells which might have caused sensitization. A single injection of Rhogam provides protection for the next pregnancy and must be given within 72 hours after delivery.

The use of Rhogam on all patients who are candidates for it offers the hope of eliminating hemolytic disease caused by the Rh factor. The criteria for giving Rhogam are: the mother must be Rh negative; the baby must be Rh positive; and the direct Coombs' test, a test for antibodies done on the cord blood at the time of delivery, is weakly reactive or negative. Although Rhogam is expensive, the cost is considerably less than the risk of having a sick baby who requires special care and exchange blood transfusions.

Care of the Infant with Erythroblastosis Fetalis

Infants with known incompatibility to the mother's blood are examined carefully at birth for pallor, edema, jaundice, enlarged spleen and liver. A severely affected infant may be stillborn or have *hydrops fetalis* in which there is extensive edema, marked anemia and jaundice, and enlargement of the liver and spleen. These babies are in critical condition and will need exchange transfusions at the earliest possible moment.

The fetus of an Rh negative mother is usually checked during gestation by frequent examination of the amniotic fluid. When a rising bilirubin titer is indicated, labor may be induced and an exchange transfusion made ready for use as soon as possible after birth.

The severely affected infants who survive without treatment run the risk of severe brain damage, called *kernicterus*. Symptoms appear after about the third day of life. At first these include lethargy, poor muscle tone and poor sucking. These may be followed by spasticity and convulsions. Death occurs in about 75% of infants with kernicterus; those who survive may be mentally retarded or develop spastic paralysis or nerve deafness. Exchange transfusions are given at once to those infants who have signs of neurological damage when first seen, although there is no proof that the damage can be reversed. Fortunately, present day ability to detect and treat this hemolytic disease before brain damage occurs has reduced the number of infants who become permanently damaged.

A severely affected, very sick infant at birth will usually be transfused without waiting for laboratory confirmation. All other suspected infants will have a sample of cord blood sent to the laboratory for a Coombs' test for the presence of damaging antibodies, Rh and ABO typing, hemoglobin and red cell level, and measurement of plasma bilirubin. A positive direct Coombs' test indicates the presence of antibodies on the surface of the infant's red blood cells. A negative direct Coombs' test indicates that there are no antibodies on the infant's red blood cells.

Treatment

A positive Coombs' test indicates presence of the disease but not the degree of severity. If bilirubin and hemoglobin are within normal limits, the infant will be watched carefully; frequent laboratory blood tests will be done. Hemoglobin below the level of 10.5/100 mg., or a rising bilirubin will be an indication for an exchange transfusion.

Exchange transfusions. Exchange transfusions require elaborate preparations and are time-consuming. The infant may be cared for in the intensive care unit, and will receive his transfusions there. It is important that the infant be kept in a warm environment at about 75° to 80°F. A servocontrolled radiant heat unit may be used for this purpose. Resuscitative equipment must be readily available: intubation equipment, laryngoscope, means for providing endotracheal suction, oxygen and resuscitative drugs. An exchange transfusion tray will contain the needles and instruments necessary for the transfusion. Disposable sets are available.*

Procedure. Feedings are omitted for 3 to 4 hours before the transfusion to avoid the risk of vomiting and possible aspiration. A polyethylene catheter is cannulated into the umbilical vein with strict aseptic technique. A sterile syringe is attached and about 10 to 20 mg. of blood is withdrawn, and replaced with a like amount of fresh Rh negative blood. This procedure is continued until approximately 500 ml. of blood has been withdrawn and replaced.

An assistant experienced in assessing newborn heart rate and condition, and familiar with resuscitation techniques, should be present. He gives oxygen if necessary, keeps the infant's airway clear, and is capable of giving resuscitation if needed. Following the transfusion, blood hemoglobin and serum bilirubin levels are measured every 8 to 10 hours. Repeat exchanges are given as indicated.

Nursing Care. After an exchange transfusion the infant is carefully observed for signs of shock or other reactions. Temperature, pulse and respirations are recorded routinely. He may be fed about 1 hour after the transfusion, or 6 hours after birth. If he is not too severely ill, he may be breast-fed by his mother then returned to his incubator. These babies need to be kept well hydrated. Intravenous feedings may be needed if the baby is premature.

Whenever the birth of a baby with erythroblastosis is anticipated, an incubator with a source of oxygen should be readied. These infants are lethargic and weak and need frequent changes of position. A careful watch must be kept for signs of impending kernicterus, such as loss of Moro reflex and decreased responsiveness.

Any infant admitted to the newborn nursery should be examined for jaundice during the first 36 hours. The nurse must keep in mind that early development of jaundice is a probable indication of erythroblastosis.

*Pharmaseal Products.

Infants who have been adequately treated, their bilirubin restored to normal levels, may be removed from their incubators to regular bassinets and returned to nursery routine. They are discharged to routine home care, just as any well newborn.

ABO INCOMPATIBILITY

A similar condition which is not as severe as the Rh incompatibility may result when a man with either type A or B blood marries a woman with type O blood. A or B are both dominant over type O, and it results in an ABO incompatibility in the infant. The infant develops jaundice after birth but responds better to conservative treatment, such as placing him under a bilirubin light. He is less likely to require exchange blood transfusions.

Hydrops fetalis is extremely rare. The jaundice can, however, become severe and kernicterus develop. Care and treatment are the same as for Rh incompatibility.

RESPIRATORY CONDITIONS

Anoxia is a condition which occurs in various respiratory difficulties of the newborn. It may occur before birth or as a result of difficult birth. At birth the infant is limp and unresponsive and has difficulty establishing respirations (See Chap 11). Mouth to mouth respiration may be necessary.

Method of Mouth-to-Mouth Breathing†.
1. Clear the patient's airway with a finger.
2. Tilt the patient's head back, and pull his jaw forward. Make certain that his tongue does not fall back and obstruct his breathing.
3. (For an infant.) Place your wide open mouth over the infant's nose and his mouth. Blow puffs of air from your *mouth only.*
4. Move your head back, and allow the patient to exhale.
5. Repeat step 3. Breathe rhythmically, approximately 16 to 20 times per minute.
6. Continue until the physician arrives and gives further instruction.

†As advocated by the Red Cross.

Atelectasis. This term indicates that the lungs are collapsed and there is no air exchange. This may be a primary condition due to failure of the lung to expand properly at birth or it may be a secondary condition due to collapse of the alveoli after expansion (See Chap. 11).

Clinical Manifestations. Small areas of atelectasis may cause no observable symptoms. Moderate degrees of atelectasis may cause mild cyanosis and little more. Extensive lung collapse causes cyanosis, labored breathing, grunting respirations and eventual exhaustion.

Treatment. The infant will need continuous observation, preferably in the intensive care unit. Humidified air and oxygen are provided. The infant will do best in an Isolette. The infant should be handled as little as possible, but he needs his position changed frequently.

Aspiration of gastric contents may be done to prevent aspiration of vomitus. Feedings should be given slowly and carefully, or feedings by gavage may be ordered to avoid undue fatigue. Although atelectasis is found in the full-term infant, it appears much more frequently in those infants born prematurely.

BIBLIOGRAPHY

Blake, F. J.: Nursing Care of Children. ed. 8. Philadelphia, J. B. Lippincott, 1970.

Bowman, J. M. and Friesen, R. F.: Hemolytic disease of the newborn. *In :* Gellis, S. S. and Kagan, B. M. (eds.): Current Pediatric Therapy. Philadelphia, W. B. Saunders, 1970.

Fitzpatrick, E. *et al.:* Maternity Nursing. ed. 12. Philadelphia, J. B. Lippincott, 1971.

Johnson, W. and Morgan, C: Management of Rh disease. Hospital Topics, 47:97, 1967.

Nitowsky, H.: Prenatal diagnosis of genetic abnormality. AJN, 71:1551, 1971.

Potter, E.: Pathology of erythroblastosis. Clinical Obstetrics and Gynecology, 7:1027, 1964.

Queenan, J.: Intrauterine transfusion for erythroblastosis fetalis. AJN, 65:62, August 1965.

Rh hemolytic disease of the newborn. Nursing Currents, 21:2, 1972.

Suggested Readings for Further Study

Boggs, T.: Proper place of intrauterine transfusions in management of fetuses with Rh hemolytic disease. Clinical Pediatrics, 9:636, 1970.

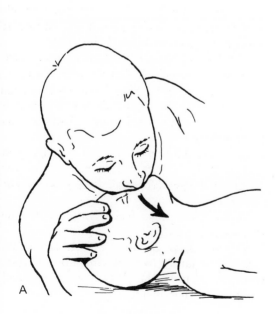
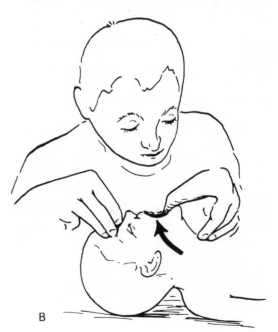

Figure 21-2. An infant receiving mouth-to-mouth resuscitation.

Dekaban, A. S.; and Kappy, M. S.: Late form of congenital rubella syndrome—thoughts on pathogenesis. Clinical Proceedings of the Children's Hospital of Washington, D.C., *26:*152, 1970.

Friendly, D. S.: Gonococcal conjunctivitis of the newborn. Clinical Proceedings of the Children's Hospital of Washington, D.C., *25:*1, 1969.

Glynn, E.: Nursing support during intrauterine transfusions. AJN, *65:*68, August 1965.

Kalayoglu, M. *et al.:* Meconium ileus: a critical review of treatment and eventual progress. J. of Ped. Surg., *6:*290, 1971.

Overall, James C. and Glascow, Lowell A.: Virus Infections of the Fetus and Newborn, Journal of Pediatrics, *77:*315, 1970.

Birth Injuries and Congenital Orthopedic Conditions

22

INTRACRANIAL HEMORRHAGE

Intracranial injury is usually the result of trauma during birth. Trauma with intracranial hemorrhage is particularly likely in difficult deliveries where the head is large in proportion to the size of the mother's pelvic outlet. Brain trauma is more likely to occur in precipitate delivery or difficult breech delivery than when the head can gradually mold in slowly progressing labor. Prolonged, hard labors may also be a cause, and skilled, judicious use of forceps may decrease the incidence of brain damage.

Clinical Manifestations

The newborn infant may be difficult to arouse, and the Moro reflex is diminished or absent. Respirations may be irregular and slow. Periods of apnea, cyanosis, failure to suck well, high-pitched shrill cry, muscular twitchings, and convulsions are all symptomatic. In mild case of hemorrhage, signs may be limited to listlessness, poor appetite and occasional vomiting. Diagnosis is based mainly on history of delivery and the clinical signs.

Treatment

The infant should be handled gently and disturbed as little as possible. He should be placed in an incubator where temperature can be regulated and oxygen supplied as needed. Continuous observation is essential; therefore, he is best cared for in the intensive care nursery. An anticonvulsive drug, such as phenobarbital, may be ordered, and Vitamin K may be given to minimize

bleeding. Sometimes cranial pressure is relieved by spinal or dural taps.

Prognosis

This is largely dependent on the severity of the condition. Death may result within the first 3 days due to respiratory failure. In the surviving infants, recovery may be complete, or such conditions as cerebral palsy or mental retardation may result.

Prevention

The best preventive measure is the use of skillful and judicious obstetrical management. Many cases of intracranial hemorrhage are avoidable.

FRACTURES OCCURRING DURING DELIVERY

Fracture of the clavicle. This is the most common form of fracture in difficult delivery. It may occur when there is difficulty in delivering the infant's shoulder. No special treatment is needed beyond a possible temporary immobilization of the arm and shoulder on the affected side. Healing occurs in a few days.

Fractures of the humerus or femur are treated with immobilization or traction. Complete healing results with good callus formation.

PERIPHERAL NERVE INJURIES

Brachial Palsy. This is a partial paralysis of one arm due to excessive stretching of the nerve fibers that run from the neck through the shoulder. It occurs when traction

303

exerted on the head during delivery of the shoulder.

In mild cases spontaneous recovery occurs within a few weeks. In cases where injury to the nerve fibers is more severe, permanent damage may result. Treatment consists in relaxation of the paralyzed muscles. This may be accomplished by the use of a clove-hitch restraint attached to the head of the crib so that the arm is abducted and rotated externally, with the elbow flexed. Later an airplane splint may be used to hold the arm in proper position, and physical therapy used. If recovery does not occur, neurosurgery may offer partial recovery.

Forceps Marks. The use of forceps generally leaves marks on the infants face. Although these may be alarming to the mother, they are only skin bruises and disappear in a few days.

CONGENITAL ORTHOPEDIC CONDITIONS

Infants with congenital orthopedic defects usually receive primary treatment on the general pediatric ward, and thus the

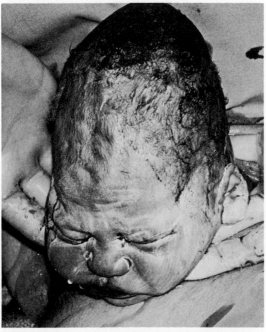

Figure 22-1. Forceps marks are visible on the newborn.

nurse should be aware of the nature and treatment of these abnormalities. The two most common and important are clubfoot and dislocation of the hip.

Congenital Talipes Equinovarus

Congenital clubfoot is a deformity in which the entire foot is inverted, the heel is drawn up, and the forefoot is adducted. The Latin *talus*, meaning ankle, and *pes*, meaning foot, make up our word talipes, and is used in connection with many foot deformities. Equinus, or plantar flexion, and varus, or inversion, denote the kind of foot deformity present in this condition. The equinovarus foot has a clublike appearance, hence the term clubfoot. (Fig. 22-2)

Congenital talipes equinovarus is the most common congenital foot deformity, appearing as a single anomaly, or in connection with other defects, such as myelomeningocele. It may be bilateral or unilateral. Etiology is not clear; an hereditary factor is occasionally observed. A theory that receives some acceptance postulates an arrested growth of the germ plasm of the foot during the first trimester of pregnancy.

Detection During the Neonatal Period

Talipes equinovarus is easily detected in a newborn infant but must be differentiated from a persisting fetal "position of comfort" assumed in utero. The positional deformity can be easily corrected by the use of passive exercise, but the true clubfoot deformity is fixed. The positional deformity should be explained to the parents at once to prevent anxiety.

Nonsurgical Correction

If treatment is started during the neonatal period, correction can usually be accomplished by manipulation and bandaging, or by application of a cast. While the cast is being applied, the foot is first gently moved into as near normal position as possible. Force should not be used. If the infant's mother can be present to help hold him while the cast is being applied, she will

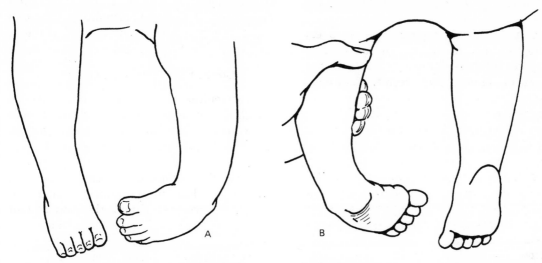

Figure 22-2.   Unilateral clubfoot; *(A)* front view, *(B)* back view.

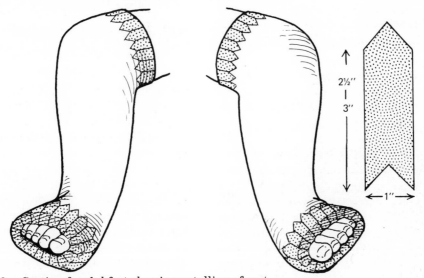

Figure 22-3.   Casting for clubfoot showing petalling of cast.

have the opportunity to understand what is being done. The very young infant gets his satisfaction from sucking, therefore a bottle of glucose water or formula will engage his attention and help prevent squirming while the cast is being applied.

The cast is applied over the foot and ankle (and usually to mid-thigh) to hold the knee in right angle flexion. (Fig. 22-3) Casts are changed frequently to provide gradual, nontraumatic correction. Treatment is continued until complete correction is confirmed by x-ray and clinical observation, usually in a matter of months.

Any cast applied to a child's body should have some type of waterproof material protecting the skin from the sharp plaster edges of the cast. One method is to apply strips of adhesive vertically around the edges of the cast in a manner called petaling. This is done by cutting strips of adhesive 2 to 3 inches long and 1 inch wide. One end is notched and the other end cut pointed to enable smooth application.

An alternative method involves the use of a Denis Browne splint. The splint is composed of a flexible, horizontal metal bar attached to two foot plates. The child's foot is attached to the foot plate with adhesive tape, and the attachment of the horizontal bar permits changing the relationship of the bar to the plate as necessary. This splint must be used for a period of time, as long as seven or eight months, until a wide over-correction is attained. (Fig. 22-4)

Following correction from a cast or a splint, a Denis Browne splint with shoes attached is used to maintain correction for another six months or so. After over-correction has been attained, a special clubfoot shoe should be worn—a laced shoe with a turning out of the shoe and the outer wedge of the sole. The Denis Browne splint may still be worn at night, and passive exercises of the foot should be carried out by the child's mother.

Surgical Correction

Children who do not respond to non-surgical measures, especially older children, need surgical correction. This involves several procedures dependent both upon the age of the child and upon the degree of the deformity. It may involve lengthening of the Achilles tendon, capsulotomy of the ankle joint, release of medial structures, and, for the child over ten years of age, an operation on the bony structure. Prolonged ob-servation, after correction by either means, should be carried out at least until adoles-cence; any recurrence is treated promptly.

If a Denis Browne splint is used instead of a cast, check the foot for irritation from adhesive tape, for swelling or for any other indication of circulation impairment from the tight strapping. Check frequently the position of the foot on the foot plate. These splints are uncomfortable until the infant becomes accustomed to them. He cannot kick the way he is accustomed to; in fact there is less freedom of movement than when casts are used. These babies have a special need for comforting and being held.

Nursing Care Following Surgery

Check vital signs until they are stable.
Observe the cast for signs of bleeding.
Elevate the affected leg.
Observe circulation and temperature of the toes.
Be alert for any signs of infection.

Nursing Care in the Hospital

The infant or small child in a cast cannot explain to his nurses that his cast is too tight, impairing circulation, or is irritating his skin. Nursing observation should include the following:

Check the color and the temperature of the toes at frequent intervals. Check ex-cessive irritability—indicating acute dis-comfort—with the attending physician.

Prevent the child from banging and denting his cast before it is dry. A clove-hitch restraint may be necessary.

Petal edges of the cast, when dry, with adhesive to prevent skin irritation.

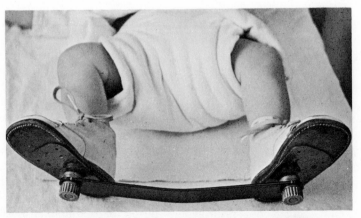

Figure 22-4. A Denis Browne splint with shoes attached.

Hold and comfort the child when possible. Better still, if his mother or father are present they can do this.

Home Care

If the mother has helped with the hospital care, her baby is going to be much better served when he goes home. His mother must continue to watch for skin irritation and for signs of pressure from a cast that has become too tight. She must be prompt for any appointments, and also understand the importance of notifying the physician or the clinic whenever the cast needs attention or if the splint appears to have slipped. The family must also be prepared to give additional emotional support until the infant becomes accustomed to the splint or cast.

Congenital Dislocation of the Hip

A defective development of the acetabulum, with or without dislocation, may be present in the newborn infant. The malformed acetabulum permits dislocation, the head of the femur becoming displaced upward and backward. The condition is difficult to recognize during early infancy. When there is family history of the defect, increased observation of the young infant is indicated. The condition is approximately seven times more common in girls than in boys and is frequently bilateral.

Diagnosis

Early recognition and treatment, before an infant starts to stand or walk, is extremely important for successful correction. Early signs include the following.

Asymmetry of the gluteal skin folds (they are higher on the affected side).

Limitation of abduction of affected hip. This is tested by placing infant on his back with his knees flexed and then abducting both knees passively until they reach the examination table without resistance. If dislocation is present, the affected side cannot be abducted beyond 45°. Sometimes a clicking sound may be elicited as the head of the femur slips over the rim of the acetabulum.

Later signs, after the child has started walking, include: lordosis, sway-back, protruding abdomen, shortened extremity, duck-waddle gait, positive Trendelenburg sign. To elicit this sign, the child stands on his affected leg and raises his normal leg. The pelvis tilts downward rather than upward toward the unaffected side.

Roentgen studies are usually made to confirm the diagnosis. Uncorrected

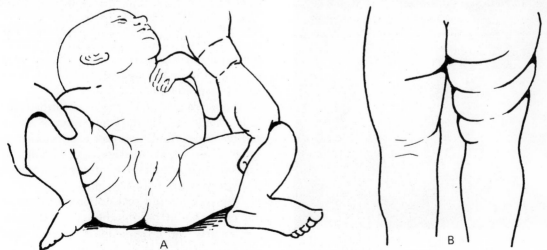

Figure 22-5. In congenital hip dislocation there is limitation of abduction of the affected leg (*A*) and asymmetry of skin folds of the thighs (*B*).

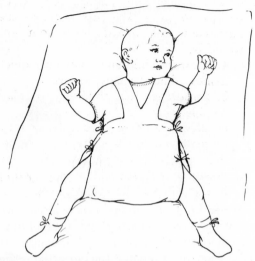

Figure 22-6. The Frejka splint is used to correct congenital dislocation of the hip.

dislocation causes limping, easy fatigue, hip and low back discomfort, and postural deformities.

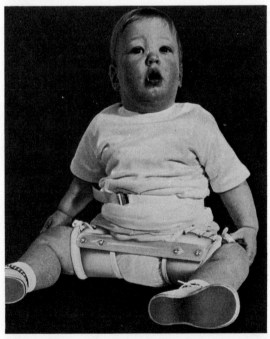

Figure 22-7. The Camp plastic abduction splint may be used with the child having congenital hip dislocation. (Courtesy S. H. Camp and Co.)

Treatment

When the dislocation is discovered during the first few months, treatment consists of manipulation of the femur into position and application of a spica cast or brace. If treatment is delayed until after the child has commenced to walk, open reduction followed by a spica cast is usually needed. After the cast is removed, a metal or plastic brace is applied to keep the legs in wide abduction.

It is important that the legs be kept in the proper position. The Frejka splint is a kind of harness attached to a pillow that holds the legs wide apart. It is applied over the diaper, so much care is needed to keep the baby's legs in position while diapers are being changed.

A metal or plastic splint is applied after the cast has been removed. A newer product made of lightweight nontoxic polyethylene plastic has foam padded edges and laced cuffs.* The splint is moistureproof, sanitary, well ventilated and can be fitted over or under the diaper. (Fig. 22-7)

The child in a cast needs careful observation of circulation, attention to his skin, and comfortable positioning. A hard mattress is needed, with pillows for positioning while the cast is drying. Complaints of pain should be heeded and reported. The cast, which extends from the upper abdomen to the toes, should be petaled with adhesive around the waist and the toes with a plastic sheet tucked under the cut-out pubic area and taped over the cast for protection from soiling and wetting.

If open reduction has been performed, the child should be watched for signs of shock and bleeding; fluids and diet are resumed as usual. The edges of the cast should be petaled with adhesive or otherwise covered to avoid irritation to the skin.

The skin around and under the edges of the cast should be watched for irritation, particularly for crumbs of plaster or food

---

*Camp Plastic Abduction Splint.

that may fall under the cast. The child may stuff a small toy or some food that he is supposed to have eaten, into the cast. The cast around the perineal area should be inspected daily for dampness or soiling, and the waterproof material washed, dried and reapplied as needed.

The child may be held after the cast is dry; with a frog-leg cast he can sit on the nurse's lap, particularly for his meals. In bed he must be turned frequently and should be taken to the playroom or perhaps on rides about the hospital on a stretcher for diversion. Parents need to learn the proper home care—learning most easily acquired through participation in the child's care before discharge.

BIBLIOGRAPHY

Raffensperger, John G., and Primrose, Rosellen, Bohlen (eds.): Pediatric Surgery for Nurses. Boston, Little, Brown, 1968.

UNIT STUDY QUESTIONS

1. The following reflexes are normal in the newborn:
    a. Moro and tonic neck reflexes
    b. grasp and stepping reflexes
    c. rooting reflex
    d. sucking reflex
    The answer is:
        1. a, b, and d
        2. b, c, and d
        3. a, b, and c
        4. all of them

2. Demand feeding has come into favor for the following reasons:
    a. frequent feedings allow the infant to be better nourished.
    b. all babies need to be fed more often than every 4 hours.
    c. the mother doesn't have to waken the baby to keep him on schedule.
    d. demand feedings for a healthy baby will best fit his individual needs.

3. Mrs. Jones has three children at home, ages 6, 4, and 2, and she is afraid they will make too much noise and the baby won't be able to sleep. The best response the nurse could make to Mrs. Jones' comment would be:
    a. allow the children to play only quiet games while the baby sleeps.
    b. encourage the children to play outside while the baby sleeps.
    c. allow the children to play as they normally would while the baby sleeps.
    d. encourage the children to play noisily so the baby will become used to it and will still be able to sleep.

4. When a nursery nurse observes a newborn with jaundiced skin during his first 3 days of life, she should:
    a. accept this as physiological jaundice and make a note on his chart.
    b. realize that jaundice in the first 2 or 3 days of life is not normal, and alert the physician.
    c. tell the mother her baby is jaundiced, and ask her if she is Rh negative.
    d. put the baby under an ultraviolet lamp.

5. How should an infant born of a mother who had rubella in the first trimester of pregnancy be treated?
    a. placed in the nursery and treated as any other infant because he will not harbor rubella virus after birth
    b. be given rubella vaccine to prevent the disease
    c. be examined carefully for any defects resulting from virus having crossed the placental barrier
    d. kept away from susceptible people until his blood can be cultured for virus, because he may shed virus even though he has no observable defects.
    The answer is:
        1. a and c
        2. b and d
        3. c and d
        4. b and c

6. A meningocele is a:
    a. defect in the vertebra.

b. malformation of the occipitocervial region.

c. protrusion of meninges through a defect in the spinal column.

d. protrusion of meninges and spinal cord through a defect in the spinal column.

7. The *goal* of *surgery* on infants with myelomeningocele is:

a. removal of a cosmetically unac-cepted deformity.

b. closure of a surface defect while preserving all functioning nervous tissue.

c. prevention of infection of the sac to avoid the underlying cause of hydrocephalus.

d. restoration of normal circulation in cerebral spinal fluid.

8. Baby Brown has an order to be fed 6 hours after delivery. The nursery nurse notices that he has excessive mucus, drooling and choking. Which course of action should she follow?

a. suction him, and try feeding as ordered.

b. suction him, and give him some sterile water to clear away the mucus.

c. suction him, and try passing a gastric tube.

d. suction him, withhold any oral feeding, and notify the physician.

9. One congenital anomaly that may have serious consequences if not discovered is an imperforate anus. To avoid overlooking such a defect, the nurse should:

a. take a rectal temperature.

b. insert a small gauge rectal tube.

c. check to see if an anal dimple is present.

d. watch for passage of a normal meconium stool within the first 24 hours.

Unit Six: The Child in the Hospital

Supportive Nursing Care 23

ADMISSION PROCEDURES

No one questions that a sick child comes to the hospital to be healed of his physical illness, if that is possible, or that the task of the nurse is to help in that process. It is equally true that we, as nurses, cannot function adequately in that capacity unless we understand the child's emotional needs—according to his age level, and in relation to him as an individual. This understanding is of considerable importance, for we know that healing takes place most readily in a positive, accepting environment. Security, acceptance and warm human relationships are the most potent of all medicines.

The fact still remains, however, that the child has come to be treated for his physical disability, with the goal seen clearly as a return to his family. We must not neglect the physical care while offering emotional support. In actual practice, it is difficult to give one without giving the other; certainly emotional support may be manifested through the kind of physical care the nurse gives.

The nurse has learned that in order to give good nursing care, she must see the child as a person in his own right, as well as a member of his family. This means many things. It means that she should know certain things about him before she enters his room. She should know his name, his nickname, and his age. She needs to know the special words he uses to make his needs and his desires understood. It is helpful to know something about his family, whether he is an only child, or whether he is the oldest, youngest, or in-between, and whether

both parents are living with him at home. This kind of information changes the "patient in for eye surgery" to "Bobby, a 4-year-old boy."

In most children's departments, the parents are asked to fill out a form giving this information on admission. It may also include items pertinent to the child's age: if a toddler, information concerning toilet training, "security blanket" or favorite cuddly toy, ability to feed self, and similar things. This sheet is then placed on the child's chart, with necessary items copied onto the Kardex file.

One cannot explain hospitalization to an infant or reassure him in words about the forthcoming experience. His best reassurance is the familiar presence of his mother through the entire procedure. She can undress him, take his temperature if she has done this before, and hold him throughout all the strange and potentially frightening admission procedures. She is his only security, his only tie to the familiar. He must not be expected to let this go, to face the unknown alone.

After an infant is admitted, the mother should be encouraged to stay with him and continue to do those ordinary things for him she would do at home, if this does not mean neglecting the rest of the family. The very young infant has not learned to differentiate his mother from others who care for him. He can rather quickly learn to relate to someone who offers him the same quality of loving interaction. The mother of such an infant needs to have her emotional health considered, however. If being with her young infant during his illness is important to her

311

(and it usually is) she should not be denied this.

Older infants and toddlers suffer most severely through hospitalization and separation from familiar environments. This has been demonstrated by Bowlby, Robertson and others.

The Toddler in the Hospital

When the toddler enters the hospital, he brings his own developmental patterns with him. If he is a normal child, he will show negativism and dependence as well as independence. In addition to this, his physical development is at the stage when his muscles must be used actively. All this makes this age a difficult period for hospitalization.

The hospital is an institution set up primarily for the treatment and the healing of the sick. At its best, it can never provide an adequate environment for a developing child. It cannot take the place of a child's home, even when that itself is far from ideal.

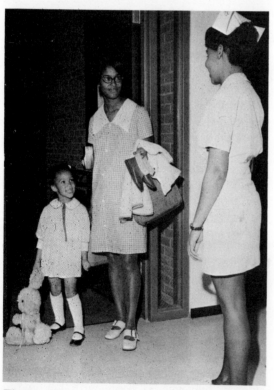

Figure 23-1. A nurse greets the child on admission.

At home, he gets recognition as a person, and personal attention from his mother or someone in her place.

A Representative Two-Year-Old is Admitted

J. is a normal two-year-old about to be taken to the hospital for admission. He knows what a doctor and nurse are through his experience in well child or pediatric clinic, or the pediatrician's office.

J. has had a warm, close relationship with his mother. He may have attended nursery school for short periods. He almost certainly has had experience with a babysitter, but he has never been away from home overnight. His growing sense of independence and self-reliance are possible only because they are firmly rooted in a comfortable sense of security. His mother—his source of strength—is never far away.

When J. enters the hospital he comes along cheerfully enough with the nurse, chattering and smiling—and holding his mother's hand. He is undoubtedly also clutching his favorite toy.

Now he is undressed, put in a crib; perhaps his mother is asked to go to the resident's office to give his history. Meanwhile, he has a rectal temperature taken, is weighed, examined, perhaps has blood drawn. By the time his mother returns he is screaming with terror, and the stage is set for an unpleasant hospital experience. Unfortunately, in too many children's departments, the child's fright is compounded by sending his mother home with the assurance that J. will adjust better if she is not here. Yes, indeed, this sort of admission still happens.

J. has entered the hospital with considerable confidence. The building is big and strange, the elevator ride perhaps a new sensation. However, his feet are firmly planted in the old and the familiar. His stuffed animal, his shoes, his clothes, and most of all, his mother, are all part of his security. Now all of that security has been removed. Is it any wonder that he is frightened?

J's trust and security can be maintained when some thought is given to what this experience means to a small child. A more insightful and thoughtful routine is here outlined.

1. The nurse meets mother and child in the admitting room and introduces herself. She makes no effort to come between the child and his mother, nor to be overfamiliar. She understands a small child's initial distrust of strangers.

2. On the children's department she takes the child and his mother to his room or place on the ward. She points out the toys and leaves mother and child together to adjust for a short while.

3. The child's mother undresses him, while the nurse stands by, observing his condition and noting anything significant. If the child is to be weighed and measured she does this with the mother's assistance.

4. If an admission temperature is desired, the mother takes this if she knows how, otherwise she holds and comforts him while it is being taken.

5. After this activity quiets down, the child can be given toys to play with, while the nurse talks with the mother. The mother is encouraged to talk freely about her child's condition, as well as about any problems troubling her.

6. It is important for the child's adjustment that those caring for him know as much as possible about his normal routine. What is he called? What words is he familiar with for toileting, as well as for other routines? What does he eat, how many naps is he used to—anything that will be helpful in keeping to his normal schedule as nearly as possible.

7. The nurse shows the mother where her child can keep his possessions, where the toilet is (if he is toilet trained), or where the clean diapers and other supplies are kept. If a urine specimen is needed, the mother is given a container and told anything necessary so that she may be the one to obtain the specimen. A child just learning toilet control experiences con-

siderable difficulty urinating in a strange place with strange people. The nurse shows the mother the playroom and lets her use her own judgment as to when the small child is ready to play there. If the mother cannot stay with the child overnight, the parents are encouraged to get him ready for bed and stay beside him until he falls asleep.

Little children are very possessive about some articles of their own clothing, especially their shoes. Some actually seem to feel that their shoes are an integral part of themselves. One little boy wore his shoes to bed, and another stamped manfully to his bath in his bathrobe and cowboy boots. A bathrobe and a pair of slippers left with the child are comforting if in plain sight. His own pajamas are a big link with home. All of these articles give him a feeling that he has not been abandoned in a strange new place. If the mother must leave, she should be encouraged to leave some personal

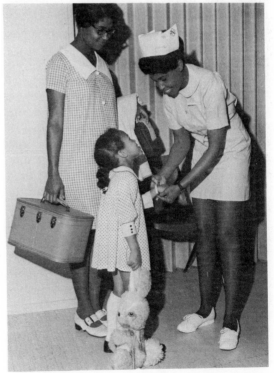

Figure 23-2. The child gets an identification bracelet.

possession of her own with her child for the same reason.

When a Mother Stays with Her Child

A mother should be allowed to stay with her child as long as she wishes. She should be allowed to stay in the room to comfort and sustain him while he has treatments. She should accompany him to x-ray, physiotherapy or other specialized treatment areas. Routines can be adjusted to allow her as far as the door of surgery and into the recovery room. Intensive care nursery personnel are beginning to understand the need of premature babies and their mothers for personal contact. Surely this need is as great for the young child.

Whether the mother remains with her young child throughout his hospital stay or only during the daytime hours, some planning for the rest of the family is necessary. If this is a planned admission, arrangements for the care of the children at home will have to be made. Relatives, friends, neighbors may help out. A babysitter or a homemaker may be available.

A nursery school may provide temporary care. In the United States, a number of hospitals provide day care for the children of their employees.* Some of these will accept other children also, particularly the children of patients. This service could be extended to day care for brothers and sisters of a sick child, if the facility is large enough and adequately staffed.

The small child may enter the hospital well prepared for the experience. Perhaps he has a need for some corrective surgery that has been postponed until he has grown some more and until his capacity for understanding was greater. Now he needs this surgery, either to make him look like others, or to improve his health, or to avoid unnecessary absences from school later.

Although these children have had ample time for adequate preparation for the hos-

---

*Child Care Services Provided by Hospitals. Women's Bureau, U.S. Department of Labor, Washington, D.C. Bulletin 295, 1970.

pital experience, many others do not have this opportunity. The toddler and the preschooler are frequently victims of their own curiosity. Most cases of poisoning occur in children under the age of five years. Accidents also bring many children into the hospital, including that most dreaded of all accidents, severe burns.

When the preschool child moves out into the larger world and enters into neighborhood activities, he encounters several risks to his health and well-being. His lack of experience leads him to take risks that frequently cause painful accidents. He is exposed to the common childhood diseases, and is quite susceptible to infections. One of these experiences may bring him to the hospital.

The child who enters the hospital in a routine manner has had advantages that the child who comes in on an emergency basis cannot have. There has been ample opportunity to prepare the non-emergency child for this experience. Many pediatricians carefully explain hospitalization to the child, but the responsibility for adequate preparation rests with his parents.

Parents, however, are not always too well informed about hospital procedures. Rumors and tales are spread around about misunderstood hospital experiences, causing anxiety among those whose task it is to reassure the child. A mother is poorly equipped to handle a situation about which she herself has serious misgivings. Her words may *sound* confident, but the child senses the uncertainty behind them. Such a situation occurred when four-year-old James was being prepared for tonsillectomy. He had been cheerful and pleasant since admission, but when the nurse prepared to give him his preoperative medication he went into panic. No one, including his mother, could calm him. He was a husky boy, and he put up a truly remarkable resistance. He fought and kicked. His mother repeatedly remarked that she could not understand it, because she had told him exactly what would happen, and he had seemed to accept it well.

After a thoroughly frightened, exhausted little boy had gone to surgery, his mother showed her own anxiety in the following words: "I have been dreading this. Are you sure he's going to be all right? A little boy in our neighborhood just died from an operation like this, and I have been worried."

One can only imagine what bits of gossip and half-understood talk the child had heard. Unfortunately, no one on the staff knew or understood the cause of his fear. James returned in good condition and was later discharged, but the emotional trauma must have been considerable.

THE NURSE'S ROLE IN PREPARING A YOUNG CHILD FOR HOSPITAL EXPERIENCE

It is obvious that some children will need to be prepared for their new experience and that all children will profit from such preparation. Perhaps the first step is to acquaint the child with routines and give him an opportunity to become familiar with hospital apparatus. At the same time, it is most important to answer his questions and to clear up his fantasies of a dreaded experience.

Such a technique could be carried out using hand puppets. If a group of children are admitted at the same time for surgery, they could have a short period together with the nurse; an individual child could profit from this puppet play also.

The nurse can have a doctor or nurse puppet on her hand, while the child wears a boy or girl puppet. A dialogue can be worked out so that the child is able to tell what he knows and voice any concern that he may have. The nurse can reinforce any teaching that the child has received, straighten out misunderstandings and generally put the child more at ease. It is much easier to put ideas into the mouth of a puppet than to voice them as your own, and the puppet can ask questions that the child may shrink from asking as his own.

One precaution must be kept in mind. Too much preparation, with too much lingering over details, may frighten the child rather than reassure him. Letting the child participate in role-playing is a manner of providing him with an opportunity to bring out his own apprehensions, and to straighten things out in his own mind.

One group of students devised a plan that worked very well. They made a two-room hospital from a carton, papered it with shelf paper and furnished a ward and an operating room, using cardboard, pipe cleaners, paper cups, small containers, pictures, and plenty of imagination. Small dolls represented Johnny, his mother, the nurse and the doctor, with one or two patients for atmosphere. A nursing student acted out a trip to the hospital, making the doll-patient go through an admission and an entire stay. The entire play lasted about 20 minutes, and attention never wavered. In fact, there were always calls of "do it again."

An opportunity for the children to handle and try out stethoscopes, blood pressure

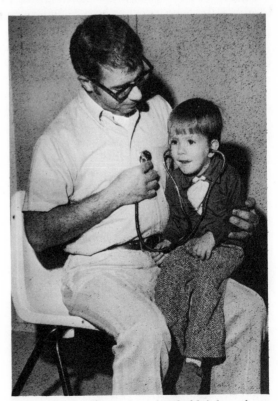

Figure 23-3. He can hear his daddy's heartbeat.

Relieving the Child's Anxiety

George was a child with an obsessive fear of needles. His one anxiety from admission onward concerned the injections he might receive. He did indeed receive an injection shortly after admission, and the nurse was unable to promise that he would not receive another in the morning.

At bedtime, George was missing. A thorough search did not reveal any George, and eventually the alarmed nurses were considering calling his mother, when someone noticed a slight shadow behind the ward door. George had been crouching there for nearly an hour, not making a sound, and quaking with fear.

In the morning, George asked incessantly, "I don't have to have a needle, do I?" As surgery was to be quite late, George was brought out to the nurse's station and was encouraged to draw pictures. One picture after another was rapidly drawn and pinned up on the bulletin board as a prized picture. Each time he asked the question "Do I have to have a needle?" the answer was a firm "Yes, George, you will have to have a needle before you go to surgery." Eventually, George accepted this fact enough to change his question to, "I will only have to have one, won't I?" When the time came to get ready for surgery, he went willingly enough, and although he could not find enough courage to hold still, he accepted the intramuscular medication without protest.

It is not only the openly terrified child, however, who is afraid. The child who is good, who makes no protest, is frequently as terrified, but is able to suppress his fears. This child may be facing a greater psychological emergency than the one who overtly (and loudly) expresses his distress.

---

cuffs and similar professional materials helps remove fear of the unknown. There are times, however, when just an understanding of procedures is not enough. A child's greatest need may be for support to help him face the inevitable.

Some children are admitted for diagnostic purposes. The convulsive child may come in for electroencephalograms, blood tests, and perhaps for more strenuous neurological tests. The child who has failed to grow properly may be tested for fibrocystic disease, or celiac disease. Perhaps the child has been admitted because of an exacerbation of a long-term illness.

These children may have been prepared for admission, but still find it very difficult to adjust to the necessary tests and procedures. Little can be done by way of explanation before admission. The nurse must play a supportive role during the unpleasant times.

Two little sisters were admitted for tests to determine the presence of fibrocystic disease. The six-year-old was permitted to stay in the same ward with her three-year-old sister to help her adjust. Both girls were subjected to the extremely uncomfortable duodenal drainage test for the presence of trypsin. At mid-morning they lay in their

beds "draining," while between the two beds, their nurse sat quietly reading to them, turning the book from time to time to show them the pictures.

This nurse showed her understanding of what nursing really means. The ward had not been tidied up, and the girls had not been bathed, but the nurse had been able to communicate her understanding and sympathy. Anyone coming into the ward could feel the confidence and trust they had in their nurse. She rightly understood that the other tasks were secondary to the main problem of providing support and understanding in time of stress.

Additional, much needed support is provided if the familiar nurse accompanies her patient when he has to leave the department for various diagnostic procedures or treatment. Any patient appreciates the presence of a familiar person when he encounters new and potentially frightening situations, but for the young person who cannot understand what is happening, a familiar person to comfort and—he reasons—to protect him, becomes an essential part of his nursing care. This kind of support is not always given the serious consideration it deserves, but it holds importance equal to any other essential procedure. Of course, in the ideal situation, the familiar person is mother—and why shouldn't she be? When free visiting hours are a reality, this usually can be accomplished.

In *The Widening World of Childhood*, the implications of injury and hospitalization to the small child are brought out with keen insight.* Three-year-old Sam, having lost the tip of his little finger in a slammed door, is helped through the subsequent hospital and surgical experience with the understanding support of his mother, his doctors and his nurses. Sam's reaction to separation from his mother during surgery and at the surgeon's office, his use of "Woody," an imaginary elf to take his mother's place, as well as the positive aspects of the experience, are brought out in a manner that provides guidance for the nurse which is probably unequaled elsewhere.

What about the child who comes into the hospital on an emergency basis? Jimmy found a peanut can in a cupboard under the sink. He hardly had time to sample the contents before his mother came and immediately began to act very strangely. He knew that he was not allowed to eat peanuts, but his mother acted as though he had committed some crime. She snatched the can away from him, spanked him, then grabbed him up and called the doctor. In no time at all, he was being sped to the hospital where more strange and terrifying things happened to him. His stomach was thoroughly washed out, a most uncomfortable procedure. He struggled manfully against this indignity, but many big hands held him firmly and his mother never did a thing to interfere. She must have been really angry.

The next thing he knew, he was undressed, taken on a sort of rolling bed up in the elevator and put to bed in broad daylight. People in white gowns and caps came with further indignities, needles to jab into him, unpleasant medications, jackets

---

*Murphy, L. B.: The Widening World of Childhood. Chap. 6, pp. 115—144. New York, Basic Books, 1962.

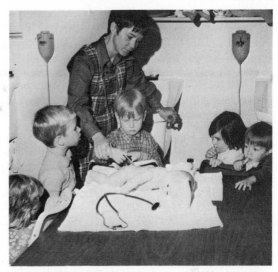

Figure 23-4. The children see how a rectal temperature is taken.

tied on to keep him in bed, strange food on trays, thermometers, stethoscopes, doctors who punched and probed. When would this nightmare end and when could he find out that it was all a bad dream?

Not right away, because Jimmy had to stay in the hospital for days and days, each day followed by a scary night away from home. For the "peanuts" Jimmy had eaten were mole pellets that contained arsenic. Fortunately, treatment was prompt and thorough, and he went home still wondering why such a little act should have brought about so much punishment.

The independence of the young child, coupled with his lack of experience, leads him into many dangers. He does not understand what these dangers are, and instead, quite innocently eats or drinks a substance not meant for human consumption. Soon he feels ill, and perhaps he becomes extremely ill. If he has swallowed lye or a strong acid, his mouth and throat are burned. He finds little support in his mother who is far more frightened than he. He is rushed to the hospital and treated in a way that does nothing to strengthen his sense of security.

Dealing with the Sense of Guilt

If this child is three, or four, or five, he

has other problems. Quite likely, he has been told not to touch, or not to go into the street, or some other prohibition has been made. Being at the stage of development where the forbidden is glamorous, he did touch, or eat, or run into danger. So now, he has strong guilt feelings to add to his misery. Anything that you, as a nurse, may have to do to him undoubtedly is understood as punishment.

We hear of parents who threaten their children with the policeman or the doctor in order to get them to obey. That this is true is evidenced by the words one hears during visiting hours. "If you don't leave that alone, I will tell the nurse and she will tie your hands down," or "Drink that or the nurse will come and give you a needle," and so on. The reaction of the parents can be better understood if one can feel their anxiety; procedures are frightening to parents too. All too often, no one has bothered to explain them. Picture how an oxygen tent or gastric suction must appear to someone who has never seen them before.

Then also, the mother may feel as guilt-laden as the child. She knows that many, perhaps most, accidents could be avoided. Over and over again she thinks, "If I had only done so-and-so, this wouldn't have happened." Perhaps the father, distraught, and not entirely free from guilt himself, adds to her distress. All too often, the parents catch snatches of conversation on the ward in which they hear themselves condemned for their carelessness. One would suppose that the burden of guilt that a parent has to carry, perhaps throughout life, would be great enough without adding to it.

Neither are nurses always guiltless in this respect. One group of students who over-heard the doctors discuss the possibility of an insecticide spray as a causative factor in a blood dyscrasia, accepted this as a proven fact, and discussed it so freely that the parents heard the discussion. Another group severely criticized a mother for neglect of her infant because of a doctor's free, but indiscreet, diagnosis. In both cases, the assumptions were false, but the damage was

done. We are apt to forget to put ourselves in another person's place.

Accepting Regression

The child who has been admitted because of an emergency, or the child who has come in without preparation for the experience, is almost certain to regress to a more infantile level. He seeks comfort and reassurance from those things that memory tells him have brought him satisfaction in the past. He may regress to thumb sucking or bed wetting. He may pick his nose, or rock himself. None of this behavior needs any comment from the nurse. She can, however, do much for him by providing him with some of the comfort he is seeking. It is sad to see little children sitting alone and idle in their cribs hour after hour, and a good nurse does not allow this to happen.

There is a distinct advantage present in working with this age group. The nurse should make the most of it. The infant or the preschooler can not understand, but this child is eager to learn and to know. Knowing gives him an excellent reason for using his own wit and imagination in participating in his own care.

The Older Child

A school age child entering the hospital for the first time is interested in learning about the world around him. If the nurse would take advantage of this interest, she should have little difficulty. For example, a child who enters for the repair of a heart defect wants to know what is going to happen to him. Take one of the small plastic hearts that the Heart Association provides and explain the anatomy, the action and the physiology of a normal heart. Point out the location of his defect, and explain how it affects the function of his own heart. Show him how it will be fixed. From there on, it should be easy to explain the reasons behind the various nursing procedures, and his cooperation can be assured. Of course he will try to cough, to turn, to accept the unpleasantness of the chest tubes, the oxygen tent and intravenous fluids—he knows all about them. Besides the plastic heart, diagrams appeal especially to this age group, and there are now on the market teaching models of the circulatory system and of other physiological processes which are fun to put in functioning order and to understand. The child nearly always is admitted early enough before surgery for the very purpose of getting him accustomed to hospital environment.

THE CHILD IN THE HOSPITAL ENVIRONMENT

Our present hospital policy of early ambulation and of letting the child out of bed whenever this does not interfere with his health or recovery appears to make the child's hospital stay more pleasant, bolsters his morale and is generally desirable. Still, it does call for more thoughtful planning on the part of the nurse in order to take full advantage of the helpful effects, while at the same time, keeping the child from overdoing. An average child is quick and alert. He is very much concerned with demonstrating his own competence, and gives himself wholeheartedly to his job. This aspect of development can be of tremendous value to the nurse, if she uses it, in her effort to develop relationships with the children under

her care. First of all, however, she must be secure herself before she can relate properly to a child.

Naturally, one does not let the child dictate his own care, but older children can understand the reasons behind the various treatments if explanations are made. When made members of the team, they usually become enthusiastic, meticulous performers. Then let the nurse beware if she breaks technique!

The Importance of Knowing About the Child

The nurse needs to have a firm background knowledge of normal growth and development if she is to give competent care. Here is a 2-year-old under her care. What should she expect of him in the way of motor skills? Should he be able to feed himself entirely, cut up his food and open his milk carton, or should she offer to help? What is the average weight of a child at this age, and how does he compare? What are normal skills for a 2-year-old boy? If it is important to know that 98.6°F is a normal body temperature, it is also important to know what is normal behavior for various age groups. No one expects the nurse to remember all the details of normal growth and development, nor should she expect this child to be like all other 2-year-olds, but her

---

Martha had been receiving a rather complicated daily dressing over a long period of time, and had come to learn every step of the procedure by rote. The ritual had eventually banished her fear, but now, a new nurse was to do the dressing, and much of her anxiety returned. The nurse, Miss Brown, recognized Martha's uncertainty and suggested that she needed the little girl's help, because she had not done this treatment for Martha before. From then on, everything went along very well. Sitting on the treatment table, Martha directed the procedure. She told Miss Brown where to find the dressings and how to set up the tray. She told her the order in which to proceed, when to put on her gloves and all the rest. Miss Brown was secure enough to recognize the child's need, and also to take advantage of the child's knowledge and ability.

A few days later, another nurse, who had not done this treatment on Martha before, had to do it. Martha now felt so much a part of the team that she confidently started to play the role that she believed to be hers. The nurse did not have enough security in herself, however, to allow Martha to participate. The first time that Martha said, "We remove that first, then we do this," the nurse said firmly, "I know how to do this, you just sit still." Then she proceeded to do the treatment in her own way. Immediately Martha's anxiety returned, and the entire procedure became a battle between the nurse and her patient. The nurse went away convinced that Martha was a most uncooperative child and reported that she would need help to hold the patient still tomorrow if she was to be able to maintain any sort of aseptic technique. This seems quite a high price to pay in order to reinforce the nurse's desire to show her authority.

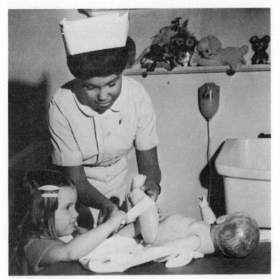

Figure 23-5. This is the way to bandage a hurt.

assignment to this particular child gives her the opportunity to check her general knowledge from the texts, and to apply that knowledge. For instance, she does not hold a drinking straw to the lips of a year-old baby and expect him to understand how to use it.

The nurse is able to give better care if she knows something of the child's physical history. Has he been a healthy child, with this his first hospital admission, or has he had repeated illnesses with many admissions? One may expect him to react differently to his present admission in response to previous experience. The child experiencing his first hospitalization may be frightened, shy, bewildered. The old-timer may take it in stride, or may be very angry and resentful.

The nurse needs to know the child's admitting diagnosis. Although certain techniques and skills are called for simply because this is an ill child, the type of illness may call for specialized knowledge and skill.

Finally, the nurse would do well to put together all the knowledge she has acquired and form it into a pattern. She should find it helpful to write it down as a composite picture of the child. As she studies this picture, what needs and problems does she expect to emerge, to be coped with when she

starts caring for him? Here is a child at a certain level of development, with a specific background, both modified by a certain disease. Mix these with his own distinctive personality, and what is likely to happen? After the nurse has become involved, she has no time to try out various approaches; she needs an immediate plan of action. Perhaps it does not fit the situation entirely, perhaps she has misjudged the child. She expected the child to respond to her loving manner, but all she received was rejection. She had devised a way to help him through an unpleasant experience, and he would have none of it. At the end of the day, she evaluates the situation, discards certain techniques and adopts a new approach for the next day. She modifies, changes, or follows through as her day's experience has taught her.

The Nursing Care Plan

Some nurses have found that making a

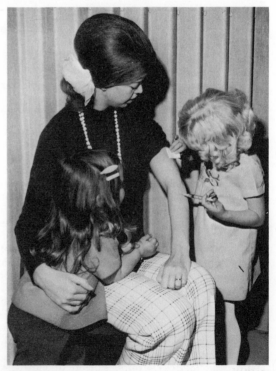

Figure 23-6. Children practice giving a "shot."

nursing care plan, using pocket-size index cards that they can carry with them, has proved helpful. One·such plan is illustrated here.

FIRST CARDS

NAME BOBBY S.	AGE 2	DIAGNOSIS MALNUTRITION
Pertinent Background	*Development*	*Comparison to Average*
1. Place in family	Present weight	% weight for age
2. Type of home	Present height	% height for age
3. Birth weight	Motor development	
4. Birth height	Speech	
5. Pertinent background material	Adaptive behavior etc.	

Add symptoms of disease that the child exhibits, comparison with textbook pictures; medications ordered with effects desired and toxic reactions; treatments and procedures scheduled, as indicated.

WORK CARDS (SAMPLE) FIRST AND SECOND DAY

Objective	Anticipated Problems	Anticipated Solution	Evaluation
1. To foster security	1. Expect him to be shy, may not relate to me	1. Kindness, but let him make advances	1. Worked well, tomorrow will try...
2.	2. May rebel against bed rest	2. Divert him by (suggest according to age)	2. Cried, would not be diverted will try...
3.	3. May refuse food and drink	3. Plan a tea party	3. No problem N.P.O. today

---

At the end of the first day, the nurse reviews and evaluates, notes new problems, discards those solved or that did not appear, and makes her work card for the next day.

FOLLOW-UP CARDS

Evaluation, Teaching, Long Term Planning

1. Evaluation of results
2. Planning for future needs
3. Plans for parent, child, nurse teaching
4. Long-term home care
5. Community resource
6. Bibliography

This kind of care plan has proved valuable to the nurse. It is also taken to clinical conferences and serves as a basis for discussion. The nurse presents the knowledge and understanding she has acquired, shares her findings with the staff, and gains added insight through the discussion centered around her preliminary study.

This certainly is not an inflexible form, to be used as it is, but a plan of some sort is very helpful. The nurse no longer thinks of this child-patient as "the patient in room

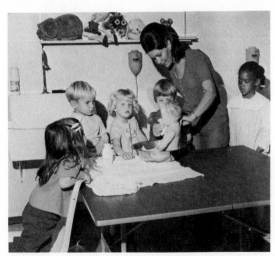

Figure 23-7. Everyone helps give the baby a bath.

415" or as "the child with malnutrition." Rather, she thinks of him as 2-year-old Bobby who has been taken from his home and put under her care.

The nurse can now care for him with some definite ideas about his needs and about how to meet them. In the course of the day, she may discover that he does not entirely conform to her expectations, and that perhaps her solutions were not entirely satisfactory, so she goes on from there. She has provided a measure of security for herself, however, before caring for Bobby, and her own confidence should provide strength for the child.

The Importance of Meaningful Observation

Caring for 2-year-old Bobby means more than this, however. He has not learned many words, and his background experience is decidedly limited. His mother has thought for him, anticipated and met his problems before he even knew that he had any. Here in the hospital, he may feel miserable, be nauseated or have a headache, or any number of other symptoms may be manifested. He cannot express them, perhaps cannot even localize them. The nurse must be the one alert enough to read the signs and to interpret them. Above all, she must remember to record them.

The doctor makes rounds at 9 A.M., and sees Bobby crying, or sleeping, or lying in an apathetic manner. He seeks information from the nurse's notes and reads, "Bed bath and A.M. care, ate poorly, sleeping." The doctor does not particularly care whether Bobby had a bed bath, he looks clean enough. "Ate poorly," what does that mean? "Sleeping," he saw that for himself. Of what use were these notes to him, telling about the child's condition, his symptoms, state of well-being?

As the nurse is the only person with the opportunity to observe the child over any period of time, the pediatrician would like to be able to rely heavily on her observations. She may not always know the significance of certain signs, but if they are different, if the child acts in any manner other than the way

he has been observed to act, she should note this. Perhaps it has no significance: that is fine. Perhaps it signifies a need to wait and see. It may be, however, a clue to the child's condition, and this no one can afford to miss.

ASPECTS OF CHILD OBSERVATION

Probably the most important role the nurse can play in her care is to be constantly observant. This means being cognizant of the child's behavior, being aware of the factors influencing that behavior, and being aware of the constancy of that behavior. These statements need to be broken down and considered separately.

Awareness of Child's Behavior

a. Observe how he behaves in all respects.
   1. Physical behavior
   2. Emotional response
   3. Intellectual response

b. Be aware of factors influencing your observations.
   1. Child's age; correlate this behavior with expected behavior for his age.
   2. His environment; be aware that he is in an abnormal environment.
   3. His previous experience; how much separation from his parents has he previously experienced? Has he ever been hospitalized before?

c. Be aware of the constancy of his behavior.
   1. Does he constantly manifest the same behavior, or is his reaction today different from that of yesterday?
   2. If his reaction is inconsistent, are there any reasons you can discover for the change? For example, does he seem sad and moody when ordinarily he is sunny and cheerful?

These general observations become more meaningful when considered from the various age levels.

The Infant

State of activity. A healthy infant is constantly active. Some are more intense and curious than others, but all are absorbed in this developmental task of their age. Illness modifies this level of activity. An important measure of the severity of the illness is the degree of impairment of activity in the infant. Does he lie quietly and manifest little or no interest in his surroundings? Do you find him in the same position every time you look at him?

State of muscular tension. The muscular state of an infant is tense, his grasp is tight, he raises his head when prone, and he kicks with vigor. When lying supine, there is a space between the mattress and his back. How does this infant compare? Does he lie relaxed, with arms and legs straight and lax? Does he make any attempt to turn his head or raise it if placed in a prone position? Does he move about his crib?

Constancy of reaction. A healthy infant shows a relative constancy of response and does not regress in his development. Was this child peppy and vigorous yesterday, but less so today? Did he respond to discomfort and painful procedures in an apathetic manner? Was he formerly interested in food, but now turns away? Does he respond to your presence or voice with his usual interest, or does he now turn his head and cry?

Behavior indicating pain.

1. A healthy baby appreciates being loved and picked up. Does this child cry or protest when handled, and seem to prefer being left alone? Perhaps he cries when picked up, but stills after being held quietly for a time, thus indicating that something hurts when he is moved.

2. A healthy baby shows activity as distinguished from restlessness. Does this baby turn his head fretfully from side to side? Perhaps he pulls his ear or rubs his head. Perhaps he turns and rolls constantly, seeming to try to get away from pain. Is he indicating by these actions the discomfort that he cannot put into words?

3. A healthy baby shows activity in every part of his body. This infant guards an arm or leg, or portion of his body, because it hurts to move it.

Physical signs of illness. Babies normally have a strong, vigorous cry. A weak, feeble cry, or a whimper indicate trouble. Nerve involvement may show in a high pitched, shrill cry. Perhaps he cries for long periods of time, refusing to be soothed. Sometimes, if the infant appears to cry excessively, a cry chart is helpful to determine just how much he actually does cry. Observe the infant every half hour, and fill in the time period with various shadings of color for his activity at the time, such as sleeping, feeding, lying quietly awake or crying. This makes your observations less subjective.

The Infant's Color. A healthy infant has a rosy tinge to his skin. His fingertips and toes are pink, his mucous membranes are pink-tinged. Is this child pale, with shadows under his eyes, or does his skin appear mottled? Does he show unusual pallor or blueness around his eyes and nose, or in his fingertips? Are his mucous membranes pale?

The Infant's Appetite or Feeding Pattern. A healthy infant has an interest in food. He exhibits an eagerness and impatience for satisfaction of his hunger. The sick infant may show an indifference toward his formula, or suck half-heartedly. He may vomit his feeding or habitually regurgitate. He may take his feeding and subsequently exhibit discomfort.

Bizarre Behavior. Any kind of behavior that differs from that expected for the level of development should be noted. Is this child overly good, or passive, in the face of strange surroundings? Does he, on the other hand, respond with rejection to every overture, friendly or otherwise? Is he overly clinging, never seeming satisfied with the amount of attention he receives?

It cannot be stressed too strongly that any *one* manifestation in itself may not be significant. The important thing is whether this behavior is consistent with this particular child, or whether it is a change from previous behavior. Perhaps he has always been pale or passive, or fussy in his feeding. Any such behavior needs to be noted, of course, but much of the significance depends greatly on the constancy of such behavior. As a nurse, can you tactfully, without alarming the parent, try to discover if he has always been a finicky eater, or been overactive, or an unusually quiet child? Of course, you have been observing and recording changes since admission to the hospital.

The Older Child

All of the previous observations are valid for the older child as well. In addition, there are a few somewhat different, or more mature reactions that may indicate an unhealthy state.

a. *Covering up for pain or discomfort.* A child seldom sees any enjoyment in illness or hospitalization. His burning desire is to get home again, and he will often go to great lengths to cover up any discomfort. Watch him sometime when he does not know that you are. Is he limping, or holding one side of his abdomen, or showing any other sign of pain? If so, what does he do when he sees you watching him? Does he straighten up and say that he was just playing? Do you take his word for this, or do you report the behavior?

b. *Extremes of aggression or passivity.* How does this child behave? Does he resist any and all advances, and strike out against playmates or adults? Perhaps instead, he accepts everything. Even more important, is this a change in behavior? How can you know unless you have been consistently observant and have recorded behavior?

c. *Reaction with parents.* Get a feeling of how a child reacts to his parents and they to him. How he reacts on the ward may be a reflection of his feelings toward his parents, or theirs to him. It may also reflect the parent's attitude to the situation of illness and hospitalization, or to the care that he now receives.

COMMUNICATING WITH CHILDREN

The nurse must realize that she is always communicating with her child patients regardless of whether they are able to understand her words or to answer her. The infant attaches his own meaning to her actions and thus forms his own evaluation of her. His background is too limited for him to realize that she is rushed or insecure when she picks him up abruptly or handles him in a hurried, impersonal manner. What she is telling him is that she is a potentially frightening person, that she does not love him. He relies entirely on his senses for information about his environment. Everyone knows that an infant can be called a rascal or any harsh name, and that he coos with delight if the tone is soothing, warm and loving.

The child who has reached the age when he can begin to differentiate between persons tends to be frightened of strangers. Anything unknown is potentially dangerous even to the adult. This phase usually begins sometime after the sixth month of life. Previously, an infant who has a background of security responds favorably to any warm, accepting person. Now, however, he has learned to recognize persons, and if he does not know them, he has no inner experience to tell him that they are friends. If you make sudden, abrupt, or loud approaches to him he is pretty sure to think that you are up to no good. If you let him stay secure in his mother's arms while he looks you over, this is helpful. You need to stay rather aloof as he makes his appraisal, and let him initiate the relationship. If his past experience with people has been good, it will not be long before he is making the advances and wanting you to respond.

This distrust of strangers may carry on through three or four years of life. If this is your first day to care for Johnny and he does not appear ready to accept you, try to be casual. Do not give him the feeling that you reject him, but let him see by your interested and warm manner with all the children that every one of them means something to you. Go slowly and gently, and do not reject him or his behavior. If he is showing rejecting or aggressive behavior, or being a "bad boy" he may be putting up a defense against his own fears. You should overlook as much of this behavior as possible. If it is such that it cannot be overlooked, either for his own or other's safety or well-being, be firm, and do whatever is necessary without showing anger or disgust.

Some nurses have considerable difficulty in accepting their own feelings while working with children. Miss Green came to her advisor greatly troubled because she felt anger and hostility toward the children when they misbehaved. Another nurse was disturbed because she could not accept the child who did not obey immediately when she spoke. The nurse needs to understand that she brings her own feelings, fears and conflicts to a new situation. Persons often feel a great inadequacy when they first have relationships with children. Perhaps they secretly feel that they are not the all-knowing, all-powerful persons the child thinks they are, and are afraid that they are going to be found out, so they in turn use aggressive feelings to cover their own insecurity. The nurse needs to understand this and be willing to accept the fact that she, too, is very human. She can still consciously accept the child, and she will find that as she grows more secure, she can learn to understand him. A good nurse must be self-accepting and self-confident, it is true, but she does not necessarily begin that way. She usually has to grow in maturity and insight.

After the nurse has honestly faced and accepted herself, she is free to turn to the child. She is no longer preoccupied with her own inner inadequacies and fears. Perhaps she does have the impulse to command and demand instant and complete obedience. She can accept this as a result of unfortunate experiences in her earlier life, but she does not need to stop there. Now she must consider the child's environment, his background and his stage of development, and will try to discover why he behaves as he does. Is it a result of his own inconsistent handling at home, or is it the urge to try toward independence that his nature demands? Perhaps it might even be a response to her own authoritarian attitude. Careful consideration should help her modify her expectations. If a child senses the nurse's genuine interest, he eventually puts forth some effort to respond.

Problems of Discipline

The entire problem of discipline in the hospital deserves careful study. It becomes one of the most frustrating and difficult problems that the nurse meets in the pediatric department.

It is quite true that the nurse can win if she fights in a battle of wills. She has everything on her side; authority, strength, size and reinforcement. What, however, is she likely to end up with after she has secured submission from the child? Surely not a child who has learned to respect authority?

There comes a time in the child's development when he both needs and desires restrictions as a help toward achieving self-control. Of course, when the nurse meets a child in the hospital she finds a person with his personality and character already deeply affected by his home environment. She meets children from widely different home backgrounds, which, of course, does not make her task any easier. A child in the hospital does present many disciplinary problems.

Restrictions—Are They Necessary?

Naturally, a definite set of rules cannot be written to fit all occasions, or to fit all children. Rules, of course, are as necessary in the children's ward as they are elsewhere, but they should be written primarily for the child's welfare and comfort rather than for the convenience of the ward (although that certainly must be considered as well).

Restrictions against children playing with wheelchairs, especially racing up and down corridors in them, are valid safety measures. If a child finds wheelchairs new and fascinating, perhaps someone can find time to push him around in one, even if he does not especially need this form of locomotion.

There may be rules or restrictions that do not seem to make very good sense and may be a carry-over from the past. Children should be allowed, and encouraged, to visit in other wards, to eat together, and to form friendships. A sign on the boy's ward that says in big letters—"NO GIRLS ALLOWED—THIS MEANS YOU," will call for an answer from the girls, "BOYS KEEP OUT." There may be "Nurses may come in except to give shots," or even, "No doctors allowed." This provides for considerable giggling, but no one would be more surprised and hurt than the boys and girls themselves, if the signs were heeded. This certainly is a harmless way to brighten life in the hospital.

Children of Other Cultures

The United States has a heterogeneous population, with people from many cultural backgrounds. Many have not adopted our culture in their homes, preferring to carry on their familiar way of life. Children from such homes are apt to adapt rather quickly to new ways, but such adaptation is usually superficial. During illness, loneliness and separation from home, they revert to their parents' teachings. This return to the teachings that are the real valued ideals of a culture is not limited to the child patient. The families have clung to their old ways because they believe in them and accept what they represent. They are understandably unwilling to let these traditions become lost to their children.

The native born North American is somewhat inclined to develop a mental stereotype of the behaviors of other peoples, and is inclined to cherish the belief that strange cultures are inferior to his own. It is natural for people to believe their own way of life is best; to a degree it bespeaks a feeling of pride and self-respect. Unfortunately too often it borders on chauvinism and a fanatical derogation of anyone different from ourselves.

When someone takes the trouble to ignore stereotypes and seeks to understand an *individual* person, he finds someone like himself with the same emotions, fears and satisfactions. He may also possibly discover that the other's culture has given him something fine that he can admire and wish for himself. The Puerto Ricans, Mexican-Americans, American Indians, the Orientals, all have something to contribute. Their contributions enrich our culture just as those of the Italians, Swedes and Irish did before them.

When a child from such a home enters the hospital, the nurse needs to make an effort to understand his background. Was his family permissive in the rearing of the small child, as many societies are? As he grew older has he been taught to be stoical in the face of pain or emotional disruption? Does his culture frown on competition or deviation from the norm?

One cannot in honesty say all American Indians are stoical or noncompetitive. Nor can one say all black children learn to feel inferior at an early age, or all lack a strong father image, or whatever the particular stereotype happens to be. So much depends on the particular family, their socio-economic position, their individual reactions to life. This is not denying cultural differences and mores peculiar to a society. In this vast country, however, even cultures become extensively intermixed and modified.

Most nurses appear to have few prejudices against children because of race or ethnic background. In the hospitals children are generally evaluated as children: passive or aggressive, peacemakers or troublemakers, mischievous or disciplined.

The child himself may have learned to look for discrimination, and react as though he were being discriminated against. The nurse should be aware of this possibility and try to understand his feelings. Gentle, persistant loving care, given in the same measure as it is to others, will eventually help him realize the falsity of his expectations.

However, there are occasions when special attention needs to be given to a child to help him realize his own worth. This was the case with Helen.

Helen was a ten-year-old black child who came into the hospital to have her diabetic status reevaluated. She came from a home where affection was present but understanding of her condition was at a rather low level. She was obliged to take over the management of her own diabetic control if she was to remain healthy.

Helen had been admitted twice before for instruction and for control, but this had not been during the pediatric rotation of the student nurse who was now to care for her and give her instruction. Miss Brown was asked to do this and was told that no one was sure how competent the child was, or how much of her previous instruction she had retained. Miss Brown had the task of discovering how much she knew and of proceeding from there.

Helen was a reserved, shy girl, who did not relate easily to new personnel. She indicated, however, that she knew how to draw up the insulin into the syringe, and how to give it. Miss Brown brought a tray containing the insulin syringe, regular and long lasting insulin, and skin antiseptic to Helen's room. Miss Brown said, "Show me how you would prepare the insulin in the syringe." Helen picked up the bottles, carefully shook them, and after deciding which one to put in the syringe first, drew them up correctly. She cleaned the site on her thigh and inserted the needle. She placed the needle in a position which was too horizontal, however, so that it would go into the tissue intradermally, instead of subcutaneously. Miss Brown, who had been giving unqualified approval, now suggested that she remove the needle and try again, explaining why. Helen did so, but again placed the needle in the wrong position. Using the greatest possible tact, the nurse removed the needle and demonstrated to the little girl the correct angle for the needle and finished the procedure herself. In spite of the praise for her excellent procedure, Helen's eyes filled with tears, and she appeared distressed that her performance had not been entirely accepted. Miss Brown was distressed over Helen's reaction. She suggested that they both practice later in the day, and use an orange to get the correct angle. This they did, and Helen soon corrected her error. Miss Brown felt that there was more involved here, however, than a mere mechanical error, and spent some time studying the situation.

Helen was a girl with extremely plain features, whose home was in a community in which she did not fit. She had received much rejection in her short life from her peers as well as from others outside her family. Miss Brown made an effort to establish a genuine friendship with this child and succeeded to the extent that Helen came out of her reserve enough to talk, and even to begin a show of interest in participating in some activities. Helen's roommate was a blonde, blue-eyed child who was both the pet of her family and of the hospital department. Her family and her friends poured in to visit, walking past Helen without even acknowledging her presence. Personnel waved and smiled to her but seldom noticed Helen. Helen seldom responded to any overtures anyway, and so she was easily ignored.

One morning, Miss Brown came into the room to find that Helen had resumed all her defenses and failed to respond to any of her overtures. Miss Brown discovered that the roommate's family had brought several gifts to her the evening before, had put a pretty bathrobe on her and a dainty cap.

Miss Brown went into action. She spent a long time giving Helen her bath, lavishly massaging her with a fragrant bathing lotion. She brushed the child's hair until it shone, and then tied it with a bright ribbon that presented suitable competition to the child's cap. The nurse's hope was that the obvious affection she showed, as well as the extra attention, would help the child accept her own worth. A conference with staff members was planned to help them realize that this child needed attention before she could respond to them. Helen went home before much else could be done, but Miss Brown became so interested that she planned to see her when she returned to the diabetic clinic, in order to show her very real interest and affection for the child.

THE HOSPITAL PLAY PROGRAM

Importance of Play for All Children

Play is the business of children. It is only by practice, by imitation of the adult world, by trial and error, that the child learns. The apparently aimless movements of the infant are actually purposeful. His incessant postural activity is his work, and a tremendous amount of energy is needed for it. In this way, he strengthens his muscles, perfects his coordination, and keeps abreast of his rapidly maturing nerve cells.

As the infant matures, every stage of development calls for the learning of new skills. This learning is physical as well as mental and emotional. The muscles must be used, and will ache if forcibly kept still for

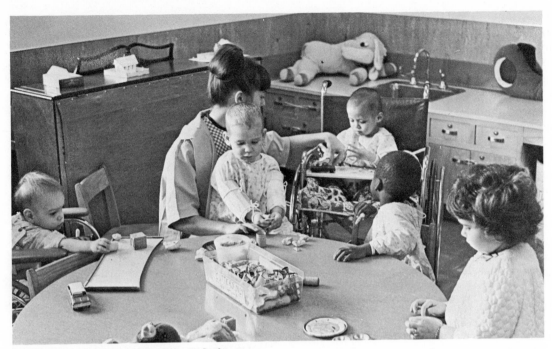

Figure 23-8.   Children in a hospital playroom.

any length of time. The mind must interpret and learn, but there cannot be any significant mental or physical stimulation in an emotionally deprived atmosphere. The infant needs approval, love, and praise to stimulate him, and to provide the all-important background of security.

It has been said that a child does not stop growing and developing when he enters the hospital. This is something to think about. Without meaning to, nurses are apt to think of the child patient as being somehow different from the children they see on the street, in the bus, or in the neighborhood. Actually, the only difference is that the child patient is restrained by his illness, or by hospital rules, from carrying out his developmental tasks in a satisfactory manner. To present for discharge a child who is healthy in mind and body is the objective of all nursing care.

In *Why Play in the Hospital,* we read, "It is, however, quite apparent that play activity is one of the most important aspects of a child's life and is the major way in which a child learns about the world around him and how to deal with other children. Any serious examination of the question will show the need for playtime in the daily activity of growing children ....We know children play in hospitals with or without the blessing of the hospital staff."*

Hospital Play Programs

The hospitalization of children has changed markedly in the last few years. Newer treatments have shortened the need for bed rest in many instances. There are, of course, still some conditions that prohibit activity, either temporarily, or on a long-term basis. A visit to the pediatric wards today, however, shows many beds empty during the daytime hours.

Hospitals have met the challenge of the child's needs in various ways. Ideally, a spacious playroom, well equipped for the particular age group, and well attended, is the answer. Newly built or remodeled hospitals can plan for these playrooms as an

*Play Schools Association: Why Play in a Hospital—How. p. 13. New York, Play Schools Association.

essential part of the children's wing. Some hospitals have met the challenge in other ways, sometimes by taking over some other room for a playroom. Naturally, these rooms are not always ideal for this purpose, but can be made to serve.

Other pediatric departments, unable to find a spare room, have used ingenuity and imagination in planning play experience. In large wards, toys, tables and chairs are provided. Toy carts, which are circulated from bed to bed, are easily made.

Sometimes, when a central playroom is used, it is very easy to forget the child who is confined to his bed back in the room. Actually, keeping a number of playroom children occupied in a constructive manner requires total concentration. Although some playrooms are large enough to allow a few cribs to be brought in, not all children on bed rest are able to tolerate the busy pace of the playroom.

There may even be some advantages in having to use the ward for play activities. The children on bed rest may participate in the same activities as the ambulatory children, and this may be quite a morale booster for them. Children on bed rest can have their beds protected by sheets of plastic and join in the finger painting, water play, or other messy activities. They can have their beds rearranged so that they feel they belong to the group.

The mobile child who can roam at will can find some diversion for himself. True, this may take the form of some unacceptable activity, but he will find something if he is unrestricted. The child confined to his bed has a serious problem. If his nurse has any interest in children, she talks to him as she bathes him, but all too often personal contact ends there. The child may be too sick to be interested in play, and clutching his favorite toy may be enough activity for him. Most children who are confined to their beds, however, need something to occupy their minds and to provide stimulus.

In some forward looking hospitals, considerable imagination is used in affording the hospitalized child opportunities for play. In one children's hospital, tricycles were being ridden up and down the corridor. Unless things got out of hand, no one was told to be quiet, or to "play in your room." One little fellow was gravely stopped by a friendly intern and presented with a traffic ticket, much to his delight.

Opportunity for active games is provided for those whose medical condition allows this. Crafts, ceramics and table games are available for those who must be quiet. Children's libraries are handy with books freely available. Provision for out of door play (or quiet observation) is a valuable aid toward restoring health. Few hospitals have broad tree-shaded lawns anymore, but playgrounds are sometimes managed. Failing these, solariums and sun decks help take the emphasis off the institutional atmosphere.

Of course, the above described active play presupposes that these children are dressed in daytime clothes. It is difficult to run around in poorly fitting pajamas, cloth slippers and a dragging bathrobe. It seems

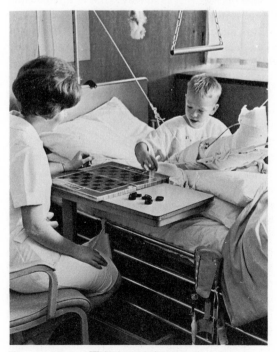

Figure 23-9.   This is nursing too.

difficult to justify the use of night clothing for children up and about. Are simple cotton suits and dresses more difficult to make and launder than hospital gowns and pajamas?

Play Experience in Nursing

It is now a commonly accepted practice to include play experience in each student nurse's educational background. This is excellent for a number of reasons, but there is one danger to guard against. The student nurse may feel that because she is not play nurse for the day, she has no obligation toward directing the child's activities. This feeling stems largely from the student's attitude toward her pediatric experience. If she has an enthusiasm for her work with children, and a genuine interest in their welfare, she not only sees this as an obligation, but as a challenge to her ingenuity and to her imagination. To rescue a child from apathy and withdrawal provides one of the greatest satisfactions known to a nurse.

A student may feel insecure and inadequate after she has finished giving the child patient physical care. She is apt to take refuge in some activity that takes her away from him. She feels sorry for the child, but she does not know what to do for him, and so she frequently finds herself busy elsewhere. She is also apt to feel guilty because of her withdrawal from the child, and the pediatric experience becomes less of a fulfillment for her.

One student made the remark that she disliked playroom experience. "It takes imagination to play with children," she said, "and I just don't have any."

Many young nurses, perhaps a majority of them, have been baby sitters during high school; either as a means of making money, or as older sisters in the family, or as an adoring aunt. Perhaps they have also had experience as camp counselors, Sunday school teachers, vacation school teachers and helpers. Why, then, are they so unsure of themselves in the hospital situation?

Perhaps this panic stems from the nurse's conception of her role, as well as her

mental image of the hospitalized child. She must again remind herself that these are *children*, quite similar to her brothers and sisters, her neighbors and friends. Illness and strangeness may cause them to put on a front of apathy, indifference, or even dullness. Down underneath is still a person with all of the instincts, capabilities, longings and potential of any child at that particular level of development. Who will bring out this hidden child for all to see? Can the nurse? What a challenge!

Below is described an incident that brings into sharp focus the possibilities for the nurse's understanding of the child. It is one of the highlights in pediatric nursing.

Play in Pediatric Nursing: An Example

Merrilee was a tot just under 3 years of age who had been through a ghastly experience. She and an older sister had been temporarily alone in their house when the whole building burned down. Merrilee was rescued, but she suffered extensive second and third degree burns on her face and on her body. Weeks of isolation in the hospital, painful procedures, and difficult, agonizing movements, had taken their toll of this little one's emotional state. She had come to prefer to be alone, showing no interest in anyone. After all, why should she? Usually, the entrance of a nurse or doctor only meant more pain.

Eventually, the time came when the urgency of physical care subsided, and concern was felt over this child's uniformly negative responses. She was encouraged to sit up in a chair and look out into the corridor, but she cried whenever she was placed facing in that direction.

Day by day, quiet, persistent effort on the part of the staff brought a slight response, but one day the breakthrough really came. A student nurse, noticing that the only unburned areas were Merrilee's feet and lower legs, thought that some play activity involving her feet would be painless and might stimulate interest. She asked the recreational leader for a hand puppet, and was given a brightly colored duck. She placed this on Merrillee's foot, and the child was entranced. She made the duck open his mouth, quack, and soon Duckie was biting the toes of the other foot.

Merrilee forgot to be shy. All day, people came to her door to see a proud child make Duckie bite her toes. She chatted excitedly and freely. Other students, not to be outdone, invented other games, and soon Merrilee was running about her room. She just naturally shrugged off any discomfort and commenced using other parts of her body. Soon she was transferred to the ward, and here one had difficulty recognizing the child who had rejected everyone. As a leader in mischief, she became unsurpassed. She related lovingly and trustingly to everyone, and was soon well on the way toward being spoiled.

Certainly it is true that one does not know instinctively how to be at ease with children simply because one is a nurse, or because one has had previous experience with children. If a recreational leader needs training, why shouldn't the student nurse have some guidance as well? It certainly is not realistic to send her into the playroom with nothing more than a "Today you are play nurse."

Suggestions for crafts, games and just "things to do" are abundant and easily found. Anyone with a little persistence can find plenty of help in pamphlets, books, magazines and newspapers. Here, it may be helpful to suggest some specific activities for various situations.

Children with Limited Opportunities for Play

The Child on Complete Bed Rest

Before any discussion of complete or strict bed rest can be attempted, it is necessary to define the term. This is somewhat difficult when dealing with children. One is much more confident when speaking of adults. An interpretation of complete bed rest should mean that the patient does nothing for himself; he is bathed, fed and turned, and encouraged to avoid excitement and strain.

How does one go about keeping a child on such strict bed rest? He lacks the experience for understanding the issues involved. He lives for the here-and-now, not for a vague and shadowy future. Do we restrain him? If so, will his resistance and resentment prove a greater strain on his heart than free movement about his bed?

It is necessary to find out how much restriction is actually meant by this term. It could mean that the child is kept in bed but is allowed to feed himself, and also allowed some quiet activities. It could simply mean that the child is not allowed to have bathroom privileges. It could also mean just what it says; the child is kept quietly in bed, is fed, bathed, allowed to do no schoolwork or anything involving the use of his arms. His visitors and his television are restricted. In such a case, he probably would be receiving some sedation to help control his restlessness. Doctors vary the meaning of the term when they use it as a prescription for different children.

After ascertaining just how much activity the child is allowed, the nurse can make her plans. At the moment, we are speaking about the child who feels physically well enough to chafe against his enforced inactivity. For the child in acute distress or pain, the condition itself limits activity. The normally active, fun-loving boy or girl who is so sharply restricted finds this a great trial, and it is one for those caring for him; yet he needs mental stimulation to prevent him from suffering considerable psychological damage. This aspect of his care is at least as important as his physical handling, and requires even more thought and planning. Frequently, it is helpful to pool the thinking and planning of all concerned in a ward or staff conference.

Suggestions for activities. The American Heart Association has suggestions available for the asking. Most of them do not take the expenditure of money but utilize common everyday materials. Many suggestions to help the child occupy his mind during the long hours of enforced idleness are available in other publications.

Fast growing plants are fun to watch. One can almost see them grow. The nurse can take an eggshell, fill it with water or dirt, and dropping a seed into it, find that it soon starts to grow. She can take an egg carton and stand the eggshells upright in it, first coloring the shells if she wishes. In water, large seeds such as melon, squash, grapefruit, grow pretty vines. Nearly any flower seed grows in dirt. A sweet-potato vine is very pretty, with heart-shaped leaves, and grows from a slice of sweet potato kept in water, or in dirt. A carrot or a beet makes a vine. For even more fun, take a large carrot, scoop out the inside, make two holes in the sides near the top for a cord or ribbon to hang it by. Fill the hollowed-out portion with water, and hang it. The carrot must be kept filled with water, however, so choose as large a carrot as you can find, because it dries out quickly.

An herb garden is fun to watch grow. Parsley grows quickly and profusely. Garlic,

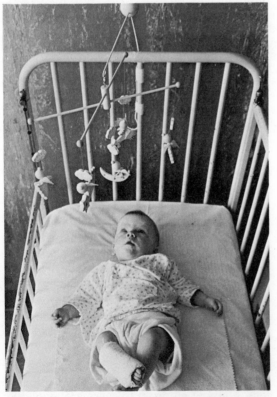

Figure 23-10. Mobiles are fun to watch.

dill, chive and other herbs can be grown in pots or planters. There is great satisfaction for a child in being able to give mother a sprig of parsley or rosemary to dress up her dinner.

Pets, of course, are a great source of satisfaction. These require care and are not always allowed. However, a small fish in a fish bowl at the child's bedside may be a great comfort to him and require practically no care on the part of the staff. One boy kept a goldfish at his bedside, and they became great friends. Eventually, when he went home after some months in a convalescent hospital, he held the bowl up to the car window all the way home so that "Jimmy" could see the scenery too. He was sure that after many months of confinement Jimmy would be as anxious to see the outside world as he was himself.

Mobiles are great fun to watch. They are fun to make as well as interesting to watch. If you live in an area where colored plastic baskets are used for marketing berries, ask people to save them for you. They make beautiful bird cages. Place one for top and one for bottom, lace them together with ribbon and hang a small paper or plastic bird inside. Hang from a hook with a gay ribbon and bow. Of course, live birds in real cages are wonderful diversions if anyone is available to care for them.

Record players and television are both fine for children's wards, but may prove too stimulating for some children. If television is provided, make sure that someone supervises the program and the reception. Too often, one walks into a room where the television is either out of focus, or the program is an adult one, totally unsuited to the audience.

Greeting cards that are sent to the child make a cheerful wall decoration, and can be put up with masking tape. If cards do not come, this may be an opportunity to use some of the greeting cards that people are always anxious to donate to the children's ward. Naturally, the cards from family and friends are more welcome, and the suggestion to schoolmates or fellow Scouts that Jimmy does not want to be left out of things may inspire short letters and cards.

Surprise boxes are an excellent tonic for the person confined to bed. A shoe box filled with small packages, one to be opened each day, gives a little spice to life, and helps the person look forward to tomorrow. If there is no family to make such a box, is there any reason why nurses cannot include making one of these boxes as a part of nursing care? The child with little stimulation from friends or family is the child needing this type of care more than the others.

The Child on Simple Bed Rest

The child on bed rest without other limitations, can have more active occupations. There are, of course, some children whose condition makes bed rest advisable or mandatory. The child may move about his bed freely, may feel well, but because of some condition may not be allowed to get up. Perhaps he has a cast that limits his ability to move about. Perhaps he has a slight fever, or a slight cold, or a condition that may necessitate bed rest but does not restrict his activity while in bed. He feels fine, but he must stay in bed as he sees the others troop off gaily to the playroom. Such children suffer from boredom, and may lose interest in life in general if some stimulus is not provided for them.

It should not be too difficult to find occupation for these children. Most of the crafts can be carried out on a sturdy table. For the school-age child of perhaps 5 to 8 years of age, crafts are interesting and may become absorbing.

A child's problem is solved. A good example of this was Bobby—a patient in a school-age ward—who, because of an infection, was placed in a room alone. He was apathetic, listless, whiny, and disagreeable. It was just before Christmas, and the whole ward was busy making decorations, but the report was that Bobby was not interested in doing any thing, and was a thoroughly disagreeable little boy.

One of the nurses decided that Bobby should be brought into the activities

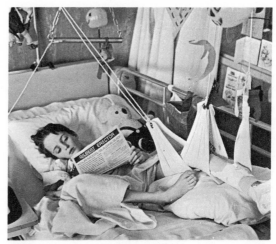

Figure 23-11. Building projects are an absorbing interest for a child on bed rest.

somehow, but she found it difficult to arouse any enthusiasm in this 6-year-old boy. Finally, she took some paper medicine cups, water paint, and plain string into his room. She painted the outside of the cup red, punched a hole in the bottom and hung it up. Bobby was interested and soon had a row of Christmas bells—red, green and gold—strung across his room. Next he made paper chains, and finally engaged in a really big project. Stencils of Christmas scenes were available, so he traced, colored, and gave pictures to his favorite people, after liberally decorating his own room with them. This was much more satisfying than putting up just any old pictures.

These activities seemed to bring back much of his old interest in life. His appetite improved, and he became much more lively. He was discharged to return shortly after Christmas, and this time he was in the ward with the other boys. He became a thoroughly typical boy, lively and full of mischief; so it seemed that he had learned that the hospital could be fun after all.

For the toddler who must have his activity restricted, a special kind of toy must be provided. Everything goes into his mouth (with potentially dangerous results) as you may discover the first time you rescue a small car, marble, or coin from starting down a small child's throat. Crayons are colorful, and to a toddler, meant to be eaten. Paper is to be torn and perhaps to be eaten as well.

Cloth books are safe, as well as stuffed animals, although even here the nurse must make sure that there are no ripped seams, because stuffing is great fun to pull out, or any button eyes to remove. Large, sturdy cars, trucks, and planes are fun.

The older child, who can be trusted with crayons, finger paints, coloring books, or with blunt scissors, can find a great deal of satisfaction and diversion, even though he must stay in bed.

Suggestions for the Child with Limited Mental Ability

Mention must be made of the child whose mental abilities are limited. He is in need of recreation as much as the normal child, perhaps more so. Try to discover the kind of toy that satisfies him, even though it is at a very low level for his chronological age. Even the child who appears to be functioning at an extremely low level may have his attention caught by a bright object hanging within his field of vision. (See also section on mental retardation.)

The nurse must consider the limitations imposed by any disease, such as the desirable amount of activity and the amount of restriction of movement. It would seem to be as important for the nurse to plan the child's recreational activity as to plan his individual nursing care. All ages, as well as all conditions, must be considered.

The Infant

The infant can of course benefit greatly from stimulation. There is seldom an occasion when the nurse should leave the infant without some type of play material suitable for his age. A cradle gym takes only a minute to fasten across the crib, and more than once an apathetic infant, having accidentally batted one of the toys with his hand or foot, has found stimulation and interest in trying again. Sturdy rattles and soft, cuddly animals are a part of the picture. If the child is at the age when he derives his greatest pleasure

from throwing his toys out, it is profitable to tie them to the crib sides.

Babies can often be put in playpens, perhaps more frequently than nurses realize. This may well provide a change of scene as well as give an opportunity to stretch those developing muscles.

Therapeutic Characteristics of Play

We must not forget the *therapeutic value of play* that is frequently important. The incident of the burned child who learned to manipulate a puppet with her feet is one example. Another one could be the manipulation of various kinds of toys for the purpose of strengthening weak muscles.

If the nurse is uncertain about what kind of toy to use, or needs to have her imagination stimulated, a visit to the occupational therapist is helpful. Nurses can make a real contribution to the sick child's well-being and ultimate recovery. The nurse must understand the importance of a relaxed, happy atmosphere in the total picture of nursing care.

Some children have very little contact with the outside world through visitors or mail. Such children look on wistfully as a more fortunate roommate opens his cards or letters. It takes but little time or imagination to drop a card in the mail, or even a cheery note. To be valuable, these should come through the mail, so that Johnny will get real mail, just like the others. That someone cares enough to send a card is excellent medicine.

We do not do *play therapy* as such, that is not our purpose. However, we are in one sense using therapy for the children. The time the child spends in the hospital should not remain empty. He does not live in vacuum, but continues to grow and to develop. We can help or hinder this growth by the opportunities that we provide for him. A play program needs thought and planning if it is to be anything more than a means of keeping the children quiet. A trained recreation leader appears to be an essential part of the pediatric staff, and the nurse can learn much from her. The "play lady" is only one person however, and is not in as close and personal contact with the individual child as is the nurse caring for him.

Group play can be of great value in helping the sick child overcome boredom or homesickness. If the ward is a noisy one, or the children appear to be over stimulated, quiet games are frequently calming. Games like "I packed my suitcase" may be effective, or the continuous story, going from child to child. One student introduced a story telling hour while giving morning baths. One child started an adventure story that was followed by fantastic adventures from the next bed, each child trying to outdo the others in imagination and fantasy. Even the shy, unhappy child found himself drawn into the company. Another time, the charge nurse was puzzled to find the ward door closed, but on opening it she discovered the reason. The nurse was bathing one child while leading a vigorous chorus of *Old MacDonald Had a Farm.* Material benefits from such thoughtfulness are apparent; the child sleeps better, eats better, and has less tendency to think about himself.

Mention has been made of *television.* Certainly it has a place in the picture, but it should be used intelligently. It has also been demonstrated that a child given something interesting or constructive to do, spends far less time as a mere observer of television.

When There Is No Existing Play Program

Much of the previous discussion has been concerned with hospitals at which a play program has been initiated. The nurse may find herself in a situation where no such program exists, and may find that the initiative for starting such a program must be her own. A well organized program is in effect in many hospitals, and the nurse easily becomes a part of it. There are still some hospitals without such a program.

There seems to be no real reason why a nurse cannot work toward such a program if she is convinced of the necessity for it. It certainly is not difficult, and need not be expensive. Play materials are easily im-

provised from the simplest articles. Pretty pictures have been made by pasting lima beans, green or yellow split peas, and red beans onto a cardboard plate in a flower design. Some of the happiest children were scaring the nurses with horrendous masks made from paper bags pulled over their heads, with eyes, nose and mouth cut out.

Socks or stockings make excellent hand puppets, or can make delightful stuffed dolls. Soap can be carved into animals by the child who can be trusted with the necessary tools. Finger paint, paste and modeling clay can be made very simply at home. Spools, cardboard, craft paper, milk bottle caps, discs from round boxes, can all be put to use to make delightful dioramas enclosed in deep shoe boxes.

Cellophane and macaroni straws make necklaces, and drinking cups make fine doll bodies. It takes more imagination than money to stock a play cupboard.

A place to keep these materials is frequently a problem. A consultation with the nurse in charge may reveal a cupboard or closet that could be used. The nurse needs to decide whether she wishes to have the materials available to the children, or whether she puts someone in charge to hand out the materials as they are needed. In any case, she should remember that the children are still in the hospital when she has left them at the end of her day. One sometimes sees all play materials put away under lock and key after 3:30 or 4 P.M. and totally inaccessible over the weekends.

Books, of course, play a large part in children's entertainment. If your hospital does not have a children's library, why not start one? One group of students started a drive among their friends and families for used books suitable for children, and soon acquired a very respectable library. A word of caution is needed. The books must be carefully screened against trash or unsuitable material. Some people see a book drive as a chance to get rid of all the old books that they have been saving for years. The children's librarian of the public library would be glad to help choose the books. A great deal of tact is necessary in dealing with donors whose generosity exceeds their judgement. Nevertheless, a children's library is a profitable venture.

Toys can be collected in the same manner. They must be sturdy, durable and suitable. At one school, the student nurses had fun with "dorm" parties, at which they mended and repainted toys. Making doll wardrobes, knitting dollhouse rugs, crocheting drapes and curtains—all were fun. In fact, one group had several sessions in which they papered rooms in a homemade dollhouse, making fixtures, rugs, curtains, and finally painted the outside of the house. When finished, it was put on a portable table and used in the ward, mainly for the children who had to stay in bed. A family was provided with the dollhouse, and the children were encouraged to make clothes for them if they wished. This proved to be a great morale booster, especially for the homesick child. The house took quite a beating however, and required frequent refurnishing

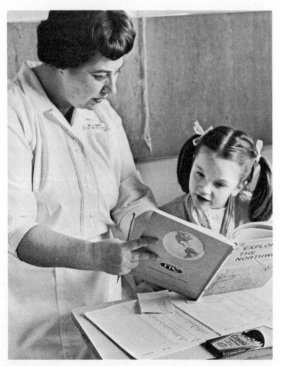

Figure 23-12. School continues in the hospital.

and repainting. The furniture can be made from sturdy cardboard and replaced frequently, or may be made from heavier material that can withstand rather rough use.

THE SCHOOL PROGRAM IN THE HOSPITAL

The school program in children's hospitals has become quite well established in many areas. Convalescent hospitals and those for chronic diseases of children have had this service for children for some time. Occasionally, teachers or tutors have come into general hospitals to help an individual child. However, the idea of teachers regularly employed by the school system and working in the children's unit of a general hospital is relatively new.

Certainly being able to keep up with his classmates is a morale booster to a hospitalized child. However, such a program for the child with a short term illness has other values as well. In addition to his illness, the hospitalized child suffers from the strangeness of his surroundings. He is separated from all that is familiar in his life. The school atmosphere of teacher, books, and lessons gives him one familiar base on which to build security. The normal, everyday school experiences seem to be psychologically helpful to a child.

Seidel, in his excellent chapter on educational needs of the hospitalized child, says this:*

"Thus the hospital team ... must be aware that a child who sits in the hospital doing nothing depresses himself and those around him ... and shares the common experience that hospital walls are a prison."

Seidel comments further "We all need a continuing sense of achievement, and if, for any disruptive reason, we are removed from our normal milieu, we need the assurance we can return to that environment unhindered."

---

*Seidel, Henry M.: Educational Needs and Programs for the Hospitalized Child. In Haller, J. Alex. ed.: *The Hospitalized Child and His Family.* pp. 57—58. Baltimore, Johns Hopkins Press, 1967

Table 23-1.   TOYS SUITABLE FOR VARIOUS AGE GROUPS

INFANTS

Cradle gym	Soft washable dolls and animals
Rattles (doughnut, dumbell, plastic keys)	Floating bath toys
	Pots and pans
Soft balls	Small plastic or wooden blocks

TODDLERS—AGE 1-2 YEARS

Cloth, plastic books (illustrations of familiar objects, preferably one to a page)	Push toys and pull toys
	Telephone
	Dolls
Nested blocks of soft plastic or wood	Musical top

PRESCHOOLERS

Record player, nursery rhymes	Floor trains
Large wooden beads for stringing	Blackboard and chalk
Housekeeping toys	Easel and brushes
Transportation toys (tricycle, trucks, cars, wagon)	Clay, crayons and finger paint
	Outdoor toys, sand box, swing, small slide
Blocks	Books (short stories, action stories)
Hammer and peg bench	Drum

KINDERGARTNERS AND FIRST GRADERS

Blocks	Blunt scissors, simple sewing sets, paste and colored paper
Dolls	
Housekeeping toys	Doll house
Dress-up clothes, tea parties	Simple puzzles
Outdoor toys	Books, records
Easels, blackboards, paint	Matching card games

OLDER CHILDREN

Paper dolls	Bicycles
Table games	Work benches, good tools and materials
Books for self-reading	
Electric trains	Puppets and marionettes
	Crafts

THOSE IN MIDDLE CHILDHOOD—9-12 YEARS

Hobby collections	Table games
Telegraph sets, short-wave radio*	Outdoor sdports
Model car, boat and plane sets	

These are but a few suggestions for appropriate toys and games for various age groups.

*Electrical appliances in the hospital (such as x-ray) may interfere with reception.

A successful school program has been in operation for several years at Doernbacher Children's Hospital, division of the Medical School Hospital of the University of Oregon. Every school-age child is enrolled in this program regardless of the length of his stay, unless his condition forbids such activity.

There are two regularly employed school teachers for a unit of about 30 children. As this hospital unfortunately does not have an adolescent unit, two additional teachers teach high school subjects to teenagers throughout the hospital. All children do regular schoolwork unless too ill. At 9 A.M., the teachers come around to each ward, bring the child's school bag to him, and get him started on his work for the day. Because of the diversity of ages and grades, individual study is the rule. Every effort is made to furnish the child with the same books and the same kind of instruction he has been receiving in school. Many children bring their school books with them. The school teachers go from child to child, moving on quietly when treatments are due. At noon, materials are collected, then after a rest period, the afternoon is given over to art work and crafts. Excellent rapport is established between nursing and educational personnel. The teachers are employed by the school system, thus school hours and holidays are observed. During the summer months, a play director and volunteers are with the children part of each day, although there is no regular school program.

BIBLIOGRAPHY

Abbott, Nancy, Hansen, Phyllis, and Lewis, Kathryn: Dress rehearsal for the hospital. AJN, *70:*2360, 1970.

Bowlby, J.: Maternal Care and Mental Health. Schocken, 1966.

Child Care Services Provided by Hospitals, U. S. Dept. of Labor: Womens Dept., 1970.

Haller, J. Alex (ed.): The Hospitalized Child and His Family. Baltimore, Johns Hopkins Press, 1967.

Murphey, Lois: The Widening World of Childhood. New York, Basic Books, 1962.

Noble, Eva: Play and the Sick Child. Levittown, N.Y., Transatlantic Press, 1967.

Robertson, James: Young Children in Hospital. London, Tavistock, 1958.

Robertson, James: Hospitals and Children. New York, International Universities Press, 1963.

What to Do When There's Nothing to Do. The staff of Boston Children's Hospital. New York, Delecort Press, 1968.

— —WHY— —Play in a Hospital— —How— —. New York, Play Schools Assn.

Physical Care of the Sick Child 24

GIVING MEDICATIONS TO CHILDREN

Giving medicines to small children is not an easy task. Even a nurse accustomed to preparing medications for adults will experience some anxiety when she contemplates giving them to a child.

Certainly the importance of the right drug in the right dosage at the correct time to the right child cannot be overemphasized. However, administering medications involves much more than this. Of equal importance to both nurse and patient is the nurse's background knowledge of the purpose for giving the drug, its expected action, its potential side effects, and the expected results to be obtained. In addition, none of this knowledge will be of much use if she does not observe the effects of the dosage on this *particular* patient.

Oral Administration

The older practice of a *medicine nurse* worked against this. The medicine nurse's contact with any one patient was brief, limited to the successful administration of the drug. Occasionally she was notified that the child had spit out or vomited the dose and she was asked to give it again.

Indeed, the medicine nurse had little, if any, opportunity to observe the effects of an administered medication on any individual patient. The nurse's duties were strictly routine and ritualistic. This could hardly be dignified by the term "nursing."

The nurse who gives her patient total care prepares herself for administering his medications as well. She checks the purpose for which the medicine is given. Reference books and drug brochures are helpful.

Frequently, research has proven the worth of certain new drugs in alleviating conditions, information that has not yet been included in the standard references. In such cases the nurse should inquire of the physician ordering the drug.

The nurse observes the child under her care for any unusual behavior following administration of any medication. She records all such manifestations, calling attention to the fact that they occurred during the period that a certain drug or drugs were being given. If the presumed reaction is severe or unexpected, she reports verbally as well to the nurse in charge of the department.

Medicine that is vomited immediately after being swallowed can usually be repeated, if the nurse can be sure it has all come up. It is well to check with the nurse in charge, however, as the child may have a hypersensitivity to the drug. When the medication is vomited after being in the stomach for a short period, the nurse always seeks direction before repeating any or all of the dosage.

Fractional Doses

Medications for children are seldom given in adult-size doses. The drug may be received from the pharmacy in the proper dosage for the child or the nurse may be required to compute a fractional dose from the standard size. This is an area where an error in computation can have serious consequences.

The simplest way to determine the amount needed of a standard strength drug is to use the fractional method of computation. Thus, the desired strength divided by the strength of the drug on hand will give

339

the necessary fraction of the full strength drug to be used. As most pediatric medicines are administered in liquid form the nurse simply gives the required fraction of the standard amount. The formula is:

$$\frac{\text{desired dose}}{\text{dose on hand}} \times \text{dilutant} = \text{amount to be given.}$$

For example, elixir of phenobarbital is made up with 20 mg. of phenobarbital in each 5 cc. of the elixir. If the order reads "give 4 mg. of phenobarbital," one would figure 4/20 x 5 cc. (1/5 x 5) = 1 cc. to be given (as this is an elixir it should be well diluted with water before giving it to a child).

After computing the dosage, the nurse should always have her figuring checked by her instructor, the charge nurse, or someone on the department delegated for this purpose. Errors in figuring are easy to make, and also easy to overlook. It is preferable for the second person to do the computation separately, then check both results.

Errors in medications. Nurses are human and can make errors. To admit an error, is often difficult, especially if there has been carelessness or laxity concerning the rules. A person may be strongly tempted to adopt a "wait and see" attitude. This, of course, is the gravest error of all. It is much easier for a nurse to accept the censure of the doctor or the head nurse, whether deserved or undeserved, than to endure the anxiety and guilt she feels while she waits to see if there are to be any ill effects. She certainly should want to avoid, at all costs, the terrible guilt that comes if the child suffers any serious consequences from her error, and which might have been avoided had the mistake been disclosed promptly.

GIVING MEDICATIONS TO INFANTS AND TODDLERS

A small baby is not too particular about the taste of his food if he is hungry. Almost anything liquid can be sucked through a nipple, including liquid medicines, unless they are quite bitter. Medications that come in syrup or fruit-flavored suspensions are easily administered this way. Another method of administering oral medications is to drop them slowly into the baby's mouth with a plastic medicine dropper. If a small medicine cup is used, remember that an infant only swallows a few drops at a time. Too much poured into his mouth may cause him to choke and perhaps to aspirate, or he may simply let the medication run out of his mouth.

When giving medicine to an infant, raise his head and shoulders from the bed, or hold him in a semi-upright position. Be certain to make a positive identification of the child. He is entirely dependent on you, and he cannot tell you if you have the wrong patient.

After giving him the medication, open his mouth to see if he has swallowed all of it. Leave him lying on his side, or with his head elevated, as a precaution against aspiration should he vomit.

Elixirs contain alcohol and are apt to make him choke unless they are diluted. Syrups and suspensions do not need dilution in themselves, but are thick, and they may need dilution to insure that the baby gets the full dose.

Although the nurse knows her patient, it is well to check the medicine card against his identification. A hastily read card, or quick recognition of a child by sight, may lead to an error, particularly with a small child who cannot protest an incorrect dosage.

The age at which children can swallow pills varies greatly. Some quite small children down them readily, whereas other, much older children gag and choke. If you have given a child a pill, make sure that he swallows it before you leave. Usually he opens up so wide that you can see way back to his tonsils.

It usually is best, however, to give a small child his medicine in solution form. If you must use a tablet, dissolve it in water. Do not use orange juice for a solvent unless specifically ordered to do so. The child may associate the taste of orange juice with the unpleasant medicine for the rest of his life. If the medicine is bitter, honey or corn syrup can disguise the taste. He may come to dislike corn syrup, but this is not going to be as important to him as the inability to take orange juice.

An interesting example of one person's use of imagination to help a child take medicine occurred with three-year-old Bobby. He was a cooperative child, but had great difficulty in taking his medicine. He absolutely refused the suspension form, and gagged over the pill. Medicine time became a time of trial. Finally someone crushed the pill, placed it between two layers of honey on a spoon, and told Bobby to take the spoon in his hand and lick it like a popsicle. Thereafter, twice daily, he sat solemnly licking his "popsicle."

There is little excuse for restraining a small child and forcing a medication down. The child can always have the last word if he chooses, and bring it up again. The danger of aspiration is very real. Of even greater importance is the antagonism and helplessness built up in the child by such a procedure. A child's dignity needs to be respected as much as that of an adult.

One does not offer a child a choice, of course, over whether to take his medicine when he really has no choice. Within limits, one can choose the most auspicious time. Small children on waking from sleep are usually bewildered and apt to be negativistic. Waiting a few minutes until the child becomes oriented to his surroundings may be all that is needed. Interrupting a child's meal is usually a poor practice.

Enlisting a child's cooperation is important of course. However, the nurse must be the authority figure here, and show by her kind firmness and matter of fact approach that there is no reason for the child to refuse.

The older child deserves explanation about any treatment or medication. He may still lack the courage to cooperate, but he understands (even if unwillingly) the necessity for the procedure, and he does not lose his sense of self respect.

TECHNIQUE FOR ADMINISTERING ORAL MEDICATION TO INFANTS AND YOUNG CHILDREN
Oral Medication

1. **Preparation**
   a. Compute a fractional dose if necessary; have the computation checked. (See Method for Computing Fractional Doses.)
   b. Prepare according to the form of medication.
      1. *Tablet.* Crush it and dissolve it in a small amount of water or glucose water. If the tablet is bitter, crush it and mix it with honey or with corn syrup.
      2. *Suspension and syrup.* Shake well. Fruit flavored suspensions and syrups do not need dilution unless it is desired.
      3. *Elixir.* Alcohol base; these must always be diluted with an equal amount of water (or more) to prevent aspiration.
   c. Heart medication. Check the apical beat before administration, and compare it with the previous reading for the rate, the quality, and the rhythm. Report any significant deviation.

2. **Administration (Infant)**
   a. Identify the infant.
   b. Pour the medication into a one-ounce disposable bottle. Raise the infant's head or hold him and allow him to suck. (Alternative.) Raise the infant's head, administer the medication with a plastic medicine dropper. Give it very slowly, and allow the infant to swallow before continuing.
   c. Ascertain that the infant has swallowed all the medication before leaving. Look in his mouth.
   d. Place the infant on his side to prevent aspiration.

3. **Administration (Child)**
   a. Crush the tablet and dissolve it in water (for a small child) or give it in corn syrup or honey.

b. Identify the child.

c. Hold the child in an upright position. Allow the child to hold medicine cup if he wants. Give it slowly.

d. If the child resists, use firmness but do not force. Never hold the child's nose to force him to swallow.

e. Allow the child to swallow before continuing.

f. Check his mouth to ascertain that the medication has been swallowed before leaving.

g. If the child vomits, estimate the amount of emesis and report it. Do not repeat the medication unless so ordered.

4. Recording

Record the time, the dosage, the route (p.o.), and the child's reaction, if it is unusual.

Methods for Computing Medication Doses for Children

1. Computing fractional dose from full strength medication:

$$\frac{\text{strength of ordered drug}}{\text{strength of drug on hand}} \times \text{dilutant}$$

(see page 340)

2. Estimated proper dosage of medications for infants and children:

Fried's Rule for infants under one year of age

$$\frac{\text{age in months x adult dose}}{150}$$

Clark's Rule for children of two years of age and over

$$\frac{\text{weight in lbs. x adult dose}}{150}$$

Young's Rule for children of two years of age and over

$$\frac{\text{age x adult dose}}{\text{age in years} + 12}$$

These *estimated rules* are primarily useful to the nurse for validating her understanding of the doctor's order. They provide only an approximate dose which must then be adjusted by the physician to fit the individual patient.

When ordering any specific drug, the physician considers the *proper* dose to be the amount required to *safely* bring about the desired action. The physician may use a formula utilizing surface area of the patient to arrive at a more accurate dosage. The above rules, however, can give the nurse an understanding of the approximate dosage for age or weight of a child. Thus she can spot any gross errors in her computation of fractional doses, or any misreading of an order.

Intramuscular Medications

Children, of course, have the same fear of needles that adults have. Students are reluctant to hurt the child, and frequently cause the very pain they are trying to prevent by inserting the needle slowly. A swift, sure jab is nearly painless, but the nurse must be prepared for the child's squirming and stay calm and sure. She should avoid trying to give an intramuscular injection alone to a small child. A second person is essential if the child is to be held firmly.

Always take time to explain to the child what you are going to do when you give him the needle. He may be too small to understand all of the words, but tell him anyway. Children appreciate being treated honestly. A child who has been told that an injection or treatment will not hurt learns very quickly that he cannot trust adult promises. Neither does it boost the child's morale to be told "Oh, you're a big boy. Big boys don't cry." The child knows the needle does hurt. Moreover, he is *not* a big boy and

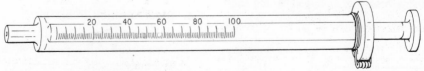

Figure 24-1.   A tuberculin, or 1-cc. syringe. These syringes are calibrated in one hundredths of 1 cc.

there is nothing wrong in crying over a hurt anyway.

Be careful, however, not to spend too much time on preparation. The child can sense your reluctance and is quick to take advantage of it with stalling tactics. He may also find it quite impossible to comply even if he wants to please you. He has a definite need for your firmness. Explain what has to be done, then go ahead and do it.

Intramuscular Injections
Principles

The point of the injection must be as far away as possible from the major nerves to avoid a serious injury to the system. (Note: a serious injury to the sciatic nerve, resulting in paralysis, has occurred following improperly placed injections in the buttocks.)

The nurse giving intramuscular injections should have a basic knowledge of anatomy, particularly about nerve pathways and muscle placement. For example, the gluteal area actually extends to the anterior superior iliac spine—which should be taken into account when measuring the buttock for an injection site.

The muscular area chosen should be sufficiently developed to tolerate the injection. (Note: infants under the age of six months have poorly developed gluteal muscles. The lateral aspect of the midanterior thigh is the preferred site for infants. Some pediatricians prefer this site for young children as well.)

The needle should be long enough to penetrate well within the muscle before depositing the medication. The plunger of the syringe should not be depressed until the needle is well within the muscle.

Equipment

A sterile syringe. A 2 cc. Luer syringe; or a 2 1/2 cc. disposable syringe; or a 1 cc. tuberculin syringe for a fractional dosage computed in one-hundreth of one cc.

A sterile injection needle 20 to 22 gauge, 1 inch in length.

A sterile container with skin preparation material.

Bandaids.

Procedure

1. Prepare the medication under sterile conditions and take it to the bedside.
2. Identify the patient from his identi-band.
3. Explain the procedure to the child.
4. Select the proper site and give the injection deep into the muscle. Withdraw the plunger slightly to check for blood in the syringe before injecting the medication.
5. Apply pressure over the site with sterile cotton, and withdraw the needle. Apply pressure and gentle massage. (Massage may be contraindicated if giving medication such as Imferon.)
6. Apply a Bandaid if there is any oozing.

Selection of the Site

A. Gluteal Area

Muscle: gluteus maximus. Area—upper outer quadrant of the gluteal area.

Method of Selection

1. Place the patient on his abdomen with his toes turned in.

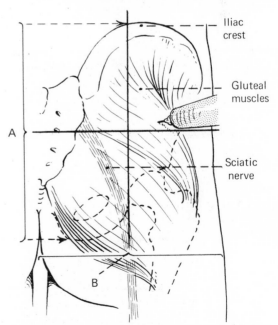

Figure 24-2. Site for an intramuscular injection into the upper outer quadrant of the gluteal muscle.

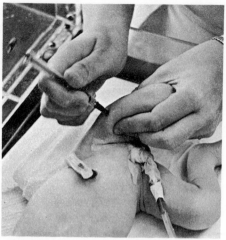

Figure 24-3. An intramuscular injection into the anterolateral aspect of the thigh.

2. Using your thumb, define the anterior superior iliac spine. Fig. 24-2. (Site for I.M. injection into the gluteal muscle)
3. Place your index finger on the head of the trochanter.
4. Define the quadrants of the gluteal mass.
5. Select the inner angle of the upper outer quadrant.

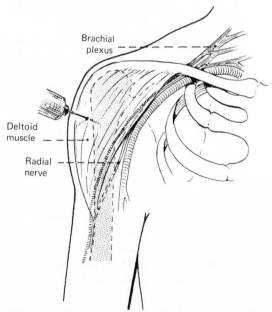

Figure 24-4. Appropriate site for an intramuscular injection into the deltoid muscle.

6. Inspect the area for induration and for trauma from previous injections. Rotate the sites as indicated.
   Note: if a suitable site cannot be found within acceptable boundaries, report this and seek instruction before giving, or use the anterior lateral aspect of thigh (or the deltoid, if approved).
7. A second person should be present to assist when giving intramuscular injections to children. The assistant should help position the child, and can restrain and divert him.
   Note: explain to child that you are helping him hold still, not punishing him.
8. Give the injection as explained in procedure.
9. Comfort the child. Apply a Bandaid as a comfort measure. The child may hold the Bandaid until ready. Allow the child to give an injection to a stuffed toy animal or a doll if he wishes, using a play syringe.

B. Area of Anterior Lateral Aspect of the Thigh
1. Place the infant on his back.
2. Measure the area from the greater trochanter to the patella. Select a site midway between the knee and the hip joint, using the lateral aspect of the thigh.
3. Give the injection as explained in procedure.
4. One nurse alone may give this injection to a small infant. Two nurses are preferable for an older infant.
5. Hold and comfort the infant following the injection.

C. Deltoid Muscle
   The use of this area is limited because of the small space available, the undeveloped muscle in young children and painfulness of the procedure. It may be useful for older children, particularly for those who have limited availability for other sites.
   Only a small area between the upper and lower portions of the deltoid muscle may be used to avoid the radial nerve. Injections should not be made into the middle or the

lower third of the upper arm. Permission should be obtained before using the deltoid area in children.

FUNDAMENTALS OF FLUID BALANCE

Maintenance of fluid balance in the body tissues is essential to health. Severe imbalance, when uncorrected will cause death, as exemplified in cases of serious dehydration resulting from severe diarrhea or from the loss of fluids in extensive burns. A brief review of fundamental concepts of fluid and electrolyte balance in body tissue will help the student understand the importance of adequate fluid therapy for the sick child.

Water

A continuous supply of water is necessary for life. At birth, approximately 77% of body weight is water. This proportion decreases to the adult level of approximately 60%, at about one year of age.

In health, the body's water requirement is met through the normal intake of fluids and foods. Intake is regulated by the person's thirst and hunger. Normal body losses of fluid occur through the lungs (breathing), the skin (sweating), in the urine and feces. In normal health, intake and output balance each other out, and the body is said to be in a state of *homeostasis.*

Homeostasis, meaning a uniform state, signifies biologically the dynamic equilibrium of the healthy organism. This balance is achieved by appropriate shifts in fluid and electrolytes across cellular membrane, and by elimination of end products of metabolism and excess electrolytes.

Body water, containing electrolytes, is situated within the cells, in the spaces between the cells, and in the plasma and blood. Failure to maintain homeostasis may be the result of some pathological process in the body. Imbalance is also the cause of disruption in water, electrolyte and acid-base balances found in many disorders. Some of the disorders associated with imbalance are pyloric stenosis, high fever, persistent or severe diarrhea and vomiting, and extensive burns.

Retention of fluid may occur through impaired kidney action or impaired metabolism.

Intracellular fluid is that fluid contained within the body cells. Nearly half the volume of body water in the infant is intracellular.

Each cell must be supplied with oxygen and nutrients to keep the body in health; also its water and salt levels must be kept constant within very narrow limits.

Cells are surrounded with semi-permeable membrane which retains protein and other large constituents within the cell. Water, certain salts and minerals, nutrients and oxygen enter the cell through this membrane. Waste products and substances produced within the cell are diffused out into the surrounding spaces.

Extracellular fluid is situated outside the cells. It may be *interstitial,* situated within the spaces or gaps of body tissue, or *intravascular,* situated within the blood vessels or blood plasma. *Blood plasma* contains protein within the walls of the blood vessels, and water and mineral salts that flow freely from the vascular system into the surrounding tissues.

Interstitial fluid has a composition similar to plasma except that it contains practically no protein. This reservoir of fluid outside the body cells decreases or increases easily in response to disease. An increase in interstitial fluid results in edema. Dehydration depletes this fluid before affecting the intracellular and plasma supply.

In the infant, about 25% body weight is due to interstitial fluid. In the adult, interstitial fluid accounts for only approximately 15% of body weight. Intracellular fluid accounts for about 45% of body weight in both infants and adults.

The infant and child become dehydrated much more quickly than the adult. In part, this is because of a greater fluid exchange caused by the rapid metabolic activity associated with the infant's growth, and in part because of the relatively larger ratio of skin surface area to body fluid volume; two or three times that of the adult.

Because of the above factors, the infant who is taking in no fluid will lose an amount of body fluid equal to his extracellular volume in about five days, or twice as rapidly as will the adult. The infant's relatively larger volume of extracellular fluid may be designed to partially compensate for this greater loss.*

Electrolytes

Electrolytes are chemical compounds (minerals) that break down into *ions* when placed in water. An ion is an atom having a positive or a negative electrical charge. Ions having a positive charge are called *cations.* Those having negative charge are called *anions.* Sodium (Na^+) is one example of a cation, chloride (Cl^-) is an example of an anion.

Cations and anions must balance each other to function properly. This does not mean they are equal in amount, but rather in equilibrium. The chemical combining activity of cations and anions is expressed in milliequivalents. One milliequivalent of any cation reacts completely with any anion to produce activity.

Important cations in body fluids are sodium (Na^+), potassium (K^+), magnesium (Mg^{++}) and calcium (Ca^{++}). Important anions are chloride (Cl^-), phosphate (HPO_4^{---}), and bicarbonate (HCO_3^-). Electrolytes have the important function of maintaining acid-base balance. Each water compartment of the body has its own normal electrolyte composition.

Acid-Base Balance

The acidity of a solution is determined by the concentration of hydrogen ($H+$) ions. Acidity is expressed by the symbol pH. Neutral fluids have a pH of 7.0, acid fluids below 7.0, and alkalines above 7.0. Normally,

body fluids are slightly alkaline. Internal body fluids have a pH ranging from 7.35 to 7.45. Body excretions, however, are products of metabolism and become acid in character. Normal pH of urine, for example, is 5.5 to 6.5.

Defects in the acid-base balance result either in acidosis or alkalosis. Acidosis may occur in such conditions as diabetes, kidney failure, or diarrhea. Hypochloremic alkalosis may occur in pyloric stenosis due to the decrease in chloride concentration and increase in carbon dioxide.

In normal health, the electrolyte and fluid balance is maintained through the intake of a well balanced diet. The kidneys play an important part in regulating concentrations of electrolytes in the various fluid compartments. In illness, the balance may be disturbed due to excessive losses of certain ions. Replacement of these minerals is necessary to restore health and to maintain life.

Fluid Therapy

Fluid therapy consists of the administration of water, electrolytes, sometimes protein and calories to restore normal fluid balance. It may be needed to make up a body deficit, to replace abnormal losses, or to maintain normal fluid balance.

Fluids may be given orally, subcutaneously, or intravenously. When an illness is not serious and the child is able to take and retain fluids, oral feedings are usually sufficient. Accurate records of intake and output must be kept to ascertain whether the child's intake and output are well balanced. Normally, these should amount to approximately the same amounts.

Oral fluids may be mixtures of glucose, water and electrolytes, for the child who is able to retain fluids taken by mouth. The child can, of course, progress to formula or full liquids and on to solid foods as his condition permits. Certain conditions, such as acute diarrhea, may be aggravated by oral intake. In such cases, parenteral fluids are indicated.

---

*Snively, W. D., Jr., and Sweeney, M. J.: Fluid Balance Handbook for Practitioners. P. 10. Springfield, Charles C. Thomas, 1956.

Parenteral Fluids

Parenteral fluids are commonly given intravenously. Occasionally subcutaneous infusions are given, but this is rarely practiced in children.

Intravenous therapy may be used to correct electrolyte imbalance, as a medium for medication, or as a method of feeding when oral feeding is contraindicated.

Intravenous Infusions for Infants

Because an infant has small veins which are difficult to enter a scalp vein may be used. Scalp veins are relatively easy to enter, and scalp vein infusions are easier to manage. Special scalp vein needles attached to small tubing are available. The area to be used needs to be shaved and cleansed with an antiseptic (Fig. 24-5). The baby should be mummied (see Fig. 24-11) for the insertion, and his head held firmly against the treatment table. After insertion, the needle should be firmly taped in place, and the plastic tubing taped to the side of the infant's head or cheek.

Sandbags are used to immobilize the head, and clove-hitch restraints are useful to prevent the infant from reaching the needle or catching his arm in the tubing.

Other sites are on the back of the hand, the flexor surfaces of the wrist and the medial side of the ankle. The antecubital space is seldom used in small children because it is extremely difficult to restrain the child so that he cannot bend his arm.

Intravenous drip must be slow for the small child, in order to avoid overloading the circulation and inducing cardiac failure. It is extremely difficult to slow a regular intravenous drip to 4 or 6 drops per minute and still have it function properly. Various adapting devices are available which decrease the size of the drop to a "mini" or "micro" drop of 1/50 or 1/60 ml., thus delivering 50 to 60 mini- or micro-drops per cubic centimeter rather than the 15 drops of a regular set. Many intravenous sets also contain a control chamber that is designed to

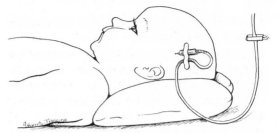

Figure 24-5. A scalp vein infusion.

deliver controlled volumes of fluid, avoiding the inadvertent entrance of too great a volume of fluid into the child's system.

None of these safeguards obviate the necessity of frequent inspection of the therapy. The drops are counted frequently and the site of injection examined. The child's movements frequently cause the infusion to slow up or to speed up, or may cause the needle to slip out of the vein.

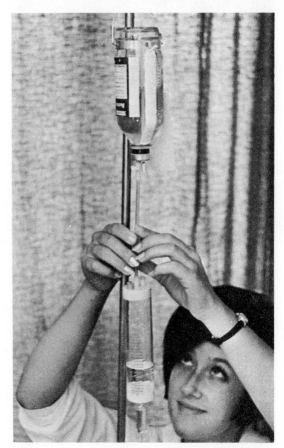

Figure 24-6. Regulating intravenous flow.

Routine recording of the rate and the amount of fluid is necessary.

The intravenous infusion therapy is uncomfortable, and the necessary restraints increase the child's frustration. If the nurse is reasonably careful, and if the needle is securely taped, the infant can frequently be held for comforting and relaxation.

When long-term intravenous therapy is contemplated, an intravenous cut-down is usually performed. This is accomplished by cutting down to the vein and threading in plastic tubing, with two or three silk sutures required to close the wound. This requires a sterile dressing and subsequent removal of the sutures.

A more recent technique that modifies this surgical procedure is the use of an especially constructed needle through which tubing can be threaded into the vein and the needle then withdrawn, thus doing away with the dissection of a cut-down.

The infant needs careful restraint to avoid difficulties at the start of an intravenous infusion as well as to prevent him from dislodging the needle later. The mummy restraint is useful when attempting the scalp vein technique, or a modified mummy leaving an arm or a foot free if another site is used. A clove-hitch restraint for arms or legs gives the infant some freedom, and at the same time prevents interference with continuing therapy, or elbow restraints may be useful. Sandbags are necessary to immobilize the head if a scalp vein is used.

Types of Intravenous Fluids

Intravenous fluids are manufactured to meet many needs—for correcting electrolyte imbalance, for supplying additional protein or carbohydrate, and as vehicles for medications. Many of these, however, still need modification if they are to meet individual infant requirements.

Mixing intravenous solutions requires considerable technical skill, the use of aseptic technique, and correct calculations. It should be attempted only under supervision until the nurse has become proficient. The addition of medication to intravenous fluid also calls for conscientious and experienced personnel.

The older child needs explanation and emotional support during intravenous therapy. Threatening a child with a needle if he doesn't eat (or drink) is encouraging his fantasies of "badness" and punishment. Quite aside from the psychological harm, such treatment rules out any possibility of cooperation from a healthy-minded child. In an emotionally disturbed child, it deepens his despair over his self-convinced lack of worth.

Explanations help clear the air of misunderstandings. For the child old enough to understand, time taken to explain in simple terms the mechanism and purpose of the procedure is time well spent. It will help greatly in obtaining the child's cooperation. Emotional support is of primary importance for any age.

An intravenous infusion does not necessarily interfere with the child's play activities. When the needle is securely placed, the child may usually be allowed up in a chair and into the playroom. His activity is allowed or limited by his understanding, his cooperation, any necessary restrictions, and the presence of an informed and watchful attendant.

ASSISTING WITH PAINFUL TREATMENTS

One of the most difficult duties a pediatric nurse has to perform is that of assisting with, or performing, painful treatments on a small child. Most nurses find satisfaction in perfecting their technique and carrying out a smooth, flawless performance. Their confidence, though, is shaken when they realize that they are causing great discomfort, with the child understanding little of the cause or reason for it. The nurse has an obligation to hide her own feelings when giving or assisting with uncomfortable or painful procedures. The child greatly needs her support at such times. This presents an excellent argument for total care, that is, for one nurse to be responsible for all

Billy, age three, had to have daily treatments which were quite uncomfortable. He was told that he could cry as much and as loudly as he wished, but that he must lie still. Every day Billy marched into the treatment room, helped to arrange himself on the table, and never moved. As soon as the doctor appeared, he opened his mouth and yelled until the treatment was finished, but he did not move. When the nurse said, "You may stop crying now, Billy," he closed his mouth, climbed down from the table and went about his business. It was all a part of the treatment.

the care a child gets during her time on the department.

The pediatric nurse on the toddlers' ward has a greater opportunity to explain than she did on the infants' division; but at best she will be imperfectly understood. Even if the toddler does grasp the words, they have little meaning for him. The big reality is that he hurts.

Sometimes the child's interest can be reached so that he can forget his fright. He must always be allowed to cry if he needs to do so. He should always be listened to, and his questions answered. It takes maturity and experience on the nurse's part to know exactly when the questions are stalling techniques, which call for firmness and action. Frequently, the nurse spends much time talking and reassuring the child, with the result that he senses the nurse's own insecurity. He needs someone to take charge in a kindly, firm manner that tells him that the decision is not in his hands. He is really too young to take this responsibility for himself.

Nurses have conflicting feelings about the merit of giving some reward after a treatment. Careful thought is necessary about this. Whenever a child is given a lollipop or a small toy following an uncomfortable procedure, he tends to remember the experience as not wholly bad. This has nothing to do with his own behavior. It is not a reward for being brave, or good, or big. It is simply a part of the entire treatment. The unpleasant is mitigated by the pleasant.

An older person can supply his own reward by contemplating the improvement in his health, but the little child does not have the background for this.

SAFETY IN THE CHILDREN'S DEPARTMENT

Parents entrust their children to hospital personnel, frequently with many misgivings. It is extremely traumatic to everyone, parents, nurses, and the children themselves, when accidents occur. The nurse needs to realize that she stands in place of the parents during their absence. Not only must she guard against the kind of accidents that can occur in the home, but also against accidents peculiar to the hospital situation.

The problem of giving adequate protection to the young children under our care in the hospital is ever present, and we must exercise greater care and vigilance than we would in our own homes. When a toddler is home, his mother is there to watch him; if he falls, she may blame herself, but she, or someone taking her place, assumes responsibility. When a young child is injured in the hospital, however, it would be an unusual mother who would not think "I wonder if they really watched him carefully enough." Nurses on the children's ward have many children to watch, so they must be unusually careful.

High chairs in the pediatric ward present one hazard for the young person just learning to stand. Nurses, and mothers too, may as well accept the fact that a toddler will try to stand in his high chair; therefore, the sensible thing to do is to prevent the accident before it happens. The simplest and most effective way is to abolish the use of high chairs in the hospital. Low chairs and tables are preferable for children who can sit steadily; a Baby-tenda is good for smaller ones. Of course, he may fall from a small chair too, but the consequences are usually not so severe.

Children love to climb, and an empty crib is fun to climb into and less fun to fall out of. A good rule is never to leave small children unattended while they are up. A familiar sight in many children's departments is to see one, two, or three children

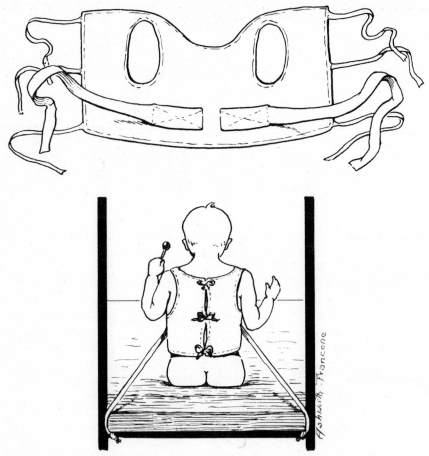

Figure 24-7. Jacket restraint to keep child in crib. Ties may be tied tightly to prevent child from standing in crib, or climbing over sides.

tagging along while the nurse goes to the linen closet or the supply cupboard; and when she takes one child to the tub room, one or two others go along and play happily beside the tub where she can watch them. Crib sides kept up, whether or not the crib is occupied, also removes the temptation to climb in.

No child in restraint, whether it is the jacket type, net crib-cover, or other, should be left unchecked for very long. Children have strangled by getting their heads between the net edge and the crib, or by becoming entangled in the jacket ties. (Fig. 24-7)

Numerous examples verify this possibility of danger. One two-year-old, after misbehaving in the playroom, was put in her crib and the restraint jacket fastened. In a fit of temper, she climbed over the cribside and was found dangling over the side with the jacket pulled up around her neck. She could easily have strangled.

A toddler was told by his doctor that he could "go home today when his mommy comes." A little later he was found wandering the halls looking for mommy to take him home. Climbing over the side of his crib he had pulled the ties off his jacket and reached the floor. Another child might have suffered a serious fall.

Nets over cribs have been used with a tie missing or have not been tied securely enough and toddlers have been caught between net and crib, with great danger of strangling.

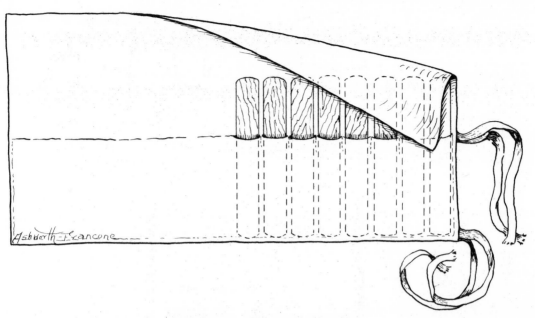

Figure 24-8.   An elbow restraint.

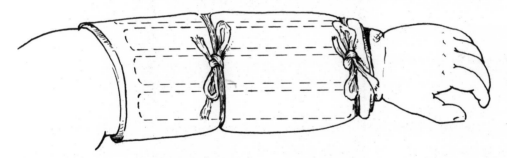

Figure 24-9.   Elbow restraint applied.

Restraints are also necessary to keep a young child or infant from interfering with treatments. To the young child all the medical and surgical treatments mean only one thing: they are uncomfortable. His instinct is to remove anything that hurts him or interferes with his comfort. The nurse should remember that restraints are not to be used unless no other way of preventing damage to his health and safety can be found. Figures illustrate the usual kinds of restraint used in the hospital to prevent the young child from ruining an important test or treatment.

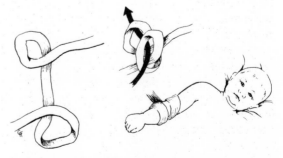

Figure 24-10.   The clove hitch restraint. To keep infant or child from reaching intravenous needle or interfering with dressings.

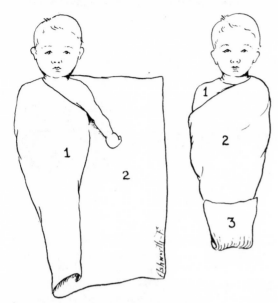

Figure 24-11. Mummy restraint.

BIBLIOGRAPHY

"Fluids and Electrolytes," Abbott Laboratories, 1969

Nelson, Waldo, Vaughn Waldo; Vaughn, Victor C.; and McKay, R. James: Textbook of Pediatrics, ed. 9. Philadelphia, W. B. Saunders, 1969.

Snively, W. D., Jr. and Sweeney, M. J.: Fluid Balance Handbook for Practitioners. Springfield, Charles C Thomas, 1956.

Suggested Readings for Further Study

Conway, Barbara, et al.: The seventh right. AJN, *70:*1040, 1970.

Dickens, Margaret L.: Fluid and Electrolyte Balance: A Programmed Text. Philadelphia, F. A. Davis, 1970.

Metheny, N. M. and Snively, W. D.: Nurses' Handbook of Fluid Balance. Philadelphia, J. B. Lippincott, 1967.

Parenteral Solutions Handbook. Berkeley, Calif., Cutter Laboratories, 1965.

Voda, Anna M.: Body water dynamics—a clinical application. AJN *70:*2594 1970.

UNIT STUDY QUESTIONS

1. The *primary* objective of treatment in severe diarrhea is
   a) to replace the water loss and restore electrolyte balance
   b) to rest the gastrointestinal tract by a period of starvation
   c) restoration of renal function by means of potassium hydrating solutions
   d) to relieve dehydration

2. An infant with meningitis has convulsions, and the doctor orders elixir phenobarbitol 30 mgm. The stock supply bottle label states: 4 cc = 1/4 gr. How much would you give the infant?

   a) 2 cc.
   b) 4 cc.
   c) 6 cc.
   d) 8 cc.

3. Digoxin comes in solution in which 1 cc = 0.05 mgm. The order is for 0.06 mgm, and the nurse gives:
   a) 0.8 cc.
   b) 1.2 cc.
   c) 1.5 cc.
   d) 2.2 cc.

Unit Seven: Overview of Growth and Development

Developmental Norms 25

THE BEGINNING FAMILY

The arrival of the first baby signals the beginning of major changes in the family relationship. The attention each parent has given to his partner, as well as to himself, is now largely diverted to the care of the new member. Traditionally, it is the mother who has her attention thus diverted. However, in most families in today's culture, the father also takes on responsibilities of caring for the baby. Parenthood certainly brings satisfactions and fulfillment to both parents; it also brings much hard work and dull routine chores.

There is still a tendency for many new mothers to devote themselves so exclusively to their infants that their husbands experience feelings of rejection. Their tendency is to forget that the new baby belongs to both parents. This trend is not as noticeable now as it was in the past. Mothers have begun to accept the partnership in all aspects of marriage, and fathers are assuming a share of the responsibility of caring for an infant — a role previously denied them for the most part.

In past society, the mores of western culture decreed that a father stand aloof from participation in matters of child care. Today, fathers see nothing demeaning in sharing the day-to-day care of the young children. They now have opportunity to experience the joys and the sacrifices of family living.

However, it is still the mother who must set the scene for smooth family functioning.

Strang states the matter as follows.* "On the mother, more than on anyone else, depends a healthy fabric of family relationships in which each member develops as a person in his own right, in which no one is the boss, in which each plays his special role in his own appropriate way."

FAMILY DEVELOPMENTAL TASKS

Each family member has his own developmental tasks, which are continually changing as the family develops. The family as an entity has its developmental learnings as well.

In the beginning family, *the mother* must learn a whole new set of skills. She has the tasks of keeping the baby clean and well nourished. She must learn to assess his physical and emotional needs, learning when to meet his needs completely and when to let him develop his unfolding powers at his own pace. While giving freely and perceptively to her infant, she must learn to receive just as freely. She must keep her individuality intact, not surrender her own unique personality.

The *preschool child* learns to share his mother's attention and love with a new baby. He needs help in developing a sense of his own worth and place in the family. He needs freedom for this, as well as recognition from his family that his judgment is

---

*Strang, R.: Introduction to Child Study. p. 31, ed. 4, New York, Macmillan, 1959.

353

immature so that safe limits must be provided for him.

The *older child* becomes subject to many outside pressures, which he in turn brings home to his family. His "all the other kids are allowed to do it" needs evaluation in terms of the values prized by his parents.

The *parents* must reappraise their traditional values in the light of present day culture. They must decide whether to cling to certain habits and beliefs because they are traditional or because they represent moral values pertinent to the society in which they live. A case in point is the furor that developed when young males first decided to let their hair and whiskers grow long. Sober reflection revealed the inconsistency in equating long hair with morality.

If the parents have evolved a philosophy of life that is meaningful and valuable to them, then they have a duty to say firmly "This is the way we do it in our family."

CONCEPTS OF GROWTH AND DEVELOPMENT

A student about to start her clinical experience in the children's department of the hospital may well have misgivings about her own adequacy. How should she handle the child? What can she do or say to give him the security he needs to speed his recovery? How can she help him fit his stay in the hospital into his overall psychological growth? Can she prepare herself to meet his needs with any degree of success? Can she really replace his parents and family? Probably no child can possibly be as happy and free in a hospital as he is at home. But it can make all the difference in the world to him, if the people in his new world understand him and can help him to adjust.

There are important steps she can take to prepare herself to enter this new experience with confidence:

1. Learn the principles of child development. What should she expect of a child at any given age? What is he physically able to do? How much can he understand, and how should things be explained to him? How able is he to cooperate, to adjust, to

show self-control? What should her contribution be? Normal child development is a give-and-take affair.

Some students have found it helpful to start a card file of normal development. After putting down the obvious facts of development—physical, social, emotional, intellectual—the cards are left open ended. The descriptions and tables on the following pages may prove helpful in making such a set of cards. But one thing must always be remembered:

No child will ever follow this idealized description of development exactly. Every child in this world is unique, a true individual with his own pattern. Any outline of development is built from statistics, it tells us what that nonexistent being, the "average child" does. One of the great joys of watching a child develop is seeing how he brings out his own special variations on the pattern. These descriptions are not meant to show what a child "should" do, but to help understand what happens, when it happens.

2. Consider what the effects of illness, hospitalization, separation from the family, fear and loneliness can be on a child at various stages in his development. How can she help to meet his needs at each point?

3. Learn what the effects of particular illnesses and nursing practices are likely to be on any *particular* child. Is an infant in the exploring age being tied down with restraints? Is an outgoing, friendly child being kept in strict isolation? Is a shy, sensitive child faced with too much confusion and boisterous neighbors?

4. Suit her nursing care to the individual child, meeting *all* his needs to the limit of her power. What alternative measures can she use to try to compensate for the frustrating restrictions that a stay in the hospital inevitably places on a child?

Contemporary Child Psychologists

An acquaintance with the work of present day child psychologists will reward the student with a better understanding of the child and of his reactions.

Erikson

Erik Erikson is a psychoanalyst who has built on the theories developed by Sigmund Freud. He describes development as a sequence of events on the biological, psychological, and social planes.

This development depends on the concept of a self-healing process within the individual which helps counterbalance the stresses that natural and accidental crises create. This self-healing process takes time when any major crisis, such as a stay in hospital, disrupts the normal development. It must be expected that even the best of children will regress to things long since left behind. For example, even a fairly old child may begin to wet his bed again when he comes into the hospital. He must not be scolded for this; hospitalization is a shock for a child. It often seems that the mainstays of his life (his mother, his father, his friends, his familiar home and routine) have been taken away from him. How can he be blamed if he begins to feel as bewildered as a baby for a time? Erikson makes the comment that "children 'fall apart' repeatedly, and unlike Humpty Dumpty, grow together again" if they are given time and sympathy, and are not interfered with.*

Erikson formulated a series of eight stages of development to help understand the way in which our attitudes to the world form and change. The first five of these stages pertain to children and youth. In each phase, the child must master the central problem before moving on to the next. He points out, however, that no victory is ever completely or forever won.

The list of stages as formulated by Erikson has become extremely popular, but it has also been much misunderstood. Erikson has especially cautioned against emphasizing the positive aspects without the negative counterparts at each stage.† Nor can these stages be given in terms of exact ages for the child. Every child has his own pace, and each stage overlaps with the ones following and preceding.

Erikson's eight stages of the development of attitudes to the world can be stated in the following fashion.‡

Phase 1 — Infancy: Acquiring a sense of basic trust while overcoming a sense of basic mistrust.

A tiny infant has no way of controlling the world, outside of his cries for help and his hope that the world will love him enough to come to his rescue. It is here that we learn our basic attitudes: can the world be trusted to give love and interest, or is it one in which only frustration, fear, and despair can be expected?

Formerly mothers were taught they must give their child the bottle only at specified times. One nurse was even overheard telling a mother that "if he cries between times, give him only water; you mustn't give milk between hours." An infant's stomach cannot read the clock, unfortunately! In the hospital it is particularly easy to forget that the child must come first and routine second. This is the infant's only experience of the world outside the home. He literally *cannot* wait, when his needs appear.

Phase 2 — Early Childhood: Acquiring a sense of autonomy while combating a sense of doubt and shame.

Even the smallest child wants to feel an individual, and needs to learn to "do it himself" even when this means taking a painfully long time, or making quite a mess. The little child needs to feel the reassurance which comes from feeding himself as much as he can, and from being allowed to crawl or walk whenever it is safe, and from handling and learning about objects in his environment.

You cannot expect a little child to draw a recognizable picture, but one little girl got great joy from making marks on a pad of paper with a pencil, just like the adults near

---

*Erikson, E. H. and Senn, M. J. E.: Symposium on the Healthy Personality. New York, Macy Foundation, 1950. pp. 91-146.

†Youth and the Life Cycle: An interview with Erik H. Erikson. *Children*, v. 7, # 2, March-April, 1960. p. 43.

‡Maier, Henry W.: Three Theories of Child Development. New York, Harper and Row, 1965. p. 31 FF.

her. One small boy was given a piece of carbon paper from a pad, when it might have been thrown into the trash. He remembered for years the delight it gave him to fill out "orders" in duplicate!

Not only does a little child need to have his independence respected, but he also has to learn about the nature of his own body and the world he lives in. Why should he be shamed for being interested in his excretions, or for touching his genital area? This phase is the time when he acquires self-respect and pride or has engrained in him the feeling that somehow he is "dirty, nasty, and bad" just for being a normal human being.

Phase 3—Play Age: Acquiring a sense of initiative and overcoming a sense of guilt.

A little child does not really play with other children, he plays by himself in the company of other children. Gradually he learns to interact with others, both younger and older. But he has his own timing for this, and no amount of pushing is going to help.

A five-year-old boy was given a toy to play with, one that involved fitting together very difficult pieces. It was far beyond his ability, and the first reaction of the adults was to take it away from him "before he ruins it." Actually, the boy got hours of amusement from rolling the pieces across the floor, even though the manufacturers never intended this!

Stringent rules sometimes are needed, but often they make no real sense. Does it really matter in what order the child eats his food? (And the ice cream is likely to be more nutritious than the salad, anyway!) The young child cannot understand clock hours, the coming and going of nurses as shifts change. A word that his nurse is going home to her own family now can help an unhappy child realize she is not deserting him because he was bad.

Phase 4—School Age: Acquiring a sense of industry and fending off a sense of inferiority.

"Oh boy, you can't do anything right!" she said critically, looking at the seven-year-old's drawing, "who ever saw a house look like that? And where's that man's neck?" Of course he cannot get all the details right, but he did get the important things. After all, doesn't *she* appreciate having her own mistakes overlooked sometimes?

Praise, not blame, is the rule of the day. Johnny and Bobby, Susie and Ann may be the same age but they do things differently. Johnny is not Bobby, Susie is not Ann, why should they be told that Bobby or Ann "would never do a thing like that"?

Phase 5—Adolescence: Acquiring a sense of identity while overcoming a sense of identity confusion.

For the first time, he discovers that he not only can but *must* make his own life. Now he discovers that he has to develop a sense of being an independent individual with his own ideas and goals. Sometimes he has to be different, simply to make people understand that he is a person in his own right. Parents or authorities may be right, but even a benevolent dictatorship is still a dictatorship.

Hospital rules said that bedtime was 8 p.m., and the lights were turned off then. One boy, with determined effort, lay awake in bed until midnight (confirmed by church bells outside), just to prove that he could spite the rules. And, incidentally, to prove to himself that his own sleeping needs were best judged by himself.

Phase 6—Young Adulthood: Acquiring a sense of intimacy and solidarity and avoiding a sense of isolation.

This means not only learning to relate to the opposite sex, but joining in with a group of his own sex. He, or she, is no longer a child, and will appreciate being treated as an adult, with both the privileges and responsibilities this involves.

Phase 7—Adulthood: Acquiring a sense of generativity and avoiding a sense of self-absorption.

For most people this means marriage and a family, but for some it may mean fulfillment in some other way (such as teaching, nursing, or a religious vocation). Social responsibilities are a key part of this phase.

Phase 8—Senescence: Acquiring a sense of integrity and avoiding a sense of despair.

Carl Jung commented that a person lives best if he feels "as if he had a million more years to live." This eighth phase is the least understood of all, for it means finding satisfaction with oneself and one's present state, without either regret for the past nor fear for the future.

As you become familiar with the manifestations of development in the infant and child, this outline takes on meaning. There are many detailed explanations and examples in Erikson's own presentation of the stages.*

Piaget

Jean Piaget is a Swiss psychologist who has brought new insight into how a child learns and develops that mysterious something we call "intelligence." He has presented these aspects of a child's development in three steps:

1. The sensori-motor phase (roughly, up to age 2).

Piaget points out that the newborn operates on a sensori-motor level linked entirely to his own desires for physical satisfaction. He feels, hears, sees, tastes, and smells countless new things, and moves his own body and limbs in an apparently random way. His purposeful activities are of the reflex type, that is, a response to the environment. For instance, while nursing at the breast he gazes intently at his mother's face; he grasps her finger, smells the nipple, and tastes the milk. Thus all his senses become involved.

It is very important for the infant to have objects presented to him that are actually far beyond his ability to manipulate. For example, the newborn does not know how to use his hands and arms. The string of bells and tingling objects stretched across his crib may seem useless. But as he waves his arms about, sometimes they strike the string and he hears the sound that is made. It is in this

way that he learns about cause and effect and can experiment on how to use his hands and fingers. It is mostly through making sense of such accidental events that the baby learns how to use objects.

In the same way, a tiny infant cannot understand words or even the tone of voice. But only through hearing conversation directed to him can he begin to pick out sounds and begin to understand. As he produces noises with his own mouth, the responses of those near him, encouraging him when he makes sounds resembling speech, playing when he makes other random sounds, help him learn to talk.

2. The period of preparation of conceptual thought (roughly ages 2-11).

Bobby has four ounces of orange juice in one glass; Johnny has four ounces of orange juice divided between two glasses. Bobby cries "He's got more than me!" Bobby is satisfied as soon as his orange juice is poured into two glasses too. Soon he gives himself "more" orange juice by pouring some of his original supply into still a third glass.

The little child has no clear conception of quantity: if it looks like more, then it *is* more. In the same way, he cannot tell you whether something happened an hour ago, a week ago, or a year ago. He may be able to find his way to the toilet, but he cannot tell someone else how to do it. Even an eight-year-old may not be able to draw a map of the route. That is why table games involving the simple movement of counters along rather simple paths with only one or two detours can keep children in this phase entertained for hours.

A little boy who was very homesick was told by his nurse "you can go home Friday" (it was now Monday). Half an hour later, he was in despair, because he had been "promised he could go home" and now they would not let him go! A simple "no, you cannot go home today" would have been more compassionate, in the long run. Children's stories always begin with "once upon a time" or "long, long ago," because time and space are something *felt* by the

---

*Erikson, E.H.: Childhood and Society. ed. 2, New York, Norton, 1963.

child, not something that can be measured.

3. **The phase of cognitive thought (roughly ages 11 and up).**

Try to find a limit to the 12-year-old's curiosity! He has just discovered the wonderful world of meaning. Now he can deal with abstractions which always eluded him before; he can begin to understand jokes based on double meanings, and how he delights in telling and hearing them! Nothing is too sacred or improper for the inquiring mind.

Freud

Sigmund Freud was an Austrian psychoanalyst whose studies of child development have become so famous that almost everyone has heard of them. Most books and psychologists today base their understanding of children at least partly on his work. His theories of development are concerned primarily with the child's sexual development and appreciation of his own body, as well as with relationships to other people in general.

Freud presented the child's body experiences as developing in coordination with his relationships to the people nearest him. Thus the gradual growth of social adjustment plays a major role in his view of development. Again, it was found most convenient to present development in a series of gradually overlapping stages.

1. **Oral** stage (the first one to two years of life). The newborn is first related almost entirely to its mother (or someone taking a motherly role), and its first experiences with body satisfaction come through the mouth. This is true not only of sucking, which we first think of as "oral," but also of making noises, crying, and often also breathing. For many years after the child has found other means of enjoyment, oral pleasures keep their enticement; candy, ice cream, and other foods become a treat, while most children retain pleasure in playing with new words and sounds. It is through the mouth that the little baby expresses its needs and finds satisfaction, and thus first begins to make sense of the world.

2. **Anal** stage (two to three years of age). This is the child's first encounter with the serious need to learn self control and to take responsibility. Toilet training looms large in so many people's minds, as evidence of the importance this phase once had for them in childhood. Once the art of self-feeding has been accomplished, the task of personal cleanliness follows almost automatically. Because it is one of the child's first experiences of creativity, it represents the beginnings of the desire to mold and control the environment—the mud pie era in a person's life!

Cleanliness and the child's natural pride in what he has created do not always go together, so that it is necessary to help direct his pride and interest into more fruitful paths. This is a very important part of learning to take part in society. Like all of children's play, play with plasticine and other modeling clays, crayons, dough, and the like, helps to put a natural interest to use, a process called sublimation.

3. **Phallic** stage (three to five years of age). It is only natural that interest will move to the genital area as a source of pride as well as of exploration. After all, to the child's concretistic mind, this constitutes the big difference between boys and girls, a difference which is gradually dawning upon him in the social sphere as well. Until now, boys and girls have enjoyed the same toys and games, and have been treated more or less alike. Now the boy begins to take pride in being a male, and the girl in being a female. In many families a new brother or sister comes along at about this time, arousing the child's natural interest in human origins. A hospital setting helps arouse questions that might be delayed or subdued at home and also provides answers the child might not have opportunity for at home.

This is an age when the child's understanding of what it means to be a boy or girl is first forming. It makes all the difference in the world, whether he is made to feel ashamed of being what he is, and told roughly to "stop playing down there," or whether his natural pride is accepted. At stake is whether he learns to feel satisfied with his own nature, or is laden with feelings of guilt and dissatisfaction all his life.

Some doll manufacturers have begun selling dolls with natural genital characteristics in place of the traditional sexless pseudo-boy and pseudo-girl dolls. For most children of this age, boys as well as girls, playing with dolls is a way of working out family relationships and expressing feelings that have been building up inside without fear of retaliation.

4. **Oedipal** stage (five years old, or often earlier). This is basically a time of conflict in the child's emotional relationships between attachment and imitation of the parent of the same sex, and the appeal of the other parent. The boy who for years has looked to his mother as the source of his emotional life as well as his physical well-being, now is confronted by his desire to be a man. The girl, who naturally wants to follow in her mother's footsteps, finds that her father also represents a real attraction. This is not only social but also sexual: It is through contact with parents that the child learns how to build a relationship to the opposite sex— what the interests, attitudes, concerns, and wishes of the opposite sex are. This is not merely a physical interest (although the bombardment of children with very crude stimuli via television contributes to this) but a need to learn the character of the other sex.

A child usually feels rather ambivalent at this age, at one time wanting the comfort and support of his own sex, and at other times disdaining it. It is also a time of beginning embarrassment, when a boy may be acutely embarrassed by having a female nurse insert a rectal thermometer but would not mind if a man did it.

5. **Latency** stage (about six to ten years of age). This is the time of primary schooling, when the child is preparing for adult life but his own initiative in adult living must remain latent, awaiting maturity. It is especially important as the time when the child's sense of moral responsibility is built up. This sense of moral responsibility, called the superego,

is largely composed of what he has been taught (through words and actions) by his parents. In a new setting it is a very difficult matter, because things which loom large in the child's life at home (eating manners, methods of washing, saying thank you, etc.) are disrupted in the hospital and he may often be confused.

In some ways a child in this stage is rather like a well brought up cat that was temporarily being housed by a neighbor. When night came, the cat walked around the room, miaowing mournfully in front of every piece of furniture. Understanding the problem, its new host gently picked it up and placed it on a comfortable chair, where it curled up and went to sleep. It did not want to do something wrong, but it needed help in knowing what was considered right in this house.

Most children want to do what is right, they desperately need the sense of security that comes from approval and praise, but very often they do not know what is expected. A few words of explanation that "this is how we do things here" may help to ease many difficult situations.

6. **Genital** stage (11 years or so). Physical puberty has been coming earlier and earlier as the century has gone by, and social puberty has been moving even earlier, as Vance Packard points out in his recent book The Sexual Wilderness. At this time, all that the child has learned in earlier stages comes together in the service of the most important biological drive, finding and relating to a mate. In earlier societies, mating and the formation of a new family unit took place at a fairly young age, while in our society we have tended to put it off for many years after puberty is reached, thus creating an extraordinary break during which physical and emotional readiness have to be thwarted. It is a time of great confusion and turmoil for most people, and one in which they are most sensitive. Privacy, the need to be alone (which is very difficult to fulfill in hospital settings), uncertainty in dealings with members of the opposite sex, all of these make group life difficult.

In many societies at about the age of 11 or 12 a boy is given an initiation ceremony into the men's world, and strict regulations forbid the feminine world from overpowering him. This may even extend to forbidding his mother or sisters to meet or speak with him! A similar ceremony takes place at a girl's first menstruation, when she is initiated into the feminine secrets of social living. A similar help in orientation is missing in our civilization.

Jung

Carl Jung, a Swiss psychologist who died in 1961, was primarily interested in the inner growth of personality. His contribution to the study of child growth and development focuses on this inner sequence of events.

Jung stresses the fact that human development follows lines which are inbuilt, natural to us as human beings. These patterns of development, which he called *archetypes*, take the place of the instincts which we find in animal life. In human life, the interaction of the child's inner personality with the outside environment is especially clear. For example, a normal child does learn to suck, to crawl, to walk, to be clean, to talk, etc. without any explicit attempt to teach him, but the details come from observing adults around him, and from consciously imitating them.

The interaction of inner development and environment has been most vividly clear in the studies of young children who have been deprived in one sphere or the other. Bowlby's studies of children in institutions, and Bettelheim's studies of children given good physical care but little or no emotional satisfaction, indicate how vital to life psychological interaction is.

During, roughly, the first three years of life the child coordinates the many experiences he has had and the learning he has assimilated to make a conscious personality able to remember, to plan, to reason, and to begin to take responsibility in directing life. The child gains a sense of being "I," a distinct person separate from the rest of the

environment. Thus the negativism of children near the later part of this period is especially important: it indicates that the child, by having the inner strength to say "no," is literally forming a mind of his own.

In the following years, the child gradually learns to make sense of his environment by associating new discoveries to his general way of approaching the world. Dreams, and nightmares, play a role in expressing developments of the personality which for one reason or another do not find a conscious outlet.

Jung lays special stress on the activity of the unconscious in giving direction to development. Life is not a haphazard process, but one in which the psychological center of the self follows a pattern in integrating experiences and forming a consistent personality.

During the first half of life, the principal psychological task is one of learning to adapt to the environment and to society, of finding one's own place in the world. This is the first half of the process of individuation, of becoming a real individual.

During the second half of life (roughly age 40 and up), the main task is to come to grips with the many areas of personality development which were left aside in the interests of making a living, a career, marriage, etc. This involves the formation of new attitudes, new values, and a discovery that the center of life is something within one's own spirit and not centered in the material world or other people.

Jung points out that in a child's development, it is not so much what happens to the child as how these happenings are treated that determine the effect they will have. One child may be used to seeing his parents naked; another may grow up in a very prudish home. Both may grow into healthy, happy human beings or into neurotic persons with serious sexual complexes, depending on whether sexual matters are treated as natural, accepted parts of life. An operation can leave a permanent scar on the child's personality, if it is treated in a cold, brusque, impersonal way, overlooking the child's natural feeling of terror. It may be accepted and perhaps even become a point of pride, if it is carried out in an atmosphere of assurance, support of the child's emotional concern, demonstration of love, and acceptance.

Apart from the work of these various psychologists, whose findings have helped to form an overall picture of the way child development progresses, many studies have been made of the specific skills and abilities of children at various ages. We shall refer to the insights of all these child specialists in the following pages.

BIBLIOGRAPHY

Bettelheim, Bruno: Love Is Not Enough. New York, Macmillan, 1970.
Duvall, Evelyn Millis: Family Development. ed. 4. Philadelphia, J. B. Lippincott, 1971.
Erikson, Erik H.: Childhood and Society. New York, Norton, 1963.
Erikson, E. H. and Senn, M. J. E.: Symposium on the Healthy Personality. New York, Macy Foundation, 1950. pp. 91-146.
Maier, Henry W.: Three Theories of Child Development. New York, Harper, 2nd ed. 1969.
Piaget, Jean: The Language and Thought of the Child. Cleveland, World, 1967.
Strang, Ruth: Introduction to Child Study. ed. 4. New York, Macmillan, 1959.
Youth and the life cycle: An interview with Erik H. Erikson. Children, 7:43, 1960.

Suggested Readings for Further Study

Piaget, Jean: Play, Dreams and Imitation in Childhood. New York, Norton, 1962.
————: The Child's Conception of the World. New York, Humanities Press, 1951.
Schiamberg, Lawrence B.: Piaget's theories and early childhood education. Children, 17:114, 1970.

Unit Eight: The Infant, 28 Days to One Year

Normal Growth and Development of the Infant *26*

The infant who has lived through the first month of life has a busy year ahead. This year he grows and develops at a faster rate than he will ever again. It seems incredible that this helpless, tiny bit of humanity, in the short space of one year, is going to become an individual with strong emotions of fear, jealousy, anger and love; that he will be able to rise from a supine to an upright position, and move about purposefully.

He is expected to gain both weight and height extremely rapidly. During the first six months, his growth is so rapid that he will double his birth weight at 5 to 6 months and add about 6 inches to his height.

The second six months will also be a period of rapid growth, but at a slightly slower rate. At one year of age, he should triple his birth weight.

Remember that the "average" child is no particular child at all. To determine whether an infant is reaching acceptable levels at the proper time, he must be judged in relation to his own birth weight and height. A baby weighing 6 pounds at birth cannot be expected, at 5 or 6 months, to weigh as much as

---

Table 26-1.   GROWTH DURING THE FIRST YEAR

WEIGHT		HEIGHT	
First 5 to 6 Months			
Birth weight (average) range	7 1/2 lb. 5 1/2 to 10 lb.	Birth height (average) range	20 inches 18 to 22 inches
Physiological weight loss during first week of life, due to loss of body fluid and inadequate intake	Up to 10% (normal loss)		
Weekly gain	6 to 8 oz.		
5 to 6 months doubles birth weight		5 to 6 months has grown 6 to 7 inches	
Second Half of First Year			
Now he slows down slightly.		grows approximately 3 to 4 inches during this 6 to 12 month period.	
Weekly gain	4 to 6 oz.		
At 12 months he has tripled birth weight and has grown 10 to 12 inches since birth.			

a baby who weighed 9 pounds at birth, but each is expected to double his own birth weight at about this time. A growth graph is a helpful aid to the nurse or pediatrician for assessing a child's progress.

Table 26-2 gives the average heights and weights of children between the ages of birth and eleven years. The table is based on the average heights and weights of a sampling of white, North American children whose growth ranges between the fifth and 95th percentile for their ages.

Table 26-2. Average Boy-Girl Heights and Weights of Children 0-11 Years

	Height (in inches)		Weight (in lbs.)	
Age	5th P	95th P	5th P	95th P
Birth	18.4	20.9	5.6	9.0
1 mo.	19.7	22.7	7.0	10.5
3 mo.	22.4	25.2	10.0	15.2
6 mo.	24.9	28.0	14.1	20.6
9 mo.	26.8	29.9	16.1	24.6
1 yr.	28.0	31.6	18.1	26.9
2 yr.	31.9	36.6	22.8	32.6
3 yr.	35.3	40.0	26.7	38.1
4 yr.	38.2	43.3	29.4	42.8
5 yr.	40.5	46.3	32.6	48.6
6 yr.	42.8	49.0	35.8	54.7
7 yr.	44.7	51.3	39.3	62.6
8 yr.	46.7	53.9	43.2	71.4
9 yr.	48.5	56.5	46.6	81.3
10 yr.	50.3	59.2	49.8	93.2
11 yr.	51.9	61.5	54.4	105.6

The Continuous Boy-Girl Growth Chart presents a graph on which to plot the individual child's growth. On this chart the age is marked off in months from birth to 1 year of age; in half-yearly intervals from 1 to 2 years; then in 1-year intervals from 2 years to 11 years. It is marked in inches and pounds only. A number of pediatricians have found this chart more convenient for office use than the more detailed charts. Other kinds of charts in common use are the Iowa Growth Chart and the Boston Children's Medical Center Anthropometric Chart.

PHYSICAL DEVELOPMENT OF THE INFANT

Head and Skull

At birth an infant's head circumference is usually slightly larger than his chest circumference. The two become approximately equal at about 1 year of age. The head of the newborn averages about 13-3/4 inches or 35 cm. in circumference. Chest circumference measures approximately the same as the abdomen, and less than that of the head.

The head increases in circumference to approximately 18 inches or 47 cm. at one year of age. The chest also grows rapidly, catching up to the head circumference at about 5 to 7 months of age. From then on it can be expected to exceed the head in circumference.

Fontanelles and Cranial Sutures

The posterior fontanelle is usually closed by the fourth month of life. The anterior fontanelle may increase in size slightly during the first few months of life. After the sixth month it commences to decrease in size, becoming closed between the ninth and 18th months. The sutures between the cranial bones do not ossify until later childhood.

Skeletal Growth and Maturation

During fetal life the skeletal system is completely formed in cartilege at the end of 3 months. Ossification and growth of bones occur during the remainder of fetal life and throughout childhood. The pattern of maturation is so regular that the "bone age" can be determined by radiologic examination of the bones. When the bone age is found to match the child's chronological age, we know that the skeletal structure is maturing at a normal rate.

Eruption of Deciduous Teeth

Calcification of the primary, or deciduous, teeth starts early in fetal life. Shortly before birth calcification begins in

CONTINUOUS BOY—GIRL GROWTH CHART

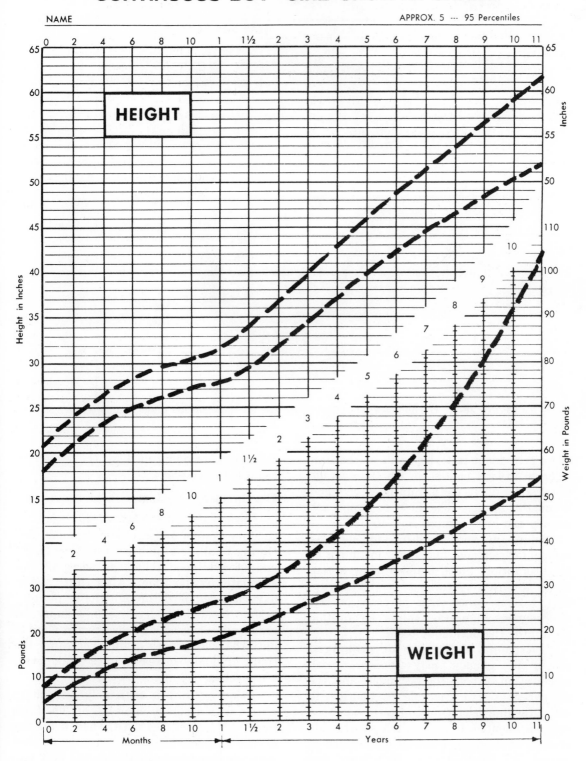

NAME

APPROX. 5 --- 95 Percentiles

HEIGHT

WEIGHT

Jaworski, A. and Jaworski, R. A.: Clin. Pediat. 7:189, 1968.

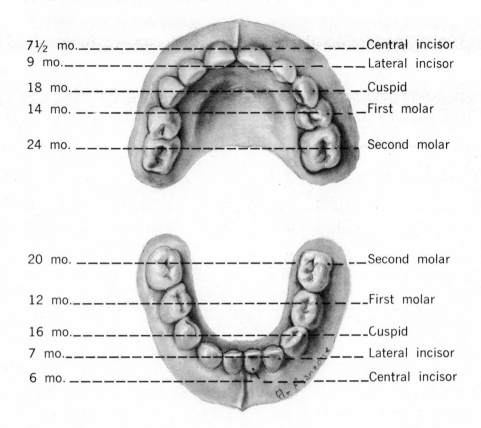

Figure 26-1.   Graph showing approximate age for the eruption of deciduous teeth.

those permanent teeth that will be the first to erupt in later childhood. On the average the first deciduous teeth erupt between 6 and 8 months of age. The first to erupt are usually the lower central incisors.

Babies in good health and showing normal development may differ in timing of tooth eruption. Some families show a tendency toward very early or very late eruption, without other signs of early or late development. Figure 26-1 shows the eruption pattern of the deciduous teeth.

Nutritional deficiency or prolonged illness in infancy may interfere with calcification of both the deciduous and the permanent teeth. The role of fluoride in strengthening calcification of teeth has been well documented. In areas where the fluoride content of drinking water is inadequate or absent, its administration to infants and children is recommended by the American Dental Association.

The Circulatory System

During the first year of life the circulatory system undergoes several changes. During fetal life a high level of hemoglobin and of red blood cells was necessary for adequate oxygenation. After birth when oxygen is supplied through the respiratory system, hemoglobin decreases in volume and red blood cells gradually decrease in number until the third month of life. Thereafter the count gradually increases until adult levels are reached.

Blood pressure is extremely difficult to obtain with accuracy in an infant. The flush method is sometimes used when a reading of the systolic blood pressure is desired. Average blood pressure during the first year

Table 26-3. HEMATOLOGICAL VALUES DURING THE FIRST YEAR OF LIFE

		Birth	1 month	3 months	6 months	12 months
Hemoglobin g/100 ml.	Average	19	14	11	11.5	12.0
	Range	(14—24)	(11—17)	(10—13)	(10.5—14.5)	(11—15)
Red cells/cu. mm. x 1,000,000	Average	5.9	4.7	4.0	4.5	4.6
	Range	(4.1—7.5)	(4.2—5.2)	(3.5—4.5)	(4.0—5.0)	(4.1—5.1)
White cells /cu. mm. x 1000	Average	17	11.5	10.5	10.5	10
Platelets/cu. mm. x 1000	Average	350		260		260

of life is 85/60. However, variability can be expected to exist among children of the same age and body build.

An accurate count of the infant's *heartbeat* requires an apical pulse count. Place a stethoscope over the left chest in a position where the heartbeat can be plainly heard, and count for a full minute. During the first year of life an average apical beat ranges from 70 (asleep) to 150 (awake), and up to 180 while crying.

Body Temperature and Respiration Rate

Body temperature follows the average normal range, after the initial adjustment to postnatal living. Respirations average 30 per minute, with quite a wide range according to the infant's activity.

Maturation and Development

As the young baby develops, his nerve cells mature, his fine muscles learn to coordinate, and he follows the developmental schedule of his peers. Naturally, his mother is full of pride if he learns to sit or stand before the baby up the street, but actually such precocity means very little. Each child follows his own rhythm of progress, within reasonable limits.

However, we need to have knowledge of average rates of growth and development for purposes of evaluation. Also, there are a few important landmarks that call for special attention, even though their absence may mean only a lack of environmental stimulation. The difficulty arising from too great dependence on routine developmental

tables is that we may take them too seriously. A mild time lag will probably mean nothing. A greater lag may call for greater stimulation from the environment, or a watchful attitude to discover how development is proceeding overall.

The following tables give accepted norms for development in motor, adaptive and social behavior, for the first year.

Normal Development at Four Weeks of Age

1. There is visual fixation and eye-following of a bright object moving within the line of vision.
2. Intent regard of the human face with diminution of body movements.
3. Body activity may cease momentarily at sounds such as a bell tinkling.
4. Head lag is still present when pulled to sitting position.
5. When placed prone on a firm surface, the baby lifts his head. Turns head from side to side.
6. Tonic-neck, grasp and Moro reflexes are still active. Hands are kept fisted.
7. Makes small, throaty sounds.

Eight Weeks

1. Social smile appears at 6 to 8 weeks. This is an important landmark.
2. There is more consistant eye-following of moving objects. Eyes follow a moving person with concentrated attention.
3. Turns head toward musical sounds. Blinks and stops movement at loud sounds.

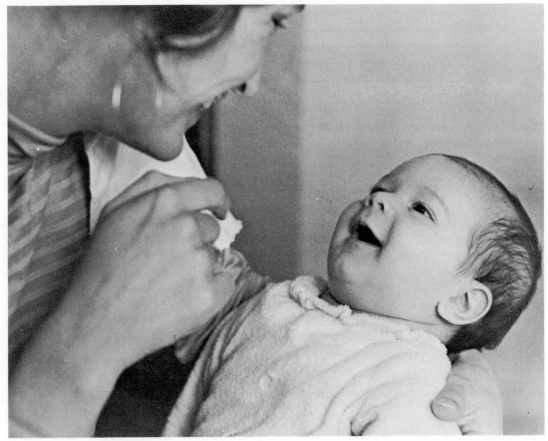

Figure 26-2. Mother and child getting to know each other. (Photograph by Peter T. Whitney.)

4. Quiets in anticipation of food when picked up.
5. Rolls from side to back.
6. Pays attention to speaking voice.

Twelve Weeks

1. Some head control when drawn to sitting position. Irregular head control when held upright; head bobbing present.
2. Active grasp attempts to make contact with offered object. When object put in his hand, holds briefly.
3. Visual inspection of objects. Stares at own hand with apparent fascination when it appears in his field of vision.
4. When placed in prone position, rests on forearms and keeps head in midline.
5. Produces vowel sounds with evident pleasure on social contact.

6. Relatively indiscriminating as to persons. If social smile is absent, look for cause.

Sixteen Weeks

1. Tonic-neck position is gradually abandoned as the predominate position during the third and fourth months. The head is generally in midline, the arms and legs symmetrical.
2. Eye-hand coordination improved, making him adept at making contact with objects within his reach. Brings objects to midline and to mouth.
3. Greatly enjoys being supported in a sitting position. Holds head steady without bobbing.
4. May begin to be responsive to emotional tone of contacts. Coos, bubbles, chuckles

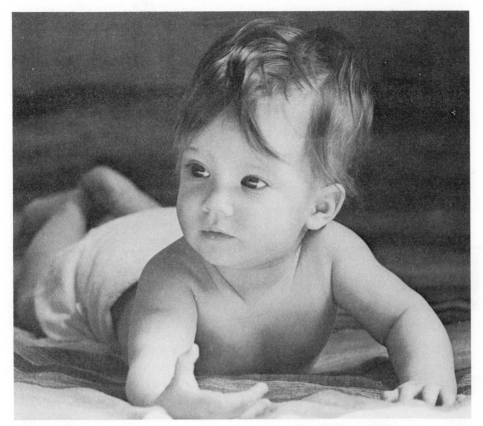

Figure 26-3. At about four months the child raises himself from a flat surface. (Photograph by Carol Baldwin.)

and laughs. Also, shows displeasure by facial expression, fussing and crying.
5. Capable of vivid smile when mother or other familiar person approaches. May sober at sight of stranger.

Sixteen weeks marks a period of developmental transition. From now on rapid cortical organization brings about important correlation of sensorimotor behavior.

Five to Seven Months

1. Commences to make repetitive vowel sounds.
2. Rolls over from prone to supine and reverses.
3. Responsive to emotional tone of contacts.
4. Enjoys shaking rattle or toys.
5. Learning to localize sound.
6. Commencing to discriminate strangers

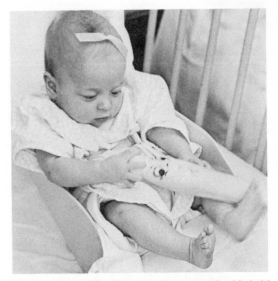

Figure 26-4. The three- to four-month-old child enjoys being propped and can focus attention on objects he can hold.

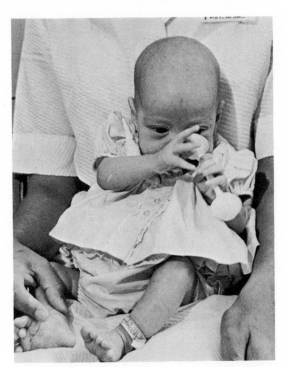

Figure 26-5. Eye and hand coordination are good at four months.

and show preference for person giving most of his care.

7. Bouncing and weight bearing when held upright.
8. Has discovered feet—eventually learns to put them in his mouth.
9. When prone, pivots in pursuit of object. (About 7 months)
10. Transfers objects from hand to hand, to mouth. (About 7 months)

Eight to Ten Months

1. Assumes sitting position without help.
2. Learns to creep or crawl with increasing dexterity.
3. Attentive to sound of own name. Makes repetitive consonant sounds.
4. Develops complete apposition of thumb and forefinger. Uses index finger for poking.
5. Can release toy by opening entire hand.
6. Starts to enjoy dropping objects at about 10 months. Watches carefully when they are picked up, tries the experiment again.

7. During latter part of period pulls self to feet and cruises sideways, holding on to chair or playpen rail.
8. If taught, can learn to clap hands, wave bye-bye, at about 10 months.
9. Feeds self food he can hold in his hand.

Ten to Twelve Months

1. Is less dependent on mother, can follow her. Apparently has developed knowledge that out of sight does not mean complete disappearance. Helps own understanding by playing peek-a-boo.
2. Imitative behavior progresses.
3. Understands "no-no!"
4. Listens intently to words. His parents may read meaning into some of the one-syllable sounds he uses.
5. Smiles at his own image in mirror.
6. Enjoys playing ball with familiar person.
7. Extends object for release into offered hand. Expects to have it returned.
8. Enjoys being center of group. Repeats performance laughed at.
9. Feeds self with fingers.

NUTRITION IN INFANCY

Except for vitamins C and D, and iron, the young infant receives the nutrients he needs for normal development from milk, either breast milk or modified cow's milk formula. A healthy, full-term infant will have stored enough iron in his tissues to supply him for about the first 4 months. His need for vitamins C and D are supplied by the addition of these to his milk diet in the form of vitamin drops or by irradiation of cow's milk to produce vitamin D. Daily amounts required for nutritional health remain constant during the first year. These are 30 mg. of vitamin C and 400 units of vitamin D.

Fluoride is needed in minute quantities for strengthening calcification of the teeth and preventing tooth decay. In areas where the water supply is deficient in fluoride, a solution of sodium fluoride can be given by mouth, or mixed vitamin-fluoride drops can be used.

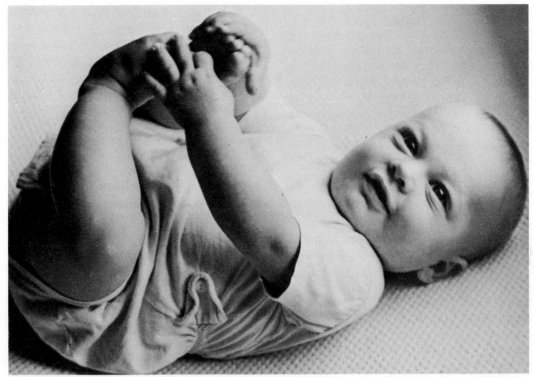

Figure 26-6. About the fifth to the seventh month the child has discovered his toes and attempts to put them in his mouth. (Photograph by Carol Baldwin.)

Addition of Solid Foods

There is no exact time or order for starting solid foods. At about 4 to 6 months the infant's iron supply becomes low and he needs supplements of iron-rich foods. Some pediatricians like to start the addition of foods other than milk during the first 4 to 6 weeks of life. The addition of cereal is particularly helpful for the young infant with a large appetite which is not satisfied with the calories provided by his intake of milk.

Cereals, fruits and vegetables are usually well tolerated. Many infants slow in accepting new foods seem to accept fruits more easily. Applesauce and raw, well ripened bananas are good starters. Strained meats are usually started early in the first year. Hard boiled egg yolk may also be added. Egg white is usually delayed until late in the first year because of the frequency of allergy among infants to egg albumen.

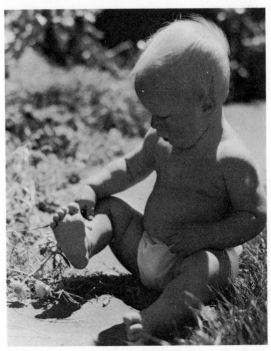

Figure 26-7. The child explores new sensory experiences. (Photograph by Carol Baldwin.)

Infant Feeding

The baby knows only one way to take food, and that is to thrust his tongue forward as if to suck, which of course has the effect of pushing the food right out of his mouth. The process of transferring food from the front of the mouth to the throat for swallowing is a complicated skill that must be learned. The eager, hungry baby is quite puzzled over this new turn of events, and is apt to become frustrated and annoyed over this routine. "What is all this nonsense, anyhow? Where's my bottle?" he is likely to protest in loud and clear terms. In fact, it is best to let the very hungry baby take the edge off his appetite with part of his formula before proceeding with this new procedure. (Fig. 26-18)

Babies like their food smooth, thin, lukewarm and bland. If a mother understands that the queer look she gets from her baby is one of astonishment, and that the pushing out of food with the tongue does not mean rejection, she can be patient.

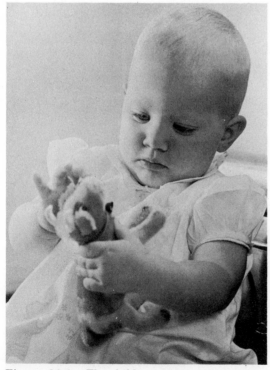

Figure 26-8. The child examines a toy using a good grasp and fine motions. (Photograph by Carol Baldwin.)

The baby's clothing (and his mother's too) needs protection when he is sitting in his mother's arms. A small spoon fits his mouth better than a large one, and makes it easier to put food further back on the tongue, but not far enough to make the baby gag. The mother needs to catch the food if it is pushed out and offer it again, but her baby soon learns how to manipulate his tongue, and comes to enjoy this novel way of eating.

Foods are started in small amounts, one or two teaspoonsful daily. The choice of mealtime does not matter. It works best, at first, to offer one food for several days until the baby becomes accustomed to it before introducing another.

When the teeth commence to erupt, the infant appreciates a piece of zwieback or toast to practice chewing on. About this time chopped foods can be substituted for pureed foods. The formula will probably be changed to whole milk or reconstituted evaporated milk around 4 to 6 months of age. The infant will soon commence to learn to drink from a cup, although he doubtless will derive comfort from sucking at breast or bottle for some time to come.

Preparation of Foods

A great variety of pureed baby foods, chopped junior foods and prepared milk formulas, are on the market, and they certainly relieve the mother of much preparation time. It should be remembered, however, that prepared foods involve a considerable expense that many families can ill afford.

The nurse can be helpful and point out that there is no magic in prepared baby food, that vegetables and fruits can be cooked and strained at home, and are just as well accepted by the baby. Cereals can be cooked, and formulas prepared at home as well. Some families prefer to spend more for the convenience and economize elsewhere, but no one should be made to feel that a baby's health or well-being depends on commercially prepared foods.

The well baby's appetite is the best index of the proper amount of food. Healthy babies

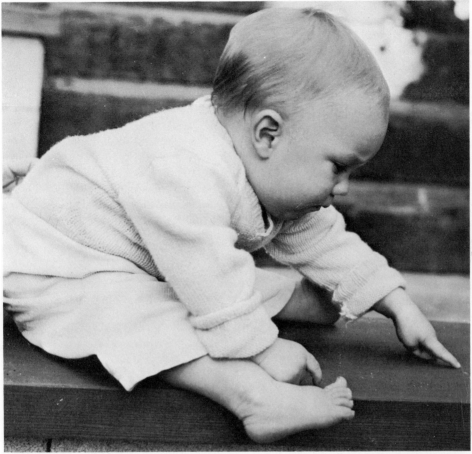

Figure 26-9.   The eight- to ten-month-old child can use his finger for poking. (Photograph by Carol Baldwin.)

enjoy eating and accept most foods, preferring those that are slightly sweet or slightly salty, but not strong-flavored or bitter. Realizing that a baby learns by imitation, we should be careful not to show our dislikes or prejudices against certain foods in his presence. If the baby does show a definite dislike for any particular food, there is no point in forcing it, because this is one of the best ways to make certain that he sees feeding time as an occasion for a battle of will power. However, a dislike for a certain food does not need to be permanent, and the rejected food may be offered again at a later date. The important point is to avoid making an issue of likes or dislikes. As has been aptly put, "A child will find it much easier to learn to like squash, for example, if he does not have a reputation as a squash hater to live up to."

Self-Feeding

The infant has an overpowering urge to investigate and to learn. He early grabs the spoon from his mother, examines and mouths it. He also sticks his fingers in his food to feel the texture and to bring it to his mouth for tasting. All this is an essential part of his learning experience. Messy, yes, but important. After preliminary testing, his next task is to try feeding himself. He soon finds the motions involved in getting a spoon right side up into his mouth are too complex for him, and he drops the spoon in favor of his fingers. But he returns to the spoon again and again until he eventually succeeds in

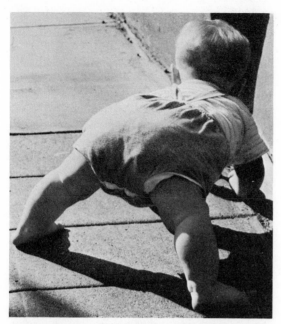

Figure 26-10. The child learns to walk on his hands and feet. (Photograph by Carol Baldwin.)

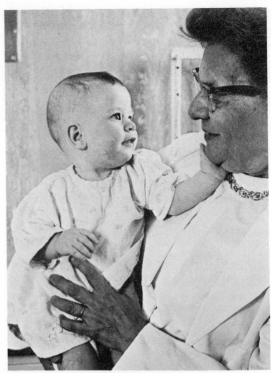

Figure 26-12. The eight-month-old child is interested and friendly with people she knows.

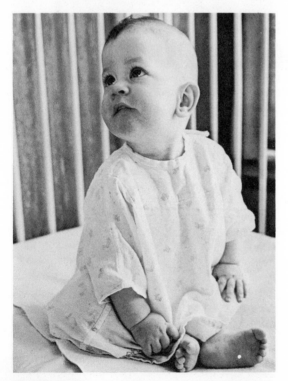

Figure 26-11. At eight months sitting alone is no problem.

getting some food from spoon to mouth at least part of the time. The nurse can help mothers understand that all this is not messing, to be forbidden, but rather it is a very necessary part of the infant's learning.

Weaning the Infant

Weaning, either from breast or bottle, needs to be attempted in a gradual manner, without fuss or strain. The infant is still testing out his environment, and an abrupt removal of his main source of satisfaction—sucking—before he has conquered his basic distrust of his environment may prove detrimental to his normal development. The speed with which weaning is accomplished should be suited to the individual infant's readiness to give up this form of pleasure for a more mature way of life.

As in all areas of childhood advancement, there must be a reciprocal balance between him and those caring for him. At the age of 5

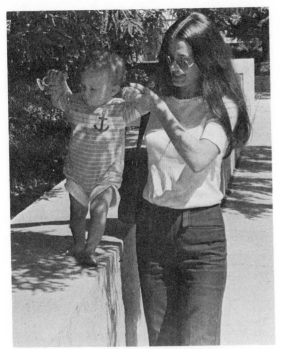

Figure 26-13. The child learns to walk. (Photograph by Peter Whitney.)

or 6 months the infant who has watched others drink from a cup will usually be ready to try a sip for himself when it is offered. He seldom is ready at this point to give up the pleasures of sucking, however, for some time to come. Some babies will gradually wean themselves. Others will be as fond as ever of sucking, and view any change with suspicion.

Forcing or urging creates more resistance and suspicion. It is better to let the infant follow his own timetable. An infant who takes his food from a dish and his milk from a cup during the day may still be most reluctant to give up his bedtime bottle. Unless the mother has strong feelings against this practice, there seems no reason to deprive him of this.

The breast-fed baby may continue nursing along into the latter half of the first year. He then can wean directly to the cup. This, says Dr. Lowenberg,* is the most

*Spock, Benjamin M. and Lowenberg, Miriam E.: Feeding Your Infant and Child. New York, Pocket Books, 1967.

natural pattern and insures the full physical, emotional and practical benefits. However, she points out, most mothers are not willing to nurse that long.

A few babies, although accepting food from a spoon, resist drinking from a cup. Fruit-flavored yogurt, custards, and other milk dishes will help fill their milk needs until they become accustomed to drinking from a cup.

The average infant who is still depending on his milk intake to supply his nutritional needs can afford to take his time about accepting solid foods. During the second half of his first year his milk consumption is not likely to be sufficient to meet his caloric, protein, mineral and vitamin needs.

The following list gives the recommended dietary requirements during the first year of life†:

Calories	100-120/kg of body weight
Protein	2-3 gm/kg of body weight
Fat	No specific quantity set
Carbohydrates	25-55% of calorie intake
Calcium	1.0 gm/day at one year of age
Iron	5-7 mg/day
Vitamin A	1500 I.U./day
Thiamine	0.4-0.5 mg/day
Riboflavin	0.5-0.6 mg/day
Niacin	6-7 milliequivalents/day
Vitamin C	30 mg/day
Vitamin D	400 I.U./day

MAINTENANCE OF HEALTH

Every infant is entitled to the best possible protection against disease, and because he cannot take the proper precautions himself, our duty is to do it for him. This care extends beyond his daily needs for food, sleep, cleanliness, love and security, to concern for his future health and well-being.

Within a very short span of time, medical science has discovered measures providing immunity against a number of serious or crippling diseases without the person having to provide his own immunity by contracting the disease itself. Because of the means at hand (which, at a very minimum of risk, assure protection against conditions such as diphtheria, smallpox, tetanus, polio and

†One kg. equals 2.2 lbs.

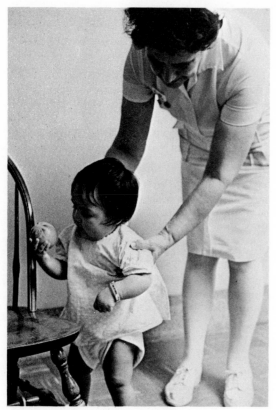

Figure 26-14. This one-year-old needs a little support and she will soon be walking.

measles) we cannot afford to take chances with our children's health with inadequate immunization.

The chronically ill child may not need to forego this protection, depending on his condition and our present knowledge; but whether he is given immunization, or protected from contact from these diseases, is a matter to be discussed in connection with the condition itself. The immunization schedule here presented concerns the healthy child.

Immunization Schedule

The Academy of Pediatrics, through its committee on the control of infectious diseases, has recommended a schedule of immunization for healthy children living under normal conditions. Children with certain chronic or acute conditions, or children who can be expected to be exposed to certain infectious conditions such as typhoid, need a modification of schedule.

The Report of the Committee on Infectious Diseases, known as the Red Book, is published at frequent intervals by the American Academy of Pediatrics. Reference numbers in the schedule refer to pages in the

Table 26-4*

Recommended Schedule for Active Immunization and Tuberculin Testing of Normal Infants and Children.

2 months	DTP · Trivalent OPV
3 months	DTP
4 months	DTP · Trivalent OPV
6 months	Trivalent OPV
12 months	Tuberculin Test · Live Measles Vaccine
15—18 months	DTP · Trivalent OPV · Smallpox Vaccine
4—6 years	DTP · Trivalent OPV · Smallpox Vaccine
12—14 years	Td · Smallpox Vaccine · Mumps Vaccine
Thereafter	Td every 10 years—Smallpox Vaccine every 3—10 years Rubella Vaccine

DTP = diphtheria and tetanus toxoids combined with pertussis vaccine. Td = combined tetanus and diphtheria toxoids (adult type) for those over 6 years of age in contrast to diphtheria and tetanus (DT) containing a larger amount of diphtheria antigen. OPV = trivalent oral poliovaccine.

*Reprinted by permission of the American Academy of Pediatrics from its Report of the Committee on Infectious Diseases, ed. 16, 1970 (Red Book).

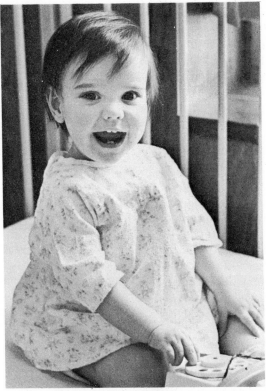

Figure 26-15. This nearly one-year-old is happy.

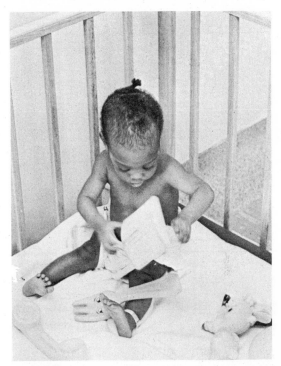

Figure 26-16. The one-year-old is interested in turning the pages of her book.

Red Book on the various infectious diseases, where more detailed information on immunization measures is given.

PSYCHOSOCIAL DEVELOPMENT

The very young infant experienced the give-and-take of life when his need for food induced him to seek it actively. When he was fed on demand he was enabled to build up his sense of trust in his world. However, he was not aware of trying to get something from another person. His only awareness was of his own need to gain comfort and to avoid discomfort, and of the satisfaction that came in response to his need.

Eventually he became aware that every felt need of his was not always met immediately on his demand. Dimly he began to sense that it was not his discomfort itself that supplied its own relief. Rather it was something outside himself that responded to his need. Gradually he learned that through

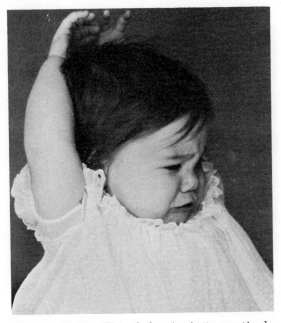

Figure 26-17. This baby is just overtired. (Photograph by Carol Baldwin.)

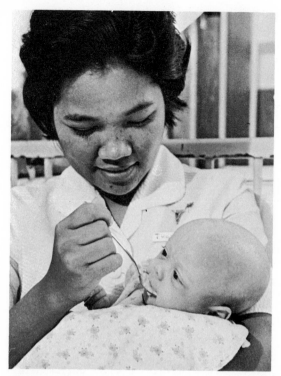

Figure 26-18. A baby tends to push his first solids out of his mouth with his tongue.

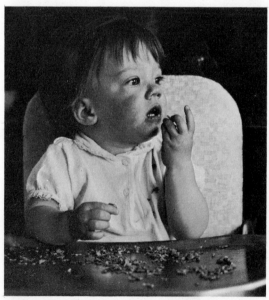

Figure 26-19. This child is feeding herself. (Photograph by Carol Baldwin.)

his own efforts, his own signals, he influenced his environment to respond to his desires. Previously he had not been aware that he and his environment existed separately and interacted.

Bettelheim puts it this way: "The importance of the entire process for the development of a self can hardly be overrated. With it, the ego expands from one that only acts into one that interacts, that responds to others and becomes slowly aware that it can modify their responses."*

An infant whose needs are consistently unmet, even though he exhausts himself in efforts to influence the outside world, will become discouraged and stop trying. After he has experienced repeated rebuffs, he concludes that he was mistaken, his own actions have no effect on the outside world. His tendency then is to withdraw within himself.

The mother who expects too much too soon from her infant is not encouraging his optimal development. Rather than teaching him the rules of life before he has learned to trust his environment, she is actually teaching him that he can gain nothing by his own activity, that the world will not respond to his needs.

Conversely, the mother who rushes to anticipate the infant's every need gives him no opportunity to test his environment. He has difficulty developing the understanding that his own actions have manipulated the environment to suit his desires.

It is said that a child who was never satisfied in infancy lives in perpetual fear lest his needs remain unsatisfied. Here we see a child whose efforts to overcome the basic mistrust of his nature failed through lack of a mutual give-and-take.

Of course, no mother is perfect, indeed a perfect mother would be totally incapable of guiding her child. She would not be able to tolerate his fumblings, his regressions. The ordinary mother is certainly going to misinterpret his signals at times. She may be

*Bettelheim, Bruno: The Empty Fortess. p. 26. New York, Free Press, 1967.

tired, preoccupied, responding momentarily to her own needs. She may not be able to cure his physical pain or to ease his restlessness. This too is learning.

As mentioned earlier, the infant's development is dependent on a reciprocal relationship between himself and his environment. The very young infant demonstrates this when he accidentally strikes his hand or foot against a hanging object and sets it moving. The movement captures his attention. After a few more accidental battings, his actions become purposeful; he fully expects the object to move when he hits out at it. If it does not respond, he very quickly loses interest and does not try again. Very early in his life he learns to expect that when he is picked up in response to his cry he will be fed, and he quiets in anticipation, even before the food appears.

Piaget speaks of intellectual development as a result of interaction between current patterns and the present stimuli. During the first few weeks of life actions such as kicking or sucking are simple reflex activities. In the next sequential stage, reflexes are coordinated and elaborated. For instance, the child's eye follows his random hand movements.

The child finds that repetition of chance movements brings interesting changes, and in the later part of the first year his acts have become clearly intentional with the expectation that certain results follow certain actions.

An infant soon learns to connect the one smiling face looking down at him with pleasurable experiences such as being picked up, fed, or bathed. His face lights up and he squirms with anticipation. At first he reacts in this manner toward anyone who smiles and talks softly to him. But in only a few weeks he learns that one particular person is the source of his comfort and pleasure.

An infant cannot apply abstract reasoning. He understands only through his senses of sight, of touch and taste. As he matures enough to recognize his mother or mother-figure, he becomes very fearful when she disappears. Out of sight has always meant, to him, out of existence. This, of course, he cannot tolerate. So he sets about the task of assuring himself that objects and people do not become nonexistent when out of sight. This is a very real learning experience he sets up for himself, for on it depends his entire attitude toward life.

It is interesting to note the manner in which an infant seeks to assure himself of the permanence of objects and persons. The game of peek-a-boo is an ancient and universal example. It is also one of the joys of infancy, as the child affirms his ability to control his own disappearance and reappearance. "The game of peek-a-boo is a replay in safe circumstances of the frightening feeling of non-being followed by the joyous affirmation of aliveness in the recognition accorded the child by the intimacy of eye to eyeness."* In the same manner by which he affirms his own existence, he confirms that of others, even when temporarily hidden and out of sight.

Emotional Support for the Hospitalized Infant

The infant in the hospital finds his development retarded to the degree that his normal pattern of living is hampered. Probably a short-term illness is not going to present him with any grave psychological problems if he is given the affection and loving care that his nature demands, and if he is promptly restored to his family. A long-term hospitalization presents different problems, even if the infant is receiving considerable attention during his stay.

What happens to the baby who lies in the hospital for long periods of time, with little manifestation of love that he can understand and little tactile stimulation? Illness in itself is frustrating, causing pain and discomfort, and forcing limitation of normal activity. None of this is understood by the infant. Add to all of this a cold, sterile atmosphere, little

*Maurer, Adah: The Game of Peek-A-Boo. Diseases of the Nervous System, February, 1967. p. 119.

cuddling or rocking, and you find that cleanliness and treatment of illness is not enough. Not once or twice, but often, a pediatrician has sent home a baby who has not been responding to treatment in the hospital, to find that the baby commenced to thrive in a home that may lack cleanliness and proper hygiene, but is rich in warmth and love.

The pediatric nurse must thoroughly understand and accept the principle that rocking and cuddling a child, playing with him, or perhaps just the watchful observation of a sick infant, are all essential elements of nursing care.

Hospitalization for an infant may have other adverse effects. The small infant's maturation moves along largely as a result of his physical development. The infant hindered by his environment from reaching out

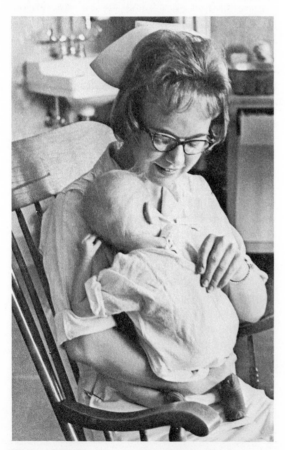

Figure 26-20. Nursing is cuddling.

and meeting the challenge presented to him by his developing senses becomes apathetic and ceases to learn. Therefore, it is natural that illness and confinement may cause regression.

The principle seems to be well understood, but it is not always taken into account; for instance when physical restraints are put on a child. Restraints are frequently necessary to keep the child from undoing necessary procedures or from harming himself. Doctors and nurses have on occasion been guilty of applying restraints when a little watchful care would have made them unnecessary. When restraints are needed, it should be compensated for by the nurse or aide with considerable evidence of affection and with any possible measures available to relieve the baby's discomfort.

The infant placed in an isolation unit suffers considerably from loneliness. He is deprived in large degree from the sensory stimulation so essential for his emotional development. All too often, the only diversion offered him is contemplation of the bare walls. This is not necessary. Toys can be sterilized after use, or if need be, thrown away. Parents and volunteers can be taught aseptic technique and then allowed to go into the unit to hold and comfort the child. Nurses also should remember that emotional support is a large segment of nursing care; they should include large portions of it in their nursing care plans.

Parent-Nurse Relationship

The nurse's relationship with the parents of her patients is most important. A mother should be allowed, and encouraged, to feed her baby, change his diaper, hold him, and to do whatever she feels capable of doing. Many parents are timid or frightened, and think that they are not allowed to do this. The nurse should ask the parent if she (or he) would like to hold or to feed the child, using tact in order not to make the parents feel guilty if they do not feel adequate in the situation.

Sometimes mothers wish to care for other infants on the ward. A mother spending considerable time on the ward, perhaps because her own infant is very ill, often feels quite useless and asks if she can fill some obvious need of some other child. Perhaps the nurse has not been able to get to a baby's feeding promptly, and he is letting the world know in no uncertain terms what he thinks of this kind of service. Perhaps he is in obvious need of a change, or is holding up his arms beseechingly to be picked up.

No blanket statement can be made about this. The nurse must first find out the rules. Some departments have strict rules against any visitor handling another child, and tact will have to be used. However, if there is no reason why the visitor should not give the little attention to others that she wants to give, and she appears capable of handling the problem, this may be quite a morale booster to her. Care must be taken, however, not to ask the visitor to help "because I am busy" or to take for granted that because she once offered to feed a baby that she will continue to do so. Abuse of this situation has sometimes been the cause behind the strict rules against allowing visitors to help.

Much has been written about the infant's need to relate to one person: his mother or a mother-figure. In hospitals where the parent is allowed to live in with the infant, this need can be largely satisfied. It does become more difficult where the mother is limited to visiting hours.

There is a trend in the thinking of present-day child psychologists to look more deeply into the concept of absolute one-to-one relationship. Mothers do work outside the home and place their infants in the care of others. With proper support, these infants do very well. In the hospital, however, the infant has discomfort, pain and strangeness to cope with, as well as separation.

Suggestions to alleviate the emotional impact of hospitalization on infants have been made. It is true that a young child needs one person with whom he can relate in a special way. Such a relationship helps the caretaker to develop a sensitivity to the individual characteristics and needs of the infant. The caretaker's response thus becomes predictable to the infant and the environment thus acquires some continuity.

Leon Yarrow* writes, "Where it is not always feasible to maintain complete continuity in person, it may be possible to minimize the degree of discontinuity experienced by the infant or young child by planning carefully the scheduling of routines, the patterns of gratification, and the modalities in which gratification is provided."

Yarrow states there are three important variables in the affectional interchange between the infant and his caretaker:†

1. The degree of emotional involvement. This is dependent on the gratification the caretaker receives from the relationship with the child.
2. The extent to which the caretaker responds to the child as an individual. How aware is she of this infant's uniqueness, how much does she respond to his individual characteristics?
3. The caretaker's acceptance of the infant for what he is.

The conclusion is drawn that one person should have major responsibility for and establish a special relationship with an infant. This could be the nurse on the day shift, who gives him the major portion of his care. In this way, the infant can identify with several mother-figures, while maintaining a special relationship with the one who has the greatest responsibility for meeting his needs.

HOSPITAL CARE OF THE INFANT

Physical Care

A child enters the hospital for one purpose only, to become physically well. However, his physical progress is greatly affected by his emotional state. It has been demonstrated that a child cannot thrive

---

*Yarrow, Leon J.: Conceptualizing the early environment. *In* Chandler, Caroline A., *et al.*: Early Child Care. p. 22. New York, Atherton Press, 1968.

†Adapted from Early Child Care, p. 21.

physically if he is emotionally disturbed or if he is allowed to stagnate mentally. *All* of his needs must be met as nearly as it is possible to do so in the highly artificial hospital setting.

In meeting the child's emotional needs, one must not neglect physical care. The basic goal remains the same: to restore the child to physical health and return him to his parents. Everyday physical routine is important. The nurse who has had limited experience in handling infants in the hospital can profit by a review of basic principles of infant care.

Bathing the Infant

A daily bath is desirable if the infant's condition allows this. The baby in the hospital should have his own bath basin, his own soap, and his individual bathing table. If the baby has no dressing or other contraindications, placing him in the bath rather

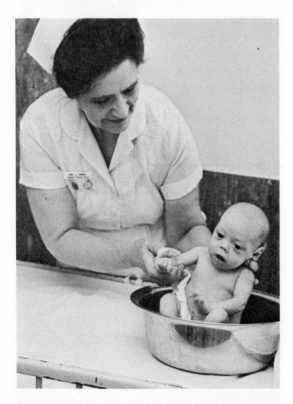

Figure 26-21. The bath basin should be set in the crib for safety.

than giving him a sponge bath can have a soothing and comforting effect.

Procedure for a Tub Bath for a Small Infant. Gather together all equipment before starting.

   large basin or small tub
   soap (a mild baby soap)
   clean cotton balls
   soft wash cloth
   large soft towel or small cotton blanket

Water in the basin should be about 95° to 100°. A bath thermometer may be used, or the temperature may be tested by the time-honored elbow test. The water should feel comfortably warm to the elbow.

Small babies squirm and move about much more than an inexperienced person might expect. A basic rule in their care is never to turn one's back on an infant when the crib side is down. A very sensible precaution when bathing a baby is to put the bath basin right in the crib and thus do away with the need for turning from the baby. Crib mattresses are plastic covered and sheets can be changed, so splashed water is no problem (Fig. 26-21).

Before undressing a baby, wash his face with clean water, using either the washcloth or cotton balls. This includes washing eyes and ears. Cotton balls are useful if any discharge is present, as a clean one can be used each time and then discarded.

If dried mucus is present in the anterior nares, a wisp of cotton may be twisted, dipped in clean water and used for cleaning the nose. This may cause baby to sneeze and bring down more mucus which can be wiped away.

Applicators have no place in the ordinary cleansing of a baby's eyes, ears or nose. Injury to the mucous membrane easily occurs as the baby squirms. Any material in the ears or nose that is too deep to remove without probing should be removed by the use of appropriate instruments in the hands of a trained person if it is important that it be removed.

The baby's scalp may next be soaped, then the baby picked up by sliding your hand

and your arm under him, grasping his head firmly as you hold it over the basin to rinse the soap away.

After drying his head, undress the baby and examine his body for rashes or excoriations. You may then soap his body all over and lift him into the basin, supporting his head and shoulders on your arm. Some nurses prefer to soap the infant with their free hand while he is in the tub, because a soapy baby is slippery and difficult to pick up.

If the baby is enjoying this experience, make it a leisurely one, and let him stay in the water for a few minutes as you take this opportunity to talk and to play with him. After he is finished, lift him out, wrap him in a towel or a blanket and pat him dry, paying attention to creases. Perhaps it should be noted that if the baby's diaper was soiled when it was removed, the feces should be wiped from his buttocks before placing him in the bath.

After the bath, the labia in girl babies should be separated and cleansed with cotton and clean water if this is needed. Boy babies have usually been circumcised and need only be inspected for cleanliness. An uncircumcised boy may have the foreskin gently retracted and any accumulation of smegma or debris washed off.* If the foreskin does not easily retract, do not force it, but report this to the pediatrician.

For the baby with healthy skin, powders, lotions and ointments are unnecessary. Powder tends to cake in the creases and cause irritation. A baby may have an allergy to the ingredients in baby lotion; in any case, a clean baby smells sweet enough without adding any trimmings.

An excessively dry skin may benefit from the application of mineral oil or a neutral lubricant. If powder is needed, corn starch is nonirritating. Various medicated ointments are available for excoriated skin areas.

A baby's fingernails need to be inspected and cut if they are long, because he can scratch his face with his aimless arm

---

*Many pediatricians now prefer that the foreskin be left alone.

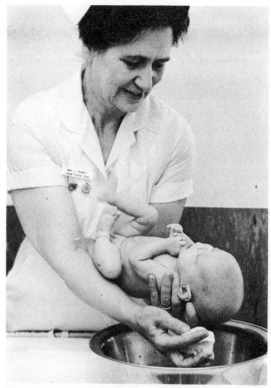

Figure 26-22. Hold the baby securely while washing her head.

movements. The nails should be cut straight across, using care to hold the arm and the hand firmly while cutting.

Bathing the Older Infant. For the older infant, the procedure is essentially the same. When the baby is old enough to sit and move about freely, he may enjoy the regular bathtub, but usually this is frightening to him. Splashing about in a small tub may be more fun, especially with the addition of a floating toy. Try to schedule your time so that this can be a leisurely process, a time for nurse and baby to enjoy together.

Sponge Bathing. For the infant who cannot be placed in a tub, a sponge bath has to be sufficient. There are several points to remember.

1. The face and head must always be washed with clean water and a washcloth before handling the rest of the body. Never does the nurse go back to the face after changing the diaper or washing the perineum without first thoroughly washing her hands.

Usually it is best to wash the face and head before undressing the child.

2. Use sufficient, *warm* water in the basin. The water can be warmer for a sponge than for a tub bath. Make an effort to keep the baby from becoming chilled.

3. After washing the child's body, wash the perineum using downward strokes, moving from front to back. Do not use a washcloth to go over the area more than once; if more than one stroke is needed, use a clean cotton ball each time.

4. Turn the baby on his abdomen if possible, and wash the rectal area last.

Naturally all precautions outlined for tub bathing are necessary here as well.

Dressing the Baby

Babies in the hospital wear cotton shirts or gowns and diapers except in hot weather when a diaper alone is sufficient. The easiest way to dress a small baby is to grasp his hand and pull his arm through the sleeve. If gowns that tie in back are used, care must be taken to see that they fit properly, are not too tight around the neck, or too loose, thus allowing the baby to get tangled in his clothing.

Diapers come in various sizes and shapes. The important point to remember is that there should not be bunched material between the thighs. Two popular diaper styles are either the oblong strip pinned at the sides, or the square diaper folded "kite" fashion. The latter kind has the advantage of being useful for different ages and sizes. (Figs. 26-23 and 26-24)

The older infant needs his diaper pinned snugly at both hips and legs to prevent feces from running out at the open spaces. The nurse needs only to clean a soiled crib and smeared baby once or twice to remember this.

Weighing the Baby

A baby may be weighed daily, semi-weekly, or weekly, as ordered. He should be weighed at the same time each day, preferably before breakfast. A regular baby scale is used. Procedure is as follows:

1. Ascertain the baby's previous weight from the record of the last weighing.

2. Place a clean diaper, sheet, or paper liner on the scoop of the scale in which the baby is to lie.

3. Balance the scale.

4. Place the baby, completely undressed, on the scale and weigh. Use a small piece of clean paper to manipulate the scales if this is the practice in the nursery.

5. In case of a significant discrepancy from the previous recorded weight, check the scale balance and have your findings checked by a second person.

6. Remove the infant from the scale, discarding the scoop liner.

7. Enter weight in the appropriate space on the chart with weight recording countersigned by a second person if necessary. (Fig. 26-25)

Taking the Baby's Temperature

In most sick baby nurseries, rectal temperatures are routine, although some favor axillary temperature taking. Each baby should have his own thermometer which should be cleaned after each use. The thermometer should be kept in a special container in the bedside stand, or in a container attached to the wall of his cubicle.

Before taking the temperature, inspect the thermometer for breakage, especially at the bulb. If the thermometer has been kept in a solution, rinse it and shake it to below 98°.

If the baby has his temperature taken rectally, hold his ankles firmly as you raise his legs to expose the rectum, and insert the thermometer into the rectum just past the bulb of the thermometer. Both the thermometer and the baby should be held firmly, and the nurse should keep her mind on the business at hand, because thermometers have been broken by kicking and squirming babies. Three or four minutes is considered a sufficiently long insertion to get an accurate temperature.

After use, clean the thermometer with a soapy cotton ball, rinse it with water, and soak it in an antiseptic solution for the

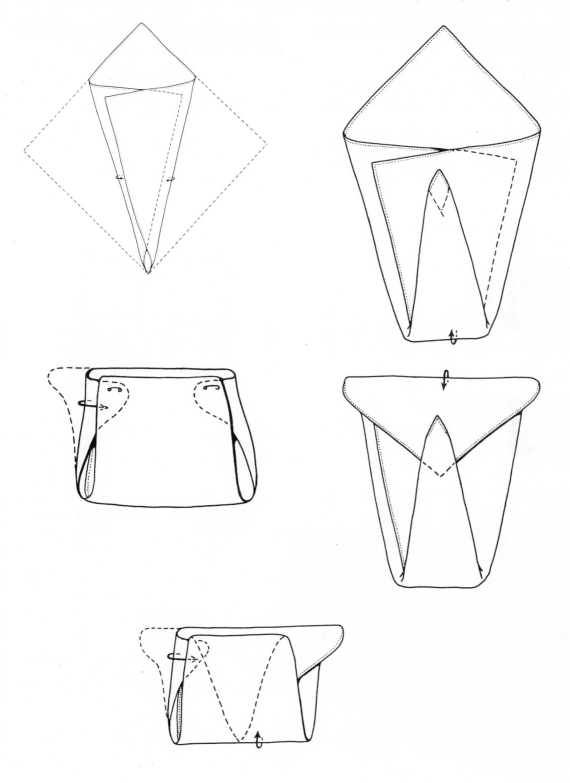

Figure 26-23. Clockwise from top left: steps for folding a diaper "kite fashion."

designated time, then dry it, and replace it in its container.

Feeding

Principles and techniques of feeding have been discussed in the section on infant nutrition. Every effort should be made to make eating an enjoyable experience for the infant. To this end, care should be taken to allow no disagreeable or painful procedures to interrupt feeding time. Only a little

consideration and forethought is necessary to accomplish this.

BIBLIOGRAPHY

Bettelheim, Bruno: The Empty Fortress. New York, Free Press, 1967.
Maurer, Adah: The game of peek-a-boo, Diseases of the Nervous System, *28*:118, 1967.
Nelson, Waldo et al. (eds.): Textbook of Pediatrics. ed. 9. Philadelphia, W. B. Saunders, 1969.

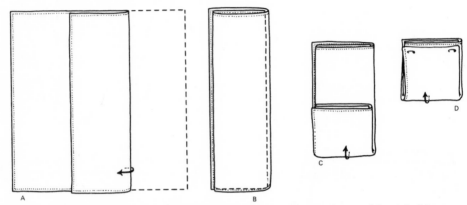

Figure 26-24.   Steps to follow for folding a diaper in an oblong fashion.

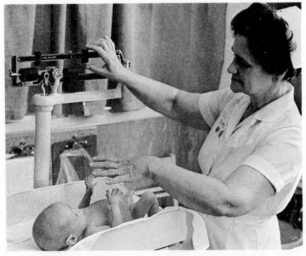

Figure 26-25.   The nurse weighs the baby.

Report of the committee on infectious diseases, American Academy of Pediatrics, 1970. [Immunizations]

Silver, Henry K., Kempe, C. Henry, and Bruyn, Henry B.: Handbook of Pediatrics. ed. 8. Los Altos, California, Lange Medical Publications, 1969.

Spock, Benjamin M. and Lowenberg, Miriam E.: Feeding Your Baby and Child. New York, Pocket Books, 1967.

Yarrow, Leon J.: Conceptualizing the Early Environment. In Chandler, Caroline A.: Early Infant Care. New York, Atherton Press, 1968.

Suggested Readings for Further Study

Bellam, Gwen: The first year of life, AJN, *69:*1244, 1969.

Nursing Care of Infants with Gastrointestinal and Respiratory Conditions

$\mathcal{27}$

MALNUTRITION

Scope of the Problem

The World Health Organization has abundantly publicized the malnutrition and outright hunger that affect more than half the world's population (see Chapter 3). Only recently, however, have people been made aware of the amount of malnutrition and hunger in the United States of America today.

Malnutrition is a term used to indicate a condition in which one or more nutrients essential for health are lacking. Malnutrition accompanies many of the chronic diseases, but the greatest number of cases of malnutrition are due to insufficient intake of essential nutrients. A deficient diet may have other than economic causes. Lack of understanding of the nutritional needs of children is one. Another is ignorance of inexpensive ways of supplying the child's needs.

Protein malnutrition results from an insufficient intake of good quality protein or from some condition in which there is an impaired absorption of protein. Clinical evidence of protein malnutrition may not be striking until the condition is well advanced.

Kwashiorkor, protein-calorie malnutrition, is a syndrome resulting from severe deficiency of protein. It is a condition accounting for most of the malnutrition among the world's children today. Its highest incidence is among children in the age period of 4 months to 5 years.

An affected child develops a swollen abdomen, retarded growth with muscle wasting, edema, gastrointestinal changes, apathy and irritability. In untreated cases, mortality rates are 30% or higher. Even when children are brought for treatment, the condition has often advanced sufficiently to keep mortality rates as high as 15 to 20% at some treatment centers. Although strenuous efforts are being made around the world to prevent it, its causes are complex.

Traditionally, these babies have been breast-fed up to the age of 2 or 3 years. The child is weaned abruptly and is then given the regular family diet, which contains mostly starch foods with very little meat or vegetable protein. Cow's milk is not generally available, and in many places where goats are kept their milk is not considered fit for human consumption.

In fact, the name kwashiorkor means in African dialect, "the sickness the older baby gets when the new baby comes." Severe protein-calorie malnutrition is one of the most serious medical problems in large areas of Africa, Asia, and Latin America. Wherever people cannot afford meat, fish, eggs or milk, or do not have access to these foods, a protein deficiency is found. If any such food does appear in the diet, it goes first to the father of the family. It is not solely an economic problem, however, but is one also of custom and belief—a situation that is

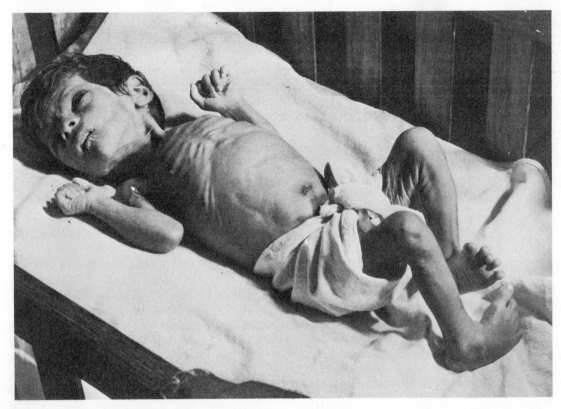

Figure 27-1. Malnutrition, which is still too frequent, is a cause of retardation. (Courtesy of the World Health Organization; photo by P. Pittet.)

extremely hard to change. In some areas meat is believed to cause worms, and milk to cause diarrhea. A reluctance to eat unaccustomed foods is not easily overcome, even among hungry people. Rice eaters in Asia have had difficulty accepting wheat when rice could not be obtained. It is said that during the potato famine in Ireland in 1845 and 1846, the Irish people, whose main dietary staple was the potato, went hungry and even starved before they would eat the maize (corn) sent from America. In some countries, snails are prized as dietary items, but it is difficult to get many Americans to accept them.

It is unrealistic, however, to educate people about proper infant diets if the essential foods are not available to them. Milk is unattainable in many areas, or, if it is available, the general lack of refrigeration lends some substance to the belief that milk causes diarrhea. Some other, economical means of supplying protein must be found. The statement is made that "when it has been brought home to mothers that their children should be properly fed with protein-rich foods, it should be made possible for them to obtain foods of this kind that are cheap, similar to familiar foods in taste and texture where this is feasible and easily prepared. In this connexion, it should be remembered (that) many African mothers are not used to buying food for their children."*

Dried skim milk has been furnished by UNICEF for the treatment of Kwashiorkor in Africa, and has been a means of reducing clinical symptoms. Some sort of acceptable protein-rich diet is necessary for the prevention and for continued use as a

*Malnutrition in early childhood: WHO Chronicle, 20:86, 1966

supplement to the usual diet. A vegetable protein mixture, made into a liquid that resembles milk in texture, and has an acceptable taste, was developed in Latin America and has proved its value. Called Incaparina, it is sold commercially, costs but a fraction of the price of milk. Its use is promoted by an educational campaign. Other countries have developed similar mixtures. Soya bean or groundnuts mixed with cereals provide a protein-rich food.

The nutritive value of mixed vegetable protein can be enhanced by adding skim milk powder or a fish protein concentrate.

These supplements are good if people will use them, but education to make use of *available* food supplements is of greater importance. Dr. Sai, a research physician in Ghana, says that children in fishing villages do not eat fish because their mothers believe fish is not good for children. Mothers should learn to use protein-rich beans by soaking them to remove their husks.* Educational programs and public health clinics are reaching numbers of people, but much yet remains to be done.

Vitamin Deficiency Diseases

Rickets is a deficiency disease caused by a lack of vitamin D. Children who live in the sunshine and wear little clothing may absorb sufficient vitamin D from the sun's ultraviolet rays, but the infant or small child in a temperate or an arctic climate rarely has opportunity to receive his antirachitic vitamin in this manner. Children of dark-skinned races also are particularly prone to rickets.

Vitamin D is not found in appreciable quantities in natural foods. Breast milk and cow's milk are poor sources; therefore, the infant needs additional vitamin D, which can be supplied through the use of fish liver oils or in water-miscible vehicles.

Rickets is a disease affecting the growth and calcification of bones. The absorption of calcium and phosphorus is diminished due to

*Michaelis, A. R.: Science for him. World Health Magazine, p. 6, May, 1963.

the lack of vitamin D, whose function it is to regulate the utilization of these minerals. Early manifestations include craniotabes (a softening of the occipital bones) and delayed closure of the fontanelles. There is delayed dentition, with defects of tooth enamel and a tendency to develop caries. As the disease advances, thoracic deformities, softening of the shafts of long bones and spinal and pelvic bone deformities develop. The muscles are poorly developed and lacking in tone, thus delaying standing and walking.

These deformities occur during the periods of rapid growth, and although rickets in itself is not a fatal disease, complications such as tetany, pneumonia and enteritis are more likely to cause death in rachitic children than in healthy children.

Infants and children require an estimated 400 units of vitamin D daily for the prevention of rickets. Because of the uncertainty of a small child receiving sufficient exposure to ultraviolet light in temperate climates, it is administered orally in the form of fish liver oil or synthetic vitamin. Whole milk and evaporated milk, fortified with 400 units of vitamin D per quart are available throughout the United States.

Certain pathological conditions such as vitamin D-resistant rickets and renal rickets are not caused by vitamin D deficiency.

Scurvy is a deficiency disease caused by inadequate vitamin C in the diet. Early inclusion of vitamin C (ascorbic acid) in the form of orange or tomato juice, or a vitamin preparation, is insurance against the development of this disease. Febrile diseases seem to increase the need for vitamin C. A variety of fresh vegetables and fruits supply vitamin C for the older infant and child, although a considerable proportion of vitamin C content is destroyed by boiling, or by exposure to air for long periods of time.

Early clinical manifestations of scurvy are irritability, loss of appetite and digestive disturbances. A general tenderness in the legs, severe enough to cause a "pseudoparalysis" develops. The infant is apprehensive about being handled, and

392 The Infant, 28 Days to One Year

assumes a "frog" position, with hips and knees semi-flexed and the feet rotated outward. The gums become red and swollen, and hemorrhages occur in various tissues. Characteristic hemorrhages in the long bones are subperiosteal, especially at the ends of the femur and tibia.

Recovery is rapid with adequate treatment, but death may occur from malnutrition or exhaustion in untreated cases. Treatment consists in therapeutic daily doses of ascorbic acid.

Vitamin A deficiency. This occurs only if the diet is severely restricted or if absorption is impaired. Children on average diets receive sufficient vitamin A to prevent deficiency manifestations, and daily supplementary doses assure ample coverage. Children on low fat diets, or those with absorptive difficulties, need large daily doses of water-miscible preparations of vitamin A.

Vitamin B Complex. The major vitamin B complex components are thiamine, riboflavin and niacin.

Thiamine insufficiency. Children whose diets are poor in thiamine exhibit irritability, listlessness, loss of appetite and vomiting. A severe lack of thiamine in the diet causes the disease called *beriberi*, characterized by cardiac and neurological symptoms. Beriberi does not occur where balanced diets are eaten which include whole grains.

Riboflavin insufficiency. This deficiency usually occurs in association with thiamine and niacin deficiencies. It is manifested mainly by skin lesions.

Niacin insufficiency. Lack of niacin in the diet causes a disease known as *pellagra*, which has gastrointestinal and neurological symptoms. Children whose intake of whole milk is adequate do not get pellagra; nor do those whose diet is well balanced. There are still some cases of pellagra in the United States, however.

Mineral Insufficiency

Iron deficiency results in anemia. The condition is not uncommon among children over the ages of 4 to 6 months whose diets lack iron-rich foods.

Calcium is necessary for bone and tooth formation. It is also needed for proper nerve and muscle functioning.

Iodine deficiency results if there are no iodine-containing foods in the diet. The condition is called goiter. Endemic cretinism (not to be confused with congenital cretinism) is also a result of iodine deficiency in certain areas of the world. It is nonexistent in the United States.

Other Causes of Malnutrition

Allergic reactions to foods may limit the child's diet to the point at which he is not getting the proper nutrients, and parents usually need a dietician's help in working out substitutes for the foods he cannot tolerate. Allergy to cow's milk has been recognized as a problem for a number of infants and children under the age of two years. Symptoms include vomiting and diarrhea, abdominal pain, asthma and rhinitis.

If milk is not withdrawn from the diet, an anaphylactic reaction with severe shock symptoms may result, and death may be the outcome. The infant with a milk allergy does well on a soybean formula such as Mull-soy,* or ProSobee.†

Diarrheal conditions, from whatever cause, or persistent vomiting, bring about a state of malnutrition requiring careful, skillful nursing.

Another condition, extremely difficult to remedy in many instances, is the marasmic state brought about in an emotionally deprived child. Diet may be satisfactory, and physical care meticulously given, but the infant who has a cold, unresponsive mother may suffer irreversible damage. A failure to thrive, when organic disease is ruled out and physical neglect is not a factor, may be the result of a lack of emotional warmth from the adult caring for the infant. This happens to the infant who is kept in his crib; whose bottle is propped; whose physical contact

---

*Trademark, Borden
†Trademark, Mead Johnson

with other human beings is confined entirely to routine care with no interchange of mutual trust and understanding. The damage is much more than physical, of course, but the malnutritional effects can be startling, and may be fatal.

The infant who is being cared for by a tender, affectionate mother is much more likely to be a relaxed, comfortable being who eats well and sleeps well. On the other hand, when the mother is tense and irritable, the baby may be fitful, cry excessively, and eat and sleep poorly.*

A National Nutrition Survey was organized in the United States by Dr. Arnold Schaefer, Chief of the Nutrition Program of H.E.W., and his deputy, Dr. Ogden Johnson. The results of the first phase of their findings were reported to the Senate early in 1969. This was a preliminary report of findings in low-income areas in only a few states.†

Cases of kwashiorkor, marasmus, rickets, scurvy and vitamin A deficiency were found among the poor of these "affluent" United States of America. Anemia due to inadequate intake of foods containing iron was also found in many children under six.

Hospital Care of the Malnourished Infant

The malnourished infant admitted to the hospital presents problems that are not easily resolved. The underlying cause must be found and eliminated or treated. If the difficulty lies in the parent's inability to give proper care, whether because of ignorance, financial difficulty, or indifference, this needs consideration, with perhaps several services involved.

The nurse responsible for the daily care of the infant has her own particular problems when attempting to meet his needs.

One such problem may be in persuading the infant to take more nourishment than he wants. Inexperienced nurses find it very difficult to persuade an uninterested infant

*Chapman, A. H.: Management of Emotional Problems of Children and Adolescents. P. 40. Philadelphia, J. B. Lippincott, 1965.
†Shaefer, Arnold E. and Johnson, Ogden C.: Are we well fed? The search for an answer. Nutrition Today, 4:2, 1969. Nutrition Today is published quarterly for health professional personnel.

to take his formula, and it can become a most frustrating experience. Infants appear to be sensitive to the handling of an inexperienced, uncertain person. Perhaps the nurse's insecurity and uncertainty communicate themselves to the child in the way she handles him. It frequently happens that an experienced nurse is successful in feeding an infant three or four ounces in a short time, while, at the same time, the inexperienced nurse who seems to be going through the same motions, persuades the infant to take only an ounce or less. The nurse need not be too discouraged, because as she and the infant become accustomed to each other, they both relax, and the feeding ought to become easier.

In addition to a lack of interest in the feeding, the infant is weak and debilitated, with little strength to suck. Intravenous or gavage feeding may be employed, but in addition it may be most important for the infant to develop an interest in food and in the process of sucking. A hard, or small-holed nipple may completely discourage him. Whereas a strong, healthy infant delights in the process of sucking itself, this infant lacks incentive and strength. The nipple should be soft, with holes large enough to allow the formula to drip without pressure. However, a nipple may be so soft that it offers no resistance and collapses when it is sucked on, or the holes may be so large that milk pours out and causes him to choke. These experiences easily frustrate a weak infant, who soon gives up any attempt to nurse.

The baby who is held snugly in the nurse's arms, wrapped rather closely and rocked gently, will find it easier to relax and take a little more. An impatient, hurried nurse nearly always communicates her tension to the child. If the nurse is tense because of other feedings she must also attend to, she should ask for help. Never does she prop the bottle in the crib. This is a dangerous practice, and it has no place in a hospital nursery.

Some of the babies may be on a two- or a three-hour feeding schedule, because most weak babies are able to handle frequent small feedings better than the four-hour ones. In this case, it is more important than ever that the feedings be given on time. Also, as sucking takes considerable energy, the weak infant tires easily. It is not good practice to take more than 20 or 30 minutes for feeding such an infant. If the baby does not take at least two-thirds of his formula, this should be reported. Accurate intake recording is essential, because these babies may need help in the form of small transfusions or parenteral fluids to furnish them with enough energy to take more oral nourishment.

Self-demand feedings, about which we hear so much, if used at all with these infants, must be used cautiously. A normal, healthy baby promptly makes his needs known if he is hungry, and will quickly fall into a routine, following the rhythmic filling and emptying of his stomach. If such a child sleeps through his feeding time only to waken an hour later in a near-famished state, he usually is the best gauge of his own needs. But the malnourished baby probably has lost the power to regulate his own supply and demand schedule.

Good Sources of Essential Nutrients

Protein. Meat, poultry, fish, milk products and eggs. Whole wheat grains, nuts, peanut butter, legumes are also good sources of protein, but need to be supplemented by some animal protein, such as meat, eggs, milk, cheese, cottage cheese or yogurt.

Vitamin A. Green leafy vegetables, deep yellow vegetables and fruits, whole milk or whole milk products, egg yolk.

Thiamine. Meat, fish, poultry, eggs, whole grain, legumes, potatoes, green leafy vegetables.

Riboflavin. Milk (best source), meat, egg yolk, green vegetables.

Niacin. Meat, fish, poultry, peanut butter, wheat germ, brewer's yeast. Although the amount in milk is small, children whose intake of milk is adequate do not develop pellagra.

Vitamin C. Citrus fruits and tomatoes, fresh or frozen citrus fruit juices, strawberries, cantaloupe. Breast milk is an adequate source of vitamin C for young infants only if the mother's diet contains sufficient vitamin C.

Vitamin D. Sunlight, fish liver oils, fortified milk and synthetic vitamin D.

Calcium. Milk is the main source.

Iron. Green leafy vegetables, liver, meats and eggs, dried fruits, whole grain or enriched bread and cereals.

Iodine. Seafoods, plants grown on soil near the sea, iodized salt.

DIARRHEA

Diarrhea in infants is a fairly common symptom of a variety of conditions. It may be mild with a small amount of dehydration, or may be extremely severe, calling for prompt and effective treatment.

Etiology

Chronically malnourished infants with diarrheal symptoms constitute a common problem in many areas of the world. This condition is prevalent in areas where clean water and sanitary facilities are lacking or inadequate.

Allergic reactions to food, particularly cow's milk, are not uncommon, and can be controlled by avoidance of the offending food. Overfeeding as well as underfeeding, or an unbalanced diet may be the cause of diarrhea in an infant. Adjustment of the infant's diet, cutting down on the sugar added to formula, or reducing bulk or fat in the diet may be necessary. Certain metabolic diseases, such as cystic fibrosis have diarrhea as a symptom.

Many diarrheal disturbances in formula-fed infants are caused by contaminated food. The infectious organisms may be salmonella, *E. coli,* dysentery bacilli, and various viruses. It is difficult to determine the causative factor in the majority of cases. Because of the seriousness of infectious diarrhea among infants, most hospitals isolate the child with moderate or severe diarrhea until it can be definitely proved that there is no infectious agent involved.

Clinical Manifestations

Mild diarrhea may show little more than loose stools, which may number from two to four to as many as ten or 12 per day. There may be irritability and loss of appetite. Vomiting and gastric distention are not significant factors and dehydration is minimal.

Severe diarrhea may develop gradually with the condition becoming progressively more serious, with marked dehydration. The skin becomes very dry and loses its turgor. The fontanel becomes sunken, the pulse is weak and rapid. The stools become greenish liquid and may be blood-tinged. They are often expelled with force. Severe diarrhea with rapid onset is usually caused by food poisoning. It starts with persistent vomiting and high fever. Extreme prostration appears early, and the mortality rate is high.

Treatment

The important factor in treatment is to establish normal fluid and electrolyte balance.

The physician may treat the mild dehydration by giving oral feedings of five per cent glucose in saline solution, or a commercial preparation such as Lytren, in place of milk or food. Sometimes a period of complete omission of oral feedings is ordered for a period of a few hours before commencing the oral electrolyte solution. As the diarrhea clears, skim milk may be offered followed by gradual additions of infant formula and food.

Mild or moderate diarrhea can convert rather quickly to severe diarrhea in an infant. Vomiting usually accompanies the diarrhea; together they cause large losses of body water and electrolytes. The infant becomes severely dehydrated, and is gravely ill. Oral feedings are discontinued completely. Fluids to be given intravenously must be carefully calculated to replace the lost electrolytes. Frequent laboratory determinations of the infant's blood chemistries will be necessary for guidance in this replacement therapy.

Nursing Care

In addition to maintaining the intravenous fluid at a correct speed and keeping accurate records of fluids, the nurse also needs to keep strict account of the number and character of the infant's stools and the amount and character of vomitus and urine. A record is kept of skin condition, the child's temperature and state of activity. Strict isolation techniques must be observed unless otherwise ordered. If high fever is present, tepid sponge baths or a cooling water mattress will be ordered.

Excoriation of the skin in the genital area must be prevented as much as possible. This area should be cleansed frequently with mineral oil or vaseline and a mild ointment applied. Leaving the diaper off, exposing the buttocks and genital area to the air is helpful. Disposable pads under the infant will facilitate easy and frequent changing. Cold cream may be applied to the child's dry lips to help prevent cracking and sores.

Meeting the infant's emotional needs will be difficult but of great importance. His mother is the one who can best fulfill the infant's needs, if she can be taught the principles of strict aseptic technique and can be relied on to maintain them.

If the infant can be picked up and rocked, this will be helpful. However, if there is a possibility that the intravenous needle may be displaced, this will not be permitted. Getting a needle into the small veins of an infant is difficult and replacement may be nearly impossible. Yet the infant's life may depend on the proper parenteral therapy.

Soothing the baby by gentle head stroking and soft speech helps him bear the frustrations imposed on him by his illness as well as by the treatment. His sucking needs may be met by means of a pacifier. When the child's mother cannot be with him, the nurse has an obligation to take her place in filling his emotional needs as much as possible.

CONSTIPATION

Many parents worry unnecessarily about the state of their infant's bowels. Breast-fed infants may go without a movement for several days without being constipated. The character of the stool, rather than its frequency, is the determining factor in constipation. A constipated stool is hard, dry and small.

Etiology

The breast-fed infant is rarely constipated. Constipation in the formula-fed baby may be the result of too little carbohydrate in the formula, or may indicate a need for more fluid intake. Obstinate, persistent constipation may indicate a gastrointestinal condition such as megacolon or a mechanical obstruction.

Treatment

Usually an increase of sugar or the addition of molasses to the formula will correct the problem. Prune juice and additional fruits are helpful. Laxatives and enemas should not be used except under a doctor's order.

COLIC

The recurrent paroxysmal bouts of abdominal pain that are not uncommon among young infants have earned for the condition the name of 3-month colic. It is a fact that the condition disappears around the age of 3 months. This knowledge gives small comfort to the parent vainly trying to sooth her colicky baby.

Etiology

Exact cause is unknown. Air swallowing and hunger have been suggested. A state of tension in the family, communicating itself to the infant is a likely factor.

Clinical Manifestations

Attacks occur quite suddenly, usually late in the day or evening. The infant cries loudly and continuously. His abdomen is tense and distended, his legs drawn up and the hands clenched. He appears to be in considerable pain. The baby may only momentarily be soothed by rocking or holding. Eventually he cries himself to sleep from exhaustion.

Differentiation from other conditions will need to be made. Allergic reaction to certain foods and intestinal obstruction or infection should be ruled out.

Treatment

No single treatment is consistantly successful. A *warm* water bottle or heating pad on low setting with the infant lying prone across it is sometimes helpful. Great care must be taken to insure the bottle or pad are not too warm for the baby's tender skin. The pad or water bottle should be placed outside his clothing, not next to his skin. The doctor may order a rectal glycerine suppository to help the infant expel flatus. Sedation such as phenobarbital for attacks that persist is sometimes useful. Attacks rarely persist after the age of three months.

Methods of feeding and of burping the infant should be examined for possible cause. However, the mother should not be made to feel guilty or inefficient in her child's care. Frequently no mismanagement in the feeding practices can be found.

VOMITING AND REGURGITATION

Vomiting is one of the commonest disturbances of infancy and childhood. It can be a symptom of a wide variety of conditions. Attention must be given toward discovering the cause and correcting it. It may be simply a matter of overfeeding or swallowing too much air.

More serious conditions can be pyloric stenosis, allergic reaction to cow's milk (see Allergies), infections or organic obstructions in any body system.

Some well nourished, active infants tend to spit up (regurgitate) small amounts of feeding rather frequently. These infants seem to regurgitate easily, especially when excited. There appears to be no particular causative factor, and change of formula seldom helps. This type of regurgitation tends to disappear as the infant grows older.

Rumination

Ocasionally an infant exhibits an unusual habit of regurgitation. He makes mouthing movements as though rechewing the material, and reswallows or spits out the regurgitated feeding. If observed carefully, the infant can be seen to gag himself with his fingers or his tongue. The infant, usually in the second half of his first year of life, is frequently one who is receiving inadequate or unsatisfactory emotional stimulation from his environment. Frequently his mother or caretaker gives the child adequate physical care but seems unable to relate to him in any warm, meaningful manner. These may be infants who are left alone in their cribs for long periods of time without interaction with people or environmental stimulation. The child appears to seek emotional satisfaction from within himself in a neurotic manner. Often body rocking, rolling and head banging are also present.

Treatment consists of providing continuous, warm relationship with a loving, maternal person. The condition can be reversed and the rumination stopped if the child is able to receive his necessary emotional support from without. However, if this is not provided, he becomes severely malnourished and eventually may die. The mother or caretaker should have counseling and emotional support in an effort to better the mother-child relationship.

PROLAPSE OF THE RECTUM

Rectal prolapse is a descent of the mucous membrane of the rectum into the anus, with or without protrusion through the anal opening. The term *procidentia* of the rectum is used when all of the coats of the rectum descend. Infants and children who suffer from severe malnutrition disturbances are prone to rectal prolapse when straining at stool in constipation, or during diarrheal episodes. Prolapse of the rectum is common in children with cystic fibrosis.

The protruding mass is bright or dark red and may be several inches in length. The protrusion may recede spontaneously, but generally needs to be replaced manually. A gloved finger, covered with a piece of toilet tissue, is gently introduced into the lumen of

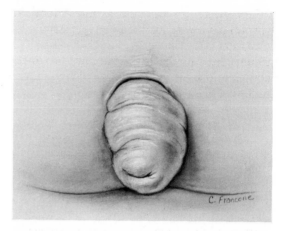

Figure 27-2. Drawing showing prolapse of the rectum.

the mass, and the mass is pushed gently back into the rectum. The toilet tissue will adhere to the mucous membrane, permitting the withdrawal of the gloved finger. The tissue will later be expelled spontaneously.

During defecation, the child's buttocks should be held firmly together. Whenever a prolapse occurs, the rectal tissue should be replaced. Treatment should be directed toward relieving the cause. For intractable cases, perineal surgery may become necessary.

INTUSSUSCEPTION

A healthy thriving baby, generally a boy, may some time after the first month of life suddenly develop extremely severe paroxysms of abdominal pain with no apparent predisposing cause. His mother may ascribe this to gas, especially when her baby resumes play after the colicky episode. Another spasm soon appears, however, and the mother realizes that something is seriously wrong.

Intussusception is the invagination or telescoping of one portion of the bowel into a distal portion. It occurs most frequently at the juncture of the ileum and the colon, although it can appear elsewhere in the intestinal tract. The invagination is from above downward; the upper portion, the intussusceptum, slipping into the lower, the intussuscipiens, pulling the mesentery along with it. (Fig. 27-3)

Incidence

The condition occurs more often in boys than in girls, and is the most frequent cause of intestinal obstruction in childhood. The greatest incidence, about 78 per cent, occurs in infants between the ages of four months to 10 months.

Etiology

The condition usually appears in healthy babies without any demonstrable cause. Its production is supposed to be favored by the hyperperistalsis and the unusual mobility of the cecum and ileum normally present in early life. Occasionally, a lesion such as a Meckel's diverticulum or a polyp may be present.

Clinical Manifestations

The infant who has previously appeared healthy and happy suddenly becomes pale, cries out sharply, and draws up his legs in a severe colicky spasm of pain. This spasm may last for several minutes, after which the infant relaxes and appears well until the next episode, which may be 5, 10, or 20 minutes later.

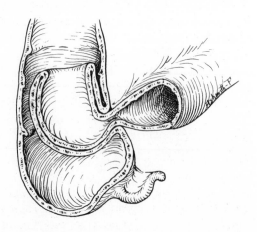

Figure 27-3. In this drawing of intussusception note the telescoping of a portion of the bowel into the distal portion.

Most of these infants start vomiting early, a vomiting that becomes progressively more severe and eventually is bile stained. The infant strains with each paroxysm, emptying his bowels of fecal contents, after which the stools consist of blood and mucus, earning the name of "currant jelly" stools.

Symptoms of shock appear quickly. Rapid pulse, paleness, and marked sweating are characteristic. Shock, vomiting and currant jelly stools are the cardinal symptoms of this condition. Fortunately, these symptoms, coupled with the paroxysmal pain, are severe enough to bring the child into the hospital early.

The nurse does not, of course, make a diagnosis; however, because she is often consulted by neighbors, friends and relatives if things go wrong, she needs to be informed and alert. Therefore, a word of caution is needed. On rare occasions a more chronic form appears, particularly during an episode of severe diarrheal disturbance. The onset is more gradual and may not show all of the classic symptoms, but the danger of a sudden, complete strangulation is present. Presumably, such an infant is already under a doctor's care.

Diagnosis

Diagnosis can usually be made by the physician from the clinical symptoms, rectal examination, and palpation of the abdomen during the calm interval when it is soft. A baby is often not willing to tolerate this palpation, and sedation may be ordered. In about half of these cases, a sausage-shaped mass along the colon can be felt through the abdominal wall.

A barium enema is not only diagnostic, but may also reduce the intussusception.

Treatment

Unlike pyloric stenosis, this condition is a true emergency in the sense that prolonged delay is dangerous. The telescoped bowel rapidly becomes gangrenous, thus markedly reducing the possibility of a simple reduction. Adequate treatment during the first 12 to 24 hours should have a good outcome, with complete recovery. The outcome becomes more uncertain as the bowel deteriorates, making resection necessary.

Early Care of Infant After Admission

The baby is of course given nothing by mouth, and intravenous fluids are started. A cut-down or catheter into the vein will probably be used.

The young baby needs very careful watching because his condition can deteriorate rapidly. Vital signs need to be checked frequently, warmth applied if symptoms of shock are present, and general condition noted. Aspiration of vomited material is a very real danger, especially as the child becomes weaker. The baby will probably not tolerate being held to any extent. Although early reduction is imperative, the baby may be in the hospital for a few hours before surgery if symptoms are not entirely clear or if he is greatly dehydrated.

Surgical technique. Surgery consists of a gentle milking of the intussusceptum back into place. This is a simple procedure, requiring a small incision, and affords an opportunity for visual assurance of complete reduction as well as identification of any possible lesion that might be present. Should the bowel be found to be gangrenous or the intussusception irreducible, resection will be necessary.

Traditionally, surgery has been preceded by a diagnostic barium enema, and it has been observed in some cases that the reduction has been accomplished by the hydrostatic pressure itself. Most surgeons prefer to follow the enema with surgery to assure themselves of complete reduction and absence of other lesions. Some surgeons, however, are relying on the reduction by hydrostatic pressure under fluoroscopic observation when the diagnosis is made early and prostration is minimal. In every case the technique is carried out by the surgeon himself, with the operating room ready for immediate surgery if reduction is not accomplished.

Technique for reduction by hydrostatic pressure should be understood by the nurse for her own satisfaction, and to enable her to explain correctly to the child's parents. The child is taken to x-ray with intravenous fluids running. A Foley bag catheter is placed in the rectum, inflated, and barium solution allowed to flow by gravity into the colon. The reduction is shown by free filling of the small intestine, disappearance of the mass, and observable improvement in the infant's condition. If any doubt exists, surgery is performed at once.

Prognosis

Early successful reduction gives complete relief with only rare recurrent attacks. Spontaneous reduction has been known to occur, but the condition is considered too dangerous to adopt a "wait and see" attitude. The mortality rate rises sharply with delay, and untreated cases are nearly always fatal.

Nursing Care

As in any abnormal condition affecting children or infants, a large portion of the nursing care is concerned with support of the parents.

Every parent is entitled to as complete and accurate an explanation as she or he can understand. The parents need to understand the condition, and its severity. Medical and nursing procedures are frequently complicated and extremely frightening to the uninformed person.

Many procedures that seem routine to the nurse do present an ominous aspect to a person who is unfamiliar with them, a fact that we too often overlook.

The baby, lying in his crib, has a tubing extending from his nose and connected to a continuous suction apparatus. Another tube extends from a bottle of fluid into a vein in his scalp. He may have still another tubing coming from his bladder into a drainage bottle. None of these may have great significance, but even the most informed nurse might have a few qualms if this child was her own.

The untrained public has certainly become more informed about medical techniques through the popular magazines, television and other media. It is still difficult to be entirely objective, however, if the affected child is your own, and thus misunderstandings are still quite common.

In situations such as this, the doctor is quite busy and concerned about the patient, and looks to the nurse to give support to the family. An explanation of the whys and wherefores can clear up some of the mystery. Perhaps a nurse's greatest asset is the ability to listen. If she is really attentive, she can show her sympathy and understanding, help correct misunderstandings, and give assurance that the child's welfare is of the greatest concern to all.

The nurse should try to make the parents comfortable, and make them feel that they are part of the group and not hindrances or unavoidable nuisances. She gives them assurance that the child will be carefully watched when they take a much needed moment of relaxation in the coffee shop or restroom, and she has someone show them where to go. She does not insist that they go, however, against their wishes.

Occasionally, a nurse falls into the trap of giving false hope or of being unrealistically optimistic. She must remember that this is a sick child, and no one can predict a recovery with certainty.

Postoperative care. Following a simple reduction of the intussusception, treatment is symptomatic. Intravenous feeding is necessary until normal bowel sounds are present, at which time feedings are cautiously resumed.

The surgical area must be kept clean and dry, and care must be taken so that it is not contaminated by urine or fecal material.

If resection has been necessary, this assumes the gravity of any major abdominal surgery. Constant gastric suction is necessary to keep the stomach and upper intestinal tract empty. Drainage must be measured, and may be analyzed for electrolyte losses that must be replaced in the intravenous fluids.

One must not forget to turn these patients frequently. The small infant cannot learn to cough or breathe deeply to keep his lungs clear. A nasal suction machine must be on hand to keep the airways clear of mucus, and activity should be stimulated by frequent turning and, if necessary, by making the infant cry. Of course this must be explained to the parents, who will probably resent measures that make the child temporarily uncomfortable. When they understand the importance of deep breathing, which in a small child, can be stimulated only by crying, and the need for changes of position to facilitate the exchange of gasses in the lungs, they can willingly cooperate.

BIBLIOGRAPHY

Chapman, A. H.: Management of Emotional Problems of Children and Adolescents. Philadelphia, J. B. Lippincott, 1965.

Jelliffe, Derrick B. and Jelliffe, E. R. Patrice: The urban avalanche and child nutrition. Journal of the American Dietetic Assn., *57:*111, 1970.

Malnutrition in Early Childhood. WHO Chronicle, *20:*86, 1966.

Michaelis, A. R.: Science for him. World Health, p. 6, May, 1963.

Shaefer, Arnold E. and Johnson, Ogden C.: Are we well fed? Nutrition Today, *4:*2, 1969.

Stare, Frederick J.: Nutritional Improvement and World Health Potential. Journal of the American Dietetic Assn., *57:*107, 1970.

Swenson, Orvar: Pediatric Surgery, vol. 1. New York, Appleton-Century-Crofts, 1968.

Suggested Readings for Further Study

Dayton, Delbert H.: Early malnutrition and human development. Children, *16:*210, 1969.

Ein, Sigmund H. and Stephens, Clinton A.: Intussusception: 354 cases in 10 years. Journal of Pediatric Surgery, *6:*16, 1971.

Nursing Care of Infants with Congenital Conditions 28

CONGENITAL CONDITIONS OF THE GASTROINTESTINAL TRACT

Cleft Palate

The child born with a cleft palate (but with an intact lip) does not have the external disfigurement that may be so distressing to the new mother—but his problems are more serious. Although a cleft lip and a cleft palate frequently appear together, either defect may appear alone. In embryonic development, the palate closes at a later time than does the lip, and the failure to close is for somewhat different reasons. The manner in which the palate normally closes is interesting.

When the embryo is about eight weeks old, there is still no roof to the mouth: the tissues that are to become the palate are two shelves running from the front to the back of the mouth, and projecting vertically downward on either side of the tongue. The shelves move from a vertical position to a horizontal position, their free edges meeting and fusing in midline. Later, bone forms within this tissue to form the hard palate.

Normally the palate is intact by the tenth week of fetal life. Exactly what happens to prevent this closure is not known with certainty. It occurs more frequently in near relatives of persons with the defect than in the general population, and there appears to be some evidence that environmental and hereditary factors may each play a part in this defect.

A cleft palate may involve the soft palate alone, or it may extend into the nose and into the hard palate. It may be unilateral or bilateral, an isolated defect, or in conjunction with cleft lip.

Management of the Defect

The goal is to give the child a union of the cleft parts that would allow intelligible and pleasant speech, and to avoid injury to the maxillary growth. Timing of surgery is individualized, according to the size, the placement and the degree of deformity. The optimal time for surgery is considered to be between the ages of 6 months and five years. Because the child is not able to make certain sounds when he starts to talk, undesirable speech habits are formed which are difficult to correct. If surgery must be delayed beyond the third year, a dental speech appliance may help the child develop intelligible speech.

Home Care Before Surgery

The infant with a cleft palate (but with an intact lip) can learn to suck without much difficulty. A rather large nipple, with holes that allow the milk to drip freely, makes sucking easier for this child, who does not get quite as much suction as a child with an intact palate. The activity of sucking is an important one for the development of speech muscles. Special cleft palate nipples, with a flange to cover the cleft, are commercially available. They are expensive and unnecessary for the average infant with cleft palate. An occasional infant, with a wide cleft, may be able to suck more easily with one of these. It may be necessary to feed such an infant with a medicine dropper. Most of these infants can learn to take milk from a spoon, slowly, at an early age.

Strained foods are introduced at the usual time and in the routine manner, within the framework of a normal diet. A little food or milk may seep through the cleft and out through the nose, and the mothers should be informed of this possibility.

Cleft lip and cleft palate centers provide teams of specialists who can give the professional services that these children need through their infancy, preschool and school years. Members of the professional team include a pediatrician, a plastic surgeon, an orthodontist, a speech therapist, a social worker and a public health nurse. The services of a child nutritionist are also available. Explanations and counseling concerning the child's diet, his speech training, his immunizations and his general health supervision can be given. Questions can be answered and misconceptions can be cleared up.

It may sound strange to speak about preparation for speech training for an infant only a few weeks of age. The babbling and cooing of a young infant is an important precursor of speech activity, and the stimulation that the parents normally give when they repeat the sounds back to him is essential. Parents normally do this, but they may be too disturbed and tense to behave in a natural manner before an infant with a palate defect. This child, however, needs to hear these sounds as a pattern for learning, even more than an infant who does not have to overcome a physical impediment.

Dental care for the deciduous teeth is of more than usual importance. The incidence of dental caries is high in children with a cleft palate, but the preservation of the deciduous teeth is important for the best results in speech as well as for appearance.

Hospital Care

The child should be in a good nutritional state and entirely free from respiratory infection when he enters the hospital for surgery. Because it is imperative that he keep his fingers out of his mouth after repair, he should have a chance to become accustomed to elbow restraints before his surgery. These restraints and a sore mouth are going to be frustrating, and because he should not cry any more than can be prevented—in order to avoid strain on the sutures—his mother should be allowed to stay with him, to hold and comfort him. If this is not possible, he should become acquainted with his nurse before surgery, and learn to accept her in place of his mother for the time being.

Directly after surgery a young child is watched with great care to prevent the aspiration of vomitus or mucus, and to prevent occlusion of the airway by his tongue. Elbow restraints are applied firmly and are checked frequently. Fingers, or any object put into his mouth, may irritate or infect the sutures, causing an imperfect repair—which may not be operable a second time.

The operating surgeon will have a routine for postoperative repair that he finds most successful. Generally, the patient is allowed clear liquids after nausea has ceased. Spoons and straws are usually forbidden, only drinking from a cup or a glass being allowed. Clear liquids that are usually accepted are Jello water, apple juice, and the synthetic, fruit-flavored drinks. Broth may be offered, but is not a popular drink with this age group. Clear liquids are allowed for a period of from three to five days, followed by full liquids for approximately ten days, after which semiliquids such as cereal, ice cream or Jello may be fed with a spoon. Some variations from this schedule may be desired by different plastic surgeons.

The sutures are not cleansed or manipulated in any way. Water, or a clear liquid after a milk drink is helpful to keep the sutures clean if the child will cooperate. In addition to vigilance in keeping toys or any objects out of the mouth, considerable care must be exercised to keep anyone with a suspicion of a cold or a cough away from the patient, whether it is a staff nurse, a family member, or some other patient. A cough or a nasal infection may well damage the best repair.

If all goes well, the child can probably be discharged about the tenth day, returning to the clinic or to his doctor's office for suture removal about the third week.

Orthodontic treatment is necessary for the majority of these children. There may be a distortion of the maxillary arch causing malocclusion, and interference with optimal growth and development of the upper jaw. Orthodontic observation and treatment is continued until the permanent teeth are in good occlusion.

Speech therapy is continued after surgery to aid the child in correcting faulty sounds learned before the defect was corrected. Parents and therapists work together with the child to help him achieve clear speech without disagreeable nasal tones.

Occasionally it is necessary to delay surgery until the fourth or fifth year of life in order to take advantage of the palatal changes that occur with growth. If surgery is delayed beyond the third year, a prosthesis will be needed to help the child develop intelligible speech. The formation of teeth is usually delayed in the area of the defect. These missing teeth can be replaced by a denture to which is attached, posteriorly, a contoured speech bulb.

Umbilical Hernia

Umbilical hernias are quite common among infants. Most of them disappear spontaneously during late infancy without treatment or manipulation. Incarceration is extremely rare, but does occur. The hernia is caused by an imperfect closure or weakness of the fibrous umbilical ring. It appears as a soft swelling covered by skin at the site of the umbilicus. The hernia consists of omentum or portions of the small intestine. It can easily be reduced through gentle pressure.

The older method of applying adhesive to strap down the hernia is ineffective and may be injurious. The application of a coin or other rigid object over the site of the hernia serves to hold the fascial ring open.

However, pain or discomfort caused by an umbilical hernia may sometimes be relieved by strapping applied correctly. Swenson* describes a method of correct strapping that may be helpful.

Use two pieces of 2-inch adhesive tape, each about 6 to 8 inches in length. Cut a 1-inch square window in the center of one of the pieces. The other piece is trimmed from one end to the midpoint by cutting a 1/2-inch strip from each side.

The skin on each side of the umbilicus where the tape is to be placed should be painted with tincture of benzoin. Apply the broad end of the trimmed tape lateral to the umbilicus leaving the narrow end free. Place the other tape on the opposite side of the umbilicus, leaving the cut window and beyond unattached. Pass the narrow tongue of the first tape through the window and pull the free ends of the tapes in opposite directions. With the umbilicus folded inward, attach the free ends to the abdominal skin. The strapping should be changed about every 2 weeks. Parents can learn to change this after the first demonstration. (Fig. 28-1)

Congenital Hypertrophic Pyloric Stenosis

Pyloric stenosis is rarely symptomatic during the first days of life. It has on occasion been recognized shortly after birth, but the average affected infant does not show symptoms until about the third week of life. Symptoms rarely appear after the second month.

Although symptoms appear late, pyloric stenosis is classified as a congenital defect. Its cause is not known. The condition appears more frequently in males with a ratio of approximately 1:200. In female infants the ratio is about 1:1000.

Pathophysiology

The condition is characterized by hypertrophy of the circular muscle fibers of the pylorus, with a severe narrowing of its lumen. The pylorus is thickened to as much as twice its size, is elongated and has a

*Swenson, Orvar: Pediatric Surgery. (revised) New York, Appleton, 1968.

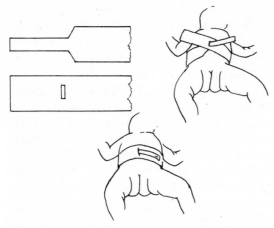

Figure 28-1. This is one method of strapping an umbilical hernia. (Swenson, O.: Pediatric Surgery. vol. 1, ed. 3. New York, Appleton-Century-Crofts. Courtesy of Appleton-Century-Crofts.)

consistency resembling cartilage. As a result of this obstruction at the distal end of the stomach, the stomach becomes dilated. (Fig. 28-2(*A*)

Symptoms

The first weeks of such an infant's life are usually uneventful; he probably eats well and gains weight. Then he starts vomiting

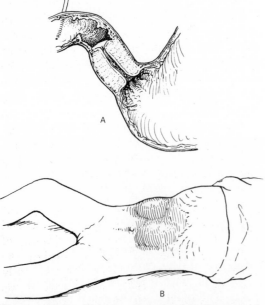

Figure 28-2. Pyloric stenosis (*A*) Narrowed lumen of the pylorus; (*B*) Visible peristalsis.

occasionally after meals. Within a few days the vomiting episodes increase in frequency and force, becoming projectile in character. The vomited material may contain mucus, but never bile, because it has not progressed beyond the stomach.

Because the obstruction is a mechanical one, the baby does not feel ill, is ravenously hungry, and is eager to try again and again. Unfortunately, the food invariably comes back.

As the condition progresses the baby becomes irritable, loses weight rapidly and becomes dehydrated. A condition of alkalosis develops from the loss of potassium and hydrochloric acid, and he becomes ill indeed.

Constipation becomes progressive because little food gets into the intestines, and the urine is scanty. Gastric peristaltic waves passing from left to right across the abdomen can usually be seen during or after feedings.

Diagnosis

Diagnosis usually can be made on the clinical evidence. The nature, type and times of vomiting, observation of gastric peristaltic waves, and a history of weight loss with hunger and irritability point in this direction. The olive-size pyloric tumor can often be felt through deep palpation by an experienced physician. Roentgenographic examination with barium swallow shows an abnormal retention of barium in the stomach and increased peristaltic waves. (Fig. 28-2 *B*)

Treatment

The condition is well-known and is suspected if a previously well infant commences to vomit his feedings. When under a pediatrician's care, either in a private office or in a clinic, these infants are carefully watched to prevent the critical degree of dehydration that was formerly so frequent. However, it still happens all too frequently that infants do not come into the hospital until dehydration and malnutrition are obvious, thus presenting an infant in very poor condition for surgical correction.

Treatment to correct pyloric stenosis is routinely surgical in the United States. The procedure commonly used is the Fredet-Remstedt operation. This procedure simply splits the hypertrophic pyloric muscle down to the submucosa, allowing the pylorus to expand so that food may pass. If performed by a competent surgeon on an infant in good condition, the operation is simple, and it gives excellent results.

In the United States, the older method of medical treatment is rarely used. This treatment consists of feedings of cereal-thickened formula, antispasmodic drugs and sedation. This treatment must of necessity be of long duration, is frequently unsatisfactory, and serves to increase the hazards to the child who is already malnourished and in poor condition. It may on occasion be used for a short time while a diagnosis is being established, but not for the child with pyloric stenosis who has lost much weight or who is already in alkalosis.

Nursing Care

Preoperative care. The infant who comes into the hospital after unsuccessful attempts at home treatment such as changes of formula and feeding techniques, is not, as a rule, in a condition for immediate surgery. He needs laboratory tests to determine his metabolic deficits and state of chemical imbalance.

Intravenous fluids are given to restore proper hydration and to correct the hypokalemic alkalosis. These are carefully calculated to restore lost electrolytes and bring the infant back into proper fluid balance.

The nurse should follow directions exactly as to the amount and type of fluid to be given. Mixing fluids, if this is required to meet the child's needs, is a very exact procedure, and should be done only by a nurse familiar with this procedure.

When the baby is in the hospital awaiting surgery, it will be very helpful if the mother is allowed to participate in his care. Both the mother and the baby are going to be happier if we can recognize their mutual needs. The nurse also needs a better opportunity to explain the purpose of waiting for surgery and the function of the intravenous fluids.

Feedings. If the baby does need a period of hospitalization before surgery, a smooth-muscle relaxant such as atropine may be ordered prior to oral feedings. Feedings may be thickened by mixing cooked cereal with the formula, and the child fed through a large-holed nipple, in the hope that some nutrients may be retained.

Recording. The nurse needs to record accurately the amount of feeding given, and the approximate amount retained, as well as the frequency and type of emesis. Urinary output is estimated or measured; the skin turgor is noted as well as the general physical appearance, state of irritability, lethargy, or any change in response to external stimulation.

Oral fluids are omitted for a specified time before surgery. Some surgeons order a stomach lavage shortly before surgery, with the nasogastric tube left in place. Preoperative medication such as atropine intramuscularly is usually ordered.

While the baby is in surgery, the mother is given a comfortable place in which to wait, and some attention is paid to her needs. She may be invited to accompany the staff on their coffee break or lunch period. If she waits in the general waiting room, some member of the staff can seek her out for an occasional friendly word. Be sure that she understands the use of the recovery room, because many parents become alarmed at a wait of several hours after the doctor has assured them that surgery is simple and of short duration.

Postoperative care. Postoperatively, the child should be positioned on his side and watched carefully to prevent aspiration of mucus or emesis, particularly during the anesthesia recovery period. When fully reacted, but restless, he may relax if his mother holds him. If so, be sure to give her a gown to protect her clothing.

The first feeding is usually given about six hours postoperatively, and generally is glucose water. If well tolerated, this feeding can be alternated with small amounts of dilute formula at frequent intervals, gradually increasing in amount and in frequency. The baby may vomit a time or two, but should progress quite rapidly toward complete recovery. Intravenous feedings may be needed until the child can tolerate sufficient oral feedings.

With early diagnosis, and surgery before dehydration and malnutrition have become severe, the child has an excellent chance for returning to a satisfactory condition in a short period of weeks, and of progressing steadily on to complete recovery. Operative fatality rate under these conditions has become less than 1 per cent.

Congenital Aganglionic Megacolon

Also called Hirschsprung's disease, this condition is characterized by obstinate constipation resulting from partial or complete intestinal obstruction of mechanical origin.

Pathophysiology

Parasympathetic nerve cells regulate peristalsis in the intestines. In Hirschsprung's disease there is a congenital absence of parasympathetic ganglion cells within the muscular wall of the distal colon and the rectum. In their absence, the affected

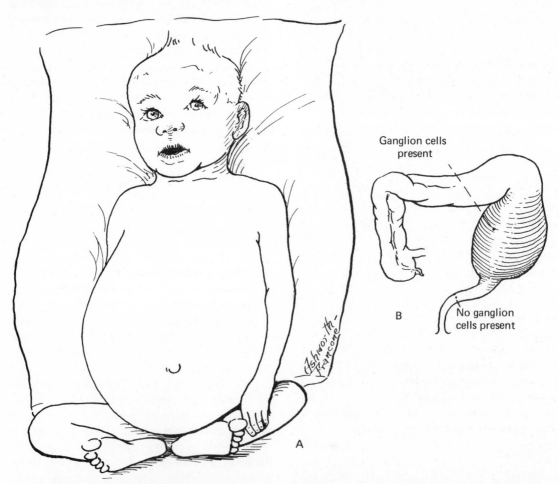

Figure 28-3. This drawing of a child with Hirschsprung's disease shows the distended abdomen (*A*) and dilated colon (*B*).

segment narrows, and the portion of the colon directly *above* the affected area becomes greatly dilated, filled with feces and gas.

Incidence

The condition may be severe enough to be recognized during the neonatal period. In other cases, it may not be diagnosed until later infancy or early childhood.

Manifestations

The *newborn* may pass no meconium during the first 24 hours. This may be symptomatic of other conditions such as imperforate anus. In any case, it is of extreme importance that accurate records be kept of the first stool, its timing and character. Failure to pass a stool within the first 24 hours should always be reported.

Other neonatal symptoms are of complete or partial intestinal obstruction, such as bile-stained emesis and generalized abdominal distention. Gastroenteritis with diarrheal stools may be present, and ulceration of the colon may occur.

Symptoms in the *older infant* or *young child* are obstinate, severe constipation dating back to early infancy. Stools are ribbonlike or consist of hard pellets. Formed bowel movements do not occur except with the use of enemas, and soiling does not occur. The rectum is usually empty, as the impaction occurs above the aganglionic segment.

As the child grows older the abdomen becomes progressively enlarged and hard. General debilitation and chronic anemia are usually present. Differentiation must be made between this condition and psychogenic megacolon due to coercive toilet training or other emotional problems. In aganglionic megacolon there is no withholding of stool or stooling in inappropriate places, and no soiling.

Diagnosis

Definitive diagnosis requires Roentgen examination following barium enema and, frequently, rectal biopsy.

Treatment

Treatment for cure requires abdominal resection. In early infancy, a colostomy is usually performed to relieve the obstruction. Resection is deferred until later infancy.

Nursing Care

The colon must be emptied of fecal material prior to diagnostic procedures, and also prior to surgery. Oil retention enemas, followed by colonic irrigation are necessary daily or at frequent intervals to empty the colon. Oil retention enemas consisting of three or four ounces of mineral or olive oil may be used.

Colonic irrigations or enemas must always consist of *isotonic saline solution*. Due to the lack of peristaltic action, the water in plain tap water enemas or soap suds enemas is retained and absorbed into the tissues, causing water intoxication. Syncope, shock, and frequently death result even after only one or two tap water irrigations. Enemas of magnesium sulfate have caused magnesium poisoning. Isotonic saline solutions should be used routinely.

Procedure for Giving Saline Enemas to Infants

1. Cleansing Enema

   #### Equipment

   An irrigating can with clean tubing.
   A catheter, size 10 to 12, French.
   Solution: isotonic saline (1 tsp. salt to 1 pint water) unless otherwise ordered. (Tap water should never be used for children unless specifically ordered.) Temperature 100° to 105°. Amount—infants 120 to 200 cc., children 200 to 300 cc.
   A lubricant.
   A bedpan.

   #### Procedure

   1. Remove the diaper or panties, and place the infant or small child on a small bedpan. Place a small pillow at his back.

2. Insert a lubricated rectal tube into his rectum for a distance of two to three inches, or less for infant.
3. Lift the can only enough to allow a flow. (Not above 18 inches.)
4. A small child will usually have better results if allowed to sit on a potty chair following the enema. Diapers should be fastened securely for an infant because returns may be delayed.
5. Clean the perineum, and replace the diaper or the panties.
6. Record the time, the amount and the kind of solution, and the results. (Note: children with sluggish peristalsis may absorb tap water through the intestinal wall into the body tissues with a resultant water intoxication that may have serious consequences. This is particularly true in aganglionic megacolon.)

2. Retention Enema

Equipment

A funnel and a small French catheter. Oil as prescribed, usually 60 to 150 cc. at 100°.

Procedure

Give slowly into the rectum. Maintain pressure over the rectum after giving, or hold the buttocks together until the urge to defecate has passed. Instruct the child to retain the solution if possible. A cleansing enema (saline) may be given in about 30 minutes if the child has not defecated.

A colonic irrigation is a potentially dangerous nursing procedure and will usually be performed by the surgical resident.

Surgery

Best results have been obtained through the Swenson pull-through procedure. In this procedure the narrowed section is pulled through and sutured to the anal opening. Modifications of the Duhamel side-to-side anastomosis are also being evaluated.

Postoperative Care

If a colostomy only has been performed, routine colostomy care is given.

Children generally tolerate this long, difficult surgery very well. The child should be closely observed until he is thoroughly awake. Vital signs are observed and recorded as in any major abdominal operation. A nasogastric tube will be left in and intravenous feedings given until bowel function is established. Temperatures should not be taken rectally. For the infant and young child, axillary temperatures can be taken. The nurse needs to be alert for rectal bleeding, abdominal distention, a rise in pulse or temperature. Any of these signs should be reported promptly. Successful surgery allows these children to grow and develop normally.

CONDITIONS OF METABOLIC IMBALANCE

The Celiac Syndrome

Intestinal malabsorption with steatorrhea is a condition brought about by various causes, the most common being cystic fibrosis and gluten-induced enteropathy, the so-called idiopathic celiac disease. In 1889, the condition of malnutrition, abnormal stools, distended abdomen and retarded growth was described and named *celiac disease*. Not until the late 1930's was it recognized that several distinct entities were being described, with cystic fibrosis and celiac disease as two conditions of differing etiology. The term *celiac syndrome* is now used to designate the complex of malabsorptive disorders.

Gluten-induced Enteropathy

The "idiopathic celiac disease" is a basic defect of metabolism precipitated by the ingestion of wheat gluten or rye gluten, leading to impaired fat absorption. The exact etiology is not known; the most acceptable theory is that of an inborn error of metabolism with an allergic reaction as a contributing factor; or possibly, an allergic reaction as the sole factor.

Severe manifestations of the disorder have become rare in the United States and in western Europe, but mild disturbances of intestinal absorption of rye, wheat, and sometimes oat gluten, are not uncommon.

Clinical manifestations. Signs generally do not appear before the age of six months, and may be delayed until a year or later. Manifestations include chronic diarrhea with foul, bulky, greasy stools, and progressive malnutrition. There is anorexia, and a fretful, unhappy disposition is typical. The onset is generally insidious, with failure to thrive, bouts of diarrhea and frequent respiratory infections. If the condition becomes severe, the effects of malnutrition are prominent. Retarded growth and development, a distended abdomen and thin, wasted buttocks and legs are characteristic symptoms.

Celiac Crisis

The chronic course of this disease may be interrupted by a *celiac crisis.* This is frequently triggered by an upper respiratory infection. The child commences to vomit copiously, has large, watery stools and becomes severely dehydrated. He becomes drowsy and prostrated, developing an acute medical emergency. Parenteral fluid therapy is essential to combat acidosis and to achieve normal fluid balance.

Diagnosis and treatment. At present the only way to determine if a small child's failure to thrive is from this disorder is to place him on a trial gluten-free diet and to evaluate the results. Improvement in the nature of the stools and general well-being, with a gain in weight should follow, although several weeks may elapse before clear-cut manifestations can be confirmed.

Response to a diet from which rye, wheat and oats are excluded is generally good, although probably no cure can be expected; and dietary indiscretions or intercurrent respiratory infections may bring relapses. The omission of wheat products in particular should continue through adolescence, because the ingestion of wheat appears to inhibit growth in sensitive persons.

Dietary program. The young child is usually started on a starch-free, low fat diet. If his condition is severe, this will consist of skim milk, glucose, and banana flakes. Bananas contain invert sugar and are usually well tolerated. Additions to the diet of lean meats, pureed vegetables and fruits are made gradually. Eventually, fats may be added, and the child can be maintained on a regular diet with the exception of all wheat and rye products.

It is not always recognized that commercially canned creamed soups, cold cuts, frankfurters, and pudding mixes, generally contain wheat products. The forbidden list also includes malted milk drinks, some candies, many baby foods and, of course, breads, cakes, pastries and biscuits, unless the latter are made from corn flour. The list of ingredients on packaged foods should be read before purchasing. Vitamins A and D in water-miscible solutions will be needed in double amounts to supplement the deficient diet.

Cystic Fibrosis of the Pancreas (Mucoviscidosis)

Cystic fibrosis is a generalized disease affecting many organs of the body. The major organs affected are the lungs, the pancreas and the liver, and the sweat, tear and salivary glands. Cystic fibrosis is an hereditary disease, inherited as a recessive trait. (See Chap. 31 for genetic condition.) When both parents carry a recessive gene for this condition, the statistical expectation is that two out of four children will carry a gene for the trait, one will be free of it, and one will have the disease. There is, however, no way to predict the sequence; any child born to these parents has one chance in four of having the disease, no matter what his siblings have inherited. The occurrence of the disease in more than 25% of the children in a small family is probably due to chance distribution.

Incidence

The disease occurs in about the proportion of 1 in 2000 live births in

Caucasian populations. In the United States it is one of the most common serious chronic conditions of children. Cystic fibrosis occurs much less frequently in African or Asian peoples.

Pathophysiology

The basic defect is not known, but is generally believed to be an inborn error of metabolism. Abnormal secretions of the mucus-producing glands throughout the body tend to accumulate; in some organs it coagulates and forms obstructions. This occurs primarily in the pancreatic ducts and in the bronchi.

Clinical Manifestations

Meconium ileus in the newborn infant may be the presenting symptom. Onset of symptoms of cystic fibrosis without meconium ileus is rather insidious. They may occur at varying ages during infancy or childhood.

A hard, nonproductive chronic cough may be the first suspicious symptom. Later, bronchial infections become frequent. In spite of an excellent appetite, malnutrition is apparent and becomes increasingly severe. The abdomen becomes distended, and body muscles become flabby. Stools are frequent, bulky and greasy, with a characteristic foul odor.

Pancreatic involvement. The pancreatic ducts are obstructed by a thick, tenacious mucus, causing the flow of pancreatic enzymes to be diminished or even absent. This achylia or hypochylia* leads to intestinal malabsorption and to severe malnutrition. The children with a moderate insufficiency do tend, however, to have a greater reduction in function as they grow older.

Because of the malabsorption of fats, the stools are bulky, greasy, foamy, and have a distinctively foul odor. Other malabsorption defects have this kind of stool however, so that this is not in itself diagnostic of fibrocystic disease. Rectal prolapse is a

*Hypochylia. Deficient secretion of gastric juice. Achylia. Absence of hydrochloric acid and rennin from the gastric juice.

frequent complication if the pancreatic condition remains untreated.

Meconium ileus. Meconium ileus is the presenting manifestation of fibrocystic disease in approximately 5% to 10% of the newborns who later develop additional manifestations. Depletion or absence of pancreatic enzymes before birth results in impaired digestive activity, and the meconium becomes viscid and mucilaginous. The inspissated meconium fills the small intestine, causing complete obstruction. Clinical manifestations are bile-stained emesis, a distended abdomen, and an absence of stool. Intestinal perforation with symptoms of shock may occur.

Treatment is surgical resection, employing one of several methods, but the mortality rate is high in spite of skillful surgery. The majority of infants who survive develop cystic fibrosis of varying degrees of severity.

Pulmonary involvement. The severity of pulmonary involvement differs in individual children, a few showing only relatively minor involvement. The degree of lung involvement determines the prognosis for survival. Present figures show that 50% of affected children die before the age of 10 years, as the result of respiratory complications. Abnormal amounts of thick, viscid mucus clog the bronchioles and provide an ideal medium for bacterial growth. Staphylococcus aureous coagulase can be cultured from the nasopharynx and from the sputum of most patients. Pseudomonas aeruginosa and Hemophilus influenzae are also frequently isolated from the sputum and from the nasopharynx. The basic infection, however, appears most often to be caused by staphylococcus.

Complications arising from severe respiratory infection are numerous. Atelectasis may appear early in the disease, and small lung abscesses are common. Bronchiectasis and emphysema develop, with pulmonary fibrosis and pneumonitis, eventually leading to severe ventilatory insufficiency.

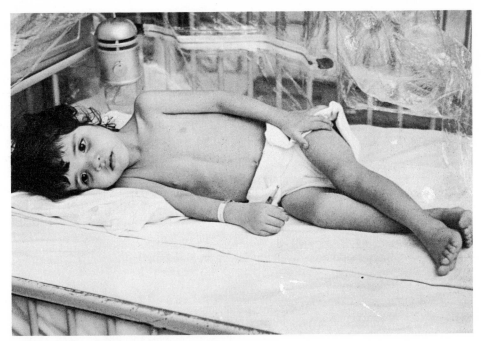

Figure 28-4.   This child has cystic fibrosis.

In the past, cystic fibrosis was a disease confined to children, because no one with respiratory involvement was known to live past adolescence. At present, with improved knowledge and methods of treatment, an increasing number are living through adolescence and into young adulthood.

Other affected organs. The tears, the saliva and the sweat contain abnormal amounts of electrolytes, and the submaxillary salivary glands are enlarged in a majority of these children. These manifestations appear to be without significance, but are useful in the establishment of a diagnosis. In hot weather, the loss of sodium chloride and of fluid through the sweat produces frequent heat prostration in these children, so that additional fluid and salt in the diet, or salt tablets, should be given as a precautionary measure.

Diagnosis and Diagnostic Tests

Diagnosis is based on family history, evidence of elevated sodium chloride in the sweat, demonstration of hypochylia or achylia, the patient's past history of failure to thrive, and on roentgen findings. A combination of high levels of sweat chloride, malabsorption or pulmonary manifestations, and a suspicious clinical history is considered sufficient evidence for a definitive diagnosis.

Sweat test for elevated levels of sodium and chloride. The sweat of affected children contains high levels of potassium, sodium and chloride. In a majority of affected children, sodium and chloride levels are elevated two to five times above normal, with a lesser degree of potassium elevation. Laboratory determination of sodium and chloride levels in the sweat provides a useful diagnostic test.

The formerly used, thermally-induced sweating method has been largely replaced by the safer and more reliable pilocarpine iontophoresis method. Formerly, a small gauze patch was taped on to the child, out of his reach, usually on his upper back; a plastic sheet or bag was wrapped around his body, and he was covered with a blanket. Sweating was induced by keeping the child thus wrapped in a warm room for a period of three-quarters of an hour to an hour.

These children, however, have a particular sensitivity to heat, and they rapidly

DIAGRAMMATIC REVIEW OF CYSTIC FIBROSIS*

Note: Since 1963, it has been discovered that achylia is not always present, although some degree of pancreatic insufficiency is always found.

The generalized disease *Cystic Fibrosis of the Pancreas*—
unknown basic defect,
genetically transmitted

↓

Exocrine gland dysfunction—
electrolyte abnormality of sweat, saliva, and tears,
chemical and physiochemical abnormality of mucous secretions,
increase in parotid secretory rate

↓

Organ involvement—
lungs, pancreas, liver, eccrine sweat glands and others

↓

Clinical Symptoms—
chronic pulmonary disease,
intestinal malabsorption (from pancreatic achylia),
occasionally, heat casualties (due to massive salt loss through sweat)
Cirrhosis of liver

↓

Diagnosis—
elevated sweat electrolytes—main test,
obstructive emphysema and chronic bronchopneumonia on X-ray of chest,
absent pancreatic enzymes,
family history

↓

Prognosis—
pulmonary involvement dominates clinical picture and determines fate of patient,
chronic lung disease frequently progressive and often leads to
fatal termination in the pediatric age group.

―――――

*After P. A. di Sant' Agnese: Ann. N.Y. Acad. Sci., *93:*495, 1962.

―――

lose fluids and electrolytes. Several fatalities from hyperthermia have followed the use of this method on ill children. If this method is to be used, the child must be carefully watched and constantly attended.

The safe, reliable pilocarpine iontophoresis method of inducing sweating utilizes a small electric current that carries topically applied pilocarpine into a localized area of the skin. Because this method is widely used, it is briefly described here.

Pilocarpine iontophoresis method. An area on the child's forearm is washed with distilled water, dried, and is covered with a 2

x 2 inch gauze square that has been saturated with a measured amount of 0.2% pilocarpine nitrate. A positive copper electrode is applied over the gauze, and a negative electrode is placed elsewhere on the same arm, and both are attached with rubber straps of the type used for electrocardiography. Lead wires are connected, and low current is applied for five minutes.

Following iontophoresis, the electrodes are removed, the gauze is discarded, and the area is again washed with distilled water. Dry gauze, which has been weighed in a glass flask, is removed from the flask with forceps, placed over the area that has been ion-tophoresed, and covered with a plastic square, firmly secured around the edges with adhesive tape. After 30 to 45 minutes, the gauze is removed with forceps, placed in the flask, weighed and analyzed in the laboratory for its sodium and chloride content.

Duodenal Aspiration Test for Tryptic Activity in Duodenal Fluid (Assay for Pancreatic Enzyme-Diagnostic Test for Mucoviscidosis)

Duodenal aspiration for trypsin activity. An index of pancreatic activity may be ascertained by measuring the tryptic activity in aspirated duodenal fluid. This is an uncomfortable procedure, quite unpleasant for the small child who must be immobilized, in a fasting state, for several hours. The tube also has a tendency to curl up in the stomach, or to become plugged with thick mucus, necessitating manipulation. Tests are frequently unsatisfactory and must be repeated. This test is important for diagnosis and treatment in a child with a positive sweat test, however. The nurse performing the aspiration should be free from other duties during the period when the tube is down, in order to give emotional support and comfort to the child.

Preparation:

1. Explain the procedure to the child if he can understand.
2. Apply restraints as needed. A mummy restraint may be necessary while the tube is passed.
3. A number 10 or 12 French catheter or small Levine tube containing three to four openings at the distal end, is passed through the child's nose, is guided through the stomach and into the duodenum. The catheter is lubricated with water only.
4. The fluid is aspirated and tested for pH reaction with nitrozene paper. If the tube is in the stomach, the reaction will be acid: duodenal fluid is alkaline.
5. The tube may be guided into the pyloric antrum under fluoroscopic control, and cautious efforts to push it through may be made by the physician.
6. After the tube has entered the duodenum (as indicated by aspirated fluid having a pH of 6 or 7 or higher), the tubing is anchored to the child's face with adhesive tape.
7. Pancreatic fluid is obtained by gravity, or by occasional gentle suction with a Luer syringe.
8. Fluid is allowed to drain into a test tube, which is preferably kept standing in ice during collection. If fluid drips freely, fractional samples may be obtained. The tubes must be changed at frequent intervals and placed immediately on ice.
9. Frequent testing of pH reaction is essential. Samples with a pH of less than 6 are not used for analysis.
10. Collection of 5 to 8 cc. of pancreatic fluid is necessary for analysis. If pancreatic failure is present, the flow may be unusually slow, and the amount collected within 60 minutes may have to suffice.
11. The aspiration procedure is extremely uncomfortable. The nurse may give support by her presence, by reading to child or by talking in soothing tone and giving assurance by her gentle touch. She may also release the restraints when she stays with child during this procedure, thus alleviating some of his discomfort.
12. After a specimen is collected, and the tube is removed, the child is comforted and given fluids, or food if he desires it.
13. Specimens are sent to the laboratory immediately and are examined within the hour. If mucoviscidosis is present, the pancreatic fluid has a high viscosity, and in some cases, it may not flow at all. The fluid is tested for the presence of trypsin by observing (in the laboratory) the effects on a gelatin substrate, using varying dilutions of pancreatic fluid.

Stool examination. The presence of tryptic activity is ascertained by the ability of a small portion of stool to digest the gelatinous coating of X-ray or photographic film. This test has only a limited value, because false, positive values may be obtained as the result of the bacterial activity.

A more useful study is made by determining the total fat content in the stools collected over a 72-hour period, during which time the child is on a diet containing a minimum of fat. When steatorrhea is present, the fecal loss of fat is greater than 5% of ingested fat. This test may be unreliable in certain circumstances.

Roentgenograms. Generalized obstructive emphysema is highly suggestive when associated with other clinical manifestations. Later in the disease, other pulmonary changes may be noted.

Treatment for Pancreatic Deficiency

The administration of commercially prepared pancreatic enzymes aid digestion and the absorption of both fat and protein. Pancreatic enzymes are given during meals, either in the form of granules, which can be sprinkled on the food, or in capsule form for older children. The pancreatic preparation should be given to all affected children, in a prescribed dosage, even if the pancreatic insufficiency appears minimal.

Dietary treatment consists of giving a diet high in carbohydrates and protein, with a moderate restriction of fats. These children have large appetites unless they are acutely ill, but they can receive little nourishment from food without a pancreatic supplement. If these children are properly treated with diet and with enzyme supplements, the stools become relatively normal, and their nutrition improves. A restriction of foods such as ice cream, peanut butter, butter, french fries and mayonnaise is advocated, but the child and his parents should not be made to feel that meals must be drab and unenjoyable. Advice similar to this might be given:

"Dick should start gaining weight and feel more peppy now that we have started his medicine. Suppose that one day a week, we let him choose his own meals, let him have anything he wants, and give him extra

digestive enzymes. Then during the rest of the week he won't mind so much waiting for his peanut butter and ice cream." A positive approach makes the whole regime appear brighter.

Because of the increased loss of sodium chloride, these children are allowed to use as much salt as they wish, even though onlookers may think it is too much. Provision for additional amounts of salt in hot weather may be made by supplying pretzels, salt bread sticks and saltines in liberal quantities.

Vitamins, in water-miscible preparations, are needed in amounts double a daily dose.

Treatment for respiratory involvement. Treatment for respiratory involvement is much more difficult. Treatment is aimed at providing respiratory drainage by thinning the secretions, and by mechanical means, such as postural drainage and clapping to move the secretions outward. Antibacterial drugs for the treatment of infection are necessary as indicated. Physical activity is beneficial as well, and should be restricted only to the extent of the child's endurance.

Inhalation treatment for thinning secretions. Prophylactic and therapeutic use of aerosol treatments is necessary for all children with cystic fibrosis. Intermittent inhalation by nebulizer of 10% propylene glycol in water or in saline, in addition to a bronchodilator drug, is necessary three or four times daily. The addition of a mucolytic agent, such as Mucomist, is especially useful during periods of acute infection.

The majority of these children profit by continuous aerosol therapy during their naptime and through the night, using a 10% solution of propylene glycol.

Humidified atmosphere. A mist tent for use during sleep is needed for every affected child. A heavy mist, raising humidity above 50%, is essential. Various types of mist tents are on the market that function through the use of a compressed air pump, but they may also use oxygen if it is necessary. An attachment for a nebulizer is provided. Children become quite accustomed to

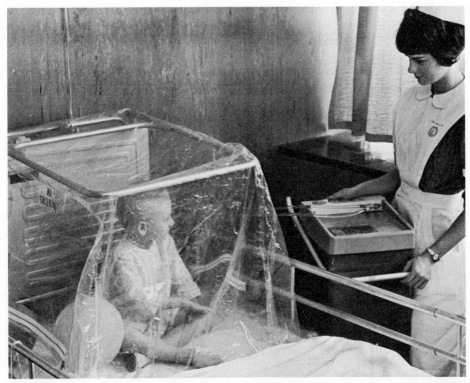

Figure 28-5. Bobby prepares for naptime in his mist tent.

crawling inside their tents for sleeping, and in times of acute distress, the use of a mist tent becomes a necessary full-time treatment.

Postural drainage. Postural drainage is performed routinely three or four times daily, even if little drainage is apparent. Clapping and vibrating of the affected areas, if done correctly, helps to move the secretions upward and outward. The nurse should become quite proficient at performing this procedure; and also needs to be able to demonstrate it to the parents. Parents should watch and practice it until they, too, become proficient.

Additional treatments. Antibiotics for the treatment of respiratory infections are used as indicated. Whether these are given as preventive medicine, or are reserved for the treatment of acute infections, is not uniformly agreed upon at present.

Immunization against childhood communicable diseases is of extreme importance for these chronically ill children. All im-

munization measures may be used, and should be maintained at the appropriate intervals.

Home Care

The home care for these children places a tremendous burden upon the concerned families. This is no one-time hospital treatment, nor is there a prospect of cure to brighten the horizon. This, of course, is true of many chronic ailments, but in the daily care of a child with cystic fibrosis, a large amount of time is spent in the performance of treatments. Parents must learn to manipulate the mist tent compressor and the nebulizer, perform postural drainage and clapping techniques. The child's diet must be planned, with the regulation of additional enzymes according to need. Great care is needed to guard against exposure to infections.

In addition to all this, the parents must guard against over-protection and against undue limitation of their child's physical

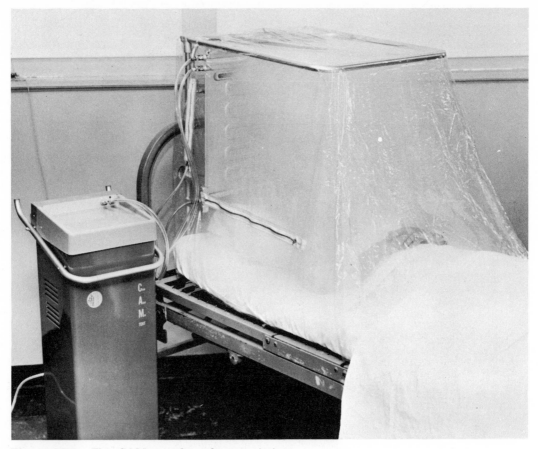

Figure 28-6.   This CAM tent shows heavy misting.

activity. Somehow, a good family relationship must be preserved, with time allowed for attention to other members of the family. This all adds up to a pretty big task.

Physical activity is an important adjunct to the child's well-being, and is a necessary help in getting rid of secretions. The child soon learns his capacity for exercise, and can be trusted to become self-limiting as necessary, especially if he has had an opportunity to learn the nature of his condition. Small children may find postural drainage fun when daddy raises their feet in the air and walks them around "wheel-barrow" fashion.

Hot weather activity should be watched a little more closely, with additional attention directed toward increased salt and fluid intake during periods of exercise.

The financial cost to the family is indeed

formidable. It is unrealistic to quote prices, but the cost is high.

Parent groups, organized in most cities, help in morale building, fund raising and educational projects. The Cystic Fibrosis Foundation is presently active in research, with established centers in a number of cities.

Camps for Children with Cystic Fibrosis

Camps for children with cystic fibrosis have been instituted in the past few years and have proved surprisingly successful. For most of the children, this has been their first experience in camping. The camps are staffed with nurses and therapists who assist with necessary treatments, such as postural drainage and inhalations. They are also available as consultants. The children

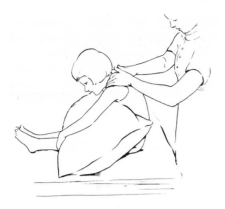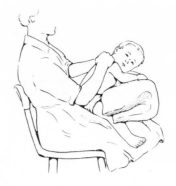

Upper lobes—posterior segments

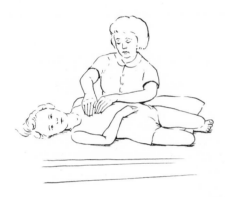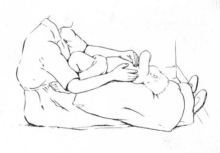

Left upper lobe—lingular segment

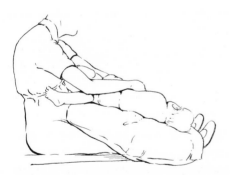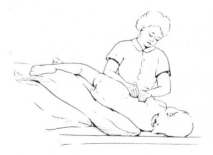

Left lower lobe—lateral segments

Figure 28-7.   There are a number of positions for postural drainage in cystic fibrosis.

participate in the usual camping activities, such as nature walks, crafts, swimming and sports. The children seem to thrive and go home enriched by the experience.

Prognosis

The prognosis at the present time is still poor. The cause of the disease is not yet

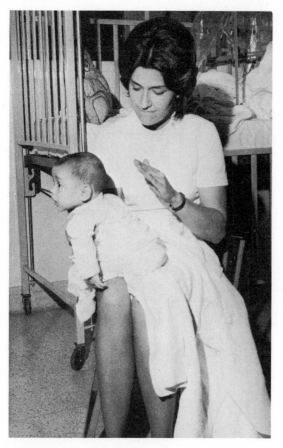

Figure 28-8. "Clapping" of the affected areas in cystic fibrosis helps move the secretion.

known, and no cure has been found. Early diagnosis and treatment are effective in prolonging life as well as enabling the child to live more normally. The severity of the disease determines the outcome, but it still must be said that few affected children live to adulthood. However, with continuing research, prospects for the future look brighter.

Wilm's Tumor

Wilm's tumor is an adenosarcoma in the kidney region and is one of the most common of the abdominal neoplasms found in early childhood. The tumor arises from bits of embryonic tissue remaining after birth. This tissue has the capacity to begin rapid cancerous growth in the area of the kidney.

The tumor is rarely discovered until it has reached a size large enough to be palpated through the abdominal wall. As the tumor grows it invades the kidney or the renal vein and disseminates to other parts of the body. Treatment consists of surgical removal as soon as possible after the growth is discovered. The medication now being used is actinomycin D given before and after surgery. Irradiation is also used post-operatively.

Prognosis is generally good for children under the age of 2 years. The use of actinomycin D has brought about a significant decrease in the mortality rate from this disorder. If the child appears well and no metastasis is evident after the age of 2, he is considered cured.

RESPIRATORY CONDITIONS

Acute Nasopharyngitis

The common cold is one of the most common infectious conditions of childhood. The young infant is as susceptible as the older child but is not generally as frequently exposed.

Etiology

The illness is of viral origin, rhinoviruses being the principal agents. Bacterial invasion of the tissues may cause complications such as ear, mastoid and lung infections. The young child appears to be more susceptible to complications than an older person.

Clinical Manifestations

The infant over the age of 3 months usually develops fever early in the course of the infection, often as high as 102° to 104°F, that is, 38.9° to 40°C. (Younger infants usually are afebrile.) He sneezes frequently, becomes irritable and restless. The congested nasal passages interfere with nursing, increasing the infant's irritability. The infant may have accompanying vomiting or diarrhea. This nasopharyngeal condition also appears as the first symptom of many childhood contagious diseases, such as

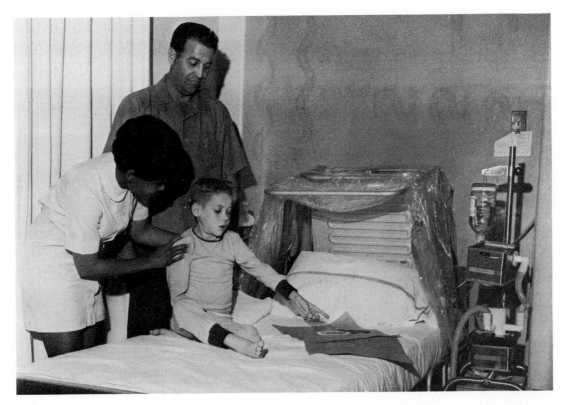

Figure 28-9. This child with cystic fibrosis proudly displays his paintings.

measles. The common cold also needs to be differentiated from allergic rhinitis.

Prevention

Because complications can be very serious for the infant, efforts should be made to keep him away from persons suffering from colds.

Treatment and Nursing Care

Nose drops will help relieve the nasal congestion. Oily nose drops should never be used because of the danger of lipoid pneumonia if aspirated. A dilute solution of Neo-Synephrine* in saline is most commonly used. Nursing care of the irritable, uncomfortable infant includes holding and rocking and soothing him.

Administering nose drops. The infant is placed across the nurse's lap with his head

_____
*Trademark, Winthrop Laboratories

lowered, or placed on his back in his crib with a folded blanket under his shoulders to allow his head to drop back. A plastic dropper with a rounded tip should be used to avoid injury to the child's nasal membrane. He should be kept in this position for a minute or two to allow the medication to shrink the nasal mucosa.

Nose drops should be administered 10 to 15 minutes before feedings and at bedtime. A bottle of nose drops should be used by only one person and discarded after its use is discontinued, as the solution easily becomes contaminated.

Acute Otitis Media

The eustachian tube in an infant is shorter and wider than in the older child. It is also straighter, thereby allowing naso-pharyngeal infections to enter the middle ear more easily. Hemophilus influenzae is an important cause of otitis media in infants.

Clinical Manifestations

A restless infant who repeatedly shakes his head or rubs his ear should be checked for ear infection. Symptoms include fever and irritability. There may be vomiting or diarrhea. Examination of the ear with an otoscope reveals a bulging eardrum. Spontaneous rupture of the eardrum may occur, in which case there will be purulent drainage and pain will be relieved.

Treatment

Antibiotics are used during the period of infection and for several days following, to prevent chronic infection and mastoiditis. Myringotomy may be necessary if improvement does not follow the use of antibiotics.

Recurrences of otitis media are common in infancy. Myringotomy to establish drainage and to obtain pus for culture is necessary in persistently recurring otitis media. Antibiotics are used as with acute otitis media. Selective antibiotics, most effective in destroying the specific organism, are used as soon as cultures have shown the causative bacterium.

Nursing Care

Emotional and physical support necessary for any ill infant should be freely given. If there is drainage from a ruptured eardrum or following myringotomy, the outer ear must be kept scrupulously clean. If ear wicks are to be inserted, the ear lobe is pulled down and back to straighten the ear canal in an infant. Ear wicks made of sterile gauze should be inserted carefully and loosely, and changed frequently. Placing the infant on the affected side helps promote drainage.

Instillation of ear drops may be ordered during the course of the infection. The procedure for instilling ear drops is as follows:

1. Turn the child's head with the affected ear uppermost.
2. Straighten the ear canal by pulling the pinna slightly down and straight back. For an older child (over three years) pull the pinna up and back as for an adult.
3. Drop warm drops into the external ear canal and hold him in position for few minutes to allow the drops to run onto the ear drum.

Acute Bronchiolitis

Acute bronchiolitis (acute interstitial pneumonia) occurs with the greatest frequency during the first 6 months of life, and is rarely seen after the age of 2 years. The majority of cases occur in infants who have been in contact with older children or adults suffering from upper respiratory viral infections.

Etiology

Acute bronchiolitis is caused by a viral infection. The causative agent in over 50 percent of cases has been shown to be the respiratory syncytial virus. Other viruses associated with the disease are the parainfluenza, adenoviruses, and other viruses not always identified.

Pathology

The bronchi and bronchioles become plugged with a thick, viscid mucus, causing air to be trapped in the lungs. The infant can breathe air in, but has difficulty expelling it. This hinders the exchange of gases, and cyanosis appears.

Manifestations

Onset of dyspnea is abrupt, sometimes preceded by a cough or a nasal discharge. There is a dry, persistent cough, extremely shallow respiration, air hunger, and cyanosis, which is frequently marked. Suprasternal and subcostal retractions are present. The chest becomes barrel-shaped from the trapped air. Respirations are 60 to 80 per minute.

Body temperature elevation is not great, seldom rising above 101° to 102°F. (38.3° to 38.9°C.). Dehydration may become a serious factor if competent care is not given. The infant appears apprehensive, irritable and restless.

Nursing Care

Nursing care includes placing the infant in a highly humidified atmosphere. At present, cold humidification is preferred to steam. Various means for providing this kind of humidity are in use, and these will be discussed later in this section.

Elevation of the child's head and chest aids his breathing. Placing the child on his abdomen provides pressure on the chest to relieve the distention, but should not be done unless the nurse can observe the infant continuously, because he is undoubtedly too weak to protect his breathing if obstruction occurs. He should be turned at least every

Case of Baby Jane

Baby Jane, four months old, was to be admitted to the sick babies' nursery with a diagnosis of acute bronchiolitis. Ruth Smith, student nurse, was assigned to get the room ready, as well as to care for Baby Jane on her arrival. The nurse was told to set up a Croupette and to prepare to maintain heavy moisture. If we follow her actions throughout the day, we may get a better picture of infant care under such conditions.

Before Baby Jane arrived, Miss Smith set up a Croupette in the crib, checking for good working order and following clearly marked directions on the Croupette itself. After this had been done, she put plenty of diapers, flannel gowns, pads and small blankets in the room, knowing that the infant would need frequent changes to prevent chilling in the moisture laden atmosphere.

Mrs. Brown and Baby Jane arrived on the ward just as Miss Smith finished setting up the unit. The mother looked apprehensive, and the nurse thought she had good reason to be. Baby Jane certainly looked sick. She had a pinched, anxious look, with a bluish pallor around her mouth. She was extremely fretful, twisting about and crying irritably, and breathing in a shallow, rapid manner.

"I just don't know what to do with her," said her mother. "She won't stop crying, she won't eat, but she still acts hungry. She looks awfully sick."

Miss Smith thought so too, but she sensed that the mother was looking to her for reassurance. "I think she will feel more comfortable if we get her in this Croupette as soon as possible. I will turn it on full while we undress her, so that she can get plenty of moisture. That should make her breathe easier. Shall I undress her for you?"

Mrs. Brown seemed relieved to have a competent nurse take over. Baby Jane was quickly put into a hospital gown and diaper, and lightly wrapped in a blanket. Her nurse cleaned the secretions from the anterior nares, using a cotton pledget moistened with water. Then she tucked the baby into the Croupette, carefully turning her on her side, with her head slightly elevated.

Baby Jane was too young and too exhausted to show any fear of the Croupette. As the moist air penetrated her nasal passages, she relaxed, breathed easier, and shortly fell asleep. Her mother also relaxed, and was happy to accept the suggestion that she go to the cafeteria for a cup of coffee.

Baby Jane required very careful nursing. In addition to maintaining moisturized air, Miss Smith kept close supervision of the sick child. As she became damp from the heavy moisture, Baby Jane required frequent change of clothing to prevent chilling. She had a great need for adequate fluid, inasmuch as a small infant can dehydrate very rapidly, and here the nurse experienced difficulty.

The baby appeared thirsty and made repeated attempts to suck her thumb, but would always pull it away angrily and cry. Miss Smith filled a nursing bottle with glucose water which she offered to Baby Jane through the tent opening. The baby sucked eagerly once or twice, and then fretfully drew away. This was repeated several times. When the doctor was informed of this he explained Baby Jane's puzzling behavior.

"Of course she is thirsty, but it is difficult for her to suck and to breathe at the same time because her nose is nearly occluded. Offer her glucose water at intervals, but do not persist if she has any difficulty. We will give her intravenous feedings to care for her liquid and nutritional needs, and this will also help to relieve her thirst."

To give a happy ending to the story, Baby Jane, who was essentially healthy and robust, recovered quite rapidly under the meticulous care she received, and went home to be once again the pride of her family. Thereafter, however, when any of the other children had a cold, they stayed completely away from Baby Jane.

hour, and needs frequent changes of clothing because of the moist atmosphere.

If he is to be fed, clean his nares as much as possible before offering a bottle. Use a relatively small-holed nipple so that he does not choke, but do not make him work hard enough to tire him. If he can be removed from his Croupette, he no doubt will fare better when he is held for feeding. If he needs to stay in his humidified atmosphere continually, be certain that his head is elevated, and hold his bottle, watching for choking or signs of exhaustion.

The nurse must remember that the baby is working hard in an effort to breathe, and can become exhausted very easily. Handling should be at a minimum consistent with intelligent nursing care. Intravenous fluids may be substituted for oral feedings until the infant is breathing more easily.

Medication is usually minimal because antihistamines, expectorants and sedatives do not appear to be useful. Antibiotics may be given to control secondary bacterial infections. Tracheostomy is not indicated in this condition.

With careful nursing care and intelligent treatment, the condition can be expected to improve within a few days. Mortality rate is low if adequate supportive care is given; it is considered to be under 1%, even in severe cases. Complications, however, can include cardiac failure, respiratory failure from exhaustion, severe dehydration from loss of fluid because of hyperventilation, and bacterial bronchopneumonia.

The Use of an Ice-Cooled Mist Tent (Croupette*)

1. Make up the crib in the usual manner. Place a cotton blanket over the sheet to absorb the increased moisture caused by humidity in the croupette (optional).
2. Unfold the frame, and set it in the crib. Open the plastic canopy and fit it over the frame, with the apron of the canopy extending toward the foot of the crib.

---

*Air-Shields, Inc. Hatboro, Pa.

The zippered side openings permit nursing care.

3. Fill the ice chamber at the back of the tent with ice for cooling the tent. (The croupette is occasionally operated without ice if the child's temperature is below normal.)
4. Fill with distilled water the jar through which oxygen or air passes.
5. Connect the designated tubing to an oxygen wall outlet or a tank, or to the air compressor motor.
6. Allow humidified oxygen or air to flow into the tent for a few minutes before placing the child in the tent.
7. Set the liter gauge at the prescribed pressure.
8. Place the child in the tent, explaining the procedure if he can understand it. Position the child on his side, with his head slightly elevated. This usually helps to alleviate respiratory distress.
9. Keep the distilled water jar filled. Clean it thoroughly when refilling.
10. When ice in the chamber has melted, the drainage tubing should be allowed to drain into a basin, and the chamber should be refilled.
11. After the child is removed from the croupette, wash all apparatus, and send the canopy to be autoclaved.

The Use of the Mistogen Tent Unit (CAM Tent)

This unit makes use of a small refrigeration unit placed at the bedside, which cools and circulates cool water through a panel (CoolXChanger) inside the plastic canopy. No ice is needed.

Directions for setting up and for operating the CAM tent accompany the unit. After the unit is set up and the canopy is in place, a gallon of distilled water is placed in the tank of the refrigeration unit. The chilled water continually circulates through the CoolXChanger and returns for re-chilling. Water does not need replacing more often than every 30 days of continual use.

When not in use, the CAM tent can be

taken down in a process that is the reverse of setting it up; the frame, the canopy, the CoolXChanger and the nebulizer may be washed, dried, and autoclaved if desired. All parts fold compactly and are hung from back of refrigeration unit for storage.

Another type of humidifier is the Mistifier.* This humidifier can be placed on the bedside stand with the outlet directed toward the patient. A plastic canopy draped over the crib with an opening to allow the vapor to enter is useful for direct inhalation. The Mistifier operates continually for about 10 hours before refilling is required, and has only to be plugged into any electrical outlet.

Bacterial Pneumonia

Pneumococcal pneumonia is the most common form of pneumonia found among infants and children. Its incidence has, however, decreased over the last several years. Staphylococcal pneumonia is still a menace to the newborn and very young infant. Streptococcal pneumonia is rarely seen in the infant.

Pneumococcal Pneumonia in Infants

Incidence. This disease occurs mainly during the late winter and early spring months. It occurs principally in children under the age of 4 years.

Pathophysiology. In infants, pneumococcal pneumonia is generally of the bronchial rather than the lobar type seen in older children. It is generally of the secondary type, following an upper respiratory viral infection.

The most common finding in infants is a patchy infiltration of one or several lobes of the lung. Lobar consolidation is unusual in infants and young children. Pleural effusion is frequently present.

Clinical manifestations. The onset of the pneumonic process is usually abrupt, following a mild upper respiratory illness. Temperature rises rapidly to 103° to 105°F

---

*Mistogen Company, Oakland, California.

(39.4° to 40.6°C). Respiratory distress is marked, with obvious air hunger, flaring of the nostrils, circumoral cyanosis and chest retractions. Tachycardia and tachypnea are present, with a pulse rate frequently as high as 140-180 per minute, and respirations as high as 80.

Generalized convulsions may occur during the period of high fever. Cough may not be noticeable at the onset but may appear later. Abdominal distention due to swallowed air or paralytic ileus is common.

Treatment. The use of antibiotics early in the disease gives prompt and favorable response. Penicillin has proved to be the most effective and is generally used unless the infant has a penicillin allergy. Oxygen started early in the disease process is important. Infants do best when placed in a Croupette. Aspirin, Tylenol or Tempra are given to reduce the fever. Intravenous fluids are often necessary to supply the needed amount of fluids.

Nursing care. The infant needs considerable emotional support in his obvious distress. Having his mother at his bedside to reach into the Croupette and stroke his head gently and talk to him soothingly is the preferable method of support. If his mother cannot be present, this will be a nursing function.

The temperature and oxygen flow rate in the Croupette needs frequent checking. The infant is usually more comfortable and finds breathing easier when his head is elevated. Suction apparatus should be at the cribside or within ready access for use to remove excess secretions if necessary.

Prognosis. With present day prompt and effective treatment, prognosis for recovery is excellent. Mortality rates have dropped to less than 1% in infants. The most common complication in infants is empyema, but this seldom occurs when adequate treatment has been started early in the disease.

Hemophilus Influenzae Pneumonia

This disease also occurs in infants and young children. Its clinical manifestations are similar to those of pneumococcal pneumonia. However, its onset is more insidious, its clinical course longer and less acute. It is usually lobar in distribution.

Complications are frequent in the young infant. Most commonly seen are empyema and bacteremia.

Treatment consists of the same measures used in other pneumonias, with emphasis on the adequate use of antibiotics.

BIBLIOGRAPHY

Fishbein, M., ed.: Birth Defects. Philadelphia, J. B. Lippincott, 1963.

Raffensperger, John G. and Primrose, Rosellen Bohlen, eds.: Pediatric Surgery for Nurses. Boston, Little, Brown, 1968.

Ravitch, M. M.: Intussusception in Infants and Children. Springfield, Ill., Charles C Thomas, 1959.

di Sant' Agnese, P. A.: Diagrammatic review of cystic fibrosis. Ann. N.Y. Acad. Sci., *93:*495, 1962.

Swenson, Orvar, ed.: Pediatric Surgery. New York, Appleton-Century-Crofts, 1968.

Suggested Readings for Further Study

Burgess, L.: Morale boosting in cystic fibrosis. AJN, *69:*322, 1969.

Johnson, Miriam E. and Fassett, Barbara A.: Bronchopulmonary hygiene in cystic fibrosis. AJN, *69:*320, 1969.

Kurihara, M.: Postural drainage, clapping and vibrating. AJN, *65:*76, 1965.

Lo Presti, Joseph M. et al.: Wilms' tumor in children. Clinical Proceedings in the Children's Hospital of Washington, D. C., *26:*81, 1970.

McCollum, Audrey T. and Gibson, Lewis E.: Family adaptation to the child with cystic fibrosis. Journal of Pediatrics, *77:*571, 1970.

Stadnyk, Sue and Bindschadler, Nancy: A camp for children with cystic fibrosis. AJN, *70:*1691, 1970.

Nursing Care of Infants with Other Conditions *29*

CONDITIONS OF THE GENITOURINARY TRACT

Acute Pyelonephritis

Pyelonephritis (pyuria, pyelitis) is an infection of the urinary tract. It is the most common renal disease in infants and children.

Incidence

Infections of the urinary tract are fairly common in the "diaper age," particularly between the ages of 2 months and 2 years.

Pathophysiology

The condition occurs more commonly in girls than in boys. Although many different bacteria may infect the urinary tract, intestinal bacilli account for the infection in about 80% of acute episodes. The female urethra is shorter and straighter than that in the male, thus being more easily contaminated with feces. Inflammation may extend into the bladder, ureters and the kidney.

Clinical Manifestations

In acute pyelonephritis the onset is abrupt with high fever for a day or two. Occasionally there is little or no fever. Vomiting is common; diarrhea may occur. The infant is irritable; convulsions may occur during the period of high fever.

Diagnois

Diagnosis is based on finding of pus in the urine under microscopic examination. It is important that the urine specimen be fresh and uncontaminated. A "clean catch" voided urine, properly performed, is essential for microscopic examination. If a culture is needed, the infant must be catheterized.

Obtaining a Clean Urine Specimen in Infants

Equipment
1. A sterile basin containing cotton balls saturated with aqueous Zephiran 1:1000 or a soap solution.
2. A plastic urine collector.* (Fig. 29-1)
3. A sterile specimen bottle. (Alternatively, the plastic collector may also be used as the specimen bottle.)

Procedure
1. Wash genitalia with soaked cotton balls using downward strokes. For girls, first separate the labis, washing away from the urethral meatus. Wash the outer surface of the perineum and the anal region. Discard cotton ball after each stroke.
2. Dry the skin. While one person holds the infant with legs abducted, the nurse firmly presses the adhesive surface of the bag down around the urethra. In girls, care should be taken to insure the adhesive adheres to the strip of skin between the vagina and the rectum.
3. Observe the infant frequently for

---

*Pediatric Urine Collector (PUC). Sterilon Company, Buffalo, New York.

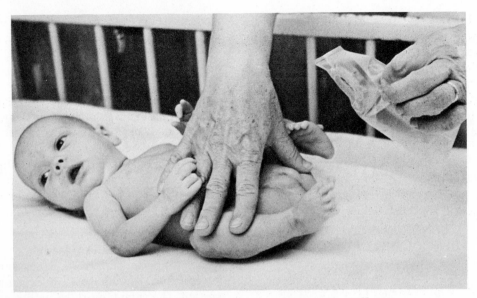

Figure 29-1. Here is one method of applying a plastic urine collector.

voiding. After the specimen is obtained, remove collector, press sides of adhesive around opening together to make a sterile container (Fig. 29-2).

4. Label and send to laboratory.

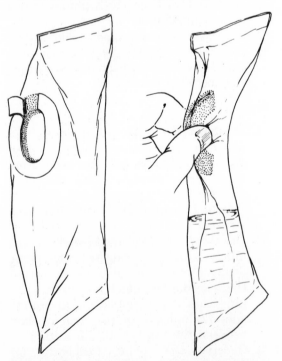

Figure 29-2. The plastic urine collector has a soft sponge around the opening (*A*) and the sides of the opening are pressed together to make the collector into a specimen container (*B*).

5. Record the time and other pertinent data.

Collection of Clean Urine Specimen from Older Children

1. Clean genitalia as outlined above.
2. A small child may sit on a potty chair and void into a sterile basin or into a sterilized potty. An older child may void into a sterile bedpan, a sterile urinal, or directly into a specimen bottle.
3. A midstream specimen is desirable, but difficult to obtain from small children. To obtain a midstream specimen, the child should start to void into an unsterile receptacle, stop the stream, and void into a sterile receptacle.

Catheterization of an Infant

A physician will usually catheterize infants. The nurse will need to prepare the catheterization tray.

Equipment

1. Tray covered with sterile towel. Contents of tray include:
   a. three sterile towels for draping
   b. sterile gloves
   c. two basins—one with soap and water, one with aqueous Zephiran 1:1000.
   d. sterile cotton balls

e. lubricant (if desired) on square of sterile gauze

f. sterile catheters size 8 to 10 French. Have more than one catheter available.

2. Culture tubes and sterile specimen bottle.

3. Extension light or other provision for clear lighting of perineal region.

The nurse will have to hold the child firmly. The presence of a familiar person to quiet the infant and distract his attention with a nursing bottle of glucose water or formula will be most helpful.

Treatment

Sulfonamides are the most widely used drugs for eradication of the affecting organism. Fluids should be given freely. The symptoms usually subside within a few days, but this is not an indication that the infection is completely cleared. Medication is usually continued after symptoms disappear.

Nursing Care

The nurse will give the infant supportive care as needed. She will need to use ingenuity in persuading the infant or young child to take the necessary amount of fluids. Glucose water or liquid gelatin dessert, is usually well accepted. The nurse should not be discouraged if only a few swallows at a time are taken. Persistence is the answer.

Chronic and recurring urinary infections are frequently associated with obstructions in the urinary tract. The urinary system should be carefully studied through the use of x-ray visualization procedures.

DISORDERS OF THE NERVOUS SYSTEM

Acute or Nonrecurrent Convulsions

A convulsion may be a symptom of a wide variety of disorders. In infants and children under the age of 2 or 3 years, febrile convulsions are the most common. These convulsions occur in association with a high fever, frequently one of the initial symptoms of an acute infection somewhere in the body. Less frequent causes of convulsions are intracranial infections such as meningitis,

toxic reactions to certain drugs or minerals such as lead, metabolic disorders, and a variety of brain disorders.

Clinical Manifestations

A convulsion may appear suddenly without warning, however frequently restlessness and irritability may precede an attack. The infant's body stiffens and he loses consciousness. In a few seconds clonic movements occur. These are quick, jerking movement of the arms, legs, and facial muscles. Breathing is irregular and there is an inability to swallow saliva.

Treatment and Nursing Care

A child whose fever or other symptoms indicate that a convulsion may be anticipated should be placed where he can be easily watched. Crib sides should be padded to prevent injury, but some space should be left at the foot of the crib so that the infant is not entirely isolated from his environment. An airway or a padded tongue blade should be kept at the bedside.

When an infant starts to convulse, the nurse should turn his head to one side to prevent aspiration of saliva or vomitus. However, the child's movements should not be restrained. Mouth suctioning, using a soft catheter, removes excess saliva. A padded tongue blade placed between the jaws of an older infant or young child prevents him from biting his tongue. Sodium phenobarbital given intramuscularly is usually ordered.

Recording

Recording should be detailed and complete. The record should include:

1. Any symptoms observed previous to the convulsion,
2. Kind of movements: rigidity, jerking, twitching, whether generalized or localized in one part of the body,
3. Duration of seizure,
4. Child's color, pulse and respiration rates and quality,
5. Any deviant eye movements or other abnormal signs.

Prognosis

An isolated convulsion may cause no harm, but repeated convulsions may result in brain damage. Most physicians will give the child a thorough physical and neurological examination following a single convulsion, and will carefully check the child's history concerning all phases of his health and of his level of development.

Febrile Convulsions

Febrile convulsions are usually in the form of a generalized seizure, occurring early in the course of a fever. Although usually associated with high fever, 102 ° to 106°F (38.9° to 41.1°C), some children appear to have a low seizure threshold and convulse when a fever of 100° to 102°F (37.8° to 38.9°C) is present.

Prevention and Treatment of Febrile Convulsions

Prompt reporting of elevated temperatures is essential for all sick children. Aspirin and tepid sponges or a cooling mattress are usually ordered for reduction of fever.

Reassurance for Parents

A convulsion is a frightening occurrence to parents. Explanations are needed to reassure them that febrile convulsions are not uncommon in small children. Parents also need to understand that the thorough examination given a child after he has had a convulsion does not mean the physician suspects some serious condition. He is seeking to *rule out* any possible cause other than the nervous system irritation caused by high fever.

Procedure for Tepid Bath to Reduce Fever
Equipment

A basin containing tepid water.
A bath blanket (two for an older child).
A wash cloth.
Isopropyl alcohol 35 per cent (only if ordered).

Technique

1. Take the child's temperature and record it.
2. Wash your hands, and assemble the equipment.
3. Undress the child, and place a bath blanket under the child (to absorb moisture and to prevent undue chilling).
4. Cover an older child with a second bath blanket.
5. Expose his arms and his chest. Wring wash cloth lightly from tepid water, sponge gently, making long, even strokes. Apply gentle friction with your hands, following the sponge. Repeat 2 or 3 times, giving attention to the axillary area.
6. Sponge the abdomen, the legs and the feet in the same manner.
7. Turn the child on his abdomen and sponge his back.
8. Sponge the inner surface of the groin and the perineal region. (Sponge the anal region last.)
9. Do not continue longer than 15 or 20 minutes.
10. Take the child's temperature every half-hour until it is reduced to an acceptable level. Note: The child's temperature may continue to fall after sponging. Wait for 30 minutes before resuming the sponge bath. The child may be left uncovered following the sponge bath if his temperature remains elevated.

Purulent Meningitis

Etiology and Incidence

Purulent meningitis in infancy and childhood is caused by a variety of agents. Among these are the meningococcus, tubercle bacillus and the *Hemophilus influenzae*. The most common form is the influenza bacillus meningitis.

Hemophilus Influenzae Meningitis

Peak occurence of influenza bacillus meningitis is between the ages of 6 and 12 months. It is rare during the first 2 months of life and seldom seen after the fourth year. Purulent meningitis is an infectious disease. Strict isolation techniques should be carried out for 24 hours after the start of effective antimicrobial therapy, or until pathogens can no longer be cultured out from the nasopharynx.

Clinical Manifestations.

The onset may be either gradual or abrupt following an upper respiratory infection. Young infants with meningitis may have a characteristic high pitched cry, fever and irritability. Other symptoms include headache and stiffness of the neck and spine. Projectile vomiting may be present. Generalized convulsions are common in infants. Coma may occur early, particularly in the older child.

Diagnosis

Early diagnosis and treatment are essential for uncomplicated recovery. A spinal tap should be done promptly whenever symptoms raise a suspicion that the disease may be present.

The spinal fluid will be found to be under increased pressure. Laboratory examination of the fluid will reveal increased protein and decreased glucose content. Very early in the disease the spinal fluid may be clear, but it rapidly becomes purulent. The causative organism can usually be determined from stained smears of the spinal fluid. It enables specific medication to be started very early, without waiting for growths of organisms on culture media.

Treatment

Treatment consists primarily in administration of medication in effective dosage. At present, ampicillin, or chloromycetin plus penicillin is the treatment of choice. Initially these medications are usually given by the intravenous route for rapid assimilation or by intramuscular injection. Later in the disease, they may be given orally. Treatment is continued for at least 7 days, and longer if there is persistent fever, subdural effusion or otitis media.

Complications

Subdural effusion may complicate the condition among infants during the course of the disease. Fluid accumulates in the subdural space between the dura and the brain. Needle aspirations through the infant's open suture lines or burr holes (in the skull of the older child) are used to remove the fluid. Repeated aspiration may be required.

Other complications of influenzal meningitis are hydrocephalus, nerve deafness, mental retardation and paralysis. The risk of complications is lessened when appropriate medication is started early in the disease.

Prognosis

Since the advent of the use of sulfa drugs and antibiotics, the recovery rate has been about 95%. However, serious and permanent complications do occur, in spite of optimal treatment.

Nursing Care

Because of the irritability associated with meningitis, noises and bright lighting should be kept at a minimum. The child should be handled as little as possible during the stage of irritability. However, frequent turning is necessary to avoid skin breakdown and upper respiratory infection. All turning and handling must be done as gently as possible. The mother or nurse may help calm the child by sitting at his bedside within his range of vision and speaking to him softly.

Nursing care includes attention to such manifestations as vomiting, convulsions, urinary retention, food and fluid intake. Prompt reporting and accurate recording is essential. When the fever is high, a cold water mattress, or tepid sponges are usually indicated. Mouth and skin care are given as needed. During convalescence, careful record should be kept of any unusual behavior, or signs of deafness, enlarging head or any abnormality.

Assisting with a Lumbar Puncture

Equipment

1. Obtain a sterile set from the central supply room. The set should contain the following:
   a. Spinal manometer and 3-way stop-cock
   b. Lumbar puncture needles
   c. Two medicine glasses
   d. A 2-cc. syringe and hypodermic needles
   e. Gauze squares
   f. Sheet for draping
2. In addition to the sterile set have the following supplies:
   a. Local anesthesia
   b. Skin antiseptic
   c. Sterile gloves
   d. Marked culture and chemistry tubes

Procedure

Bring the child to the treatment room and place him on his side with the lumbar region at the edge of the examining table. Restrain his legs by wrapping them in a sheet if necessary. Flex the child's knees and bend his head forward and hold the child's head within a circle of your arm and with your other arm under his flexed knees. (See Fig. 29-3)

The doctor will paint the area with antiseptic and infiltrate the skin and subcutaneous tissues with local anesthesia. He will then insert the lumbar puncture needle. When fluid appears in the needle he will attach the manometer and measure the pressure. He will then collect fluid for chemical determination and culture. After the needle is withdrawn, a bandage is applied over the site, and the child returned to his crib.

SUDDEN DEATH SYNDROME

Sudden "crib deaths" have received considerable attention because of the unresolved mystery which still surrounds this sudden death in infancy. The sudden death syndrome cannot be rigidly defined at

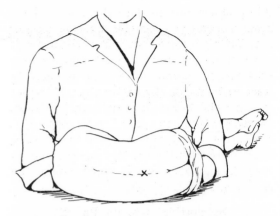

Figure 29-3. Positioning the child for lumbar puncture.

present. Bergman *et al.* give this definition "The sudden, unexpected and inexplicable death of an infant." They add "A thorough postmortem examination fails to show cause of death."*

The infant is put to bed in apparently good condition—at most perhaps with a slight head cold, but is found dead several hours later. In actual fact, this is not a new phenomenon, nor is it limited to any one culture or country. It occurs principally in infants under 6 months of age, with its peak incidence between 2 and 4 months. Many more such deaths occur between midnight and morning and during the cold months of the year, than at other times of day or in the warmer months.

It is estimated that the incidence may be as high as one out of 350 babies. Certain antenatal factors do appear to have a bearing on the incidence, such as low maternal age, maternal cigarette smoking, and birth order. It is observed more frequently among second-born and less frequently among first-born than might be expected. Low birth weight is related to crib death to a statistical degree.†

Considerable research has been done on

---

*Bergman, A. B., Pomeroy, M. A., and Beckwith, J. B.: The psychiatric toll of the sudden infant death syndrome. GP, *40:*99, 1969.

†Valdes-Dapena, Marie: Crib Death. Medical World News, Pediatric Issue, January 1970.

this problem but to date the results have been inconclusive. There have been a number of theories put forth, but it has been difficult to substantiate any of them. Autopsies have shown some inflammation of the respiratory tract in many of the infants but does not appear to be sufficient to account for death. Whether a common cause will be pinpointed or whether various causes will be found is not clear at present. Current thinking tends towards a combination of factors obtaining or acting simultaneously.

Supportive Help for Parents

The most important task for physicians and nurses faced with such death is the support and reassurance of the parents. Quite naturally they will look for a reason or will blame themselves for some possible neglect. Reassurance on several points can be given with complete honesty.

1. Nothing the parents did or did not do has any bearing on this tragedy. It could be neither predicted nor prevented according to our present state of knowledge.

2. There is no evidence that these deaths occur because of suffocation or infection. Death is believed to come swiftly, without suffering for the baby. It appears to be a silent death; crying is not known to occur before death.

3. Sudden death syndrome can and has occurred in the best of circumstances, to infants of the most capable parents.

4. There is no evidence at present that this is a genetic disease.

A national parents' group has been organized with chapters throughout the country. This is the National Foundation for Sudden Infant Death, Inc. with head offices at 1501 Broadway, New York, N.Y., 10036. Its reason for being is to give support and comfort to affected parents, to educate the public, and to support research.

SKIN CONDITIONS

Miliaria Rubra

This condition, often called prickly heat, is common in infants who are exposed to summer heat or are overdressed. It may also appear in febrile illnesses and may be mistaken for the rash of one of the communicable diseases. The rash appears as pinhead-sized erythematous (reddened) papules. It is most noticeable in areas where sweat glands are concentrated, as in folds of the skin, the chest and about the neck. It usually causes itching, making the infant uncomfortable and fretful.

Treatment should first of all be preventive. Mothers should be taught to avoid bundling their infants in layers of clothing in hot weather. A diaper may be all the clothing the child needs. Tepid baths without soap will help control the itching. Calamine lotion (plain without phenol) applied to the rash is also helpful.

Diaper Rash

Diaper rash is a common occurence in infancy. Bacterial decomposition of urine produces ammonia which is very irritating to an infant's tender skin. Diarrheal stools also produce a burning erythematous area in the anal region. Infants who become easily irritated in the diaper area may have inherited a sensitive skin. Other causes may be: prolonged exposure to wet or soiled diapers, (aggravated by the use of rubber or plastic covers); incomplete cleansing of the diaper area, especially after a bowel movement; sensitivity to certain soaps or to plastic pants; and use of strong detergents with incomplete rinsing for washing diapers and crib bedding.

Treatment. Exposure of the diaper area to the air helps to clear up the dermatitis. The use of one of the various ointments sold for this purpose is also helpful. A and D Ointment* and Desitin† are two preparations sold over the counter. When the area is excoriated and sore, the physician may prescribe an antibiotic ointment.

Care of Diapers. Diapers washed at one of the diaper services are sterilized there; this prevents the growth of ammonia-forming

---

*Trademark, White
†Trademark, Leeming

bacteria. Diapers washed at home should be rinsed thoroughly, and an antiseptic such as Diaparine added to the final rinse. Drying diapers in the sun, or in a commercial dryer also helps destroy the bacteria.

Acute Infantile Eczema

Infantile eczema is a atopic dermatitis considered to be at least in part an allergic reaction to some irritant or irritants. It is fairly common during the first year of life after the age of 3 months. It is uncommon in breast-fed babies before they are given additional foods.

Etiology

Infantile eczema is characterized by
1. A hereditary predisposition. Also, those infants who have eczema tend to have hay fever or asthma later in life.
2. Hypersensitivity of the deeper layers of the skin to protein or proteinlike allergens.
3. Allergens to which the child is sensitive may be inhaled, ingested, or absorbed through direct contact. Examples are house dust, egg white, and wool.

Clinical Manifestations

Eczema usually starts on the cheeks and spreads to the extensor surfaces of the arms and legs. Eventually the entire trunk may become involved. The initial reddening of the skin is quickly followed by papule and vesicle formation. Itching is intense, and the scratching the infant does makes the skin weep and crust. The areas easily become infected by hemolytic streptococci or by staphylococci.

Diagnosis and Treatment

The most common allergens concerned in the manifestation of eczema are:
Foods: egg white, cow's milk, wheat products, and orange and tomato juice.
Inhalants: house dust, pollens and animal dander.
Materials: wool, nylon, and plastic.
However, diagnosis is not simple. The infant may show skin-test sensitivity to one or many allergens but still show no improvement when they are eliminated. Factors other than allergy appear to be involved. These may include the sensitive nature of the skin of an infant, which reacts more quickly to marked changes in temperature and to other environmental factors.

Dietary Treatment. An elimination diet may be helpful in ruling out offending foods. A basic diet, consisting of only hypoallergic foods, is started. Some form of milk or milk substitute should be included, as well as vitamin supplements. If the child's skin condition shows improvement, other foods are added one at a time, and the effects are carefully noted.

Great care must be taken not to foster undernourishment. One child with severe eczema was kept on such a strict regime that he was in an extremely poor nutritional state and became susceptible to infection. The infection cleared when someone with common sense placed the emphasis on building up the child's nutritional status; and the emotional satisfaction this gave the child enabled him to express his needs in other than physical symptoms. Needless to say, an elimination program must always be under the strict supervision of a competent physician.

Hyperallergic Foods. The protein in egg white is such a common offender that most pediatricians advise against feeding whole eggs to any infant until late into the first year of life.

Cow's milk seems to cause or aggravate eczema in many infants. Prolonged or intense heating of protein alters it in such a way as to make it less allergenic. Because of this fact, evaporated milk may be tolerated when regular bottled milk is not. Some babies tolerate goat's milk well, but many do best on feedings of hypoallergenic milk substitutes. These are prepared from soya (soy bean) or hydrolized casein. However, it should be kept in mind that *breast* milk rarely causes allergic reactions.

Hypoallergic milk substitutes are

prepared by commercial firms and appear to be nutritionally satisfactory. Some of these are:

Mullsoy—Borden Company (soya)
Soyalac—Loma Linda Company (soya)
Prosobee—Mead Johnson Company (soya)
Similac Isomil—Ross Laboratories (soya)
Nutramigen—Mead Johnson Company (hydrolyzed casein)
Meat-base formula—Gerber Company

Inhalant and contact allergens should be avoided as far as possible. In the infant's sleeping room window drapes, dresser scarfs and rugs should be removed, and furniture washed off frequently. He should not come in contact with feather pillows; stuffed toys should be carefully chosen. Sadly, it may be necessary to provide new homes for household pets.

Treatment

Smallpox vaccination is definitely contraindicated for the child with eczema. In fact, he must be kept away from anyone who has recently been vaccinated. A serious

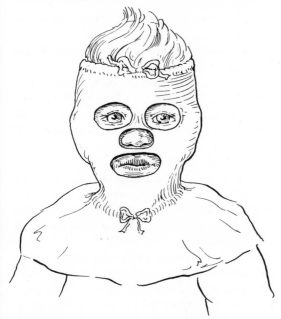

Figure 29-4. To prevent his scratching eczema of the face, the child is protected with a facial mask.

condition called *eczema vaccinatum* results when an infant with eczema is vaccinated or is exposed to the vaccination of another person. The infant becomes seriously ill and mortality rates have been high.

In the presence of infection, antibiotics will be ordered, preferably by mouth. Sedatives and antihistamines help control the itching and calm the infant. Antihistamine ointments and local anesthetics should not be used.

Daily care of the infant with eczema. Coping with the care of an infant with eczema is an exhausting task. The mother can be assured that most cases of infant eczema clear up by the age of two, but this assurance does little to relieve the present situation. Whenever possible, hospitalization should be avoided because these infants pick up infections in the hospital very easily. There are times when hospitalization seems to be indicated, either to give the child more intensive care or to relieve an exhausted parent. Great care must be taken to shield the child from infection while giving him the comfort and emotional support he desperately needs.

Physical care. The infant is apt to express his discomfort through scratching and rubbing the itching areas. He must be prevented from scratching and making his condition worse, but restraints should be used only when no alternative will work. He does not need any more frustration than he is already experiencing. Bulky wet packs of cool Burow's Solution will help alleviate the itching. These packs should not be wrapped in plastic or bandages but may be pinned together loosely or tied with straps.

An ointment such as Lassar's paste is soothing and protective of areas that are not infected. Coal tar ointment is effective in clearing up a dry, noninfected area. When tar ointments are used, exposure to sunlight should be avoided, as tar ointments contain a photosensitizing substance causing irritation in the presence of sunlight. Ointments should be applied with long, smooth strokes for the soothing effect. After an ointment has been applied, the area should be bandaged with strips of soft cotton cloth and held in place with 2-inch Ace bandages.

A face mask may be needed to hold wet dressings in place or to ensure retention of ointments applied to the face. A mask is made by cutting holes in a piece of cotton material to correspond in location to eyes, nose and mouth. The holes should be hemmed to avoid fraying. The mask is made to go around the head and is held in place with tapes or drawstrings. Care should be taken to avoid friction or binding. (Fig. 29-4)

Use of Restraints. When restraints must be used, elbow restraints are probably the most effective. Fingernails and toenails should be kept short. Mitts put on the child's hands will help prevent scratching. (See (Figs. 24-8 and 24-9)

Colloid baths. Tub baths using tepid water, cornstarch and baking soda are soothing. For a small infant tub, use about one fourth cup of baking soda and one fourth cup of cornstarch mixed together. Oatmeal baths are also used. Cooked oatmeal is put in a cheesecloth bag and squeezed through the bath water. A commercial preparation called Aveena may be used in place of the home-cooked oatmeal. Use according to directions.

The child is bathed in one of these colloid baths for about fifteen minutes. Soap should not be used. He should be dried by light dabs, not by rubbing.

Emotional Support

The infant with eczema needs at least as much cuddling and affection as the healthy child. Deprived of normal avenues of sensory stimulation, he needs opportunity to develop his mental and physical abilities, as well as to achieve emotional satisfaction.

His frustration may be relieved by use of a pacifier to provide additional sucking pleasure. Soft, smooth toys can occupy his hands and divert his attention from his discomfort. If old enough to creep or walk, he needs opportunities to do so. Some mothers may be fearful or repulsed by the child's unattractive appearance. They will need help to view their child as a normal child with a distressing, but temporary, skin condition.

BIBLIOGRAPHY

Bergman, Abraham B., Pomeroy, Margaret A., and Beckwith, J. Bruce: The psychiatric toll of the sudden death syndrome. GP, *40:*99, 1969.

Millichap, J. G.: Febrile Convulsions. New York, Macmillan, 1967.

Nelson, Waldo, Vaughn, Victor, and McKay, James, ed.: Textbook of Pediatrics. ed. 9. Philadelphia, W. B. Saunders, 1969.

Suggested Readings for Further Study

Pomeroy, Margaret R.: Sudden Death Syndrome. AJN, *69:*1886, 1969.

Valdes-Dapena, Marie: Crib death. Medical World News, January, 1970.

UNIT STUDY QUESTIONS

1. Which of the following developmental activities would you expect of a three-month-old infant?

   a. rolls over from prone to supine position

   b. stares at his hand when it appears in his line of vision

   c. reaches out and grasps small toy when offered him

   d. has a purposeful, social smile

   The answer is:

   1. a, b, and d
   2. a and d
   3. a, c, and d
   4. all of them

2. At six months of age the *average* infant:

   a. is commencing to discriminate faces

   b. bears some weight on his feet when held upright

   c. can sit with slight support

   d. is learning to localize sound

   The answer is:

   1. a, c, and d
   2. b and c
   3. all of them
   4. none of them

3. A nine-month-old infant begins to suck his thumb. The nurse's understanding of this is based on the knowledge that:

    a. an infant requires a certain amount of sucking unrelated to the quantity of food taken

    b. an infant turns to his own body for gratification of needs if these satisfactions are not gained from outside himself

    c. an infant this age has greater caloric requirements than earlier

    d. an infant this age may be starting to cut teeth and requires such activity for proper eruption of teeth

    The answer is:

    1. a and b
    2. a, b, and c
    3. a, b, and d
    4. all of these

4. Before his first birthday, the infant should receive the following immunizations:

    a. DTP only (diphtheria toxoid, tetanus and pertussis vaccine)

    b. DTP, live measles and mump vaccine

    c. DTP, trivalent oral poliovaccine

    d. DTP, smallpox and live measles vaccines

    One correct answer.

5. In the hospital the infant's mother should be held to the following rules:

    a. Keep strict visiting hours because too much attention is not good for the baby.

    b. Refrain from picking up and holding the sick baby.

    c. Keep out of the nurse's way, and do not try to care for the baby while he is in the hospital.

    d. Hold and cuddle the infant unless contraindicated, change and feed him, stay with him when he receives uncomfortable treatment if desired.

6. The treatment of infants with bronchiolitis consists of:

    a. encouraging fluids and elevating the infant's head and shoulders

    b. Croupette, encouraging fluids

    c. broad spectrum antibiotics and oxygen

    d. high humidity, oxygen and broad spectrum antibiotics

7. Which of the following signs may indicate possible pyloric stenosis?

    a. vomiting soon after birth
    b. vomiting that is bile stained
    c. absence of stools
    d. vomiting 2-3 weeks after birth

8. Which of the following names is associated with the operative procedure for pyloric stenosis?

    a. Gross
    b. Blalock
    c. Wagenstein
    d. Ramstedt

9. The vomitus of an infant having pyloric stenosis is the color of his formula because:

    a. The obstruction is above the opening of the common bile duct.

    b. The liver does not secrete bile, since its functioning is impaired.

    c. The obstruction at the cardiac sphincter prevents the flow of bile to the stomach.

    d. The stenosis of the common bile duct prevents bile from flowing properly.

10. The pathology involved in cystic fibrosis involves the

    a. pancreas, lungs, salivary and sweat glands

    b. pancreas and lungs
    c. pancreas and sweat glands
    d. lungs and salivary glands

11. The most common allergies causing eczema are sensitivity to:

    a. cow's milk, orange juice, egg white
    b. cow's milk, orange juice, egg yolk
    c. cow's milk, certain vegetables, egg white

    d. cow's milk, orange juice, certain vegetables

12. What criteria should the nurse use in selecting toys for a baby with eczema?

    a. washable, safe, soft and having a smooth surface

b. suitable for the bath and for the child's age

c. suitable to child-development achievement but free from allergic substances

d. free from allergic substances and washable

13. The sudden infant death syndrome:

a. is caused by neglect on the part of the parents

b. can be predicted and prevented

c. is caused by suffocation due to respiratory infection

d. has not yet been laid to a particular cause

14. Treatment for febrile convulsions in infants consists of:

a. tepid sponge bath, suctioning, sedation

b. cold sponge bath, tongue blade between teeth

c. turning child on back and restraining to prevent injury

d. padding crib sides

The answer is:

1. a and d
2. b and d
3. a and c
4. c and d

Normal Growth and Development of the Toddler 30

The average toddler gains somewhere between 4 1/2 and 6 pounds a year. However, some children who enjoy excellent health are just too busy exploring their environment to put on much weight. The appetite slows down accordingly, as the child's sphere of interest expands and his discoveries become ever more engrossing.

DEVELOPMENTAL SCHEDULE

A definite timetable of development cannot be set with any certainty for the second year. Even children in the same family differ in rate of development. Every child has his own pattern, depending on his personality as well as on the opportunities allowed him for testing, exploring and learning.

Twelve Months

1. Moves about with great alacrity on hands and knees, or using hands and feet. Some children prefer to slide along in a sitting position, using one foot as a propeller.

2. Pulls self to standing position, may stand alone.

3. May walk in toddler fashion, unsupported. Many normal children are satisfied with their present method for getting places in a hurry and put off walking for a few months longer.

4. Is learning to drink from cup held by another person.

5. May use specific sounds such as "dada" and "mama" to indicate parents. Normal children differ markedly in the age at which they begin to talk. Some children wait many months longer before they feel the urge to talk. It seems to be a matter of temperament and personality. These normal or bright children who are late talkers generally use phrases rather than single words when they are ready to speak. One example is the 20-month-old child who had not previously talked and who startled his mother one night by looking up solemnly and saying "turn on light."

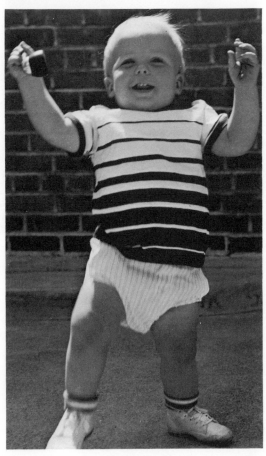

Figure 30-1. The toddler is proud of his ability to stand alone. (Carol Baldwin)

437

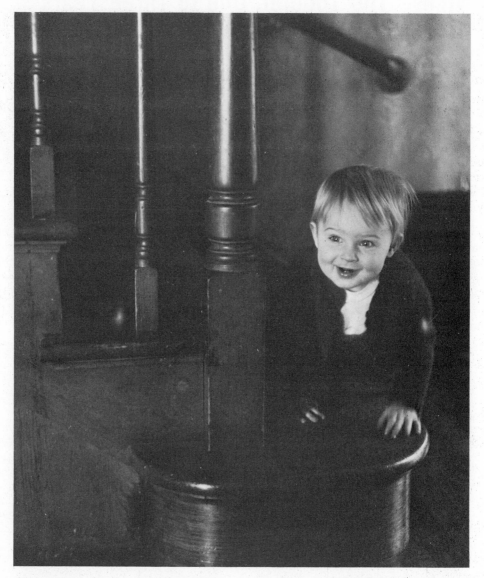

Figure 30-2.   The toddler explores the stairs on his own. (Carol Baldwin)

Fifteen Months

1. Most children are walking well by their 15th month.
2. Creeps upstairs.
3. Can stoop to pick up an object and right himself
4. Enjoys throwing a ball; is able to release the ball with a forward thrust
5. Can build a tower of two blocks
6. Scribbles spontaneously
7. Indicates wants by pointing or sound
8. Explores drawers and closets within his reach
9. Likes to imitate housework
10. Can put a ball in a box, or place a small object in a bottle

Eighteen Months

1. Runs, but with a stiff, propulsive gait
2. Walks upstairs with assistance, creeps down
3. Likes to pull a wheeled toy as he walks

4. Can seat himself on child-size chair; climbs into adult chair
5. May be able to build a tower of three blocks. This may take repeated practice.
6. Turns pages of a book, two or three sheets at a time
7. Holds a cup with both hands to drink
8. Likes to do little errands around the house
9. Self-absorbed—does not see others as individuals like himself.
10. Dislikes sudden changes; backs away, runs to hide, or screams and struggles
11. Sense of guilt is nonexistent

Two Years

1. The two-year-old is motor minded. Greatly enjoys gross activity; can run well
2. Kicks a ball forward and can throw overhand
3. Loves rough and tumble play
4. Dances, sings, jumps, laughs heartily
5. Builds a tower of four to six blocks; can place three blocks in a row
6. Can match a round block and round hole
7. Can string large beads on string with a firm tip, such as a shoelace
8. Can snip with scissors
9. Turns pages of book one by one
10. Looks for missing toys
11. Pushes chair to desired location and climbs to get at object out of reach
12. May have many or few words. Uses jargon mixed with words. Enjoys stories, expecially rhythmic ones, such as Mother Goose.
13. Senses "oneness" as against "many" or "more"
14. Points to a named body part
15. Has a proprietary interest in persons and things. Takes a favorite toy to bed.
16. Dawdling is characteristic

Two and One Half Years

1. Can pedal a tricycle
2. Jumps in place
3. Can stand on one foot for one second
4. Can build a bridge with blocks

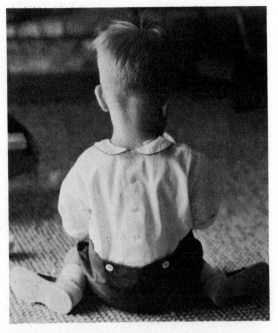

Figure 30-3. A favorite sitting position is easily achieved by the toddler. (Carol Baldwin)

5. Imitates vertical and horizontal lines. Can copy an O
6. Puts on shoes, but does not tie laces
7. Washes and dries hands
8. Accepts mother's absence for short periods
9. Plays interactive games such as tag

A review of a child's development from the neonatal period through the toddler age shows a steady, orderly progression. Timing is variable, depending on a number of factors. Opportunity, enrichment of environment, acceptance and sense of security, as well as the child's own personality, all have their effect. However, in the normal child, maturation proceeds in an orderly manner, even though exact timing is unpredictable.

NUTRITION

This is the age period when most feeding problems appear. There are several reasons for this.

1. The child's growth rate has slowed down. As Dr. Lowenberg puts it, "Nature has other much more complicated plans for

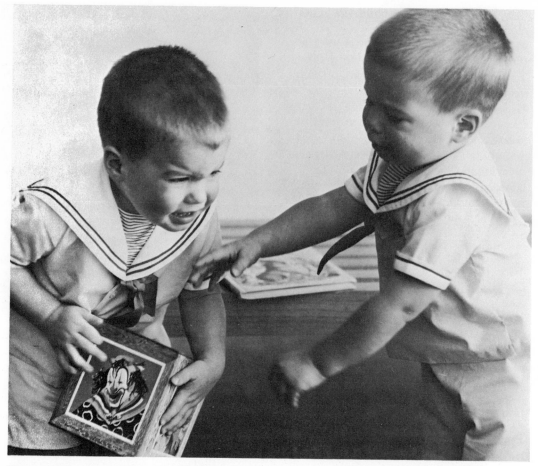

Figure 30-4.   The child is self-centered and possessive at an early age. (Carol Baldwin)

him. Eating and growing now take second place."*

2. The child has a strong drive for independence. He is beginning to acquire awareness of himself as a person. This compels him to assert his will, to prove to himself and others that he is an individual in his own right.

3. A child's appetite varies in regard to the kinds of food offered him. He is apt to go on "food jags," desiring one kind of food only for periods of time. "There's no need," says Dr. Lowenberg, "to get into wrangles with a small child about his variations in appetite. This is fortunate," she says,

"because even if there were a need there is no use. Arguments will only increase his obstinacy."†

Certainly a small child needs a well balanced diet. Proteins, carbohydrates, minerals and vitamins are essential for his health and sense of well being. As has been pointed out, however, arguments and force-feeding only increase his obstinacy and turn him into a "feeding problem." Some ideas for helping a small child remain well-fed and happy are listed here.

1. Serve small portions. Dr. Lowenberg recommends small portions, less than the child will probably eat. Let him ask for seconds. This will bolster his beginning sense

---

*Spock, Benjamin M. and Lowenberg, Miriam E.: Feeding Your Baby and Child. p. 232. New York, Pocket Books, 1967.

†Ibid.

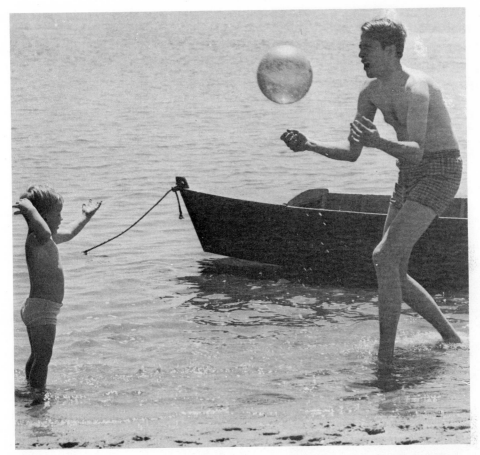

Figure 30-5. The child enjoys his father's participation in play. (Carol Baldwin)

of autonomy as well as remove the need to rebel.

2. Keep in mind that there is no *one* food that is positively essential to health. There is enough variety in any food category to allow substitution for a disliked food.

3. Toddlers like their food warm or cool, not hot or cold. Simply prepared foods are preferred.

4. Most children are stimulated to eat better when they eat with the family. They are great imitators, accepting or rejecting the foods as they see the other family members do.

5. Foods a child can pick up in his fingers are helpful. However, when the child wants to use a spoon or fork, he should be allowed to try.

6. Parents should *let* a child eat, not *force* him to eat. Forcing is often done in subtle ways: Be a good boy and eat your spinach to please mother; Eat your meat, it will make you strong like your big brother; Just one more bite.

When a child has eaten all he wishes he should be allowed to leave the table. If he has refused most of his food, has been finicky and negativistic, calmly remove the plates and make no comment. Be firm about withholding additional food until the next meal or snack period. No healthy child will ever starve himself.

7. Dawdling at mealtime is a common problem in this age group. It can reasonably be ignored, with an allowance made for a child's lack of feeding skill. If this period stretches on to unreasonable lengths, or becomes a play for power, the food can be calmly removed without comment.

8. Making desserts a reward for good

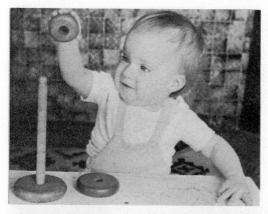

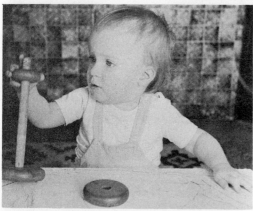

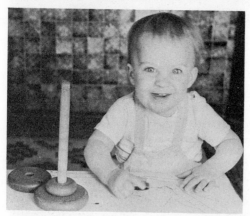

Figure 30-6. The toddler can take round blocks from the pole and put them on. (Carol Baldwin)

manners or eating habits is poor practice. It only gives added value to the dessert while making vegetables or other foods undesirable. Desserts should be served casually as a usual part of the meal.

Other useful reminders include the fact that small children use up more food than they can eat at any one meal. Regularly planned snacks are usually needed. Well-chosen snacks are milk, crackers and peanut butter, cheese cubes, pieces of fruit. Dishes should be easy to handle and scaled to the proper size for a small child's use. Unbreakable dishes will save much aggravation when inevitable accidents happen.

DENTAL HEALTH

One factor in the production of sound teeth is adequate nutrition. However, the actual process of dental caries is linked chiefly to the effect of the diet on the oral environment. Tooth decay is a problem among children. It is said that the average child has two carious lesions (cavities) by the age of 2 years.

Tooth decay is caused by bacteria acting mainly in the presence of sugar and forming a film, or dental plaque, on the teeth. Persons who frequently eat sweet foods accumulate plaque easily and are prone to dental caries. This is particularly true of foods that have prolonged contact with the teeth, such as lollipops. Sugars that are eaten in conjunction with other foods, as at mealtime, are somewhat neutralized by the buffering capacity of other food and are therefore less injurious to tooth enamel. It is probably a good policy to limit candy and other sweets to mealtime as much as possible. The child should also be taught to rinse his mouth or brush his teeth after meals.

Home Care of Temporary Teeth

At about the age of 2 years, it is a good idea to commence teaching the child to brush his teeth. The child of this age is particularly interested in copying every thing he sees being done. Having watched his parents or other children brush their teeth he wants to do this also. Brushing should be done after meals and snacks. At first plain water may be used until he has learned how to spit out toothpaste. The use of fluoride drops in areas where the drinking water is not fluoridated strengthens tooth enamel and helps prevent tooth decay.

Thumb-sucking

It is now generally agreed by dentists that thumb-sucking before the age of 5 or 6 years is harmless. Persisted in after the permanent teeth come in, it may cause a forward displacement of the front teeth.

Visits to the Dentist

It is well to take the child to the dentist somewhere around the age of 2 years. The first visit, and perhaps the second or third, will be for the purpose of acquainting the child with the dental office, and for making friends with the dentist. Thereafter, a dental check-up about twice a year is usually recommended.

TOILET TRAINING

Learning control of the bowels and bladder is an important component of the socialization process. This includes the disposing of body waste products in a place considered proper by society. A great sense of shame and disgust concerning body waste products has been built up in Western culture.

The young child, however, has no such sense of shame. The emptying of bowel and bladder gives him physical relief. During infancy he has operated on the pleasure principle, accepting immediate satisfaction as his right. Now, just as he is beginning to learn that he has some power over his environment, that he can make certain events happen or can prevent them, he is asked to forego some of his gratifications. One of these is the satisfaction of emptying his bowels and bladder when he feels the urge to do so, regardless of time and place.

Erikson says that the child must now learn "to *will* what *can* be, and to convince himself that he *willed* what *had* to be.* In other words, he must now not only learn to conform to please his mother, but in addition, in order to preserve his integrity, he has to convince himself that of his own free

*From Maier, Henry W.: Three Theories of Child Development, ed. 2. p. 37. New York, Harper and Row, 1969.

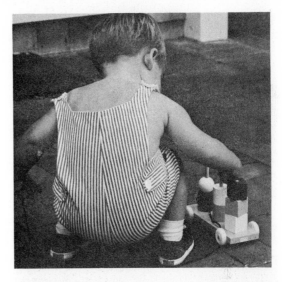

Figure 30-7. The child of two is capable of complete absorption. (Carol Baldwin)

will he accepted the dictates of society. He already knows that he has the ability to refuse to cooperate with his mother's wishes, which, after all, make no sense to him at all.

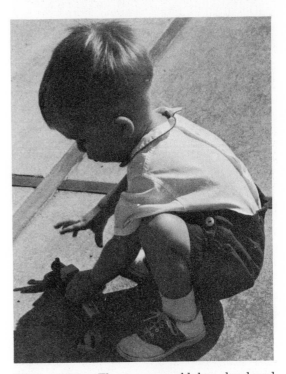

Figure 30-8. The two-year-old has developed good hand and eye coordination. (Carol Baldwin)

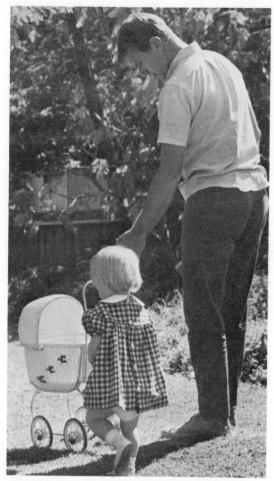

Figure 30-9. The little girl imitates her mother. (Carol Baldwin)

Timing the Toilet Training

In order for it to be possible for a child to cooperate in toilet training, he must have developed to the stage where he is able to control his sphincter muscles. Control of the rectal sphincter comes first. He also must be able to postpone his urge to defecate until he reaches the toilet or potty, and he must be able to signal his need *before* the event. This maturational development seldom takes place before the age of fifteen to eighteen months, and may be later.

At the start of training the child has no understanding of the uses of the potty chair, but if his mother wishes him to sit there he is willing to please her, for a short time. If his bowel movements occur at approximately the same time every day, he will one day have a bowel movement in the potty. He has no sense of special achievement as yet, but he does like the praise and approval he receives. Eventually he will learn to connect this approval with bowel movement in potty and is happy that he has done something on his own volition to please his mother.

Rules to Observe in Bowel Training

1. Use of a potty chair in which a child is comfortable with his feet on the floor is generally preferable. Most small children are afraid of a flush toilet.*

2. The child should be left on the potty chair for only a short time. If he has had a movement, approval should be shown, if not, nothing is said. He does not yet understand what it is all about.

3. It should be understood that during the beginning stages, the child very likely will have a movement soon *after* he leaves the potty. This is *not* willful defiance, and no mention need be made of it.

4. It is probably better to empty the potty unobtrusively after the child has resumed his play. He has cooperated and given his mother the product she desires. The fact that she immediately throws it away may be quite confusing and delay his desire to please her.

5. The ability to feel a sense of shame and self-doubt appear at this age. This should not be capitalized on, nor should the child be teased over his inability or reluctance to conform. This may indeed make him doubt his worth and shake his self-confidence. Erikson states, "Many a small child, shamed beyond endurance, may be in a chronic mood . . . .to express defiance.†

6. The parent should not expect perfect results all the time, even after control has been achieved. There are many reasons for lapses. The child may become so absorbed in his play that he ignores the signals until it is too late. Or he may have a temporary bout of loose stools. It is even possible for the best

---

*See Fraiberg, Selma: The Magic Years. p. 94. New York, Scribner, 1968.

†Erikson, Erik H.: Childhood and Society. p. 253.

natured child occasionally to feel aggression, frustration, or anger and use this method of "getting even." It is best to take no notice of such occasional lapses. If they are frequent and persistent, an effort should be made to discover the cause.

Bladder Training

This is a more difficult procedure, and complete control, especially at night, may not be achieved before the fourth or fifth year. Generally the first indication that readiness will soon occur is when the young child commences to connect the puddle on the floor with something he did himself. The next step happens when the child runs to his mother and indicates his need to urinate—after it has happened!

Not until the child has matured sufficiently to control his bladder sphincter until he can reach the desired place is there much benefit to be gained from a serious program of training. One indication of this level of maturation is manifested when the child stays dry for about 2 hours at a time.

Each child will follow his own individual pattern of development. No parent need be embarrassed or shamed because her child is still having accidents. Of course, it is possible for a parent or caretaker to ignore the signs of readiness—no one should expect the child to train himself.

Toddlers who have been admitted to the hospital regress to a more infantile state, particularly when separated from their families. It is also true that the toddler just learning sphincter control is still dependent on familiar surroundings and his mother's support. For this reason, some pediatric personnel automatically put toddlers back in diapers when they are admitted. This does not make good sense. Under the right circumstances and especially with his mother's help, many of these children can maintain control. At least they should be given a chance to try.

PSYCHOSOCIAL DEVELOPMENT

The toddler develops a growing awareness of himself as an entity, separate from other persons or objects. Erikson states

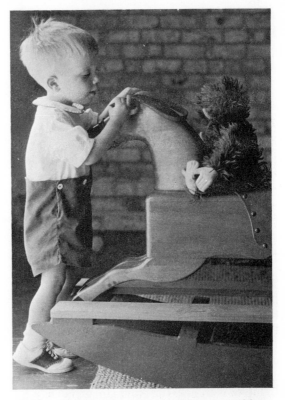

Figure 30-10. The two- to three-year-old indulges in imaginative play. (Carol Baldwin)

that "from a sense of self-control without loss of self-esteem comes a lasting sense of goodwill and pride" while "from a sense of loss of self-control and of foreign *overcontrol* comes a lasting propensity for doubt and shame."*

However, the young child, intoxicated with his newly discovered powers, and lacking in experience, tends to test his independence to the limit. This age has been called an age of *negativism*. Certainly his response to nearly everything is a firm "no," but this is more an assertion of his individuality than of his intention to disobey. Frequently he is already pulling off his clothes for the bath, or running toward the lunch table, while enthusiastically saying "no!" As Fraiberg writes, "We do not squash the new found spirit of independence, but we direct its pursuit along other lines, encouraging it where it can be useful in personality growth and exercising

*Op. cit. p. 254

reasonable restraint and prohibition where it is not."*

Other characteristics of this age are *ritualism* and *dawdling*.

Ritualism is a compromising device employed by the young child to help him develop security. He must follow a certain routine; he makes rituals of simple tasks. At bedtime he must have all toys in accustomed places, his caretaker must follow an accustomed practice. This passion for a set routine is not found to the same degree in every child, but it is a device that provides a comfortable base from which to step out into new and (to him) potentially dangerous paths.

Dawdling serves much the same purpose. The young child has to make a decision between following the wishes and routines of his parents, and asserting his independence by following his own desires of the moment. Being incapable of making such a choice he compromises and tries both. If the matter is of any importance, the course for the parent to follow is to help the child along the way he should go, in a firm and friendly manner.

Temper tantrums. The child's urge to do it himself naturally results in many frustrations. Add to this the fact that he is reluctant to leave the scene for necessary rest, and one can see that frequently the frustrations become just too great. Even the very best of mothers may lose patience, showing a temporary lack of understanding. The only reaction the child can show to this is rebellion, which he is likely to employ with as much enthusiasm as he would use in any other situation. This too is a phase he must live through as he works toward becoming a person.

Reasoning with a child, scolding or punishing while he is completely mastered by his rage is useless. Someone he trusts needs to be nearby, calm and patient until he gains control of himself. After the storm is over, she helps him relax by diverting his attention, but she does not yield the point or give in to the child's whim. This would be

telling him that he can get whatever he wants by throwing himself on the floor and screaming. Unfortunately, he would only have to learn, painfully, later in life that he cannot control others in this manner.

Admittedly, it is not easy to handle a small child who throws himself down in a fit of screaming rage in the middle of the supermarket or the sidewalk. Nor are the comments of onlookers at all helpful. The best a mother can do is pick up the child as calmly as she can and carry him away to cool off.

Discipline

Unfortunately, the word discipline has come to mean *punishment* to many people. One definition of *to discipline* is "to train or develop by instruction and exercise especially in self-control."† All small children need discipline, the need for punishment is much less frequent.

The toddler learns self-control very gradually. The development from an egotistic being whose world exists only to give him satisfaction into a person who understands and respects the rights of others is a long, involved process. He cannot do this alone; he must be taught.

We can expect to see the first faint signs of responsibility for his own acts even in the two-year-old. He lacks inner controls and is dependent on the adults to set limits. He still goes for the forbidden thing, but realizes he is disobeying, even to the extent of repeating, "No, no, mustn't," while he reaches for his father's valuable book. He understands very well what he must not do, but his desire is still too strong for him to resist. With proper guidance, he will soon incorporate the restraints into himself and develop control, or as we say, a conscience.

In the meantime he needs much help. When he hits or bites another child, he is taken away from the situation. When he tries to "read" daddy's expensive book, it is taken away from him, gently but firmly.

*Fraiberg, Op. cit. p. 66.

†Webster's Seventh New Collegiate Dictionary. p. 237. Springfield, Mass, G. and D. Merriam Co., 1969.

The child needs to experience a sense of wrong-doing in order to develop self-control. This statement can be misunderstood. He should not have an excessive burden laid on him so that his self esteem is lowered to the point where he "can do nothing right," and thereafter does nothing at all. Neither is he helped when all lapses of behavior are treated indulgently or overlooked. In this case, he will have great difficulty learning self-control.

THE TODDLER AS A FAMILY MEMBER

When a New Baby Arrives

The toddler who is a first child has had his parents' undivided attention. It is difficult to prepare a child just emerging from babyhood for the arrival of a new sibling. Even a tot can feel his mother's abdomen and understand that is where the new baby is, but this does not prepare him at all for the real baby when it arrives. This real life baby takes his place in his mother's attention.

Frequently the toddler will regress to more infantile behavior. If he has given up his bottle he goes back to it, if he is well on the way to being toilet-trained he goes back to wetting and soiling.

There can be no question that the new infant creates considerable change in the home, whether he is the first child, or the fifth. Certainly the parents of a first child have a great deal of adjustment to make and are inclined to depend on "the book" as the ultimate authority. Dr. Spock gives excellent advice when he tells young parents "Don't be afraid to trust your own common sense ....take it easy, trust your own instincts,

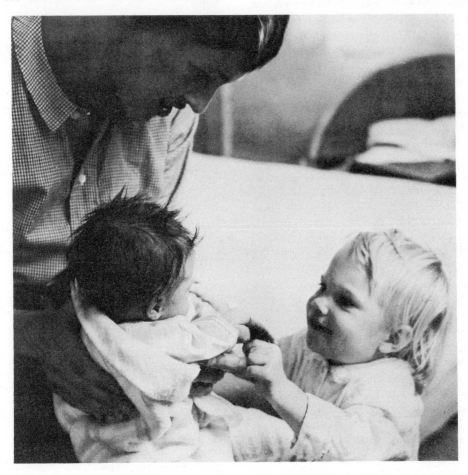

Figure 30-11. The toddler meets the new baby. (Carol Baldwin)

and follow the directions that your doctor gives you."

In homes where the previous baby is being displaced by the newcomer, some preparation is necessary. It is well to move the older child to his larger crib some time before the new baby appears so that he can take pride in being "a big boy now." Preparation of the toddler for a new brother or sister is helpful, but should not be very intense until just before the expected birth.

Probably the greatest help in preparing the child of any age to accept the new baby is to make him feel that this is "our baby," not just "Mommie's baby." If he can help care for the baby according to his ability, this contributes to his feeling that he is still important in the family.

The displaced toddler almost certainly feels some jealousy. With careful planning, mother can reserve some time for cuddling and playing with the toddler just as she did before. Perhaps he may profit from a little extra attention for a time. Anything to make him realize that his mother loves him just as

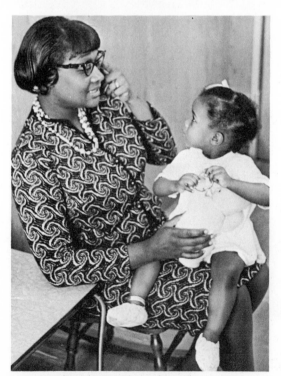

Figure 30-12. The hospitalized toddler is content when her mother can stay.

much as ever, and that there is plenty of room in her life for both children would be helpful.

The small child should not be made to grow up too soon. He may regress and go back to some of his babyish behavior. He should not be shamed or reproved, but understood and given a bit more love and attention. Perhaps the father could occasionally take over care of the new baby while mother devotes herself to the older child.

Older children in the home may at times also feel resentful of the time and attention the new baby requires, especially if they are required to give too much of their time in caring for the younger ones. This needs consideration too. With care and understanding, the experience of having a new baby in the home can become a rewarding one for all.

THE TODDLER IN THE HOSPITAL

Much of the emotional effect of hospitalization has been discussed in the Chapter on Nursing Care of Children. The goal of a hospital pediatric staff must be to get the child well and back into his home as quickly as possible. It must never be forgotten that despite our best efforts, we can never really take the place of the home, or become "mother substitutes."

While we do have the child in the hospital, however, we have a duty toward him. We must try to meet his needs here and now, under the existing circumstances. In order to meet his needs, we first have to understand them.

Naturally, a healthy child is not admitted to the hospital as a patient. He may have pain, or be uncomfortable and ill at ease. He may have little incentive to carry on with his previous zest for living.

His development continues, however. When his illness keeps him from obeying the demands of his nature, he becomes cross and irritable. If he must be confined to his crib, he becomes increasingly restless.

Disciplinary Problems

Whenever a nurse feels that she must

punish a child for non-conforming, she forgets one basic fact. The child is already being punished pretty severely by his environment and by his discomfort. The nurse should think carefully before adding to this unpleasantness.

Certainly a sick child needs discipline. A sick child who is pampered and indulged, and is perhaps allowed to follow his own immature impulses, is just as unhappy as he makes others. He would be grateful for limits set, if it is done with love and understanding.

The disciplinary problems of this age group are many and varied. The answers are not so clear. No two children come to the hospital from the same environment. Some have been ill for a long time and have been overindulged. Others have been severely disciplined or even rejected. Every child has a different capacity to withstand frustration, depending on his personality, his background, and upon his state of health.

Eating Problems

One problem that seems to loom large in nurses' minds is that concerned with the toddler's eating habits. How to get the child to eat? A worthwhile exercise for the nurse is to sit quietly for a moment and let her mind wander back to a time when she was away from home, perhaps for the first time. Perhaps she can remember visiting her grandmother or other relatives and being quite proud that she was big enough to stay without her mother. But after her mother left, things seemed very strange. She was lonely, perhaps homesick, or tired and confused. Even the way grandmother cooked foods seemed different. She could not eat.

Many small children are considered to have eating problems at home. They no longer need food with such intensity as they did during their first year, and this being the age for dawdling, they dawdle. A mother becomes anxious or frustrated or angry. In any case, the child learns that this is an opportunity for a scene, and he dearly loves scenes. This is his big opportunity, such as he had never anticipated. His mother can urge, bribe, coax and scold, but the most she can do is to put food into his mouth. She cannot make him swallow it. If she does succeed, he can always bring it back again!

Mealtime thus becomes a hectic time in many households. Frequently a mother says to the nurse, "To make him eat, try giving one bite to his doggie then one bite to him," or "Pretend that the spoon is a steam shovel

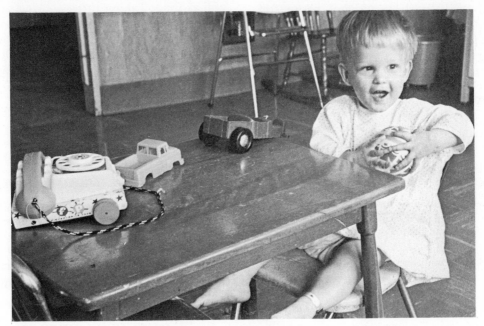

Figure 30-13.   At eighteen months of age even being in the hospital can be fun.

delivering down the little red lane," or even, "Be cross with him and he will eat." Food thus has assumed an importance out of all proportion to its value, and the nurse is left with an added problem.

Eating as a social function. In hospitals we frequently tend to forget that eating is a social function in our culture. Many a toddler who sits in his crib playing with his food would eat with relish if he were placed at the table with his contemporaries. We know this, and go as far as to provide small tables and chairs, but again and again we see a little one still in his crib with his breakfast set up in front of him because someone found it easier to give him his tray there than to get him up.

Why can't he get up for breakfast? Would something serious happen to him if he were to get up before his bath? Few children have to stay in their cribs all of the time, but even if a child must be confined to his bed, he can be pulled over nearer to the more fortunate ones for companionship.

Family-Style Meals

Some pediatric wards serve meals family-style around a big table. A fortunate few allow the nurse to eat with the children. In hospitals where this is not the practice, children can eat with their friends, perhaps in another ward. However, nurses do find eating problems in the toddler ward. The child eats poorly and the mother urges the nurse to "make him eat."

Tactics for Helping the Hospitalized Child Enjoy His Meals

1. Do not put a plate piled high with food before the toddler. This is enough to discourage him at the start. Give him small portions and, if possible, let him have a second helping if he wants it.

2. Let the child eat with his fingers when he finds utensils hard to use. Don't worry about a mess; it can always be cleaned up.

3. A little calculated neglect at mealtime often works wonders. When you hover over him urging him to take just one more bite, the attraction of saying no becomes irresistible. If it appears to make no difference to you personally whether he eats or

not, there is no need for resistance, because there is nothing to resist. He can then permit himself to be influenced by the attractiveness of the food. He is also free to fall under the influence of his peers at the table, one of whom, it is hoped, is a good eater. An adult at the table eating in a businesslike manner may be a beneficial influence.

4. Serve the dessert along with the rest of the meal. It is not important whether he eats it first or last. Hospital desserts for children are usually as nourishing as other foods.

5. If the child is accustomed to other foods, such as Mexican tortillas or Italian spaghetti, find out if the hospital will allow his mother to bring in these foods. Many hospital administrators realize that a small child finds it particularly difficult to eat strange foods, especially when illness takes away his appetite.

"Push fluids" is an order that is frequently quite difficult to carry out in the toddler's department. A small child cannot take much fluid at one time. Persistence seems to be the answer. Fluids should be offered in a small cup or glass.

A morning tea party with small cups and a pot to pour from provides entertainment as well as fluid. Taking turns pouring prolongs the party until everyone has had a turn. The pot may need many fillings, but the fluid chart is going to look much better. Often we find that it takes just a little imagination to help solve the problems of little people.

BIBLIOGRAPHY

Erikson, Erik M.: Childhood and Society. ed. 2. New York, Norton, 1963.
Fraiberg, Selma: The Magic Years. New York, Scribner, 1959.
Maier, Henry W.: Three Theories of Child Development. New York, Harper, 1965.
Spock, Benjamin M. and Lowenberg, Miriam E.: Feeding Your Baby and Child. New York, Pocket Books, 1967.

Suggested Readings for Further Study

Breckenridge, Marian E. and Murphy, Margaret Nesbitt: Growth and Development of the Young Child. ed. 8. Philadelphia, W. B. Saunders, 1969.

Genetic Inheritance *31*

In 1865, an Austrian monk, named Mendel, discovered the principles of genetics through experiments with common garden peas. It is said, "in the succession of events leading to genetics, the Mendelian revolution was primary."* However, the significance of his discoveries was overlooked for many years. It has been only within the 20th century that his principles have been rediscovered and employed in science and medicine.

Before Mendel's time, it was believed that the characteristics of parents were blended together in their children. Mendel proved that this blending does not occur, but rather that the characteristics would reappear unchanged in later generations. (Fig. 31-1) This so-called unit of inheritance was only one of Mendel's discoveries. Mendel is credited with laying down the foundations of genetics.

BASIC GENETICS

All living organisms, whether human, animal, or plant, are composed of living cells that contain all the material necessary for the maintenance and propagation of the particular species. Each cell contains a number of small bodies called *chromosomes*. Chromosomes are threadlike structures occurring in pairs, each pair attached at the center by a *centromere*. Apparently these centromeres do not carry genes but rather function in the distribution of chromosomes to the daughter cells on reproductive division of the cell.

*Dunn, L. C.: Old and New in Genetics. National Foundation—March of Dimes Reprint Series, 1964.

The normal number of chromosomes in a cell differs according to the species. For example, mice have 40 chromosomes in each cell, the cells in corn contain 20 each, while humans have 46 chromosomes in each body cell. These 46 chromosomes consist of 23 essentially identical or homologous pairs. One member of each pair will have been contributed by the father, one by the mother, to the single cell formed by the union of sperm and egg at the time of mating. Twenty-two of these pairs are alike in both male and female. These are called autosomes. The remaining pair is the pair of *sex chromosomes* that differ in male and female.

Chromosomes are large enough to be seen through a microscope, and after chemical treatment can be photographed. In 1960, a group of investigators in human cytogenics adopted a standard system for the identification of groups of chromosomes, arranging them into seven numbered groups, according to size and appearance. (Fig. 31-2) Some pairs can be easily distinguished from others in their group; many cannot. For example, chromosome pairs 4 and 5 in group B cannot be distinguished from each other.

Karyotypes

Photographs of the 46 chromosomes are enlarged, the individual chromosomes are cut out, matched in pairs and grouped. These *karyotypes* are used to locate chromosomal malformations and translocations (the change in position of a segment of chromosome to another location on the chromosome or to another chromosome). Karyotypes of normal chromosomes show them properly paired. In some abnormal

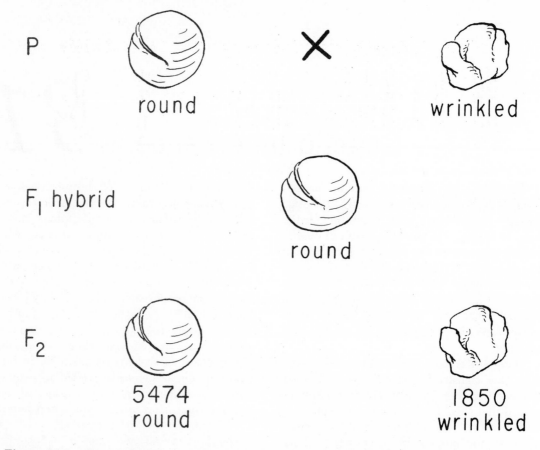

P

round   X   wrinkled

F₁ hybrid

round

F₂

5474
round

1850
wrinkled

Figure 31-1.   One of Mendel's experiments shows that the round seeds are dominant over the wrinkled in the second generation, but the wrinkled seeds appear again in the third generation.

conditions translocations occur, such as in one form of trisomy 21. In *translocation trisomy 21,* there appears to be one extra chromosome in Group C, and one chromosome missing from group D.

The more common trisomy 21 (Down's syndrome, or mongolism) has three chromosomes in the 21 or 22 position, making a total of 47 chromosomes instead of the normal 46. Deletions and duplications can occur during *meiosis.* One condition, the *cri du chat** or cat cry syndrome, shows partial deletion of the short arm of number 5 chromosome.

Determination of Sex

All egg cells from the female carry a pair of female chromosomes, called the X

*See p. 468

chromosomes. Sperm cells, however, carry one X (female) and one Y (male) chromosome paired together. It appears to be a matter of chance whether the egg, which always has an X chromosome, will be fertilized by a sperm carrying an X chromosome or by one carrying a Y. (Sperms and ova are the only human cells which have half the normal chromosomal complement.) In the former case the offspring is a girl. The Y chromosome is dominant over the X, so that if the Y enters into the union, the result is always a male child. In any event, it is the father's sex cell that determines the child's sex. (Fig. 31-3)

Cells reproduce by division, each parent cell producing two daughter cells, each of which in turn produces two new cells. It is in this manner that the single cell produced by

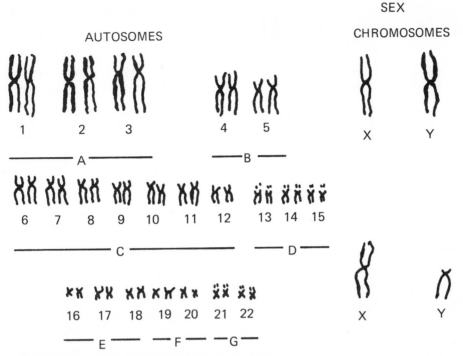

AUTOSOMES

SEX CHROMOSOMES

Figure 31-2. Arrangement of normal chromosomes into a standard karyotype.

the union of sperm and ova eventually multiplies to produce a human child.

The term *mitosis* indicates the type of somatic cell division by which the body grows and replaces discarded cells. Mitosis can be divided into four stages: prophase, metaphase, anaphase, and telophase. (Fig. 31-6)

Meiosis is a special type of cell division

occurring only in sex cells in which the chromosome divides into halves. This new sex cell, the *zygote*, thus contains the standard number of 23 pairs of chromosomes. (Fig. 31-6)

The processes of mitosis and meiosis are extremely complicated. The student is advised to consult textbooks on human genetics for more detailed information. Two of these are Sutton's *Introduction to Human*

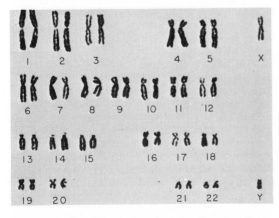

Figure 31-3. Karotype of normal male. Compare sex chromosomes (*right*) with those of female in Fig. 31-5. (Courtesy of Dr. Kurt Hirschhorn)

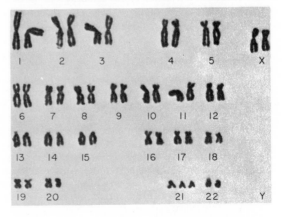

Figure 31-4. Karyotype showing Trisomy 21. Note 3 chromosomes in 21 position. (Courtesy of Dr. Kurt Hirschhorn)

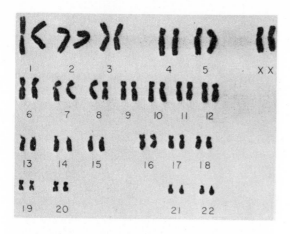

Figure 31-5. Normal female karyotype. (Courtesy of Dr. Kurt Hirschhorn)

Genetics, * and Thompson's *Genetics in Medicine.*†

Genes

Within the chromosomes are the ultramicroscopic bodies called *genes*. "The gene is a unit carrying genetic instructions from one generation to another with mathematic regularity; the instructions are called the genetic code."

In order to have any understanding of the hereditary nature of certain illnesses, it is necessary to have at least a rudimentary

*Sutton, H. Eldon: An Introduction to Human Genetics. New York, Holt, 1965.
†Thompson, James S., and Thompson, Margaret W.: Genetics in Medicine. Philadelphia, 1966.

The Genetic Code*

1. The gene, discovered by Mendel, is a unit carrying the genetic instructions from one generation to another with mathematic regularity; the instructions are called the genetic code.

   a. Form:
     (1) DNA: The genetic code is now known to be held in the nucleus of the cells in tightly coiled strands of deoxyribose nucleic acid (DNA).
     (2) Chromosomes: Dark, rod-like structures in the nuclei of all cells containing the genes; they are largely composed of protein and DNA.
   b. DNA: Everything characteristic of a living entity—its size, shape, and orderly development—that can be passed to progeny is recorded by an arrangement of molecules in its DNA.
     (1) Structure: Each unit of the DNA macromolecule consists of a nitrogenous base, a sugar, and a phosphate; the repeating unit of the DNA macromolecule is called the nucleotide. DNA consists of two stacks or strands of nucleotides twisted to form a double spiral or "helix."
   c. Protein synthesis: DNA governs the production of both the enzymatic and non-enzymatic proteins of the body and records in code form the amino acid arrangement which must be followed to synthesize a particular protein.
     (1) Only four nitrogenous bases exist in DNA, arranged in such a way as to avoid ambiguity; they become the code or symbol for an amino acid.
     (2) Major protein synthesis takes place in the special cytoplasmic structures called *ribosomes*. Information is replicated from DNA in another type of nucleic acid, ribonucleic acid (RNA). It carries information from the DNA of the nucleus to cytoplasmic sites; thus it is called the *messenger* RNA.
     (3) Major protein "assembly lines" of the cells are located in the ribosomes. Messenger RNA carries the program needed to manufacture one type of protein to the ribosomes.
   d. Amino acid activation: The synthesis of protein revolves around the formation of peptide bonds between amino acids; the major source of energy for this process is ATP (adenosine triphosphate). The activated amino acid must be in the place programed for it on the "assembly line." A code-reading escort, transfer RNA, must read the coded instructions.
   e. Genetic biology: Many disorders arise because the ribosomal template from which enzymatic proteins form is defective. DNA controls the configuration of the template.

---

*From Jacob, Stanley and Francone, Clarice: Structure and Function in Man. ed. 2. Philadelphia, W. B. Saunders, 1970.

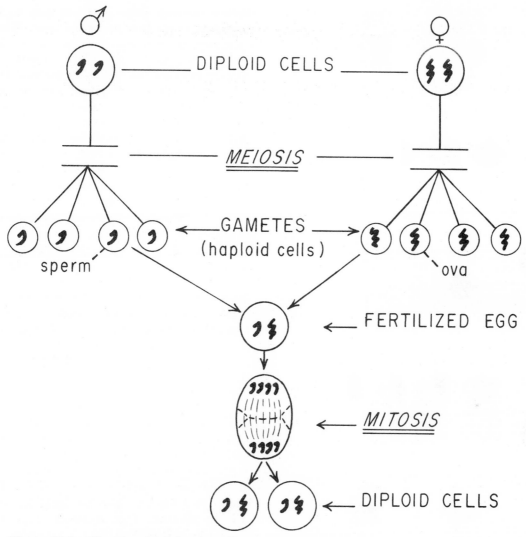

Figure 31-6.   The type of cell division that sex cells undergo is meiosis. Once fertilized, the egg divides, as somatic cells do, by mitosis.

knowledge of certain aspects of human genetics. Genes carry biochemical codes which determine which traits we will inherit, but any gene can be altered by mutation or chromosomal rearrangement. The science of genetics studies the way activities of the genes transmit both normal and abnormal traits from generation to generation.

Mutation in a gene means essentially a fundamental change in its structure, resulting in the transmission of a trait different from that normally carried by the particular gene. The cause of mutations is not well understood at present, although it is accepted that exposure to high radiation is one cause. As far as is known, most mutations result in undesirable traits.

Chromosomes may also become displaced or malformed, thus producing disease or defects in the offspring of affected persons. Trisomy 21, known also as Down's syndrome, is one example. Trisomes may also appear in other chromosome positions, such as chromosomes 13-15 in the D_1 position, Trisomy D.

Inheritance

When any two members of a pair of genes carry the same genetic instructions, the

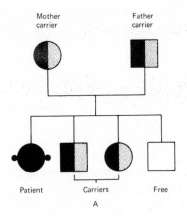

A

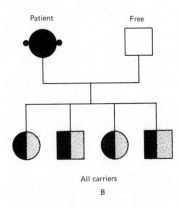

B

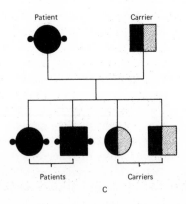

C

Figure 31-7. Autosomal recessive pattern inheritance. (*A*) Both parents carriers—ratio of one patient, two carriers, one free from disease. (*B*) One parent patient—one parent free from disease, all children carriers—no clinical disease. (*C*) One parent carrier, one parent has disease—ratio of two children with disease, two carriers.

person carrying these genes is said to be *homozygous* for that particular trait. When each member of a pair of genes carries different instructions, the person is *heterozygous* for the trait. One member of a heterozygous pair of genes will be the dominant gene. Thus, a trait or condition appearing in a heterozygous person will be called an *autosomal dominant trait*. (Sex-linked dominant traits will be discussed later.) A gene carrying different information for the same trait which is not expressed (e.g., blue eyes vs. brown) is called a recessive. Inheritance patterns for autosomal recessive traits are shown in Figure 31-7. However, if both parents express the recessive trait, all their children will have the same trait or condition, because each parent must have two genes for the trait and the children cannot possibly escape inheriting two also. Some examples of recessive diseases are thalassemia and cystic fibrosis.

A dominant gene may be defined as one that is expressed in only one of a chromosome pair. A recessive gene is only detectable when present on both chromosomes. One example of a dominant inheritance is the condition of osteogenesis imperfecta.

In autosomal dominant inheritance, the affected parent will usually transmit the dominant allele* to half his children, who will be affected. This, however, may not *always* be the ratio of 1:1.

GENETIC ANOMALIES
Inborn Errors of Metabolism

The concept of an inborn error of metabolism is that of a genetically controlled enzyme deficit leading to an interruption of a metabolic pathway. Inborn errors of metabolism are inherited as autosomal recessive traits. Examples are diabetes mellitus, phenylketonuria, galactosemia.

Mental Retardation
History

Mental retardation is doubtless as old as the human race, although it is difficult to

*Allele—forms of a gene found at the same locus on homologous chromosomes.

find evidence of its existence in ancient medical writings. The first treatise found devoted entirely to mental deficiency was written by Paracelsus, a Swiss medical writer, in about 1530. He also wrote the first clear medical description of cretinism.

Another Swiss physician wrote in 1614, "In infants this dullness of the intelligence soon becomes evident, when they are educated, and forced to learn some things, and especially at the time when they are taught to read....only by....much exertion can they recognize the letters of the alphabet, put syllables together, and form complete words from them."* As Cranefield comments, "This passage....assuredly shows that the notion that the 'high-grade' defective, whose deficit is revealed only when he goes to school, is not a new one."†

In the late 1800s, several pioneers in the study of mental retardation believed that the retarded could lead more normal lives in society through education and training. Jean Itard had worked with the "wild boy of Aveyron" at the end of the 18th century. The boy was undoubtedly a mental defective who had wandered away from his home, rather than one who had been raised by animals, as it was then believed. Although the boy never learned to speak, Itard inadvertently showed that intelligence can be improved and raised to a higher level of function through motivation and individual attention.

Edouard Seguin (1866) based his entire program of sensory and motor training on Itard's work. Seguin was a great force behind the establishment of special schools for the severely retarded. Other well known names are those of Maria Montessori, who established methods of special education for the mentally defective in Italy, and Samuel Howe, of Boston, who treated Laura Bridgeman and trained the teacher of Helen Keller.‡ Howe, Seguin and others created

small, homelike institutions for retardates located in the hearts of the communities. They were so successful in restoring their charges to normal society that of the 465 residents admitted to Howe's Massachusetts School for Idiotic and Feebleminded Youth, over 18 years 365 had been discharged and returned to the community.

Unfortunately, as time went on, the function of institutions for the retarded changed to an emphasis on "sheltering the deviant from society," which in essence meant isolating them from the community. Still later, the emphasis changed to "protecting society from the deviant," still isolating the retarded.§

White and Wolfensberger give a graphic illustration of the "evolution of dehumanization in U. S. public institutions for the retarded." (Fig. 31-8)

In recent times a greater understanding of the mentally deprived has done much to make institutions places of learning and development rather than detention homes. Much, however, remains to be done. In the United States, the Kennedy administration was instrumental in encouraging considerable research and experiment in the care of the retarded, with amazing results. Unfortunately, some of the most promising new programs have been practically abandoned or inadequately carried out due to lack of funds for training workers and possibly due to some disinterest among potential workers.

In 1968 a declaration of rights of the mentally retarded was proclaimed by the International League of Societies for the Mentally Handicapped. This clearly states the rights of the mentally retarded and is reprinted in full on page 460.

THE MENTALLY RETARDED CHILD

The term mental retardation is used freely, but not always with a clear understanding of its meaning. Definitions

*Phillips, Irving, ed.: Prevention and Treatment of Mental Retardation. p. 5.
†Ibid.
‡Helen Keller was sensorially deprived as she could neither see nor hear, but she was intellectually gifted.

§White, Wesley D., and Wolfensberger, Wolf, P.: The evolution of dehumanization in our institutions. Mental Retardation, 7:5, 1969.
#Ibid, p. 8.

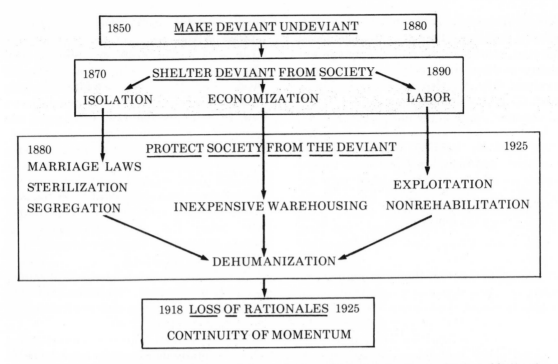

Figure 31-8. Graphic summarization of the evolution of dehumanization in U. S. public institutions for the retarded. (Courtesy of White and Wolfensberger, Mental Retardation, 7:5, 1969)

formulated within the past few years have done much to clarify our concepts of mental retardation.

"Mentally retarded are children and adults who, as a result of inadequately developed intelligence, are significantly impaired in their ability to learn and adapt to the demands of society."*

Another definition is equally helpful.

"Mental retardation refers to subaverage general intellectual functioning which originates during the developmental period and is associated with impairment in adaptive behavior."†

Impairment in adaptive behavior is reflected in maturation, learning and in social adjustment. Actually, mental retardation is a relative concept that depends on

---

*From: A Proposed Program for National Action to Combat Mental Retardation. A Report of the President's Panel on Mental Retardation. Washington, U. S. Government Printing Office, 1962.
†Heber, R. I.: Modifications on the manual on terminology and classification in mental retardation. Amer. Jour. Mental. Defic., 65:499, 1961.

the prevailing educational and cultural standards of society. A person who may function adequately in a society that demands proficiency in certain skills, may be utterly unable to cope with the demands of a complex culture.

Intelligence itself is measured in terms of ability for abstract thinking. It includes causal reasoning, spatial comprehension, verbal expression, visual and auditory memory, and other adaptive adjustments.

Methods for attempting to measure intelligence were first formulated in France in the early 20th century, in an effort to screen out mentally deficient persons from the general population. Alfred Binet and his colleagues developed tests for measuring intellectual levels that have been modified and revised by Terman and others. These tests measure one aspect of intelligence, but do not necessarily indicate the degree of social adjustment or the maturational level. Other measuring devices, such as the Bender-Gestalt, or the Draw-A-Man tests, attempt to reach a *gestalt*, or organized pattern of experience. All of these tests have real value, particularly if no one test is relied upon for the total measure of a child's ability to adapt to his environment. No test has been able as yet to solve the problem of innate intelligence versus social deprivation, the so-called nature-nurture problem.

Norms of Intellectual Ability and Adaptive Behavior

While keeping the limitations of predictive tests in mind, some idea of what to expect from a person in terms of intellectual ability and social adaptation is necessary. Labels are important insofar as they affect the education that a child is offered. A label has negative value if it is used to hold a child within a given area, such as severely or moderately retarded, without frequent attempts to discover whether he can make further progress. His developmental level must take into account his mental, physical, emotional and social adjustment.

Leland* reminds us that subaverage intellectual functioning of a person does not of necessity indicate a low IQ, but rather indicates that when within a group of persons doing an intellectual task, the individual does not do as well as the average. It must be remembered that as society becomes more complex, and intellectual requirements on the individual more demanding, persons who formerly were accepted as behaving on an average level may no longer be considered to do so.

"Thus," Leland concludes, "the real test of a classification scheme must be on how well it serves the individual being classified. If it tends to merely label him .... it must be a false scheme."

Terms Used for Measuring Extent of Mental Impairment

The older terms of moron, imbecile and idiot carry high emotional import, and are no

---

*Leland, Henry: Relationship between "Intelligence" and mental retardation. Amer. Jour. Mental Defic., *73:*534, 1969.

longer in good usage. Preferred terms are mildly, moderately, severely and profoundly retarded. Terms such as educable, trainable and dependent are still in common use, but these terms tend to set limits that may influence attempts to help the child reach a higher potential.

Etiological Factors in Mental Retardation

Prenatal Causes

Inborn errors of metabolism. For example, phenylketonuria. Very early detection may lead to measures preventing serious mental damage.

Prenatal infection. For example, toxoplasmosis. Microcephaly, hydrocephalus, and other brain damaging conditions may result from intrauterine infections.

Intrauterine growth retardation. The cause is not clear. A higher incidence of mental retardation is found in this group than in the general population.

Teratogenic agents. For example, maternal irradiation or drugs. It appears that most drugs pass through the placental barrier, and that some of them may have an adverse effect on a developing fetus.

Genetic factors. For example, Down's syndrome. Inborn variations of chromosomal patterns result in a variety of aberrations, the most commonly known being mongolism (Down's syndrome).

Perinatal Causes

Birth injuries, anoxia, and difficult birth have all been etiological factors in brain damage. It is possible, however, in some instances, that prenatal factors were already present.

Postnatally Acquired Mental Deficiency

Poisoning; for example, lead poisoning. Children who develop encephalopathy from chronic lead poisoning usually suffer significant brain damage.

Infections and trauma; for example, meningitis, convulsive disorders, hydrocephalus, and other brain damage, are

Declaration of general and special rights of the mentally retarded

Whereas the universal declaration of human rights, adopted by the United Nations, proclaims that all of the human family, without distinction of any kind, have equal and inalienable rights of human dignity and freedom;

Whereas the declaration of the right of the child, adopted by the United Nations, proclaims the rights of the physically, mentally or socially handicapped child to special treatment, education and care required by his particular condition.

Now Therefore

The International League of Societies for the Mentally Handicapped expresses the general and special rights of the mentally retarded as follows:

ARTICLE I

The mentally retarded person has the same basic rights as other citizens of the same country and same age.

ARTICLE II

The mentally retarded person has a right to proper medical care and physical restoration and to such education, training, habilitation and guidance as will enable him to develop his ability and potential to the fullest possible extent, no matter how severe his degree of disability. No mentally handicapped person should be deprived of such services by reason of the costs involved.

ARTICLE III

The mentally retarded person has a right to economic security and to a decent standard of living. He has a right to productive work or to other meaningful occupation.

ARTICLE IV

The mentally retarded person has a right to live with his own family or with fosterparents; to participate in all aspects of community life, and to be provided with appropriate leisure time activities. If care in an institution becomes necessary it should be in surroundings and under circumstances as close to normal living as possible.

ARTICLE V

The mentally retarded person has a right to a qualified guardian when this is required to protect his personal wellbeing and interest. No person rendering direct services to the mentally retarded should also serve as his guardian.

ARTICLE VI

The mentally retarded person has a right to protection from exploitation, abuse and degrading treatment. If accused, he has a right to a fair trial with full recognition being given to his degree of responsibility.

ARTICLE VII

Some mentally retarded persons may be unable due to the severity of their handicap, to exercise for themselves all of their rights in a meaningful way. For others, modification of some or all of these rights is appropriate. The procedure used for modification or denial of rights must contain proper legal safeguards against every form of abuse, must be based on an evaluation of the social capability of the mentally retarded person by qualified experts and must be subject to periodic reviews and to the right of appeal to higher authorities.

ABOVE ALL—THE MENTALLY RETARDED PERSON HAS THE RIGHT TO RESPECT.

October 24, 1968.

From Mental Retardation. 7:2, 1969.

frequent sequelae of central nervous system infections.

Impoverished early environment. The degree of stimulation the infant receives in early life is an important factor in intellectual development. It is generally accepted that irreversible impairment to a child's ability to respond to his environment may result from complete emotional rejection in early life. Certain physical disabilities may so hamper a child that he cannot respond normally to his environment. The child severely affected by cerebral palsy who cannot talk, walk, or care for himself, may have no damage to his intellectual capacity, but his motor disabilities effectually hinder his ability to learn.

Meeting the Needs of the Mentally Handicapped Child

The most important need of any child is for understanding parents, and the mentally handicapped have this need in at least as great a measure as do normally bright children. Perhaps the greatest change we need to make is in the way we view these children. These are not children set apart or different; they are our children, just as all the others are. An unfortunate condition makes them slower to develop, and places a limit on their learning, but they are still our children. Not until we really grasp this point, both intellectually and emotionally, can we be of help to them.

Counseling the Family

One of the meanings of counseling is "Interchange of opinions as to future procedure: consultation: deliberation."* This is just what the nurse hopes to do. She accepts the parents as they are, and she starts from there. This implies that she understands what happens when the knowledge comes that their child is mentally retarded.

---

*The American College Dictionary, p. 276. New York, Random House, 1964.

The Mildly Retarded Child (Educable). This child is a slow learner, but is capable of acquiring basic skills. He may learn to read, to write, and to do arithmetic to a 4th or 5th grade level. He is slower than the average child in learning to walk, talk, and feed himself, but his retardation may not be obvious to casual acquaintances. With support and guidance, he usually can develop social and vocational skills adequate for self-maintenance. He has a mental age of 6 to 10 years; his intelligence quotient is 51 to 70.

The Moderately and Severely Retarded Child (Trainable). The moderately retarded child has little, if any, ability to attain independence and academic skills. He has a noticeable delay in motor development and speech, but is capable of responding to training in self-help activities. He may be able to learn repetitive skills in sheltered workshops. Some may learn to travel alone, but few rarely become capable of assuming complete self-maintenance. Mental age range is from 2 to 6 years. IQ score, 20 to 50.

The Profoundly Retarded Child (Totally Dependent). This child has a minimal capacity for functioning, and has need of nursing care. He may eventually learn to walk, and develop a form of primitive speech, but is not capable of self-care and needs continued nursing care. Mental age range from 0 to 2 years. IQ score, 0 to 20.

As our understanding of mental retardation progresses, and as newer teaching methods develop, fewer persons need to remain at this level. Exciting results have occurred in terms of learning some degree of self-help, such as toilet training and self-feeding. There remain those, of course, so severely damaged that even this amount of learning appears to be unattainable.

The first reaction of most parents to this tragedy is one of disbelief: this cannot be, there must be a mistake. When forced by obvious facts to accept the condition, a search for a reason begins. Sometimes the concept of punishment enters in; perhaps this pregnancy had been rejected. Probably all women have a few moments of unhappiness over their thickening figure, curtailment of previous activity, morning sickness; but if the result of the pregnancy is an imperfect child, there are apt to be feelings of guilt. Many other presumed causes, frequently unrealistic, are found, because the shame of not being able to produce a perfect child must be dealt with in some manner.

Some rejection of this child is nearly inevitable, but this is also unacceptable. It may be compensated by over-protection or over-concern to the point of making the child unnecessarily helpless, with perhaps some of the anger and frustration taken out on the normal children.

Another method of coping with this intolerable problem is to set the child apart as someone special, someone sent to teach them love, humility and charity. If parents are to become effective, they have to face their reactions, until they can accept the child as a member of their family, to be helped, loved, disciplined and accepted just as the others.

The nurse, however, should not expect the parents to pour out their feelings to her, nor should she expect to assume the role of a professional counselor—a role for which she has neither the training nor the experience. She should be ready to listen, to observe, to help formulate a plan of care, and to use her knowledge and skills as they are desired and accepted. As she works with the family, her acceptance of them makes her an understanding partner, a partner in whom one can confide and with whom one can discuss problems. If the family and the nurse find the problems are beyond their ability, the nurse should know where they can seek expert help.

The Nurse's Role

In practical, everyday terms, what is the nurse's role? She may go into the situation prepared to discuss long-term goals and overall plans, but she is quite likely to find that the immediate, practical problem of getting the child to eat is absorbing the mother's attention, and that the mother is impatient with abstract goals until she has been able to cope with today's problems. Therefore, the nurse must begin with the problem at hand.

All but the most profoundly retarded children go through the sequence of normal development, with delays at each stage and a leveling off of ability much earlier as they reach the limits of their capacity. A retarded child, however, proceeds according to his mental age rather than according to his chronological age. Thus, a six-year-old retardate may be functioning on a mental level of two years, and the expected behavior must be, essentially, that of a two-year-old.

The most important requirement for the nurse is an adequate knowledge of the important landmarks of normal growth and development, in order to understand the progressive nature of maturation. One of the first expectations of normal development is that the infant's nervous system will have matured sufficiently at six or eight weeks to enable him to smile purposefully: that is, he smiles in response to pleasure and refuses to smile when he does not wish to do so. Failure to have developed this far is a cause for concern. Whether the abnormal maturation is the result of environmental conditions or from a lack of intellectual ability, there is still cause for concern. The next section makes some suggestions about helping the child to cope with the basic skills of everyday living.

Teaching Self-Help to the Child

Teaching a mentally retarded child the basic self-help skills does not differ in principle from teaching any young child. If we can accept this child as "anychild," and not just a strange creature, we can free ourselves of all fanciful imaginings and set about meeting his needs according to his present stage of maturation. In actual fact, one should not need any particular set of rules for this child, but because the physical image does distort our judgement, a reinforcement of the application of knowledge of growth and development usually proves helpful.

An outline similar to the following may be a helpful aid in setting up a program of self-help.

Preparation for Program

1. Study the child for the effects of any superimposed physical handicaps. The incidence of muscular disability, a physical anomaly or cardiac disease, is higher than in the average child population. The presence of these handicaps modifies the child's rate of development whether or not he has limited mental ability.

2. Estimate the child's present stage of mental development. If, at the age of six, he shows the developmental level of two-year-old, be prepared to start at a two year level.

3. Know the average development expected of the various age groups. It is difficult to start from a two year level unless you have a good understanding of the normal development of a two-year-old.

4. Keep in mind the one factor that makes this child different from the average child: his lack of ability for abstract reasoning. This prevents him from transferring learning, or applying abstract principles to varied situations. He has to learn by habit formation.

5. Remember the three Rs of habit training—Routine, Repetition and Relaxation.

6. Watch for any signs of readiness, and take advantage of them.

Procedure

Helping the Child Learn Toilet Control

Looking for signs of readiness. The average child shows this progression in toilet training:

AGE	
One year	regular time for bowel movements.
15 to 18 months	can achieve bowel control.
about 18 months	intervals between urination of one to three hours.
1-1/2 to 2 years	can achieve daytime control—must be reminded.
2 to 3 years	asks for toilet usually, may lose control in unfamiliar surroundings.
3 to 4 years or later	night control for many, but not all.

The attempt to assess the child's maturational level does, of course, take into consideration all of the developmental skills, as well as the child's environment. Has he made any attempt to walk, or has he been kept in his crib with no opportunity or encouragement?

If the mother is uncertain of the child's urination pattern, it might be helpful if she keeps a "wetting" chart for a few days.

Habit formation. Place the child on the toilet at regular intervals of approximately two hours during the daytime. It may be best to do this according to his "wetting" pattern, or it may be more effective to establish a habit before and after meals, in mid-morning, mid-afternoon, and at bedtime. Taking the child to the toilet should always be accompanied by a verbal explanation—simple, direct and friendly.

Establishing a *place* is important. If the toilet chair is moved from room to room, or if the child is placed on it while he eats, or plays, or watches television, he is not learning toilet habits. He also needs to learn that society accepts the toilet room only, as the proper place for elimination.

Routine and repetition are obvious factors. *Relaxation* is not so easily attained. It is very easy for the procedure to assume undue importance until it becomes an obsession, making everyone tense, including the child. It undoubtedly will be a long time before he succeeds in urinating at the proper time, rather than directly after he is taken off. Expressed appreciation when he has achieved, a relaxed "better luck next time" when he has not, helps keep this experience in proper proportion. About five minutes is long enough for an individual try, but if child resists, it is better to put this off for a while longer.

As with the average child, the proper clothing helps. Diapers are associated with wetting and soiling, whereas keeping training pants dry can be a source of pride. Keeping in mind that even the profoundly retarded child may reach the mental age of two, we may find that we are setting our sights too low for a particular child.

Helping a Child Learn Dressing Skills

Readiness. Any child learns to *undress* before he learns to *dress*, because manipulation of clothing is a complex skill. Records of attempts to teach aborigines who have never worn clothing to put arms and legs in the proper openings, to manipulate buttons or zippers, show how incredibly difficult this type of learning is.

The first task is to teach the child how (and when) to remove clothing, which may be more difficult than it sounds if he has formed the habit of removing shoes or clothes whenever he fancies.

When ready to teach dressing, make the experience as simple as possible. Clothing that is easy to put on, and that is placed in a predetermined order for dressing facilitates learning. Perhaps a brightly colored label to show which is the back might be useful. He probably will learn more easily if practice is with clothing itself, rather than with especially designed material for learning buttoning, tying, and so forth, because the transfer of learning from the form to his clothing may prove to be a difficult step.

Mental Age for Dressing Skills

1 year	Tries to help by co-operation, such as holding out an arm or a leg. Can remove socks.
1-1/2 years	Removes easily accessible clothes. Tries to put on shoes.
2 to 3 years	Puts on simple clothing, perhaps backwards, shoes on wrong feet. Tries to button large, easily accessible buttons, manipulate zipper.
3 to 4 years	Can dress self except for help with difficult clothing. Can button and use zipper.

It is important to remember that most mentally retarded children do increase in mental age, slowly, and to a limited level. Therefore, every child needs to be watched for evidence of readiness for a new skill, regardless of the label of mental ability.

Motor Skills

Motor abilities for retarded children follow normal developmental curves at a lower level and higher chronological age.

Norms for acquisition of motor skills in the general population are:

Mental Age for Motor Skills

1 month	Exhibits tonic-neck and startle reflexes.
4 months	Grasps objects if placed in his hand. Holds head and chest up when on abdomen.
6 to 7 months	Transfers objects from hand to hand—sits with some support—rolls over.
9 to 10 months	Transfers self to sitting position, usually pulls himself to his feet, can creep.
18 months	Walks alone, pushes chairs or objects around.
2 years	Runs, although unevenly. Turns pages of book.
3 years	Rides tricycle, climbs. Walks up and down stairs in adult manner.

Teaching the acquisition of motor skills is largely concerned with the provision of opportunity, enrichment of the environment, provision of approval of attempts, and acceptance. A child placed on the floor finds it easier to roll over than when he is lying on a soft mattress. A bright, attractive object, just out of reach, may some day catch his eye and provide an incentive to move toward it. An opportunity to observe other children attempting new motor skills sometimes provides inducement toward trying similar feats.

Providing an Enriched Environment

Environmental stimulation is essential for everyone's development. If we think that the retarded child does not need this enrichment because "he could not learn anyway," we are discouraging further development. As a matter of fact, the retarded child needs much more environmental enrichment than does the average child who can help provide his own stimulation.

Things to look at: attention getters

Mobiles, moving gently in the air, are attention catchers. Bright-colored paper butterflies or birds, or more complex objects such as airplanes or boats, strung on wires or on heavy strings of varying lengths—these can be simple for the nurse to make, or may even become an absorbing hobby for her.

Cradle gyms can be made by stringing all sorts of objects on heavy cord: painted spools, plastic lids, painted toilet paper rolls, large wooden beads. (Fig. 31-9)

Pictures, large, simple, brightly colored, pasted in cloth scrapbooks, on cardboard, or pinned up in easy sight.

Bright and interesting stuffed toys, large enough to be noticed.

Things to handle, hear and manipulate

A *sensory box* can be made up from everyday objects that can be handled for texture, form and size.

Furry object, smooth plastic, velvet, silk or satin, burlap.

Large smooth stones, sponge, sand, soap.

Small horn, bells on string, music box.

Small cars, planes.

Active manipulation

Painted tin cans of various sizes, colors.

Colored spoons to pick up and to lay down.

Hand puppets.

Bongo drums, made from coffee cans with plastic tops.

Clothes pins to drop into large plastic, cut-down bleach bottles.

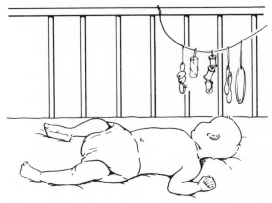

Figure 31-9. A cradle gym can be easily made from objects found in the home.

Clay, play dough.
Water play. Funnels, squeeze bottles, cups.
Gum drops for learning to chew.
Cereals such as Cheerios for hand, eye coordination.

This list grows easily with a little imagination and practice.

Discipline for the Retarded Child

Discipline, in the sense of teaching acceptable and unacceptable behavior, is as important for the retarded child as it is for any other. There are some special considerations for dealing with these children, because of their limited ability to adapt behavior to varying circumstances.

Discipline should always be consistent, and should enable a child to know what to expect. Language should be simple, direct and concise.

A positive approach, relying heavily on example and demonstration, gets much better results than a constant "don't touch" or "stop that." Obedience is an essential part of discipline, especially for the child with faulty reasoning ability, but the objectives of discipline should be considerably broader if peace and happiness are to be achieved.

One way to help prevent resentment and stubborn behavior is to set up a daily schedule and adhere to it as nearly as possible. Because of his impaired ability to reason and transfer learning, the child needs routine for his support. Reminders of the next item coming up on the schedule are frequently needed, such as "After you put your blocks away, we will have dinner;" at the same time, giving a hand to get him started. Laura Dittmann, in her excellent writing about discipline for these children, tells of three-year-old David, a mongoloid child.

"Even at 3 he can be as stubborn as a ton of cement when it comes to leaving one thing and starting the next. He twinkles and smiles, but won't budge.... When his mother insists that he get out of the bathtub he...howls and hits at her arms as she reaches for him.... She lifts him out, singing a song about bedtime and slippers. And David gets absorbed in rubbing the soft fur of his slipper and forgets all his objections. If his mother became confused about her requests and let David win, bathtime the next night might be even more difficult. By the time David is 12, possibly no one can get him to do anything."*

*Dittmann, L.: The Mentally Retarded Child at Home. P. 36. Washington, U. S. Government Printing Office, 1959.

If firmness and consistency are essential, so are kindness, love and understanding. Time out for a kiss for the hurt finger, rocking for a tired child, understanding of hurt feelings; these are part of the day as well.

If punishment is needed, it is important that it follows the deed directly, with cause and effect made as clear as possible to the child. Taking him away from the group for a short time, quietly but firmly, may help him quiet down and gain self control. Retaliation can confuse and anger him. If he is using "bad" behavior in order to get more attention, more praise and approval for good behavior may take away the need for misbehaving.

The Other Members of the Family

What happens to the siblings of the retarded child? The problems created by the presence of a retardate in the family can be severe, even in well-adjusted families in which the slow one is accepted, with allowances made for his inadequacies.

Undoubtedly, the proper care and training of a slow child take a disproportionate amount of his mother's time. It is natural for the others to feel some neglect, wishing that they could get the same sort of attention, and could themselves be helpless once in a while instead of always being called upon to be the responsible ones.

Some children do, in fact, regress to the behavior level of their retarded sibling in an attempt to get their share of attention. Parents, in turn, find it difficult to understand why the normal children cannot consistently feel the same amount of concern for the slow one's progress.

In homes in which shame is felt over the retarded child, social life is frequently sharply disrupted. The children cannot bring friends home, the older siblings hesitate over their dates. Even in homes in which the retarded child is accepted, his irresponsible behavior may create embarrassment for the rest of the family and their guests.

The nurse working with the retardate needs to be aware of these various natural reactions, showing herself friendly and interested in the other children. As she becomes familiar with the family, she should be able to help by her understanding and acceptance, as well as friendly counsel.

Home Care Versus Institutional Care

Today, there is a tendency to keep these children at home rather than place them in institutions. As more and better opportunities for help, education and guidance arise in the community, more families gain confidence in their ability to care for their retarded children in their own homes.

There is much to be said for home care for the retarded child. The individual attention, security, and the sense of belonging, of being a member of a family, are all important factors in the child's progress toward a higher level of adjustment. No institution, however progressive and expertly staffed, can entirely supply the experience a child gets in his own family.

The solution—home or institution—is not this simple, however. The profoundly retarded child may indeed take too much time and strength from the mother to allow her to give even adequate attention to the rest of her family. The retarded child may be uncontrollable, and become a great nuisance in the home and neighborhood. Parents may feel that any benefits received by the child by staying in his own home ask sacrifices entirely out of proportion for the other family members.

Each family must, of course, make its own decision. The nurse can listen, can present facts, and help find necessary information, but she should never attempt to persuade or push her own views. Such a situation is emotionally charged, and whichever way the family decides, there are undoubtedly going to be moments when they are going to wonder if their decision was the right one. Their regret can only be intensified if they believe that they made a decision against their better judgment.

Institutions in general are moving away from accepting children before the age of two, many waiting until the child is five or six. An infant is a fairly helpless person, requiring considerable care whether he is bright or dull. Therefore, the burden on the parents grows heavier as the child grows older.

Whether the child is cared for at home or not, parents may be greatly encouraged over the intense interest being shown for these children. Research centers are exploring new possibilities, homes for the retarded are receiving money for newer appliances, better surroundings and, most important, are attracting well-trained, sympathetic personnel intent on applying newly understood principles and practices.

Continuing Care

Mental disability is becoming the first cause for institutionalizing children, according to statistics provided by the Children's Bureau.* These are children who are handicapped emotionally and physically; however, the number of children in institutions for the mentally retarded increased nearly 15% between 1960 and 1964. It is hoped that our newer emphasis on programs for the mentally retarded can bring about a decrease in the child population in mental institutions.

Among the general population of the mentally retarded, it is estimated that not

---

*America's Children and Youth in Institutions— 1950-1960-1964. Washington, U. S. Government Printing Office, 1965.

more than 10% to 25% are in the profoundly, severely and moderately handicapped group, with an IQ below 50. The trainable members can benefit from special education in schools in which it is provided. The profoundly retarded become increasingly difficult to handle as they grow older and larger, because they still need total care. Most of them must eventually be institutionalized, but there have been attempts to train even these children. Training includes placing the children on flat surfaces on which they can roll about, or in supported sitting positions for a period each day, providing sensory stimulation such as using a few certain words to the child and repeating these words constantly while making sensory application, such as "shoe" while placing it on the child's foot. Success has been reported with some children who have learned to crawl, to sit, and, in some cases, to stand and to walk.

The educable child is often not discovered to be retarded until he starts school, and is not able to keep up with his class. Special classes can do much to help these children adapt to social living; many achieve quite good adjustment, and may be absorbed into society with little discrimination.

CONDITIONS IN WHICH MENTAL DEFICIENCY IS COMMONLY PRESENT

Many conditions in which mental deficiency is present are so rare that only a few are mentioned here. For a complete list of known mental deficiency disorders, a text specializing in such disorders should be consulted. Following is a list of conditions of mental deficiency occasionally seen in the hospital.

In anencephaly the cranial vault is largely absent, the brain being represented by a vascular mass. Extrauterine life is impossible, although some infants have lived for a few hours after birth.

Apert's syndrome is a disorder in which the child's head is pointed anteriorly. There may be syndactyly (webbing of adjacent fingers or toes). It is inherited as an autosomal dominant trait.

In cretinism there may be entire absence of the thyroid gland from birth or a complete absence of thyroid secretion from the gland. The condition is described on page 470.

Cri du chat, or the "cat cry" syndrome, is due to a partial deletion of the short arm of a number 5 chromosome. These children have a catlike cry in infancy and are microcephalic and severely mentally retarded. Parents of such children should seek genetic counseling before planning for more children.

Cornelia de Lange syndrome, a rare syndrome of unknown cause, is characterized by mental deficiency, small and malformed hands and feet, continuous eyebrows, and a thin down-turning upper lip.

Galactosemia is a condition caused by an inborn error of metabolism. When untreated, mental deficiency results. See page 472.

Gaucher's disease. The rather rare *infantile* form of this condition causes slowed development. These infants have respiratory and other problems and seldom survive their first year. The chronic form of Gaucher's disease appearing in later childhood or adult life is not associated with mental deficiency.

Hurler's syndrome (gargoylism) is an autosomal recessive metabolic disturbance present at birth, although most of the clinical signs appear later in infancy. The skull may be deformed, the neck short and the tongue enlarged. Kyphosis also develops. The enlarged head, grotesque faces and deformed hands in this condition account for the designation of gargoylism. Without laboratory studies the condition may be mistaken for cretinism. Because of the retarded mental and physical development, prognosis is poor.

Maple syrup urine disease, a rare autosomal recessive condition, is characterized by an odor of maple syrup to the urine, difficult feeding, and progressive mental and neurological deterioration. The infant rarely lives longer than a few months without treatment. A special diet low in certain amino acids has been successfully used to arrest the progress of this disease in some cases.

Lawrence-Moon-Biedl syndrome is an autosomal recessive disorder. Obesity, polydactylism (supernumerary fingers or toes) and mental retardation are present. Hypogonadism is occasionally found.

Microcephaly. Arrested growth of the brain is the cause of the small skull found in this condition. Severe mental retardation is present. This condition is not to be confused with premature closure of the sutures of the skull. The latter condition can be remedied by early surgery to open the sutures and allow brain growth.

Phenylketonuria is described on page 471.

Down's syndrome and other trisomies are discussed below in detail.

Trisomies

Down's syndrome (mongolism) is the most common of the chromosomal anomalies. Approximately one in 600 to 700 births is a child with Down's syndrome. The condition was first described by Langdon Down in 1866, but its cause was a mystery for many years. In 1932 it was suggested that a chromosomal anomaly might be the cause, but the anomaly was not demonstrated until 1959.

Down's syndrome has been observed in nearly all countries and races. The term mongolism is not an appropriate name for the condition, and is gradually going out of use. The majority of individuals with Down's syndrome have trisomy 21 (Fig. 31-4): a few have partial dislocation of chromosomes 15 and 21. All forms of the condition show a variety of abnormal characteristics. Mental status is usually within the moderate to severe range of retardation with the majority moderately retarded.

The most common anomalies include: brachycephaly (shortness of head); retarded body growth; upward and outward slanted eyes (almond-shaped) with epicanthic fold at inner angle; short, flattened bridge of nose; thick and fissured tongue; hair may be dry and coarse; hands are short, with an incurved fifth finger and a single palmar crease; wide space between first and second toes; very lax muscle tone (these children can assume relaxed positions difficult for normal persons); frequently there are heart and eye anomalies; susceptibility to leukemia greater than in the general population.

Not all of these physical signs are present in all individuals with Down's syndrome. Some may have only one or two characteristics; others may show nearly all. Females with this syndrome have greatly reduced fertility. A few affected females have had children. Males appear to be completely sterile.

Types of Down's Syndrome

Standard Trisomy 21. In this condition, the affected person has 47 chromosomes, with an extra chromosome on the 21 or 22 chromosome (it is not possible to differentiate between the two). When an extra chromosome is present, a large number of

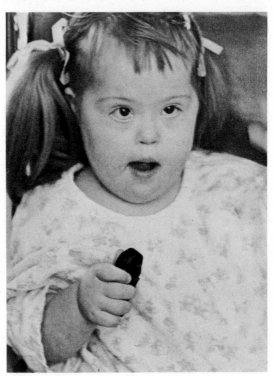

Figure 31-10. Mongolism may be a fact of life for this child, but of equal importance is the love and acceptance she receives.

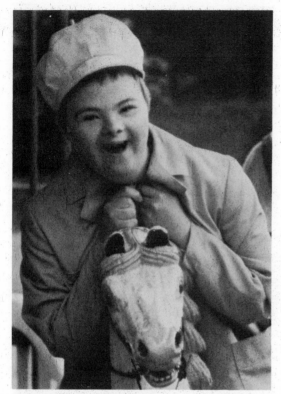

Figure 31-11. The typical facies of Down's syndrome is easily distinguished. (Courtesy of WHO; photo by E. Madelmann.)

genes are present in threes instead of the normal, balanced pairs. The additional genes may be entirely unrelated in their action; thus the individual may show many seemingly unrelated effects.

Trisomy 21 with 47 chromosomes is the most common form of Down's syndrome. This form appears most frequently in infants born to older women.

Translocation of chromosome 21. In this form the total number of chromosomes is a normal 46, but a portion of another chromosome has been interchanged with chromosome 21. These children are usually born to young mothers. There is some indication that this type may be inherited.

Mosaicism, a rare type, shows a mixture of two types of cells in the body, some with 46 and others with 47 chromosomes.

Other Trisomy Anomalies

Trisomy 18 (E Syndrome). This is less common than trisomy 21, but more severe.

Most affected infants die by the age of 6 months. These children have low-set abnormal ears, overlapping fingers, congenital heart defects, mental retardation, and other abnormalities.

Trisomy 13—15 (D Syndrome). This has many characteristics similar to trisomy 18. Fig. 31-13 shows such an infant.

Abnormalities of the sex chromosomes do appear, but are not necessarily associated with mental retardation. Some of these sex chromosomal anomalies are discussed in other chapters.

Sporadic Cretinism

Cretinism (hypothyroidism) is associated with either a congenital absence of a thyroid gland or with the inability of the infant's thyroid gland to secrete the thyroid hormone. This disorder rarely appears in more than one member of the family. Little is known as yet concerning the cause of this disorder. The condition appears sporadically in the United States, but is endemic in certain goitrous regions of other countries.

The infant appears normal at birth, clinical signs and symptoms not being fully developed before 3 to 6 months. The symptoms are very similar to those of Down's syndrome and may cause some confusion. However, Down's syndrome is nearly always recognizable at birth. There are other dissimilarities: the eyes are not slanted but appear puffy. The voice is hoarse; the skin is dry; there is slow bone development. Two common features of cretinism are obstinate constipation and umbilical hernia. Radioactive iodine given by mouth fails to reach a normal concentration in the thyroid gland, and examination of the blood shows a low level of protein-bound iodine (PBI).

Prognosis. Without treatment those cretins who live become mentally deficient dwarfs. Treatment consists of the administration of desiccated thyroid tablets orally. This must be continued throughout the individual's lifetime, with adjustments made in the dosage as needed. Sodium L-thyroxine given orally is also effective. If treatment is begun as early as possible and in adequate dosage, physical growth will proceed normally, and mental development should be relatively normal.

Phenylketonuria

Phenylketonuria is a recessive hereditary defect of metabolism that if untreated causes severe mental retardation in most but not all affected children. It is an uncommon trait appearing in about one out of 10,000 births. In this condition, there is a lack of the enzyme that normally changes the essential amino acid, phenylalanine, into tyrosine.

As soon as the newborn baby with this defect begins to take milk, either breast or cow's milk, he begins to absorb phenylalanine in the normal manner. However, because of his inability to metabolize this amino acid, phenylalanine builds up in his blood serum to as much as 20 times the normal level. This takes place at such a rapid pace that increased levels of phenylalanine appear in the blood after a day or two of ingestion of milk. Phenylpyruvic acid appears in the urine of affected babies somewhere between the second and sixth week of life.

The majority of the children with this condition develop severe and progressive mental deficiency, apparently because of the high serum phenylalanine level. The infant appears normal at birth but commences to show signs of mental arrest within a few weeks. It is therefore imperative that these infants be discovered as early in life as possible and placed immediately on a low phenylalanine formula.

Diagnostic Tests

Blood Test. A blood test devised in recent years gives good results as early as the third or fourth day after birth but is of no value until the infant has received dietary protein, which is present in his milk feedings. This screening procedure, called the Guthrie inhibition assay test, utilizes blood from a simple heel prick. It is standard procedure in most newborn nurseries, being performed just before the infant is discharged. A positive Guthrie test should always be

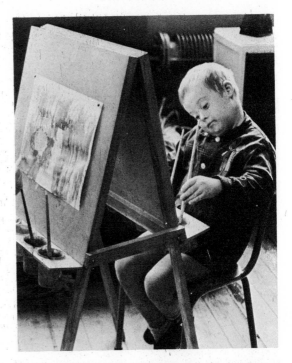

Figure 31-12. The child with Down's syndrome may express himself best in painting. (Courtesy of WHO; photo by D. Henrioud.)

followed by a blood test for tyrosine level. As many babies go home from the newborn nursery before they have ingested much milk, a urine test done a few weeks later is a good precaution.

Urine Tests. Phenylpyruvic acid appears in the urine in this condition after the first or second week of life. The presence of this acid can be detected by a simple urine test. A few drops of 10% ferric chloride when placed on a wet diaper causes a blue-green spot to appear immediately if phenylpyruvic acid is present. Variations of this test include the following.

Test tube test. Two or three drops of 10% ferric chloride added to about 5 cc. of urine turns the urine blue-green.

Phenistix test. A paper strip (Phenistix) that has been impregnated with ferric salt is dipped in urine or pressed against a wet diaper. The color reaction of the Phenistix is the same as that for the ferric chloride test.

For any of these tests, the blue-green color starts to fade quickly, sometimes within 30 seconds. Color reactions from other

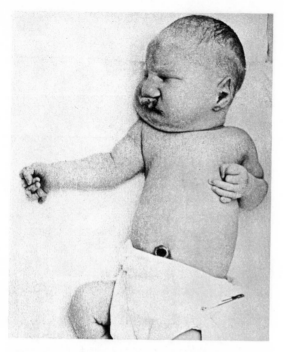

Figure 31-13. Autosomal trisomy is one type of chromosomal error not associated with mongolism.

An infant with trisomy 13–15 has multiple anomalies. Characteristics include cleft lip, extra digits arising next to the fifth finger, cerebral and cardiac defects, and other anomalies.

chemicals giving a false-positive reaction are usually longer lasting.

Filter paper test. A strip of ordinary white filter paper may be placed in the infant's diaper or dipped in urine. When dried, it is sent to a testing laboratory. This is more useful for home testing, for filter paper urine gives results for several days following use.

One disadvantage of relying upon the urine test is that most newborn infants have left the hospital before the test can be useful. In statewide programs, envelopes containing filter paper and directions are given to mothers leaving the hospital or mailed to mothers whose babies were delivered at home. Unfortunately, the busy mother may forget or fail to sense the importance of the testing, and damage occurs before the condition is diagnosed.

Manifestations of the condition are neurological. Many of these children develop

aggressive and disagreeable traits. Convulsions may occur and eczema is common. There is a characteristic musty smell to the urine.

Treatment is dietary. A formula low in phenylalanine should be started as soon as the condition is detected.* Best results are obtained if the special formula is started before 3 weeks of age. A low phenylalanine diet is a very restricted one. Foods to be omitted are breads, meat, fish, dairy products, nuts and legumes. The diet should be carefully supervised by a nutritionist.

Much confusion exists concerning the efficacy of the continued low phenylalanine diet. Most children who have had such diets since before 3 weeks of age develop intellectually on a par with their siblings. However, as controlled studies using untreated affected children of like age are not done, it cannot be proven that these observed treated children would not have developed as well without treatment.

In one study† lasting over several years, only those children who had been diagnosed and placed on the dietary regime before 3 weeks of age developed IQ's comparable to their siblings. Children who had been late treated or untreated had a lower mean IQ than their siblings. Some late treated made gains in intelligence, but the overall conclusions were that a low phenylalanine diet initiated after 8 months of age does not usually result in normal intelligence. It can be safely assumed that normal intelligence is rare in phenylketonuria. Infants of phenylketonuric mothers may show a high level of phenylalanine at birth and should be carefully watched.

Galactosemia

Galactosemia is a recessive hereditary metabolic disorder in which the enzyme necessary for converting galactose into glucose is missing. The infants generally

---

*Lofenlac is a low-phenylalanine formula produced by Mead Johnson.
†Kang, Ellen Song, *et al.*: Results of treatment and termination of the diet in phenylketonuria (PKU). *Pediatrics, 46:*881, 1970.

appear normal at birth, but experience difficulties after the ingestion of milk—whether breast milk, cow's or goat's milk—because one of the component monosaccharides of milk lactose is galactose.

Early feeding difficulties, with vomiting and diarrhea severe enough to produce dehydration and weight loss, and jaundice, are primary manifestations. Unless milk is withheld early, other difficulties include cataracts, liver and spleen damage, and mental retardation, with a high mortality rate early in life.

The earliest diagnostic finding is the presence of galactose in the urine, but if vomiting or refusal to eat have been present, the test may be negative. Galactose tolerance tests have been used, but may present definite hazards to the infant. Recently, a blood test using the Guthrie inhibition assay method, has proved a reliable diagnostic test. It can be performed in conjunction with a test for phenylketonuria.

Treatment consists of omitting galactose from the diet, which, in the young infant, means a substitution for milk. Nutramigen and soybean preparations such as ProSobee or Mulsoy, are satisfactory substitutes.

BIBLIOGRAPHY

America's Children and Youth in Institutions 1950-1960-1964. Washington, D. C., U. S. Government Printing Office, 1965.

Bensberg, Gerald J., ed.: Teaching the mentally retarded. Atlanta, Southern Regional Education Board, 1965.

Carlson, Bernice Wells, and Ginglend, David R.: Play Activities for the Retarded Child. New York, Abdingdon, 1961.

Dittman, Laura: The mentally retarded child at home. Washington, D. C., U. S. Government' Printing Office, 1961.

Dunn, L.C.: Old and New in Genetics. National Foundation—March of Dimes Reprint Series, 1964.

French, Edward L., and Scott, J. Clifford: How You Can Help Your Retarded Child. Philadelphia, Lippincott, 1967.

Heber, R. L.: Modifications on the manual of terminology and classification in mental retardation. American Journal of Mental Deficiency, *65:*499, 1961.

Hello World. (pamphlet) President's Committee on Mental Retardation, Washington, D. C., U. S. Government Printing Office, 1968.

Hymans, Jacqueline C., and Shearin, Dorothy B.: Partial deletion of short arms of chromosome. American Journal of Diseases of Children. *109:*85, 1965.

Jacob, Stanley, and Francone, Clarice: Structure and Function in Man. ed. 2. Philadelphia, W. B. Saunders, 1970.

Kang, Ellen Song: Results of treatment and termination of the diet in phenylketonuria (PKU). Pediatrics, *46:*881, 1970.

Kugel, Robert B.: Combating retardation in infants with Down's syndrome. Children, *17:*188, 1970.

Leland, Henry: Relationship between "intelligence" and mental retardation. American Journal of Mental Deficiency, *73:*533, 1969.

Phillips, Irving, ed.: Prevention and Treatment of Mental Retardation. New York, Basic Books, 1966.

Redding, Audrey, and Hirschhorn, Kurt: Guide to human chromosome defects. Birth Defects Original Article Series, The National Foundation—March of Dimes, *4:*1, 1968.

Shreiber, Mary, and Feeley, Mary: Siblings of the retarded. A guided group experience. Children, *12:*221, 1965.

Sutton, H. Eldon: An Introduction to Human Genetics. New York, Holt, 1965.

Thompson, James S., and Thompson, Margaret W.: Genetics in Medicine. Philadelphia, W. B. Saunders, 1966.

Man Into Superman: The promise and peril of the New Genetics. Time Magazine, p. 33, April 19, 1971.

Care of the Burned Child   *32*

Among the many accidents that occur in the lives of children, burns are the most frequent and frightening, exceeding even accidental poisonings in mortality rates. One tragic factor in this situation is that nearly all childhood burns are preventable, a fact which causes considerable guilt feelings on the part of the parents and the child. Failure to explain dangers to the child, carelessness on the part of an adult, the child's disobedience, all enter into the picture.

COMMON CAUSES OF BURNS

Scalds from Hot Liquids

This is a frequent type of burn in small children. Contributing factors may be:

1. A dangling cord from an electric percolator. The toddler pulls the cord to find out what is on the other end.

2. Pans of hot liquid on the stove. Handles are made for the purpose of pulling, or so the toddler reasons.

3. Cups of hot tea or coffee, and bowls of soup; all can cause painful burns if spilled on a child. An infant pulling on a tablecloth, or a toddler reaching for the teacup handle, may pull the hot liquid down over himself.

4. Small children left alone in bathtubs have frequently turned on the hot water tap, or older children have done it for them. Dangerous and fatal burns have occurred in this manner. It is never safe to leave a small child alone to play in the tub.

Burns from Fire or Heat

This type of burn is next in frequency. The contributing factors are:

1. Matches, which have an irresistible attraction for many children. Usually the child has been warned against playing with matches, so he will seek a place where he will not be detected—as a small closet or other place away from his mother.

2. Children's clothing. Many of the materials used in making children's clothing are highly inflammable and thus easily set afire. The child in panic runs for help, fanning the blaze.

3. Burning buildings. This is not a common cause of childhood burns. Small children, however, left alone in a home are helpless if a fire breaks out, whether the cause was a child's mischief, an adult's carelessness, or some unforeseeable event.

Electrical Burns

Although not common in children, nurses do see infants or toddlers with severe facial or mouth burns requiring extensive plastic surgery, from biting on electric cords—unfortunately without first removing the plug from the socket.

PREVENTION OF BURNS

Regret and self-blame are almost always present for the parents of a burned child. If the mother had not gone to answer the phone or the doorbell while the toddler played in the tub, if she had been careful to turn the pot handles in *always*; this would not have happened. The mother thinks she should have remembered how irresistible matches are to children, and should have tried harder to teach the dangers of playing with fire.

As nurses, our primary task is to teach preventive practices, as well as to set proper examples ourselves. Generally, however, the first time a nurse in the hospital hears about a burned child is when she is asked to prepare a room for his reception as a patient.

The nurse caring for a burned child must be prepared to put into use some of the most specialized and precise nursing skills. In order to do this, she needs, first, an understanding of the principles of physiological action involved; second, understanding of complications to be watched for; third, and most important of all, principles of management and nursing care concerning the burned child.

TYPES OF BURNS

Burns are divided into types according to the depth of tissue involvement; whether superficial, partial thickness, or total thickness.

Superficial or first degree burns. The epidermis is injured, but there is no destruction of tissue or of nerve endings. Thus there is erythema, edema and pain, but prompt regeneration.

Partial thickness or second degree burns. The epidermis and underlying dermis are both injured and devitalized, or destroyed. There is generally blistering, with an escape of body plasma, but regeneration of the skin occurs from the remaining viable epithelial cells in the dermis.

Total thickness or third degree burns. Epidermis, dermis, and nerve endings are all destroyed. Pain is minimal, and there is no longer any barrier to infection, or any remaining viable epithelial cells.

Fourth degree burns. Some authorities list as fourth degree burns any burns with destruction of deeper elements than skin or subcutaneous tissue; that is, nerves, blood vessels, muscle, or bone.

FIRST AID TREATMENT FOR BURNS

Ice cold water or ice packs are excellent emergency treatments for burns. The immediate application of ice compresses or ice water to burn areas appears to inhibit capillary permeability and thus suppress edema, blister formation and tissue destruction.* Present recommendation calls for application of cold to the burn area for at least 30 minutes, or until the pain subsides. Immersion of a burned extremity in cold water alleviates pain and may prevent further thermal injury.

Superficial burns can usually be treated on an outpatient basis, as they heal readily unless infected. The area should be cleaned, an anesthetic ointment applied and covered with a sterile bandage or dressing. An analgesic may be needed to relieve pain.

Treatment for Partial- and Full-Thickness Burns

It is not always possible to distinguish between partial- and full-thickness burns. In the presence of infection a partial-thickness burn may be converted into full thickness; also, with extensive burns, there is often a greater amount of full-thickness burn than had been estimated.

Total-thickness burns require the attention, skill and conscientious care of a team of specialists. Children with mixed second- and third degree burns, or with third degree burns involving 15% or more of body surface, require hospitalization.

PHYSIOLOGICAL MANIFESTATIONS AND TREATMENT IN SEVERE BURNS

First Phase—48 to 72 Hours

Hypovolemic shock is the major manifestation in the first phase of massive burns. As extracellular fluid pours into the burned area, it collects in enormous quantities, depleting the body. Edema becomes noticeable, and symptoms of severe shock appear. Intense pain is seldom a major factor.

The physician's primary concern is to replace body fluids that have been lost or immobilized at the burn areas. Because there is a distinct relationship between the extent

*Kravitz, Harvey: First-aid therapy for burns— cool it! *Clinical Pediatrics,* 9:695, 1970.

TABLE FOR ESTIMATING PROPORTIONS OF BODY SURFACE*

Age	Head (%)	Trunk (%)	Upper Extremities (%)	Lower Extremities (%)	Total % of Body Surface
Birth	19	34	19	28	100
1 year	17	34	19	30	100
5 years	13	34	19	34	100
10 years	11	34	19	36	100
15 years	9	34	19	38	100
Adult	7	34	19	40	100

*Lund, C. C., and Browder, N. C.: The estimation of area in burns. Surg. Gynec. and Obstet., *79:*352, 1944.

of the surface area burned and the amount of fluid lost, the physician needs to estimate the percent of the skin area affected. The "rule of nines," which affords a rough guide, estimates body surface area in approximate areas of nine. For a small child, whose head surface area is larger, and whose leg surface area is smaller than that of the adult, modifications are made. The table gives an idea as to how percentages of burned areas are calculated.

Intravenous fluids for the maintenance and the replacement of lost body fluids are estimated for the first 24 hours, with one-half of this calculated requirement to be given during the first 8 hours. The patient's needs may change rapidly, however, necessitating a change in the rate of flow, the amount, or the type of fluid. The physician must check frequently and carefully the urinary output, the vital signs, and the general appearance of the patient. Frequent hematocrit and hemoglobin readings indicate needs for blood transfusion or plasma.

Adequacy of the patient's airway must be assessed in terms of a possible need for a tracheostomy, and an aseptic environment must be rigidly maintained.

Nursing Care

Burn units have been organized in hospitals in several areas of the country. Also, Shriner's Hospitals for Burned Children are functioning in several localities, providing total care for burned children. The burn units are usually self-contained, with treatment and operating areas, hydrotherapy units and patient care areas. Personnel wear gowns, caps and masks. If visitors are admitted to the unit, they also must scrub, gown and mask.

In hospitals where there is no specific burn unit, a private room with a door that can be closed should be set up as a burn unit. "Reverse isolation" exercising the strictest aseptic technique must be observed.

Supplies to be Stocked for a Burn Unit

1. Sterilized sheets, towels, nurse's and doctor's gowns. "Burn packs" are usually available from central supply.
2. Sterile gloves. Sterile disposable gloves are useful, because many are going to be used.
3. Face masks and caps for personnel. Some hospitals include special shoe coverings.*

Clean Equipment to be Kept in the Room

1. Clinical thermometer, container, antiseptic solution.
2. Blood pressure cuff and stethoscope.
3. Intravenous pole.
4. Wall container of hexachlorophene soap for nurses' and doctors' scrub, orangewood sticks, and paper towels in rack.

*Hospital techniques and equipment for aseptic care vary, but the principles of asepsis remain the same.

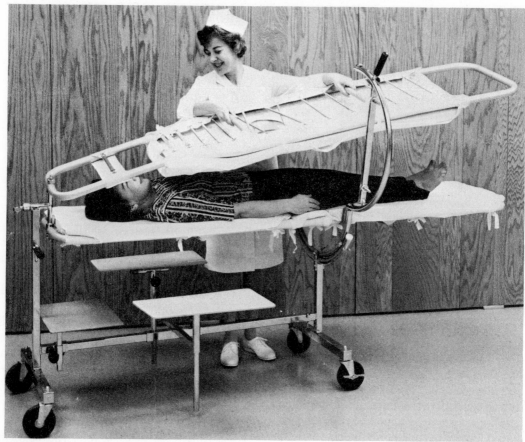

Figure 32-1.   A Stryker frame may be used with the burned patient to facilitate rotating him from front to back. (Courtesy of the Stryker Corporation)

5. Laundry bag or hamper, paper bag in wastebasket.
6. An antiseptic solution for damp dusting of furniture, and rags for dusting.
7. Routine equipment, such as a wash basin.
8. A large cradle to be covered with sterile sheets and placed over the child's body, keeping the covers away from his damaged skin.
9. A Stryker frame, or Circl-OElectric bed to facilitate rotating the patient from front to back.

Procedure Trays Ready for Immediate Use

1. Cut-down tray with intravenous fluids.
2. Blood plasma readily available.
3. Catheterization tray with a Foley catheter. For a child of six, size 8-10 Foley. Sterile water, a syringe and a needle for filling a Foley bag.

4. Emergency tracheotomy tray on a stand-by basis. Pediatric tracheotomy tube, the size according to age.
5. Nasogastric suction machine, clean and in working order. Nasal suction catheters, size 14-16 French.
6. Source of oxygen, pediatric-size face mask for emergency use.

Immediate nursing care is demanding, with many things to be done at once, a fact which makes it important that, if possible, more than one nurse be available. The nurse in a sterile gown, a mask and a cap, can help to place the patient on the sterile sheet spread over the bed, and can adjust the cradle over his body.

The room temperature should be kept around 80°F, because evaporation of water through the denuded areas, and even

FLUID BALANCE CHECK SHEET

Sol. #1	Gtt./ Min.	cc./ hour	time started	time finished	flow checked
250 cc. D/5/W (or ordered solution)					
500,000 units aqueous penicillin	12	48	9:00 AM		30 Min.

		INTAKE			OUTPUT		
Time Checked	Gtt./Min.	cc. in Bottle	cc. Given	Urine cc.	Emesis	Checked by	
9:00 AM	12	250	0			S N	
9:30	12	226	24			S N	
10:00	12	202	48	20		S N	
10:30	12	178	72				
11:00	12	154	96	25			
11:30	12	130	120				
12:00	12	106	144	25			

through the leathery burn eschar, proceeds rapidly, with a consequent thermal evaporative loss.

First, in order of importance, is the assistance in starting intravenous fluids, and assisting in performing the cut-down procedure. Temporary fluid, such as 5 percent dextrose in water may be started until the child's needs have been calculated, then the ordered intravenous fluid must be prepared and hung. Aqueous penicillin or other antibiotic may be ordered for addition to the intravenous fluid.

Strict monitoring of all intake and output is essential, including the amount of fluid the child has received at any given time, the rate of flow, the time the present bottle was started and when it is due to be finished, and the contents of the present bottle. The bottle itself must be clearly labeled, with an indication of any additions to the original contents, such as antibiotics.

The physican carefully estimates the amount and kind of intravenous fluid necessary, relying on the nurse to keep an accurate record. A flow sheet, kept at the bedside, may be some variation of the above example.

Urinary Output

After assisting with the insertion of a Foley catheter, the nurse should connect the catheter to a sterile drainage tubing and allow drainage into a sterile, closed, calibrated container. Urinary drainage is recorded every hour, and specific gravity recorded. After the first hour, volume of urine should be relatively constant. Any change in volume or specific gravity should be reported.

MINIMUM URINARY OUTPUT (NORMAL)

Age	24 hr. intake	Excretion/hr.
0-12 months	200-500 cc.	8-20 cc.
1-12 years	500-800 cc.	20-33 cc.

Vital signs should be checked and recorded at frequent intervals, ranging from every 15 minutes to every half to full hour, as the circumstances demand. Observation should include:

1. Patency of the airway. Check for difficult breathing, stridor, and sternal retractions.
2. Pulse rate, rhythm, and character. State whether it is rapid, weak, or irregular.
3. Body temperature, to be taken rectally if possible.
4. Blood pressure.
5. Restlessness, anxiety, excessive thirst, or presence of pain.

Oral Fluids and Medications

Oral fluids should either be omitted or kept to a minimum for the first day or two. Acute gastric dilatation is a common complication of burns, and can become a serious problem. The child's thirst, which is usually severe, should be somewhat relieved by the intravenous fluids, and sips of water may be allowed. The child needs considerable emotional support, however, to help him through this stage.

Antibiotics, if used, will probably be added to the intravenous fluids. Tetanus antitoxin or toxoid should be ordered according to the state of the child's previous immunization. If his inoculations are up to date, a booster dose of tetanus toxoid is all that will be required.

Emotional Support for the Child and His Parents

Immediately following such a traumatic accident, the child undoubtedly will be in a state of physical and emotional shock, to the extent that he is not acutely aware of what is happening around him. As his doctors and his nurses are going to be extremely busy giving him vital physical care, they may find it easy to forget the frightened child's emotional needs. A few minutes explanation of what is going to happen now, a kind and supportive attitude toward the child, is of great importance to him, even though he himself makes little response.

The parents probably need greater support than their child during the first hours, but they may get very little. No one has much time for them; they must stay out of the way. In fact, they will be quite willing to stay out of the way of such mysterious and frightening procedures.

Thoughtful concern for their comfort can be given by nurses not directly involved in the burned child's treatment, until the doctors can be free to explain and to counsel. A few friendly words from time to time, a smile in passing, an invitation to accompany some of the nurses on their coffee break, or just a willingness to listen—all this is welcomed by the parents, themselves in a state of emotional shock.

Continuing Care

After the initial fluid therapy has brought the burn shock under control, and after the extracellular fluid deficit has been made up, the patient faces another hazard with the onset of the diuretic phase. This occurs somewhere within the period of 24 to 96 hours after the accident. The plasma-like fluid is picked up and reabsorbed from the "third space" in the burn areas, and the patient may rapidly become hypervolemic, even to the point of pulmonary edema. This is the principle reason for the extremely close check on all vital signs, and for the close monitoring of intravenous fluids, which must now be slowed or stopped entirely.

The nurse needs to be alert for any signs of the onset of this phase, in order to notify the physicians at once. Clues to the onset of the diuretic phase include:

1. Rapid rise in urinary output. May go up to 250 cc. per hour, or higher.
2. Tachypnea, followed by dyspnea.
3. Increase in pulse pressure; mean blood pressure may also rise. Central venous pressure, if measured, will be found to be elevated.

If pulmonary edema becomes evident, vigorous action may be necessary, such as the use of rotating tourniquets, positive pressure respiration, and venesection. Morphine may be ordered.

Daily patient care through the first phases requires attention to positioning in order to help prevent contractures. This includes proper body alignment, the use of a footboard, keeping the head, the arms, and the legs in good position, as much as possible.

Frequent turning to prevent lung congestion and skin breakdown is extremely important, and extremely difficult. A Stryker frame, or a Circl-OElectric bed on which a child may be turned quickly and painlessly, may be used. Children are, however, apt to become very frightened when being turned on the Stryker frame, requiring much reassurance and support.

Emotional Support for the Attending Staff

Constant nursing of a burned child is an exceedingly traumatic emotional experience, as well as a most exhausting physical one. The child needs to have one individual to give him the support so important to his welfare, and the explanation and demonstration of complicated procedures takes a disproportionate amount of time if these must be repeated to constantly changing nurses. The nurse on each shift who has the care of the burned child needs a great deal of support from the personnel on the department.

Frequent checking to determine her needs, whether it is some article from outside the room, help with a procedure, or a few minutes relief, is most welcome. She needs prompt relief for meals, and coffee breaks are of great importance in order to get her away from the situation for a short time.

Second Phase (48 Hours to Two or More Weeks)

Many surgeons prefer to treat burns by the open, or exposure, method. The tough outer covering that forms over the burned area—called eschar—makes a satisfactory initial covering. When the burned crusts commence to separate from the underlying tissue, wet dressings and soaks will help loosen the eschar in preparation for skin grafts.

Infection is rarely a problem during the first 48 hours, if the proper aseptic en-

vironment is maintained. Normal skin bacteria invade the broken skin under the most careful management, however, so that every burn is potentially infected. Frequent incidence of *Staphylococcus aureus* and *Pseudomonas aeruginosa* infection are observed during the second phase in spite of stringent attempts at prevention of cross-contamination.

Topical applications of silver nitrate, 0.5%, to second and third degree burns reduce the severity of secondary infections. Thick gauze pads saturated with 0.5% silver nitrate are applied to the burn areas, and held in place if necessary with bandage. Catheters incorporated in the dressings facilitate moistening, which should be done at 2- to 4- hour intervals. Dressings are changed 2 or 3 times daily as ordered. Electrolyte imbalance may result due to silver nitrate therapy, therefore careful monitoring and electrolyte replacement are necessary. Silver nitrate stains the linens and equipment, as well as nurse's gowns.

Another method for treating burns is the use of Sulfamylon* ointment. Using a sterile glove, the nurse applies Sulfamylon cream to the burn area, much as one would spread butter. In fact, the process is called buttering the burned areas. The cream is washed off in the daily bath, and the burned areas rebuttered with Sulfamylon. Sulfamylon suppresses bacterial growth and allows viable areas of skin to regenerate and fill in.

Occlusive dressings are not used as frequently as in the past, but they are occasionally necessary. Sulfamylon treatment delays eschar separation, so that the application is sometimes stopped for a few days while wet saline packs or occlusive dressings are applied.

Early debridement of the eschar to allow early skin grafting is considered important in the control of infection. After the initial shock phase, daily tub baths help remove the eschar. Gentle washing with a sterile washcloth or gauze during the bath hastens the

---

*Trademark, Winthrop

process of debridement. Use of a whirlpool is also helpful.

Nutritional Needs

The child who has received extensive deep burns must receive special attention regarding his nutritional needs. The nutritional problem is much more complex than simply getting a seriously ill child to eat. He is in negative nitrogen and caloric balance from a number of causes, including the following:

1. Poor intake, from anorexia, ileus, Curling's ulcer, or diarrhea.
2. External loss, due to exudative losses of protein through the burn wound.
3. Thermal losses from the burn itself; heat loss from the radiation of heat and from water loss, responsible for large caloric losses.
4. Hypermetabolism, from fever, infection, and from the state of "toxicity."

A diet high in protein, for healing and for replacement, high in calories, and essentially bland in character, is an essential component of therapy. Great efforts must be made to interest the child in foods essential for tissue building and repair. Large servings are not acceptable because of anorexia as well as the physical condition of the child. This is one time when all the imagination and the ingenuity of the nurse and the dietitian are needed to the utmost degree. Foods rich in protein, high in caloric value, and easily digested are needed, but are going to be of no value if the child refuses to eat them. Colorful trays, foods with eye appeal, and any special touches to spur a child's appetite, should all be tried. A number of hints are suggested in the section The Care of the Chronically Ill Child.

Some kinds of useful food are:

Flavored milk shakes, ice cream shakes.
High protein drinks containing eggs and extra dried protein milk.
Hard candies, ice cream, milk and egg desserts.
Pureed meats, and vegetables.

With the best efforts of nurses, dietitians, and of the child himself, the burn patient can seldom eat an amount of food sufficient to meet his increased needs. Tube feedings are frequently necessary as supplements to the daily intake. The dietary department can make up a supplementary formula that will meet the child's needs.

Great care must be used to avoid making tube feedings a threat—"Unless you eat, you will have to have a tube"—or a punishment—"You didn't eat all your food today." The child must understand what is to be done and why. For instance, "Johnny, you need extra food, more than you can eat by yourself, to help your skin heal and to help make you strong again. Let's put this tube into the doll's mouth (or nose) and watch. It goes right down into her stomach. See? Now, I'll pour some of this drink into the tube— down it goes! Do you want to try doing it? Now you know just what happens when you swallow the tube. It will make you gag a little bit, but it won't hurt."

Foods are "blenderized" into a liquid state for tube feedings.

Complications

Curling's ulcer. Curling's ulcer is a gastric or duodenal ulcer that frequently occurs following serious skin burns. It can easily be overlooked when the attention of nurses and doctors is directed toward the treatment of the burn area and prevention of infection.

Symptoms are those of any gastric ulcer, but usually are rather vague, concerned with abdominal discomfort, with or without localization, or with relation to eating. Appearance of an ulcer, if it occurs, is during the first six weeks.

Blood may be present in the stools, an occurrence which, combined with abdominal discomfort, may be the basis for a diagnosis. If desired, roentgenograms can confirm the diagnosis.

Treatment consists of a bland diet, the use of antacids such as Maalox or Amphogel, and antispasmodics. Extensive hemorrhages are rare if the condition is recognized and treated.

Rehabilitation Phase

Occupational and physical therapy are frequently combined for the child in order to help maintain his normal functions, as well as to provide near normal situations for the child's continued growth and development.

One child's burns involved his chest, his axilla and his upper arm. It became essential for him to use his right arm in a variety of ways to prevent both contractures and permanent deformities, but Donny saw little sense in causing himself so much discomfort. Little by little, he was encouraged to use his arm for pushing along a wheeled toy, for crayoning, for cutting pictures, and for similar activities. The real inspiration was the solitary fish in a small bowl. Bright yellow stones came in a bag for Donny to drop in, one by one, to provide a foundation, and every day he raised his arm to drop food into the bowl. Soon he became proud that he could feed his fish with his right hand, and willingly gave the fish loving care. (Fig. 32-2)

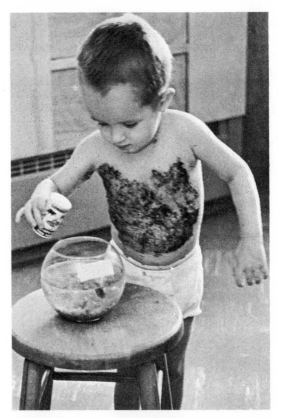

Figure 32-2. Feeding the fish is one way of motivating the child to move his right arm after chest and axillary burns.

Burn Bath (Tub Bath When Ordered)

Equipment

Isolation gown; mask and cap if used.
Two sterile sheets, plastic or Koroseal.
Two pairs of sterile gloves (if dressings are to be used).
Ordered solution for bath (pHisoHex, Ivory Snow, saline, etc.).
A bath thermometer.
A waxed paper bag (for soiled dressings).

Procedure

1. Clean the tub thoroughly with pHisoHex or with hexachlorophene soap.
2. Fill the tub with enough water to cover the burned area.
3. Check the temperature of water (105° to 110°).
4. Add the desired solution or Ivory Snow (about 1-1/2 oz.).
5. Put on a gown, a mask, and a cap (if one is to be used).
6. Cover a stretcher with a sterile sheet, place the child on the sheet and wrap it lightly around him.
7. Move the child to the bathroom. If the child has dressings, put on gloves and remove the outer layers. Remove your gloves.
8. Put on clean gloves, and place the child in the tub, lowering him very slowly and carefully. The child may be very frightened, and may need much emotional support.
9. Support child as necessary while he is in the tub. Never leave a child alone.
10. Leave the child in the tub for the designated time. (Not longer than 15 to 20 minutes.) His dressings will soak off.
11. Place on sterile plastic, cover with sterile sheet on stretcher and lift the child onto the stretcher, wrapping the sheet around him.

12. Return him to his room, place him on a clean, sterile sheet on his bed.
13. Apply dressings (if any are to be used) using sterile technique.
14. Record the type of bath, the condition of the burned areas, and the child's response to the treatment.

Burn Soaks or Wet Packs

Equipment

A sterile basin.
Solution as ordered.
Sterile gloves (2 pairs if dressing is to be changed).
A sterile bulb syringe.
An isolation gown. A mask and a cap (if they are to be used).
Sterile dressings (if the dressing is to be changed).

Procedure

1. Wash hands, and assemble the equipment.
2. Put on a gown (and a cap and a mask).
3. Open a sterile basin, and add the solution.
4. Unwrap a sterile bulb syringe (if the dressing is to be moistened but not changed).
5. Put on gloves. If the dressing is to be changed—
   a. remove the outer layers, and place them in a waxed bag,
   b. change gloves,
   c. soak gauze in the solution, and cover with dry, sterile dressings.
6. If the dressings are to be moistened only—
   a. put on gloves, fill a syringe with solution and moisten the dressing. Sterile plastic or Koroseal may be laid under area.
7. Record the time, the child's response to his treatment, and the condition of the burned area if the dressings were changed.

Débridement and Grafting

Eschar requires approximately 7 days to two weeks to slough off spontaneously, so débridement is frequently done mechanically in surgery under light anesthesia. If the area is clear of infection, grafts may be applied at the same time. Blood for transfusion should be ready because there may be considerable bleeding, especially if large areas are debrided.

Skin grafts. Grafts may be either homografts or autografts. A *homograft* consists of skin taken from another person, and is eventually rejected by the recipient tissue, sloughing off after a period of three to six weeks. It provides a temporary dressing after debridement, and has proved a life-saving measure for children with extensive burns. Skin from cadavers is often used; it can be stored and used up to a period of several weeks, and permission for this use is seldom refused.

An *autograft,* consisting of skin taken from the child's own body, is the only kind of skin accepted permanently by recipient tissues, except for the skin from an identical twin. It is usually impossible to obtain enough healthy skin to cover a large area; therefore, homografts are of great value for immediate covering. If the donor site is kept free from infection, and grafts of sufficient thinness are taken, the site should be ready for use again in 10 to 12 days.

After grafting, donor as well as graft sites are kept covered with sterile dressings.

Billy's Story

The story of Billy, who spent nearly a year in the hospital with 60% burns, gives a vivid picture of what such a disaster can mean to a small child.

Six-year-old Billy's behavior in the hospital was quite characteristic of the behavior one may expect to find in a severely burned child of this age group. For many weeks, he was in a private room with constant attendance while it seemed that painful or unpleasant procedures were almost constantly being performed. He fought back with all of his ability. He screamed and raged at everything done in his room, and at everyone doing it. He was terribly afraid of being turned on the Stryker frame, turning pale and trembling whenever this was done. If the attendant was not accustomed to his care, he would assure her that the security straps were not to be used, or that he was not to be turned any more, and became enraged when he could not control his environment.

His voice, when he was not shouting with rage, became a whine almost impossible to understand, a circumstance that only made him more angry.

Long* remarks about the similar behavior found in many severely burned children. It makes nursing the child so difficult and so exhausting, both emotionally and physically, that the nurse assigned to his care needs a great deal of support. These children need the ministrations of some one person in order to build up confidence and security. It is considerably less traumatic to a child if the person entering the room in the morning is secure in her knowledge of the physical care needed, as well as in her knowledge of this particular child.

Billy's slow progress proceeded over a period of months, until the entire process became a way of life for him, although he never fully accepted it. His burned areas were temporarily covered with homografts, but there was extremely little skin to use for autografts, and much scar tissue and many adhesions with contractures resulted.

After many months, some of Billy's problems had been solved, but many others remained. One was of fluid intake. Imagination on the nurse's part helped. One day, Billy became so intrigued with being allowed to pour his own drinking water from a light pitcher into a one ounce medicine glass, and reading the amount on the calibrated side, that he spent an hour pouring and shouting, "Another 45 cc., now 30; here's 60 more. Did you write that all down?" His nurse spent many hours finding drinks that he would take, such as weak tea and carbonated drinks, and occasionally he would consent to drink some chocolate milk.

Billy was now in a four bed room, and here he had considerable difficulty adjusting. The necessity of almost constant attendance had made him extremely selfish. He could not share either his nurses, the television, or the playthings. He would ask other boys to show him their toys, and frequently refuse to return them if they took his fancy. Long, patient, loving discipline was necessary before this little boy could learn to live with the others. Sometimes his rage at life was turned against his roommates who could do so many things he could not, and he would destroy their possessions. Gradually, he learned. He still required many hours of daily care, with wet packs over certain areas, with elastic bandages to his legs, and special shoes whenever he was up, and he needed much help generally. The nurse still needed to check orders carefully because he would solemnly insist that certain procedures were no longer being done.

Physical and occupational therapists worked with Billy daily. In spite of his severe handicaps, he learned to do much. His arms were contracted in a fixed position, but his wrists were flexible, and he learned to feed himself with little difficulty. The therapists taught him the ability to raise himself from a lying position to a sitting one and to a standing one without the use of his arm muscles. He learned to put on his bathrobe by backing into it. These skills were not easy to acquire, and he never volunteered information concerning what he could do, while on the ward. His normal mischievousness began to assert itself, although it found little scope in his restricted surroundings. It seemed to his nurses that it consisted mainly in misleading them about his treatments and routines. If he became bored with physical therapy, he would solemnly assert that he was not to go today, and was believed. When the messenger came for him, he was not ready. The gleam in his eye when she came told of his satisfaction in having for once "fooled the nurses."

Billy started schoolwork with the teacher before his discharge, although his attention span was short, and he had difficulty disciplining himself to any serious work. He was an intelligent boy and could probably learn quickly once he had established the necessary habits. His greatest thrill in the hospital came when he was transferred from his Stryker frame to a regular hospital bed, "just like normal people use," he said.

Eventually, it was time for him to go home. His mother came to the hospital to learn how to care for him, and to take him home. He had been home for short periods of two or three days before, but this time it was for "keeps," until he needed surgery at a later date.

Billy faced tremendous problems at home. A normally active little boy, with lively brothers and sisters, he would find life far different from the home life that he remembered. The problems must have seemed tremendous to his parents too, but they were willing to try. The nurse in the community would have to give them much support and help. Billy still had a long road ahead.

---

*Long, R., and Cope, O.: Emotional problems of burned children. New Eng. J. Med., *264:*1121, 1961.

BIBLIOGRAPHY

Sister Mary Claudia: T.L.C. and sulfamylon for burned children. AJN, *69:*755, 1969.

Henley, Nellie L.: Sulfamylon for burns. AJN, *69:*2122, 1969.

Long, R. and Cope, O.: Emotional problems of burned children. New Eng. J. Med., *264:*1121, 1961.

Suggested Readings for Further Study

Minckley, Barbara B.: Expert nursing care for burned patients. AJN, *70:*1888, 1970.

Accidents and Accidental Poisoning *33*

ACCIDENTS

In the United States as well as in many other countries, accidents kill more children than any single illness. Throughout the entire world, deaths from childhood accidents appear third on the list of causes of child mortality. In the United States the most common cause of home accidents among children from the ages of one to five is accidental poisoning.

The nurse, as an educator and leader in public health practices, must be acutely aware of these facts. She must first examine her own conduct. What sort of example does she set in the home, in the hospital ward and in the community?

It is rather frightening to consider that whereas the death rate from disease among small children has been drastically reduced in recent years, the accidental death rate has not been. Motor vehicles appear first on the list as a cause of accidental death, and home accidents appear second. A short discussion of the various kinds of accidents that occur in the home and the hospital can help fix certain preventive measures in our minds. As has often been pointed out, the best treatment for accidents is prevention.

Incidence

The age group in which most accidents occur is that of the toddler and the preschooler. The toddler's urge to explore, coupled with his lack of experience, leads him into innumerable dangerous situations. Painful burns occur when he pulls the pan or the cup down to his level to discover the contents. That electric cord, dangling so invitingly, must have something at the other end; what can it be? Anyhow, electrical outlets are intriguing and meant to be poked (to the imaginative mind of an 18-month-old child).

A healthy toddler is constantly on the go during his waking hours. It is indeed difficult to keep up with him, or to foresee all possible dangerous situations. Warning a small child of potential danger is of little value, because his memory span is short, and he has had no background experience to reinforce the warning.

The public has become quite well aware of the dangers of suffocation when discarded refrigerators and plastic bags are within easy access of the curious child. There are many hazards outside the home also.

Swimming pools are very popular as well as enjoyable, and swimming is excellent exercise. The very young child has no fear of water unless he has had an unpleasant experience that has frightened him. A newborn baby makes instinctive swimming movements, as indeed he did swim effortlessly before birth. Of course, at that period he had no need to breathe.

Very young children can be taught to swim before they develop any fear of water. An infant can be taught to paddle himself to safety if he is pushed or falls into a body of water.

In her excellent book *Teaching an Infant to Swim*, Virginia Hunt Newman explains her

487

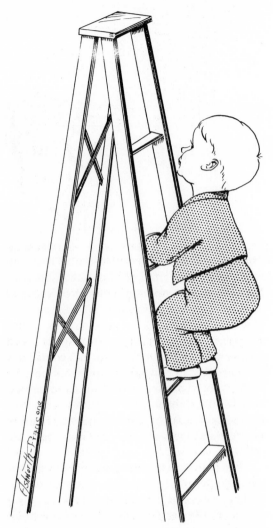

Figure 33-1.   The child's natural desire to climb and explore can lead to accidents.

method for teaching water safety to infants. She emphasizes over and over that one does *not* leave an infant or tot unwatched around a pool or at the beach, regardless of whether he has learned water safety. However, many tots do wander out of sight, and the occurrence of drownings among infants and young children is tragically high. According to the National Safety Council, the two-year-old child is the one at greatest risk from drowning among young children.

Covers for swimming pools, high fences and locked gates are all good preventive measures. But occasionally someone forgets to lock the gate, or the child climbs the fence. Certainly if the toddler knew how to handle himself in the water, this *could* prevent another drowning.

Automobile Safety

Children are injured in car accidents just as adults are. The adult is somewhat protected by a seat safety belt and safety features in the modern car.

Toddlers, however, need special appliances geared to their size. There are many toddler seats and safety belts on the market. The parent needs to check over these carefully for the one that appears to provide the best protection. The next step is to make sure the safety appliance is used properly.

Aspiration of Foreign Bodies

The severe consequences following aspiration of a foreign body are well known. Unfortunately, this still occurs among older infants and toddlers. Safety pins, thumb tacks, or any variety of small metallic objects have been aspirated. Often this is not known at the time, and the object may be lodged in the trachea or the larynx for a considerable length of time. One child was admitted to the hospital in acute respiratory distress with a probable diagnosis of laryngotracheobronchitis. The distress was so severe that an emergency tracheotomy was performed. The following day examination revealed a small open safety pin lodged in the larynx, which on extraction appeared to have been there for some time. The mother then recalled two episodes of choking and coughing within the past 2 weeks, with increasing hoarseness, but no one knew about the pin. Edema at the site had prevented visualization of the pin.

Any child being seen for respiratory symptoms of wheezing, hoarseness, or croupy cough, should be examined with the possibility of aspiration in mind, even though there is no history of foreign body aspiration.

If the object is lodged in the larynx, a severe degree of dyspnea may make a tracheotomy necessary before a laryngoscopic examination is done.

Vegetable matter, such as popcorn, peanuts, seeds or pieces of raw vegetable are easily aspirated by a toddler. These are extremely difficult to remove because they swell in the moist atmosphere of the respiratory system, and crumble into fragments when grasped with an instrument for removal.

Objects that become lodged in a bronchus may cause complete obstruction, with inflammatory swelling, atelectasis and emphysema.

Objects that are not removed from the air passages eventually cause death in a majority of cases. Particularly tragic are those instances when small children have fed particles to the tiny baby in the home, entirely unknown to the parents. One such young infant died, despite every possible treatment for an unidentified respiratory difficulty, which an autopsy proved caused by a particle of vegetable material in a bronchus. Such accidents are so totally unexpected that they may never be considered.

Peanuts and popcorn are not safe food for toddlers. Children are fond of finger foods, and raw carrots or other raw vegetables are colorful and of pleasing texture to a child of three or four. Toddlers cannot be trusted to chew them well enough, and even a three-year-old should not be allowed to run around while eating chewy foods.

If an object has been aspirated, treatment consists in removal by direct laryngoscopy or bronchoscopy. Secondary infection is treated by antibiotic medication as indicated. The most effective treatment, however, is prevention.

ACCIDENTAL POISONING

"This year an estimated 500,000 children will be victims of accidental poisoning. Ninety per cent of all cases reported involve children under five years of age." So reports

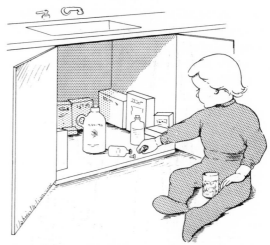

Figure 33-2. The toddler playing with cleaning agents stored within his reach is in danger of accidentally poisoning himself.

the National Planning Council for National Poison Prevention Week.*

When the nurse sees the child come into the hospital terribly frightened and frequently in pain because of someone's carelessness, she wonders how this can be allowed to happen. Yet doctors and nurses are far from blameless. Not only are they frequently careless themselves, but they are too often apt to forget their duty as teachers. Often it would take only a few words of caution to make parents more alert and thus avoid tragedy.

The commercial products of today bring an ever increasing supply of potential poisoners into the home. Mothers are accustomed to storing cleaners, polishes, deodorants and other housekeeping aids in cupboards, convenient for use. We are of course grateful for all of these materials that make the work at home easier, but we have not kept pace in our consideration of the dangers involved in their careless storage.

In the same manner, medications today have been of the greatest help to all of us; yet here again, we have not been alert to their potency in the hands of small children.

There is a strange phenomenon relating to medicines and small children. A person

*Flier "Locked up Poisons Prevent Tragedy." Distributed Spring, 1971.

can coax, or bribe or threaten a small child in a vain attempt to get him to swallow some tasteless or even flavorful medicine, and only a short time later, find the same child stuffing a handful of pills into his mouth.

This is exactly what did happen to one small girl. She had been placed on routine barbiturates for mild seizures, but her mother had great difficulty getting her to take the medication. One day, however, when her mother was away, she climbed to the medicine cabinet and swallowed about half of the contents of the bottle. This was not discovered until several hours later when the

baby sitter was unable to rouse her from an unduly long nap.

Many of these incidents do seem almost unavoidable, or at least so unlikely as to be totally unanticipated. In the light of the increasing complexity of materials in the home, and the known exploratory instincts of little children, one needs very nearly to anticipate the impossible.

Cardinal Safety Measures

There are a number of safety measures we all need to know and understand so thoroughly that they become part of our daily routine. Here are a few.

---

1. Use your prescription drugs only for the purpose for which they were ordered. This is difficult to do when you have paid a high price for the medicine. Perhaps his sister took this medicine last month for her cough, so let's give it to Johnny before we call the doctor. The prevailing practice in the United States of marking prescriptions by number only, and omitting the name of the drug from the label, increases the danger of giving the wrong medicine. Perhaps Johnny is allergic to the ingredients of this medicine, or possibly his cold is far different from his sister's. All too frequently drugs are removed from their original containers for one reason or another, even though correctly labeled—so it is possible that it is not even the medicine you gave his sister. It just is not safe. Keeping drugs in case they "come in handy" only adds to the store of potential poisons that children can get into.

2. Discard your unused drugs, but not in the garbage or rubbish. Many children, as well as pets, have been poisoned from eating pills or drinking liquids found in rubbish containers. Pills can be dissolved and flushed down the household drainage system, and liquids may be discarded in the same manner.

3. All medicines should be kept under lock and key. Even a locked cupboard may not always be safe from an active, exploring youngster, however. It is helpful if cabinets are high out of easy reach and locked, but a determined child can find a way. There are on the market cabinets that require considerable ingenuity to open. This is good, but another problem presents itself. If a medicine is being used routinely, it is quite a nuisance to unlock a cabinet for every administration, and, all too often, the medicine is left out in a convenient place while it is in use.

If grandmother comes to stay for the weekend, she might put her sleeping pills in the drawer by her bedside, just the way she does at home. Uncle John is a diabetic, so when he comes he puts his urine reagent tablets conveniently on the bathroom shelf. After all, who would want to swallow them? Johnny would.

Aunt Ruth comes to call and lets Susy play with her purse, completely forgetting the bottle of Dexedrine she carries with her, and so it goes. Here, even locking the medicine cabinet did not help.

4. Store all household chemicals such as cleansers, polishes, and insecticides, out of easy reach. Parents do not always realize that most cleaning agents (which are not meant for consumption) are potentially poisonous. They must sacrifice a measure of convenience for safety.

5. *Never* put any product not intended for eating or for drinking in a food or a beverage container. The temptation to do so is great, but the temptation to the toddler to eat or to drink from the bottle or the cup is greater. Always act as though anything in a food container carries a sign saying "eat me" or "drink me" to the young explorer in Wonderland. After all, he has just learned the purpose of eating utensils and how to use them.

6. Tell your children honestly that you are giving them medicine and not candy. Every year, children come into the hospital after having eaten flavored or candied medicine, because the adults in their lives have told them in the past that it was candy in an effort to get them to take the medication.

The new method of flavoring children's drugs has been a great boon to mothers. Sweetened fruit flavors often disguise the taste to the extent that medicine becomes quite acceptable. Unfortunately, a small child has no compunction about helping himself to more.

These are only a few of the modern hazards of which we must be aware.

Internal Manifestations of Poisons

There is no place that sharpens this awareness as well as a hospital in which one sees children who have swallowed every imaginable substance. Parents need to know that many of the cleaning substances and furniture polishes contain kerosene, which can cause a fatal pneumonia if swallowed. Ant buttons, rat killers and insecticides contain arsenic, strychnine or other chemicals that are just as lethal to the child as they are to the pest one is trying to eliminate.

Esophageal Burns. Many children come into the emergency ward after having swallowed corrosive acids or alkalies, either in commercial form or in solution. The preparations for cleaning toilet bowls or for opening drains are often kept on the floor or in a low cupboard for easy access when needed.

A child who has been burned by a corrosive substance presents a most tragic figure. Two children were admitted to the same hospital one summer, each having picked up a pop bottle on a hot day and having rapidly swallowed its contents. Each bottle contained a considerable amount of lye solution that someone had placed in it.

Although separate incidents, both children suffered severe esophageal burns with almost complete occlusion of the esophagus. Both required extensive surgery with months of hospitalization and considerable follow-up. This story can be repeated over many times in numbers of children's wards throughout the world.

Any children who get a corrosive substance as far as the mouth need to be examined for burns. Most children who swallow such substances have some burning and scarring of the esophagus. Many children of five or six are still entering the hospitals for repeated dilatations following lye ingestion during the second year. Fortunately, the discovery that the use of corticosteroids early after ingestion markedly reduces the amount of scarring has resulted in widespread use of these drugs with less serious after effects.

Pulmonary Irritation. All petroleum distillates are irritants, the principal manifestation being pulmonary irritation. The resulting pneumonitis appears to be the result of aspiration either during ingestion or during the vomiting that follows. Vomiting should never be induced, although it is seldom possible to prevent spontaneous vomiting. If much of the substance has been ingested, the physician may elect careful gastric lavage. Children are usually kept in the hospital for a period following kerosene ingestion because of the extreme likelihood of pneumonitis. In a majority of cases, the petroleum distillate that has been ingested is kerosene, although cases of gasoline ingestion have been reported.

Poisonous Medications—Aspirin

If one moves on to consider the poisonings by medications, aspirin is found to be the chief offender. Many parents do not seem to recognize this particular danger, and because a majority of households contain aspirin, or compound analgesic tablets containing aspirin, children have ready access to it. The orange-flavored children's aspirin tablets are very tasty. Drug companies are now making safety caps for bottles of children's aspirin, but no cap can be entirely childproof. The bottles are still poor playthings for children.

Safe Dosages. The readiness with which parents give aspirin to their children for any disorder contributes to the hazards. Although a majority of aspirin poisonings are of acute origin, some of them are the result of accumulated doses given by parents

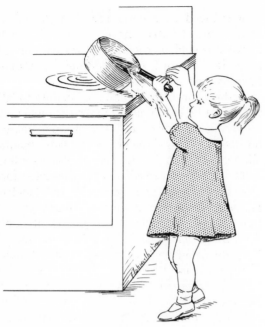

Figure 33-3. The handles of pans on the stove should always be turned away from the reach of the toddler.

who are ignorant of the safe dosage or of the cumulative effects. A safe dosage for the average child under the age of five is one grain of aspirin for each year of life, given not more often than every four hours. Thus a six-month-old child might receive one-half grain. Some children may be allergic to aspirin, however, and thus an average dose could

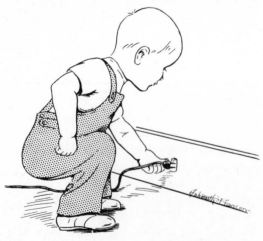

Figure 33-4. Electrical wall outlets should be covered with safety caps and electric cords should be kept out of reach of the toddler.

have an extremely dangerous effect. This does not mean that the physician may not prescribe larger doses than the average for specific conditions, but it should be given under his guidance. All of this seems to point up the dangers inherent in giving even aspirin without a physician's order.

Some drug companies are now using child-resistant safety caps on bottles of adult medicines. This is excellent practice. However, it is extremely difficult to devise any sort of container that a bright, ingenious toddler cannot find a way to open. There is still need for *all* medications to be kept locked up when small children are around.

Chronic Lead Poisoning in Children

During the late 1930s, people of the United States became greatly alarmed over the finding of hundreds of children in our country suffering from chronic lead poisoning. Investigation showed that nearly all of the children had licked, chewed or eaten lead-base paint from walls, furniture or toys. Damage to these children was extremely serious. The death rate was high, those who lived suffered severe disabilities, most prominently brain damage.

Laws were passed prohibiting the use of lead-base paint on indoor walls and furniture. Believing the problem to be solved, people turned their attention to other matters. Only recently has it been discovered that lead poisoning in our city children is frequent, according to the Children's Bureau reaching epidemic proportions in some places.

Who are the children at risk? The largest number of chronic lead poisonings occur in children between the ages of 1 and 6 years of age, living in old, deteriorating homes. Small children, who will chew or eat everything, eat the plaster and paint flaking from walls, woodwork and window sills. In 1960 there were over 30 million occupied housing units in the United States that had been built before the use of leaded paint was outlawed.* This means that most of the children ex-

*Lin-Fu, Jane S.: Childhood lead poisoning—an eradicable disease. *Children, 17:*2, 1970.

posed live in the core areas of our big cities, in substandard housing.

Although titanium has replaced lead pigments in interior paints, recent surveys show that a high per cent of houses in many slum areas still contain dangerous quantities of flaking lead paint applied years ago.

Many cities do have building codes designed to protect tenants from exposure to lead-base paint. However, building codes in many areas have been poorly enforced. Indifference, lack of new and adequate housing are two reasons, among others. Laws and codes are enacted and enforced only when the public is concerned enough to make sure they *are* enforced.

Effects of chronic lead poisoning. Children who chew on plaster or other objects containing lead-base paint ingest the lead ions which are carried by their blood streams throughout the body. Various symptoms appear with even low levels of lead. However the same symptoms are signs of other conditions as well, and are usually not recognized as signs of lead poisoning. Symptoms are loss of appetite, anemia, malnourishment, listlessness, among others. Because the brain is especially vulnerable to lead deposits, the more serious and irreversible effects are convulsions, mental retardation, cerebral palsy, and other nervous conditions.

Treatment. Satisfactory treatment consists primarily in *prevention.* The use of a chelating agent EDTA (Edetate Calcium-Disodium) has reduced the fatality rate. A chelating medication literally draws certain metals from their combination with the tissues and accelerates their excretion from the body. Unfortunately, ingestion of lead is seldom suspected until symptoms become severe. Among those who have been treated successfully, most go back to the same environment, or one similar and become reexposed.

Blood levels of lead should not exceed 0.04 mg./100 g. Clinical symptoms do not appear until the level reaches 0.06 mg./100 g., but damage may occur before symptoms are recognized. Although fatality rates have been reduced, a large number of children who have been treated have been left with handicaps such as recurrent seizures, mental retardation and cerebral palsy. Optic atrophy has also occurred.

Education of the public, of people in all walks of life, is the most important means of removing this disease. PTA groups, neighborhood meetings, television and news media all need to join in. In one city, screening tests, such as those offered for the detection of diabetes have been given by the Health Bureau. Volunteer groups of young people have helped publicize the hazards of such conditions. The Lead Industry Association in 1969 published a booklet titled "Facts about Lead and Pediatrics." This is available to those interested in helping to stamp out the menace to children.

Detection of such hazards in our communities has been the problem. This means going to houses and living places in suspected areas and removing pieces of flaking plaster and paint. As a practical procedure, this is usually done only after a child living in such a home has been found to have lead poisoning.

An x-ray device has recently been invented which, when placed against a wall, can detect the presence of lead immediately. This will cut out the need for time-consuming, complicated laboratory tests on the bits of plaster. When these machines become generally available, we should all make it possible for our local health bureaus to purchase a sufficient number to test every urban dwelling place. We can also make it our business to see that building codes are effective and enforced.

FRACTURES AND HEAD INJURIES

Childhood fractures differ from those of adults in that they are generally less complicated, heal more quickly, and usually occur from different causes. The child has an urge to explore his environment, but lacks the experience and the judgement to recognize possible hazards. In some instances, parents may be negligent in their

Household Chemicals

Happiness is a Safe Home*

Leslie Fisher

Emergency Health Services

The following evaluation of household chemicals is based on the Final Report of the National Commission on Product Safety, presented to the President and Congress, June 1970.

A one-year-old toddler swallowed about three tablespoons of furniture and scratch cover polish in a moment when his aunt left the bottle unguarded. The petroleum distillates collected in his lungs. He died 40 hours later of chemical pneumonia.

Another one-year-old child dipped his finger into the soap dispenser of an automatic dishwasher and tasted the undischarged detergent. His mother, a few feet away, heard him scream and quickly flushed his mouth at the tap. He spent two days in Children's Orthopedic Hospital's intensive-care unit for treatment from alkali burns and blisters of the mouth. His parent's quick action possibly saved his life.

Everything in the Mouth

Because young children are so curious, household chemicals pose a major hazard: every liquid or chewable substance is something for them to sample.

The chemical burns children suffer from strong detergents are particularly painful. Surface burns to lips and mouth are the most frequent, but some injure the eyes. When the caustic material reaches the esophagus or stomach, the effect can be fatal. At the least, serious burns leave extensive scars. Without frequent surgical dilations, the scar tissue may close the esophagus. Burns were suffered by 16 percent of 157 cases we studied.

Furniture polish may produce chemical pneumonia if even a small quantity gets into the lungs.

Dr. Charles C. Edwards, Commissioner of the Food and Drug Administration, estimated that ingestions of potentially harmful household substances range from 500,000 to one million a year. The figures are based on the tabulations of the National Clearinghouse for Poison Control Centers.

Two Worst Offenders

After dishwasher detergents and petroleum-based furniture polishes were studied, Dr. Edwards stated: "Over the years, two categories of household products have caused a greater degree of hospitalization than others. These are caustics and corrosives, and petroleum products."

Parents often are aware that a household chemical may be hazardous but they are unfamiliar with the degree of hazard.

Many household chemicals look like food, are attractively packaged, and pleasantly scented. Types of liquid furniture polish resemble milk, strawberry soda, or lemon soda.

Since almost anything within reach of tiny hands frequently will go into an infant's mouth, repackaging with child-resistant spouts might reduce the hazard. Single-use packets or a substitution of solids for liquid or powdered forms might also help.

Substitute Ingredients

Most important, many products can use less hazardous ingredients without loss of function. According to testimony from Cornell Aeronautical Laboratory, all brands of dishwasher detergent, regardless of causticity, are of approximately equal effectiveness. Yet alkalinity (pH value of solutions) ranges from that of lye to that of milk of magnesia. Highly caustic soda ash can be replaced by sodium tri-polyphosphate. Although the phosphate costs slightly more, less caustic brands using phosphates sell for the same price as alkaline detergents. Phosphates, however, constitute a growing source of water pollution. If there can be no salutary tradeoff between these factors, a substitute may have to be found.

The unreasonable hazards presented by household chemicals, particularly strong alkaline dishwasher detergents and petroleum-based furniture polishes, can be substantially reduced by standards requiring reformulation and protective packaging as well as by more effective warnings.

(The New York State Health Department participated in the foregoing study and provided data on injuries from household poisons.)

---

*Reprinted with permission from *HEALTH NEWS* (February 1971), a copyrighted monthly publication of the New York State Department of Health.

supervision, but frequently the young explorer is just too fast for them.

Some Major Causes of Fractures in Children

Falls from high chairs and cribs
Falls from grocery carts in supermarkets
Rolling off beds or flat surfaces
Falling out of cars
Falls due to motor imbalance (cerebral palsy, convulsive disorders)
Birth injuries
"Battered child" syndrome

Head Injuries. Because young children frequently land on their heads when they fall, head injuries are common. A fracture of the skull in itself is not of major significance, because there is no muscle pull; the important aspect is in the brain damage that may result from pressure or hemorrhage.

Older children also experience head injuries from playground, bicycle, or car accidents. A simple, linear closed fracture requires no specific treatment; parents are advised to keep the child quiet and to watch for indications of concussion or brain injury.

A depressed fracture may necessitate decompression or craniotomy. Subarachnoid hemorrhage is associated with nearly all cases of cerebral contusion or laceration, causing grave pressure symptoms. A child who has sustained a head injury must be watched for neurological signs indicating brain injury. Significant signs include the state of consciousness, either an increasing or a decreasing pulse rate, a rise or a fall in temperature, the kind of respiration, and restlessness. Eye signs, such as nystagmus or inequality of pupils, and bleeding from ears, nose or mouth, must be noted and reported.

A quiet environment is important; bed or crib sides should be padded to protect the child from injury, but mechanical restraints are generally considered harmful. A patent airway must be maintained, with a tracheotomy if it is necessary. While attending these needs, ordinary daily care should not be neglected. Diaper changes, mouth and skin care, and smooth bedding

are all important comfort aids. The voiding pattern should be watched because the child's restlessness may stem from a full bladder.

Fracture of the Clavicle. A toddler who sustains a fractured clavicle usually does well with a figure-of-eight flannel bandage for shoulder immobilization. The bandage should be tightened daily and changed frequently, with careful examination of the skin for breaks or abrasions. A small child usually recovers quickly (within approximately four weeks). An older child may require a cast applied in the same manner.

Fractures of the humerus or the elbow. These are relatively rare in children. They may be treated by a hanging cast, immobilized by a bandage, or at times, by traction. (Fig. 33-5)

Fracture of the Femur. In children this is most frequently a transverse or spiral fracture of the shaft of the long bone. A small child under the age of three is placed in Bryant's traction for best results. The use of Bryant's traction entails some risk of compromised circulation and may result in contracture of the foot and the lower leg, particularly in an older child.

For an application of Bryant's traction, two overhead bars are passed horizontally over the crib, pulleys are attached to each bar, and the child's legs are suspended from these at right angles to his body. Weights are applied in sufficient amounts to keep the buttocks just clear of the bed. (Fig. 33-6) The child's legs are wrapped with elastic bandages that must be removed at least daily, the skin inspected, and the legs rewrapped. Skin temperature and the color of his legs and his feet must be checked frequently for circulatory embarrassment. Severe pain should not be present; if it is noted, it should be reported because it may be an indication of circulatory difficulty.

An older child seems to respond best in Russell's traction. A child in either type of traction tends to slide down until the weights rest on the bed or the floor. He should be pulled up to keep the weights free, and the

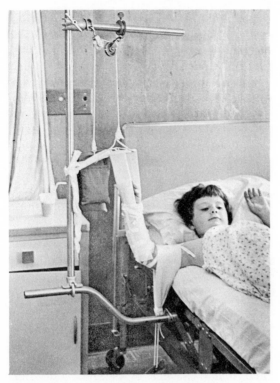

Figure 33-5. The child having a transcondylar fracture of the distal humerus may be treated with the use of a hanging cast.

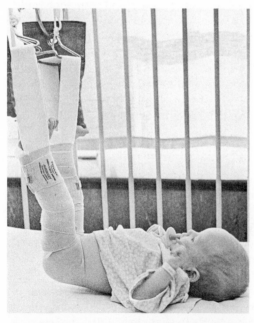

Figure 33-6. The small child who sustains a transverse or spiral fracture of the long bone may be placed in Bryant's traction.

alignment should be checked frequently. An older child may coax his ward mates to remove the weights or the sandbags used as weights. When a child is in Bryant's traction, the nurse should be able to pass her hand between the child's buttocks and the sheet. A small child adjusts to this position with surprising ease. In fact, an infant cheerfully assumes the most unusual positions, such as turning over on his abdomen while he is still in traction. He is not the one who is likely to develop pressure areas on the back of his head or his shoulders, but an older child may do so. A child is not apt to complain of any specific pain, but becomes irritable, so that the adult in his life must seek the cause. A toddler is quite likely to regress to the use of diapers, especially if he has just completed toilet training. He may have great difficulty using a bedpan when he has just learned to sit on a potty-chair, so diapers are quite likely indicated. He may also regress to the nursing bottle again, especially in the hospital. It is not uncommon to see a two- or even a three-year-old child in the hospital carefully nursing his bottle. Just be sure that he has a plastic bottle.

The social, emotional and developmental problems need consideration if a child, regardless of his age, is immobilized by a cast or by traction. It certainly interferes with his normal developmental activities. This same handicap can interfere with an adult's ability to earn a living, but a child may actually suffer impairment of normal growth and development. The child of two or three who must use his large muscles is definitely frustrated. Early childhood is a time for learning balance, motor coordination, and similar physical developmental skills. Socially, a deformity or a defect may bring ridicule or teasing from other children, causing a loss of self-approval.

An infant or toddler has neither developed a body image, nor is he inhibited by emotional barriers, so he may adapt more readily and make maximum use of any opportunities for development. In fact, he may accept his disadvantage as a normal way of life and go on from there. For instance, Bryant's traction may inhibit a small child so little that he may endanger his own recovery. It is an older child who is more likely to suffer emotionally from the inability to move freely and to control his own activities. Of course, a toddler brings along his own special problems to the hospital, which are so important that we must never overlook them. He still depends on his mother for ego strength, and is the poorest candidate of any for hospitalization if this means that he is separated from his mother.

The child may find overprotection and oversolicitude to be a problem as well. Parents and nurses tend to do those things for him that he could, and would, do for himself if given the opportunity and motivation. Children manage to feed and to help themselves in many difficult situations. They may need greater attention, understanding and approval for a time to sustain their ego, but this is not spoiling them, and the adult must watch for indications that a child is ready for a greater measure of independence.

ABUSED CHILDREN: THE BATTERED-CHILD SYNDROME

Throughout history, the rights of parents over their own children have been unquestioned. Minor children have been at the mercy of cruel, neglectful, or indifferent parents, with a conspicuous lack of supervision or inquiry from any authority. The right of the head of the family to govern his household in any manner he saw fit has always been jealously guarded. Society was not child-oriented; indeed, society in general appeared indifferent to the rights of the child.

Eventually, as societies became more complex, the state stepped in to curtail or to limit parental rights when these did not serve the common interest. For instance, because it was economically unsound for large numbers of persons to grow up illiterate, laws were passed requiring parents to send their children to school, wherever the state provided the school and the teacher.

Other absolute rights of parents over their children were curtailed as time passed. The belief persisted, however, that mothers instinctively loved and protected their children, and, if necessary, gave their lives for them. As our culture became more child-oriented, fathers no longer considered it necessary to show their authority by stern, uncompromising discipline. Society settled down into the comfortable belief that children were well protected, even pampered, except possibly a few from really depraved homes. It has come as a shock to our affluent society to discover that apparently respectable, ordinary people can be accused of mistreating their own children.

One of the earliest persons to focus our attention on this problem was Elizabeth Elmer, writing in a social work journal in 1960.* She cited several previous articles in which the possibility of skeletal trauma in inadequately explained conditions was discussed. In particular, she mentioned Silverman, who, in 1953, referred to physical trauma as "the most common bone 'disease' of infancy," and who also made note of the strong resistance of attending doctors to any implication of parental mismanagement.†

Professional interest was aroused, and many studies have since been conducted throughout the United States. The problem has been shown to be serious. In one study, 71 hospitals reported 302 cases of abuse. Of these children, 33 died, and 85 suffered permanent brain injury.‡ Similar findings have occurred in widespread areas throughout the country.

The term *battered-child syndrome* was used to characterize a clinical condition in young children who have received serious physical abuse at the hands of an adult, usually the parent. At present, the term is used to designate children who are the victims of passive as well as active abuse.

---

*Elmer, E.: Abused children seen in hospitals. *Social Work, 5*:98, 1960.
†Silverman, F.: The roentgen manifestation of unrecognized skeletal trauma in infants. *J. Roentgen., 69*:413, 1953.
‡Kempe, H. et al: The battered-child syndrome. *J.A.M.A., 181*:17, 1962.

Active abuse is manifested in such conditions as:

1. Brain injuries, subdural hematomas, skull fractures.

2. Soft tissue injuries, such as bruises, lacerations, or burns.

3. Fractures of the long bones, rib fractures; x-rays frequently show multiple fractures in varying stages of healing.

Passive abuse may include:

1. Poor nutrition, failure to thrive, severe malnutrition.

2. Poor physical condition; neglected safeguards against disease, poor skin condition, lack of proper medical attention.

3. Emotional neglect; rejection, indifference, deprivation of love.

4. Moral neglect; allowing children to remain in an immoral atmosphere, particularly if the child is old enough to comprehend.

The Children

The majority of these children are young, under the age of three years. Frequently, one particular child is singled out for this type of treatment. The child may be a child with a behavior problem (whether he has a problem because of the treatment, or whether the abusive treatment occurs because of his behavior is usually uncertain). In any case, each kind of behavior intensifies the other, causing an exceedingly vicious cycle.

When an obvious injury has occurred, parents bring the child into the hospital with a vague history of accident. An older child has pulled a blanket out from under the baby; the child caught his arm or his leg in the crib sides; the child was climbing and fell on his head. X-rays of these children frequently reveal several older fractures in various stages of healing.

There are rarely any witnesses to the accident, and the child cannot speak for himself, or is too terrified to do so. Only occasionally does a husband or a wife admit to knowledge of abuse at the hands of the other.

In the hospital these children are not likely to look to their parents for protection or assurance. They "endure life as if they are alone in a dangerous world with no real hope of safety."*

The Parent

What kinds of parents are involved in these tragic situations? No particular level of society is exclusively involved. The child may come from a neat, well-kept home, or from a poor home.

The parents are frequently young, immature persons, unready to accept the responsibilities of parenthood. They may be interested in their own comfort and pleasure, rejecting a child who gets in the way. Their immaturity may manifest itself as jealousy, the abusing parent wishing all the love and attention for herself.

Other parents are aggressive and hostile, continuously angry and unable to control their anger. Usually such parents have a background of severe rejection and deprivation in their own early childhood, which in turn they inflict on their own children.

Another kind of parent is the dependent and timid person, wanting someone to tell her what to do, how to do it, and when to do it. These parents appear unable to direct their own lives, and are utterly helpless with their children.

Examples of abuse and neglect are numerous. Bobby, not yet three, was brought into the hospital with severe facial fractures, acquired, it was claimed, by climbing and falling. Much later it was acknowledged that he had been beaten for wetting himself. When a doctor, not knowing the background, stopped to look at his black eye, Bobby was observed to flinch as though expecting a blow.

Another baby, found alone and in a filthy state, neither sat, smiled, nor responded to any show of friendliness. In his dehydrated, emaciated state, he gave the appearance of having less than normal intelligence. Intensive physical and emotional support turned our Jimmy into a smiling, laughing and playing infant, apparently well on the way to catching up with his peers.

---

*Morris, M. G., *et al.*: Toward prevention of child abuse. *Children, 11;*55, 1964.

All stories do not end so happily. Many small children sustain permanent physical or emotional injuries. Many do not survive, and others go home only to return with fresh injuries, usually to a different hospital. What can be done about this?

Legal Action

In 1963, the Children's Bureau announced that the first step in a national program protecting children from physical abuse had been taken. The Children's Bureau proposed to supply to all states suggested language for laws requiring all cases of child abuse be reported to police authorities by the doctor who sees the child.

The purpose of the suggested law was not to punish parents, but to identify children in danger so they could be protected. Many doctors, although suspecting abuse in a child patient, were fearful of reporting such cases and thus face the possibility of lawsuit. Judges have been notoriously reluctant to remove children from their homes, especially if proof beyond reasonable doubt cannot be furnished. Too often these children have been restored to their homes to become the recipients of intensified fury from their parents because of the physician's report, making the physician understandably reluctant to cause added misery.

The proposed law would give the reporting doctor immunity from criminal or civil suit. Mandatory reporting also relieved the physician of the responsibility of deciding whether to report suspicious cases. Physicians were also reminded that privileged communication between patient and physician should not apply in these cases. Clearly the duty of the physician is to the child.

Helping the Family

The nurse who receives and cares for a badly neglected or abused child in the hospital faces a nearly impossible task in trying to remain impartial. As she sees the results of actions of adults on whom the child is utterly dependent, her rage mounts. When the mother of a child who died as the result of such treatment is declared "innocent" in court, the nurse relives the difficult days of caring for a small being with sad, hopeless eyes, who accepted pain and suffering without protest, and who, in her eyes at least, made no effort to live. This nurse feels only anger and resentment that such a mother could "get away with it"; she cannot calmly and reasonably see the whole picture.

Punitive measures, however, do nothing to diminish the number of cases of child abuse, nor do they change attitudes. Whereas the approach to the problem was formerly seen as an attempt to save the child from his home, we are now starting to see that the greater need is to save the home for the child, if at all possible. We are concerned for the welfare of the child and of his parents. We still believe that most parents want to be good parents, but find that many are unable to assume adequate parental roles without outside help.

A very good case can be made for the belief that child welfare or child protective agencies are best fitted by training and experience to be the agencies receiving reports of child neglect or abuse. These agencies, of course, must then have adequate means for receiving and investigating calls at any time, day or night. They must also have authority to remove a child from a dangerous situation, or they must work together with law enforcement officers when necessary.

Understanding, skillful case work may save the home for the child, even when temporary placement of the child outside of the home is necessary. Some homes, perhaps many, can never be made safe for the child without radical changes—changes that may not be possible.

An interesting use of homemaker services has been of value. Mature, friendly women with a real interest in people, working closely with child welfare workers, can frequently help parents by their understanding support and example. They can also evaluate family situations, and clarify the need for intervention in confused situations. Many of the inadequate parents are frightened by their own actions, and are asking to be protected from their own compulsive behavior.

As nurses, we must acquire a deeper understanding of the complex issues involved in this frightening aspect of life. We have a definite responsibility to these children to protect them from personality damage as well as from physical harm. If we are interested in preventing the child from growing up into an abusive, antisocial adult, we must recognize the need for help early, before there has been irreversible damage.

The Children's Bureau-proposed law stated that report of physical injury inflicted on children should be made "thereby causing the protective services of the State to be brought to bear to protect the health and welfare of these children and prevent further abuse."*

Since the Children's Bureau recommendation in 1963, all states in the United States have enacted laws that provide some measure of protection for children. All states offer immunity from legal liability for the person authorized to report, although the majority qualify this by adding the term "if in good faith."

The persons authorized to report, as well as the agency to receive the report and take action, vary from state to state. One reporting agent is always the physician, others include nurses, social workers, etc. A few authorize any person knowing of any

*Helfer, Ray E., and Kempe, C. Henry (ed): The Battered Child. p. 238. Chicago, The University of Chicago Press, 1968.

case of child abuse, if reported in good faith. Not all states make reporting mandatory with a penalty for not reporting known or suspected cases.

Although much intelligent work has been done with the abusing parent, Dr. Helfer, one of the editors of *The Battered Child*, writes "Physical, nutritional or emotional abuse is one of the most common maladies of the young child." The book, *The Battered Child*, lives up to Katherine Oettinger's foreword: "This book, I am sure, will be invaluable in setting forth the essential medical, social and legal framework through which this problem must be faced."

BIBLIOGRAPHY

Elmer, E.: Abused young children seen in hospitals. Social Work, *5:*98, 1960.
Fisher, Leslie: Happiness is a safe home. New York, Health News, *42:*14, 1971.
Helfer, Ray E. and Kempe, C. Henry, ed.: The Battered Child. Chicago, The University of Chicago Press, 1968.
Lin-Fu, Jane S.: Childhood lead poisoning—an eradicable disease. Children, *17:*2, 1970.
Morris, M. G.: Toward prevention of child abuse. Children, *11:*55, 1964.
Newman, Virginia Hunt: Teaching An Infant To Swim. New York, Harcourt, Brace and World, 1967.

Suggested Readings for Further Study

Helfer, Ray E.: A plan for protection: the child-abuse center. Child Welfare, *49:*486, 1970.
Paulson, Morris J. and Blake, Phillip R.: The physically abused child: a focus on prevention. Child Welfare, *48:*86, 1969.

Illness in the Toddler Group 34

EYE CONDITIONS REQUIRING TREATMENT OR SURGERY

Cataracts

A cataract is an opacification of the crystalline lens. Congenital cataracts may be hereditary, or may be complications of maternal rubella during the first trimester of pregnancy. Cataracts may also develop later in infancy or childhood from eye injury or from metabolic disturbances such as galactosemia or diabetes.

The degree of opacity determines whether surgery should be performed. If the cataract is small and does not significantly impair vision, it is not usually removed. Following surgery eyeglasses will be needed to provide light refraction. Surgical results are not as successful as in the adult patient. 20/20 vision may not be attained.

Glaucoma

Glaucoma may be of the congenital infantile type, occurring in children under 3 years of age; juvenile glaucoma, showing clinical manifestations after the age of 3; or secondary glaucoma, resulting from injury or disease. Increased intraocular pressure due to over-production of aqueous fluid causes the eyeball to enlarge, the cornea to become large, thin, and sometimes cloudy. Untreated, the disease slowly progresses to blindness. Pain may, or may not, be present. Goniopuncture, which provides drainage of the aqueous humor, is effective in relieving intraocular pressure in a large number of cases. Goniotomy may improve the function of the filtration angle if it is defective.

Strabismus

Strabismus is the failure of the two eyes to direct their gaze at the same object simultaneously. Binocular (normal) vision is maintained through the muscular coordination of eye movements, so that a simple vision results. In strabismus, the visual axes are not parallel, and diplopia (double vision) results. In an effort to avoid seeing two images, the child suppresses vision in the deviant eye, causing a condition of amblyopia ex anopsia (dimness of vision from disuse of the eye).

A wide variation in the manifestation of strabismus exists; there are lateral, vertical, and mixed lateral and vertical types. There may be monocular strabismus, in which one eye deviates while the other eye is used, or alternating strabismus, in which deviation alternates from one eye to the other. The term *esotropia* is used when the eye deviates toward the other eye; *exotropia* denotes a turning away from the other eye.

Treatment is dependent on the type of strabismus present. Occlusion of the better eye in monocular strabismus, to force the use of the deviating eye should be carried out early, and should be continued constantly for a period of weeks or months. The child should be stimulated to use the unpatched eye by such occupations as puzzles, drawing, sewing, and similar activities.

Glasses can correct a refractive error if amblyopia is not present. *Therapeutic*

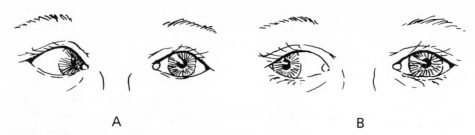

A   B

Figure 34-1. Strabismus: (*A*) esotropia, (*B*) exotropia.

exercises (orthoptics) to improve the quality of vision may be prescribed to supplement the use of glasses or surgery.

Surgery on the eye muscle to correct the defect is necessary for those children who do not respond to glasses and exercises. Many children need surgery after amblyopia has been corrected. Early detection and treatment of strabismus is essential for a successful outcome.

Eye Injury and Foreign Objects in the Eye

Eye injuries are fairly common, particularly in older children. Ecchymosis (black eye) is of no great importance unless the eyeball is involved. A penetrating wound of the eyeball is potentially serious—BB shots in particular are dangerous, and require the attention of an ophthalmologist. With any history of an injury, a thorough examination of the entire eye is necessary.

Sympathetic ophthalmia may follow perforation wounds of the globe, even if the perforations are small. Sympathetic ophthalmia is an inflammatory reaction of the uninjured eye, showing photophobia, lacrimation, pain and some dimness of vision. The retina may finally become detached, and atrophy of the eyeball may occur. Prompt and skillful treatment at the time of the injury is essential to avoid involvement of the other eye.

Small foreign objects such as specks of dust that have lodged inside the eyelid may be removed by rolling the lid back and exposing the object. Cotton-tipped applicators should not be used for this purpose because of the danger of sudden movement and of possible perforation of the eye. If the object cannot be easily removed with a small piece of moistened cotton or soft clean cloth, the child should be taken to the physician.

Eye Infections

A condition called properly *external hordeolum*, but known commonly as a *sty*, is a purulent infection of the follicle of an eyelash, generally caused by Staphylococcus aureus. Localized swelling, tenderness and pain are present, with a reddened lid edge. The maximum tenderness is over the infected site. The lesion goes on to suppuration, with eventual discharge of the purulent material. Warm saline compresses applied for about 15 minutes three or four times daily give some relief and hasten resolution, but recurrences are common. The sty should never be squeezed. Antibiotic ointment may help prevent accompanying conjunctivitis and recurrences.

Hospital Care for Child with Eye Surgery

A person suffering from any kind of sensory deprivation may experience difficulty in keeping contact with reality. A child who must have his eyes covered is particularly vulnerable. The implications of not being able to see are not always appreciated by nurses who have not themselves experienced this. A young child who wakens from surgery to find himself in total darkness may well go into a state of real panic. If one observes such a child closely as he is returned to the ward, the panic may be quite evident; he trembles, and starts nervously if he is touched or spoken to. In hospitals that still limit visiting hours, eye surgery is seldom considered a condition serious enough to allow a mother to stay continuously. His mother may be at the bedside when he returns from surgery, but who is there beside him when he hears strange voices the next morning—but sees no one?

Preparation for the event, should, of course, be carried out as well as it is possible to do so, but the small child has no background experience to help him understand what actually is going to happen. The darkness, the pain and the discomfort, and the total strangeness of the situation, can be overwhelming.

Restraints should not be used indiscriminately, but the majority of small children do need some reminder to keep their hands away from the sore eye, unless someone is beside them to prevent them from rubbing or from removing eye dressings. Elbow restraints are useful, although they do not prevent rubbing the eye with the arm. Flannel strips applied to the wrists in clove-hitch fashion can be tied to the cribsides in such a manner as to allow freedom of arm movement, but to prevent the child from reaching his face.

Special care should be taken by the nurse to speak to the child before touching him, and thus to make him aware of her presence. The child does need tactual stimulation though, so after speaking and identifying herself, the nurse would do well to stroke or to pat him, to pick him up, if this is allowed, or in some other way let him feel her presence.

If a nurse expects to have the care of a blind person, or one who must have sight covered, it becomes important that she find out from first-hand experience what the loss of sight means. She should cover her eyes for a period and learn the difficulties involved in finding her way about, or in ordinary self-care.

A Three-Year-Old has Eye Surgery

The nursing care described in the study below was carried out by a student during her clinical experience in child care. It illustrates the kind of experience that may be valuable in furthering the student's understanding of children; it shows, through the eyes of the child and of his nurse, the responses to hospitalization that are evoked in a small child; and finally, it attempts to illustrate the ways in which the traumatic effect of sensory deprivation, (in this case, a temporary loss of sight because of eye dressings) may be minimized. The study has been put into a compressed form, with names and details slightly changed.

This was a nursing care study concerning a child's response to hospitalization and surgery for the correction of exotropia of the right eye. The purposes of the study were outlined:

1. To observe the effects of hospitalization on the child,
2. To attempt to make the experience a maturing one for the child.

The reasons for choosing a patient having eye surgery took into consideration the fact that deprivation of sight, even though temporary, is frightening to a young child who cannot understand its temporary nature. The strangeness of the hospital environment may further intensify this fear, and lead to a feeling of abandonment. Therefore, this kind of patient should profit from pre-hospital preparation and from intensive care during the hospital experience.

Nursing Care Study

Gail's clinical experience included doing a care study. She spent a morning in the pediatric eye clinic observing eye examinations. Upon discovering that appointments for elective surgery were made three or four months in advance, it appeared unrealistic to choose her patient from among those in the clinic at that time. Therefore, with the assistance of the clinic personnel, she chose a three-year-old boy, Gary D., from the list of eye surgery cases scheduled for the following two weeks.

The preliminary planning. Gail called Mrs. D., Gary's mother, by telephone, and explained the purpose of her proposed study. Mrs. D. appeared interested and pleased; together, they made an appointment for Gail to visit Gary at home. Mrs. D. had told her son about the hospitalization, but welcomed the opportunity for Gary and herself to become acquainted with his future nurse. She also had several worries about the forthcoming experience that she wished to discuss.

Following the telephone call, Gail spent several hours in the library, reviewing the norms of growth and development for a three-year-old, and read articles about the effects of hospitalization on a young child. She also familiarized herself with the condition of exotropia and its surgical correction.

Gail wished to discuss her participation in the home visit with someone qualified to make meaningful suggestions. For this, she chose the mental health instructor.

Further preparation included a visit to both surgery and the recovery room to familiarize herself with the physical setup, in order to feel at ease in her support of the patient. She also observed anesthesia induction in a young patient. Gail had no previous surgery experience, and she felt that this was very important.

The home visit. In preparation for the visit, Gail had made drawings that she thought would be of interest to a small boy about to enter the hospital. They included a boy on his way to the hospital, riding to the ward in an elevator and being admitted, and also pictures of a nurse and of a doctor. She believed that explanations to a three-year-old should be limited to a consideration of immediate events; therefore, she did not, at that time, depict hospital experience beyond admission.

Keeping all of this in mind, she made plans for the home visit as close to admission date as possible; this was to be two days before admission. Realizing that a small boy would be shy, Gail spent the first several minutes chatting with the family—his brothers and his sisters and his mother; then she invited Gary to look at her pictures. Gary, who preferred to be called Buddy, quickly overcame his shyness and chatted freely about his tricycle, a television program that he had been watching, and his red fire truck. He told Gail that he was "going to the hospital to get my eyes checked," and looked at her pictures with mild interest.

Gail had brought her nurse's cap, which she now showed him, and told him she would be his nurse. Then she put the cap on her head and wore it throughout her visit. She also showed him a patient gown and slippers similar to those he would wear. Gail had taken a blindfold along, intending to play "blindfold" with him, making a game of trying to identify objects and voices. She now decided, however, that this could be played more naturally with his family, and after explaining her purpose to Mrs. D., it was agreed that the entire family would play the game with him during the next two days.

Hospital admission. Gail met Buddy and his mother at the admission desk, and took them in the elevator to the pediatric department. Buddy was at ease with her, and was able to identify the surroundings from the pictures he had been shown. She showed him around the ward, making a point of taking him to the toilet room, because his mother had felt he would be too shy to ask, and might regress to wetting himself.

Buddy was called to the eye clinic, so his mother and Gail took him in a wheel chair, which he greatly enjoyed. Upon their return, Gail put on a surgical gown, a cap and a mask to show him how she would look tomorrow in surgery and in the recovery room. She told him she would go with him "to get his eye fixed," but he would be asleep when it happened. She worried over the "sleep" concept, not wanting to make him afraid of sleep, but she could not think of any way to avoid it. Buddy played with his toys, and accepted all of this quite casually—perhaps because of the casual way in which it was presented. Surgery was scheduled for the early morning, otherwise she might have chosen to wait until morning for this part of the preparation. After being tucked in, however, he slept through the night without waking.

Operative day. On the morning of surgery, Buddy was happy and full of energy, playing peek-a-boo with Gail and apparently enjoying the novelty of his surroundings. Just before the time for his preoperative sedation, she told him about it, saying it would hurt a little. He was cooperative and did not appear frightened. He did cry, however, and Gail picked him up, holding him for a little while.

In the surgery department Gail left him to change into surgery garb. She found him asleep, and unconscious of her return. She knew, however, that some children do not respond to sedation this quickly—in which case her precaution of showing Buddy how she would look in operating room garb could be helpful.

Anesthesia induction was by endotracheal tube, and Buddy relaxed smoothly. Surgery consisted of a shortening of the medial rectus muscle and a lengthening of the lateral rectus muscle of the right eye; an intricate process which took two hours. Both eyes were covered, and Buddy was taken to the recovery room.

When Buddy wakened from anesthesia, Gail recorded that he was "very irritable, nauseated, and sleepy." He was returned to his room where his mother waited, anxious to know his condition and the results of the surgical procedure. The eye surgeon described the surgery in some detail, and Gail was able to report Buddy's good condition.

An injection for the relief of his nausea made Buddy very angry, but he soon relaxed and slept most of the remainder of the day, secure in the presence of his parents and his friend, the nurse. He again slept through the night.

First postoperative day. When Buddy wakened, Gail was at his bedside and, putting her hand on his arm, said "Buddy, this is Gail." He smiled and stretched out his arms to her, and she "gave him a big hug, and told him I loved him." She felt that her preparation had been helpful and furnished a link between a frightening experience and the outside world.

Buddy was eager for breakfast, drinking his milk so fast "his tummy didn't like it." This disturbed him, but after Gail explained that his stomach was empty and that food would make it feel better, he ate all his breakfast, accepting the necessity of having to be fed, although Gail thought he did not like it. Gail told him the doctors were coming to remove the dressing from the unaffected eye, only minutes before they came. They removed both dressings, checked the operated eye, and replaced that dressing. He accepted the procedure well, but his eye was sore and he cried for a while after they left.

Gail had prepared a box of toys of a variety of shapes, sizes and textures for sensory satisfaction, for him to manipulate while his eyes were still covered. Buddy had not wakened sufficiently for this, but Gail now produced it, and he enjoyed playing with the toys, stringing the large beads to show her how well he could do. She stayed with him throughout the day, reading to him, giving him necessary physical care, and playing with him. His parents were with him during the evening and tucked him in for the night. Again, he slept well.

Second postoperative day. Gail had told Buddy she would not be with him until the evening. When she came, he jumped down from his mother's lap, showed Gail his toys and strung some beads for her. His mother said that he had sat on her lap since she had come, cried because Gail had not come, and had wet his bed during afternoon nap (a most rare occurrence for him). Gail felt that he had interpreted her absence as rejection, although she had tried to prepare him. She stayed with him through the evening, and put him to bed for the night, staying, until he went to sleep.

Day of discharge. Buddy was discharged shortly after breakfast on the third morning. Before leaving, he and Gail made arrangements to visit at his home about 10 days later. Gail wished to discover if there was any noticeable change in his behavior, how he would react to her, and what parts of his experience he remembered, as well as how he interpreted the experience.

Second home visit. Buddy was playing outside when Gail arrived. He ran to the car, greeted her, and immediately started telling her about what he was doing. Buddy's mother and his older sisters thought that he was much more active than he had been before his hospital experience. They thought he was more forceful, and played more roughly with his younger sister. Gail wondered if this might be interpreted as a release of emotions built up during his hospital experience.

Gail found that Buddy's parents were greatly pleased with the interest she had shown, and with the results of their son's surgery. He had not talked much about the hospital experience, but frequently referred to "my nurse." He appeared to remember very little about his discomfort or the nausea following surgery.

Buddy sat on Gail's lap during her visit, gave her a present, and asked her to come again. A few weeks later, she visited him in the eye clinic, finding him friendly and cheerful, happy over her visit, but casual in his manner, showing his ability to put the entire experience into proper perspective.

The meaning of the experience to the nurse. This can best be expressed in Gail's own remarks.

"With a three-year-old, it is a very difficult task to explain an operation as a health-giving device. Instead of explaining the operation to Buddy, I told him the strange and new things he would see. I feel this worked out satisfactorily. He didn't have any severe emotional reactions to the operation, and he established a new relationship outside of his family group.

The most important result for me is the truly satisfying relationship that has been established between Buddy and myself. It is something I have never had with a young child before. I feel a relationship like this can help children through a traumatic experience. They must have this constant feeling of security and love, because everything is strange and frightening to them."*

---

*Original nursing care study carried out by Gail Womack, junior nursing student at the University of Oregon School of Nursing.

Eye Dressings and Instillations

An "eye tray" is usually kept in the treatment room on the pediatric department. The treatment room nurse has the responsibility for refilling all trays and checking expiration dates for medications or solutions, sterile trays and dressings. The tray for eye care contains routine solutions for pupil dilatation, such as atropine and homatropine, vials or ampules of sterile saline solution, and other eye drops or ointments in common use.

The eye dressing tray should contain
1. Sterile eye pads
2. Sterile cotton balls
3. 4 x 4 gauze pads (flats)
4. A small sterile basin
5. Sterile scissors and small forceps
6. Adhesive tape
7. Container for water

The nurse may be expected to instill eye drops, particularly before eye surgery. When preoperative eye drops or drops prior to eye examination are ordered, timing must be exact. She will also have occasion to apply eye ointments and do eye dressings, as ordered by the physician.

Instillation of Eye Drops

A small child cannot understand the necessity for having anything put in his eye, and cannot be expected to cooperate. It is usually necessary to apply a mummy restraint (Fig. 24-11) and have a second person hold the child's head still. The lower lid should be pulled down gently and the drops instilled into the inner canthus. Care must be used to prevent touching the eyeball with the dropper.

If a multiple dose bottle of solution is used, a clean dropper must be used for each patient. When the solution is in a sealed dropper vial, individual bottles for each patient will help prevent the spread of any infection.

RESPIRATORY CONDITIONS

Tonsils and Adenoids

A brief description of the placement and the functions of tonsils and adenoids may be helpful before the difficulties of infection and the indications for removal are discussed.

A ring of lymphoid tissue, called Waldeyer's ring, encircles the pharynx, forming a protective barrier against upper respiratory infection. This ring consists of groups of lymphoid tonsils.

The faucial tonsils, the commonly known *tonsils,* are two oval masses attached to the side walls of the back of the mouth between the anterior and posterior pillars.

The pharyngeal tonsil, known as *adenoids,* is a mass of lymphoid tissue in the nasal pharynx, extending from the roof of the nasal pharynx to the free edge of the soft palate.

The lingual tonsils are two masses of lymphoid tissue at the base of the tongue.

There is a normal progression of enlargement of lymphoid tissue in childhood between the ages of two and eight or ten years, regressing during the pubertal period. If the tissue itself becomes a site of acute or chronic infection, it may become hypertrophied to the extent of interfering with breathing, causing partial deafness, or it may become in itself a source of infection.

Tonsillectomies and adenoidectomies are not done as frequently today as in the past. No conclusive evidence has been found that a tonsillectomy, in itself, improves a child's health by reducing the number of respiratory infections, increasing the appetite, or improving his general well-being. Studies tend to show that incidence of colds may increase following removal of the tonsils. It is generally agreed that absolute indications for removal of tonsils are: frequent attacks of acute tonsillitis; recurrent peritonsillar abscess (which has become rare); chronically infected tonsils with enlarged cervical nodes, which fail to yield to antibiotic therapy; and hypertrophy of tonsils to the extent of interfering with swallowing and breathing. Systemic disturbances, such as rheumatic fever or glomerulo-nephritis, are not considered as indications for tonsillectomy, unless the tonsils can be proved to be the source of an infection that fails to yield to antibiotic treatment.

Adenoids are more susceptible to chronic infection. Indication for adenoidectomy is hypertrophy of the tissue to the extent of impairing hearing or interfering with breathing. An increasingly common practice is to perform an adenoidectomy alone, if tonsil tissue appears to be healthy.

Care of the Child Admitted for Tonsillectomy

Tonsillectomy is postponed until after the age of four or five years, except in the rare instance when it appears urgently needed. Often, when a child has reached the acceptable age, the apparent need for the tonsillectomy has disappeared. When the decision has been made to remove the tonsils, a period of two or three weeks following an acute infection should pass, although this is not always possible. On occasion, a surgeon, after several cancellations of surgery because of new infections, may decide that it is safer to operate while the child is relatively free from infection, rather than risk any more acute episodes. This may be demonstrated on the ward when the nurse reports a mild temperature elevation during the preoperative period. Normally, surgery is cancelled, and the child is sent home. When the child has been unable to maintain a period of two or three weeks free from throat infection, however, the otolaryngologist may agree to remove the tonsils, provided that no evidence of present acute respiratory infection is found.

Preoperative Care. In many hospitals, the child has had blood and urine tests performed before admission; if this has not been done, the nurse should make certain that the ordered tests are performed and the results entered on the chart. Written permission for surgery is then obtained, and the parents are notified of the time surgery is scheduled.

One unfortunate occurrence in busy hospitals ought never to be—that of a failure to notify the parents of an advance in surgery time, so that the parent arrives to find her child has already left the ward. A concerned parent is justifiably angered, as

she visualizes her child's fright and insecurity. A most graphic illustration concerns a mother who had been given a definite time for her child's surgery the previous evening by the surgeon. An earlier case was cancelled, however, before the schedule was sent to the ward, and so the ward personnel were entirely unaware that the mother had been told a later time. Notification of scheduled time by telephone, if the information is not available when parents are on the ward (with care to notify when changes in scheduling occur), will prevent this from happening most of the time; especially if parents are advised to come at least an hour before scheduled surgery time, to allow for the period when the child is under sedation.

Emotional preparation for surgery has been discussed throughout this book. Acting out the forthcoming experience, particularly in a group, with the use of puppets, dolls, and play doctor or play nurse material helps the child to develop security. The amount and the timing of preparation before admission depends somewhat upon the child's age. The nursing care study discussed later in this chapter is applicable to any type of elective surgery.

On the morning of surgery, the child is given no food or fluids, a fact that may well traumatize the child emotionally if he has to watch the others getting their breakfast trays. If surgery is to be late, there is no reason for keeping the child in his bed. He will be happier and better adjusted if he can spend this time in the playroom, with someone responsible for helping him resist the temptation to drink, if he should forget. As this is the age during which primary teeth become loose and fall out, the child should be checked carefully for loose teeth before surgery.

Postoperative Care. Immediately following a tonsillectomy, the child is placed in a partially prone position, with his head turned to one side, until he is completely awake. This position can be accomplished by turning the child partially over and by flexing his knee on which he is not resting to hold him in position. Pillows placed under the chest and abdomen may embarrass respiration, and so are usually forbidden. A recovery room is generally available for patient care until recovery from anesthesia, but if the patient must return to the ward immediately following surgery, he should be carefully observed until fully reacted; after which, he may be placed in a semiupright position.

Vital signs are checked every 10 to 15 minutes until the child is fully reacted, then every half-hour or every hour. The nurse should be aware of the normal rate of pulse and respiration for the child's age, in order to interpret the vital signs correctly. Any unusual restlessness, frequent swallowing, or rapid pulse may indicate bleeding and should be reported. Vomiting of dark, old blood may be expected, but bright, red-flecked emesis or oozing indicate fresh bleeding. A tracheal suction machine, ready for use, should be at the bedside. Suctioning by the nurse must be performed with great care, and not extend beyond the front of the mouth.

Fluids are encouraged as soon as the child's nausea has subsided. The thirsty child may be eager to drink, but the painful swallowing will probably quell his enthusiasm, and encouragement will be needed. Jello water, fruit-flavored, uncarbonated drinks are allowed, with the oft-promised dish of ice cream in the afternoon.

The child is discharged on the day after surgery if no complications are present. Parents are advised to keep him in bed for two days, and fairly quiet for about a week. Soft foods and nonirritating liquids should be given during the first few days. The parents are advised that a transient earache may be expected about the third day. If bleeding should occur, the pediatrician or clinic should be notified at once.

The following care study illustrates the physical care and emotional support a child needs before and after a tonsillectomy.

A Six-year-old has a T and A

Dick, a six-year-old boy admitted for tonsillectomy, was met in the pediatric admitting room by the student nurse who was to care for him throughout his hospital stay. She introduced herself to Dick as Carol B., and explained that she would be his nurse. Dick was disturbed and reluctant when the admitting nurse attempted to take his temperature. After Carol explained the procedure and showed him the thermometer, he accepted this manner of temperature taking.

Following a preoperative examination by the admitting pediatric intern, Carol took Dick to the laboratory for the routine blood check, which included an RBC, a WBC, and tests for bleeding time and clotting time. She explained to Dick that the technician would stick his finger to get a little blood, and she told him why. His only question was, "How will she take the blood out?" He cooperated well, but felt the need to cry, and was comforted by the nurse and his mother.

On the way to the pediatric department, Carol and Dick discussed what the ward looked like, why he was to sleep in a crib, and the delights of the playroom. The first thing he wished to do on his arrival was to crawl into the crib to find out what it felt like, accepting it as a novelty. He delighted in the playroom, played with the other children, and accepted his mother's departure calmly.

Although Dick had been prepared for the surgery experience by his parents, Carol talked with him about the next day's routine. She explained about the preoperative sedation, telling him it would be like the "shot" he sometimes got in the doctor's office. She told him the ride to surgery would be on a stretcher, showed him the stretcher and let him lie down on it. They examined a face mask together; Dick pretended to be a doctor, put the mask on, and listened to his own heartbeat with a stethoscope. Miss B showed him an oxygen mask, and explained that tomorrow he would wear one like it; there would be a sweet smell of ether, and he would get sleepy. Dick tried on the mask, and wanted to know where the ether would come from. After supper, Dick got into his crib, and Carol read him stories until bedtime.

In the morning Dick's mother arrived early, and shortly after her arrival he received his preoperative medication of Demerol 50 mg., atropine 0.2 mg., and Seconal 25 mg., given intramuscularly. Dick was invited to give a doll an injection, which he did with considerable vengeance. Rather than becoming drowsy, he reacted by becoming overactive and noisy, which embarrassed his mother. Carol assured her that sometimes children were stimulated in this manner, and that her son was not being naughty or uncooperative. Nevertheless, there was some difficulty in keeping him on the stretcher.

In surgery, Dick quieted and responded to the anesthiologist's explanation of the mask and the stethoscope by saying, "I know all about that; the nurse told me already." After the initial inhalation, anesthesia was given by intubation, and surgery was carried out smoothly.

In the recovery room Dick was placed in Trendelenburg's position. Carol noted that his color remained good, his skin was warm, his pulse was about 120, and that there were no signs of bleeding. In about two hours, he had recovered sufficiently to be returned to the ward, where he climbed into his crib and immediately went to sleep. Carol watched him carefully, checking his pulse every hour. The postoperative course was uneventful; Dick wakened at intervals, showed no signs of bleeding, and had only a small amount of dark brown emesis. He took fluids in satisfactory amounts, but he refused ice cream.

The night nurse reported an uneventful night, and in the morning Dick seemed glad to see Carol. He talked freely, recounting the events of the previous day until he "went to sleep," and asking in detail what happened after that. He particularly wanted to know, "What did they do with my tonsils after they took them out?" and, "What did my tonsils look like?"

Carol stayed with Dick until his parents came to take him home, reading to him and answering his many questions. Dick said goodbye with a smile, seeming to feel that he had made friends, and appeared not to have found the experience emotionally damaging.

Conditions of the Larynx and Bronchi

Spasmodic Laryngitis

Spasmodic Croup may occur in children between the ages of two and four years. The cause is undetermined; it may be of infectious or of allergic origin, but certain children seem to develop severe laryngospasm with little, if any, apparent cause. The attack may be preceded by coryza and hoarseness, or by no apparent signs of respiratory trouble during the evening. The child awakens after a few hours sleep with a bark-like cough, increasing respiratory difficulty, and stridor. He becomes anxious and restless, and there is marked hoarseness. There may be a low grade fever and mild upper respiratory infection.

This condition is not serious, but is quite frightening, both to the child and his parents. The attack subsides after a few hours; little evidence remains the next day when an anxious mother takes him to the doctor. Attacks frequently occur two or three nights in succession.

Treatment. Humidified air is helpful in reducing the laryngospasm. Taking the child into the bathroom and opening the hot water taps, with the door closed, is a quick method for providing moist air—provided that the water runs hot enough. The pediatrician may prescribe syrup of ipecac in a dosage sufficient to produce vomiting, which usually gives relief. If repeated attacks occur, phenobarbital at bedtime may relax the child enough to prevent a recurrence.

Acute Laryngotracheobronchitis

Laryngeal infections are not uncommon in small children, and they frequently involve tracheobronchial areas as well. Acute laryngotracheobronchitis may progress very rapidly and become a serious problem within a matter of hours. The toddler is the most frequently affected member of the one to four age group. This condition is usually of viral origin, but bacterial invasion may follow the original infection. It generally follows an upper respiratory infection with fairly mild rhinitis and pharyngitis.

The child develops hoarseness and a barking cough, with a fever which may reach 104° or 105°F. As the disease progresses, laryngeal edema becomes marked, and child's breathing becomes difficult. The pulse is rapid, and cyanosis may become marked. Congestive heart failure and acute respiratory embarrassment may result.

Treatment. The child is placed in a supersaturated atmosphere, such as that obtained in a croupette or some other kind of mist tent. The older croup tents, using hot steam, are rarely used. Greater relief is obtained from the use of a cold mist, and the danger of burns is avoided. The mist may be used with air under pressure, or with oxygen.

Close and careful observation of the child is important. Observation includes checking his pulse, his respiration, his color, listening for hoarseness and stridor, and noting any state of restlessness.

Type of Respiration. Pull down the covers, and watch the child breathe. Observe the amount of chest movement, shallow breathing and retractions. Listen with a stethoscope for breath sounds. Listen for the amount of stridor, indicating difficult breathing.

Heartbeat. Listen for the rate, quality, strength, and regularity of the pulse. A rapid, weak pulse may indicate impending cardiac difficulty.

Voice and Color. Increasing hoarsness should be reported. Cyanosis of the extremities or an increasing pallor are signs of impaired oxygenation of the blood, and should be reported promptly.

Difficult swallowing may limit the airway as well as prevent sufficient fluid intake.

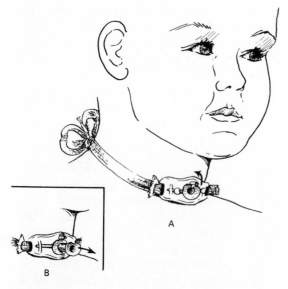

Figure 34-2. A tracheotomy may become necessary if the child has respiratory difficulty. Note the tracheostomy tube in place (*A*) and the inner cannula unlocked and partially removed (*B*).

Increasing restlessness and anxiety, are frequently signs of impending heart failure.

Intravenous fluids are usually needed, but they must be carefully monitored to prevent overloading the circulation and placing additional strain on the overworked heart.

Not all children with this type of infection become as acutely ill as their symptoms imply, but the possibility is present, and it should be understood. The majority of these infections are of viral origin, and do not respond to antibiotics.

If a tracheotomy becomes necessary because of any respiratory difficulty, the surgeon will try to perform this in the operating room, under more ideal conditions than can be obtained at the bedside. The decision as to when to perform a tracheotomy is a delicate one. Tracheotomy is a procedure not to be performed lightly or for insufficient reasons. The waiting period becomes a difficult one for the nurse, especially because her observations are used as partial basis for decision. The parents' anxiety, and her own feeling of helplessness add to her concern.

The nurse who is watching the child needs support from the other members of the nursing staff as well as from the physicians. She should not try to demonstrate her self-sufficiency or worry about the picture she may present to others. Her concern is for her patient, and she should seek help and advice without hesitation.

An emergency tracheotomy set is kept readily available for use if it is necessary, but because much better results can be obtained if the surgery is performed in the operating room—without the pressures of a last minute emergency procedure—the child will be taken there if possible. When the child is in surgery, the nurse will prepare his room for his return. The bed can now be changed completely, the mist apparatus cleaned and checked for maximum efficiency, and the plastic tent may be checked for tears or holes.

The tracheal suction machine is set up at the bedside, checked for working order, and equipped with suctioning materials.

An adequate supply of linen, as well as all nursing equipment, is then brought into the room, because a child who has had a tracheotomy should never be left alone.

Nursing Care of the Tracheotomized Child

Directly following surgery, excessive secretions in the trachea can be troublesome. The tube will need frequent aspiration, and this can be quite frightening to the child. A second person to hold him, or a mechanical constraint may be necessary, particularly at first, when the tube is aspirated. As the secretions become less troublesome, aspiration is not so frequently needed.

The nurse caring for the child must remain in a position from which she can observe his face at all times when the tracheostomy tube is in place, and she must not occupy herself with any duties that might distract her. When the child is turned, she should place her own chair at the other side of the crib, or turn the crib around. It is generally considered unwise to allow the child to lie on his abdomen, because of the danger of occluding the airway.

This constant vigil can become monotonous and tiring, and she may find it difficult to maintain her alertness. She should be relieved at intervals of two hours or less, for a period of relaxation.

The child seldom needs continual restraint while under constant observation, and certainly will be more comfortable if he can move about. His mother's presence may be soothing and comforting, depending on whether the mother can respond in a satisfactory manner, or is herself too frightened to give support.

As the child improves, he can be allowed to sit in his crib or up in a chair, and he should experience no difficulty eating. If no complications arise, recovery is generally rapid and the tracheostomy tube may be removed without difficulty. The child may have become dependent on the tube, and may panic on its removal. The surgeon may order the tube plugged for intervals until the

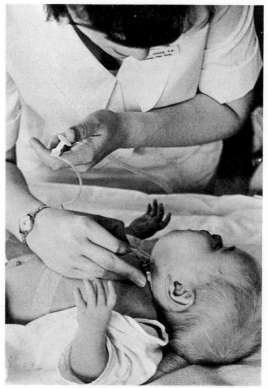

Figure 34-3. Frequent suctioning of the tracheostomy tube is necessary.

child becomes accustomed to breathing normally. Mortality rate has been considerably lowered during the last few years, with prompt treatment, antibiotic therapy to prevent secondary infection, and careful management.

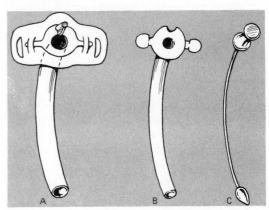

Figure 34-4. A tracheostomy tube is composed of three main parts: (*A*) the outer cannula, (*B*) the inner cannula of the tube, and (*C*) the obturator, used for inserting the outer cannula.

Equipment for Suctioning a Tracheostomy

Sterile

1 container (labelled) containing solution. Solution used: Zephiran Chloride 1:1000; or iodine 1:500,000 (8 gtts. 0.19% iodine in 200 cc. water); or normal saline; or sterile water.

1 container (labelled) containing hydrogen peroxide.

Whistle-tip catheter, size according to the size of the tracheostomy tube used.

Y connecting tube.

Sterile glove (if used). Note: procedures vary. Washing hands before suctioning may be considered sufficient.

Extra tracheostomy tube (to be kept at bedside).

2 Kelly forceps or a Trousseau dilator (to be kept at bedside).

Pipe cleaners.

Obturator from the tracheostomy set in use.

Nonsterile

A suction machine.

Procedure for Suctioning Tracheostomy Tube

1. Wash your hands and put on a sterile glove, if one is to be used.
2. Remove the inner cannula and drop it into hydrogen peroxide.
3. With the suction turned on and with the Y tube open, use your gloved hand to insert the catheter to a point 1/8 inch beyond the cannula.
4. Control the suction by covering the open arm of the Y tube with your finger. Remove the catheter slowly, using a rotary movement. Limit aspiration to 15 seconds.
5. Aspirate solution through the catheter to clear mucus.
6. Pause between aspirations to allow the patient to rest and to allow air to enter the tracheostomy tube.
7. Repeat suctioning as necessary.
8. Clean the inner cannula, insert it and lock it in place.
9. Aspirate the solution through the catheter, and leave the catheter in solution or in a sterile towel, or remove and use a fresh catheter for each suctioning.
10. Remove your glove, and turn off the suction.
11. Comfort the child.

Suctioning the Bronchial Tree.

1. If "deep" suctioning is required, specific orders should be written indicating how deep the catheter should be passed.
2. To aspirate the left bronchus, turn the child's head to the right. To aspirate the right bronchus, turn the head to the left.

Care of the Tracheostomy Tube

1. Unlock the inner cannula, remove it and clean it with hydrogen peroxide, using pipe cleaners to remove the mucus from inside the cannula. Rinse well under running water, and replace it in the outer cannula and lock it in place.
2. Check the ties on the tracheostomy tube to make sure that they are secure.

Precautions

If the tracheostomy tube is displaced or removed, hold the wound open with a Kelly forcep or with a Trousseau dilator until the physician arrives to reinsert the tube. When suctioning, if the catheter meets with an obstruction at the end of the cannula or if the child appears to receive no benefit after suctioning (although tube appears free of mucus) the tracheostomy tube may actually be out of the trachea.

No child is to be left alone at any time with a tracheostomy tube in place, except on the written order of the attending physician.

Care of Equipment.

1. Set up clean sterile equipment every 8 hours and p.r.n.
2. Thoroughly wash equipment and return it to central supply. Most tracheostomy

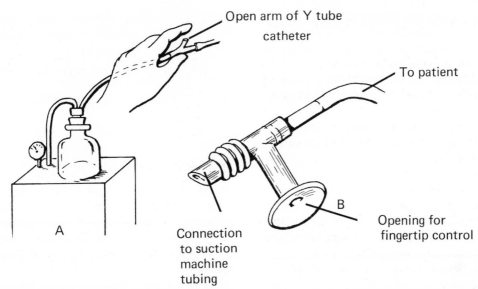

Open arm of Y tube
catheter

To patient

Connection
to suction
machine
tubing

Opening for
fingertip control

A

B

Figure 34-5. Suction catheters are used for tracheal and nasopharyngeal aspiration. Note (*A*) the Y-glass connector with fingertip placed over its open arm to create a vacuum; and (*B*) the regu-vac suction catheter to permit use of a regulated suction technique by fingertip control.

tubes do not have interchangeable parts; make sure that the correct outer cannula, inner cannula and the correct obturator are returned together.

Helping Physician Change Outer Tube

The nurse does not change the outer tube, but assists the physician when the tube is to be changed.

The equipment needed includes a sterile tracheostomy tube (inner and outer cannula, and obturator) of correct size.

Sterile gloves for physician.

Usual equipment for suctioning.

Procedure

1. Position child with neck hyperextended.
2. Restrain child as necessary; mummy restraint usually needed.
3. Standing at child's head, hold head securely between hands while tube is being changed.
4. Suction child following procedure.

BLOOD DYSCRASIAS
Anemia

Anemia is a common childhood blood disorder. It may be the result of an inadequate production of red blood cells or of hemoglobin, or from an excessive loss of either red cells or of hemoglobin. The following are examples of the more common types of anemia found in childhood; there are many others.

1. Inadequate production of erythrocytes or of hemoglobin, as in iron deficiency anemia and in anemia of chronic infection.
2. Excessive loss of red cells, as in hemorrhage.
3. Hemolytic anemia associated with congenital abnormalities of erythrocytes or hemoglobin, as in thalassemia or sickle cell disease.
4. Hemolytic anemia associated with acquired abnormalities of erythrocytes or hemoglobin, from drugs, chemicals, or bacterial reaction.

Iron Deficiency Anemia

Iron deficiency anemia is a common nutritional deficiency among young children. It is a hypochromatic, microcytic anemia, i.e., the blood cells are smaller than normal, and deficient in hemoglobin, common between the ages of 9 and 24 months. The full-term newborn has a high hemoglobin that decreases during the first 2 to 3 months of life. However, considerable iron is reclaimed and stored, usually in sufficient quantity to last for 4 to 9 months of life.

A child needs to absorb 0.8 to 1.5 mg. of iron per day. As only 10% of dietary iron is absorbed, a diet containing 8 to 10 mg. of iron is needed for good health. During the first years of life it is often difficult for a child to obtain this quantity of iron from his food. If the diet is inadequate, anemia quickly results.

Other causes, particularly in the older child, may be occult blood loss due to lesions of the gastrointestinal tract such as peptic ulcer or Meckel's diverticulum. In areas where hookworm is present, this may be a cause.

Babies with an inordinate fondness for milk, sometimes taking an astonishing amount, have their appetites satisfied, and show little interest in solid foods. Mothers sometimes misunderstand the learning of the infant requires transfer from sucking to chewing and swallowing motions, and think the baby is showing a dislike when he pushes his food out with his tongue. Babies need time to adapt to the new manner of taking food, and a mother needs considerable patience and persistence. A baby undoubtedly is going to register his surprise and his impatience with this attempt to satisfy his hunger, but he learns quickly and will become an enthusiast for the newer method, especially if he can still have his comforting bottle.

Infants and toddlers have come into the hospital with a history of taking 2 to 3 quarts of milk daily and accepting no other foods, or at best, only foods with a high carbohydrate content. (Some confusion may exist: the belief that milk is a perfect food, so why not let him have all he wants?) Examples are many; the nine-month-old who doesn't care for vegetables and fruit but enjoys pancakes with the family, and so forth.

Many of these children, however, are undernourished strictly because of the family's economic problem. Much work is needed to help provide necessary nutrients for the nation's children. It is not an economic problem alone but also a need for proper nutritional knowledge and a need to learn ways to use money for food to the best nutritional advantage.

A few children have a hemoglobin so low, or their anorexia so acute, that they need additional therapy. An iron dextran mixture for intramuscular use (Imferon) is available, which is markedly efficient in bringing the hemoglobin to normal levels. A special technique for administering this medication, called the Z track method, is necessary to avoid leakage into the subcutaneous tissues.

Home Care. The most important aspect of treatment for this condition is education for the parents. They need to understand the importance of iron in their child's diet, and the foods that are best for meeting this need. One mother was quite severely criticized in the pediatric outpatient clinic because of her child's anemic condition. "Mrs. Black," said the pediatrician, "you simply have to give your child more foods that contain iron." Mrs. Black looked at him in bewilderment and exclaimed, "But doctor, after liver—what?"

A nurse has a splendid opportunity to teach good nutritional habits in such a situation—habits that may improve the health of the entire family. She can guide the mother to the green and the yellow vegetables, to the use of egg yolk, and to iron-rich fruits such as peaches; in addition, of course, to liver. Some of the pamphlets published by commercial food companies are excellent for teaching parents, and perhaps can refresh the nurse's memory as well. These give the iron and the vitamin content of foods, and list the requirements for various age levels.

Prognosis is excellent for restored health in iron deficiency caused by poor iron intake with dietary correction. If untreated, anemia becomes progressive, with possible resultant cardiac failure.

Procedure for the Use of the Z Track Method in the Administration of Iron Dextran (Imferon)*

Iron dextran is recommended for use solely in the treatment of iron deficiency anemia—situations in which the oral administration of iron is unsatisfactory or impossible. Imferon is absorbed rapidly from the muscle, but slowly from the subcutaneous tissue. Injected into, or leaking into, subcutaneous tissue, it is broken down and stored as hemosiderin. Use of the Z track method of injection is of great importance to prevent leakage:

1. Use one needle to withdraw Imferon from the ampul, and another needle for the injection.
2. A needle long enough to insure injection into the muscle tissue must be used.
3. Use a gauge 19 or 20 needle for the injection.
4. Allow enough air to remain in syringe to void the syringe and the needle completely of any iron dextran so that there is no tissue staining when the needle is withdrawn. The use of 0.5 cc. of air is recommended for an adult. Less air should be necessary when given to an infant.
5. Inject iron dextran only into the upper outer quandrant of the buttock, never into the arm or some other exposed area.
6. Before injecting the needle, retract the skin laterally, displacing it firmly to one side. The skin should be held in this position until after the injection.
7. Insert the needle and withdraw the plunger to check against entry into a blood vessel.
8. Inject the medication and a small amount of air from the syringe.
9. After the injection, wait 10 seconds before withdrawing the needle or releasing the skin.

_____

*This information is from the brochure of distributors of IMFERON (Lakeside Laboratories) and from private correspondence with them.

10. Withdraw the needle, and release the skin.
11. Rotate sides, using opposite buttocks.

Sickle Cell Disease

Sickle cell disease is an hereditary trait occurring primarily but not exclusively in the Negro race. It appears as an asymptomatic trait when the sickling trait is inherited from one parent alone (heterozygous state). When inherited from both parents (homozygous state) anemia develops. A rapid breakdown of red cells carrying hemoglobin S, an abnormal hemoglobin, causes a severe hemolytic anemia. The sickling trait occurs in about 10% of American Negroes: there is a much higher incidence in parts of Africa. The disease itself has an incidence of 0.3 to 1.3%. The tendency to sickle can be demonstrated by laboratory tests. In those who carry one gene for the *sickle cell trait*, hemoglobin level and red cell count is normal, and the child is asymptomatic.

Clinical symptoms of the disease itself do not usually appear before the latter half of the first year of life. Sickle cell disease causes a chronic anemia with hemoglobin levels of 6 to 9 g./ 100 ml., or lower. Easy fatigability and anorexia are the usual manifestations of any form of anemia. The frequent sickle cell crises, however, make the disease a serious one.

Sickle cell crisis may be the first clinical manifestation of the disease, and may recur frequently during early childhood. This disturbance presents a variety of symptoms. The most common symptom is severe, acute abdominal pain, together with muscle spasm, fever, severe leg pain that may be muscular, osseous, or localized in the joints, which become hot and swollen. The abdomen becomes boardlike, with an absence of bowel sounds, making it extremely difficult to distinguish the condition from an abdominal condition requiring surgery. The crisis may have a fatal outcome caused by cerebral, cardiac or hemolytic difficulties.

Treatment. The child should be kept in optimum health between crises. Small blood transfusions help to bring the hemoglobin level near normal, but the increase is only temporary. Treatment for crises is supportive and symptomatic and bed rest is indicated. Analgesics are given for pain and dehydration and acidosis is vigorously treated. Oral intake of iron has no effect on the disease. The spleen becomes greatly enlarged, but in later childhood may become small and fibrotic and is rarely palpable in childhood.

Prognosis is guarded, depending on the severity of the disease.

Thalassemia

Thalassemia (*Mediterranean anemia*) is a serious hereditary blood disorder appearing principally in persons of Mediterranean origin, such as Greeks, Syrians and Sicilians, and in their descendants. In this condition, hemoglobin formation is faulty, and red blood cells are of abnormal size and shape and are rapidly destroyed.

The hypochromic, microcytic anemia resulting from this disorder is not present at birth but appears after a few months of life. As in sickle cell anemia, it is manifested as a major or a minor trait. Clinical manifestations in a minor trait are minimal, limited to a slight pallor and occasionally a slight enlargement of the spleen. These children remain unaffected by the slight anemia, but genetic counseling may be indicated. Should such persons marry individuals carrying the same trait, one in four of their children can be expected to have the major form. Unfortunately, the expectation of one in four offspring developing the hereditary condition is misleading to many persons, who think that if one child is defective, the next three will not be. Too often, it has not been made clear to them that there is no order of succession. Regardless of the condition of his siblings, any child's chance of having the major form is 25%.

Thalassemia major produces a severe irreversible anemia requiring frequent transfusions, and shortening the affected person's lifespan. Although life expectancy is somewhat better than has been supposed, a person with this disorder rarely lives beyond the third decade.

Clinical Manifestations. Early in the disease, it may be difficult to distinguish it from other types of anemia, including iron deficiency, or from other hemolytic disorders. The nature of the disorder is confirmed by an examination of the blood of the patients' parents.

Pallor, poor appetite and fever may be early manifestations. Splenomegaly appears early, and may reach disabling proportions. The most striking changes are skeletal, and exceed those of other hemolytic anemias. Changes in the facial bones give a characteristic appearance, and there is a tendency toward protusion of the teeth.

Another characteristic is the muddy, bronze color of the skin, caused by hemosiderosis, after months or years of transfusions. Growth becomes markedly retarded, and cardiac enlargement is common.

Treatment. Transfusions are required at frequent intervals with an effort to maintain hemoglobin at or above 6 gm./100 ml., with care taken to avoid overloading. In certain cases, splenectomy may be helpful.

Prognosis is very poor. With careful treatment, some children may live to adulthood, but at best, must lead lives of limited activity. The most serious problem presented is the prevention or control of cardiac failure.

Acute Leukemia

Leukemia is a fatal malignant disease involving all the blood-forming organs, and is characterized by a rapid and abnormal proliferation of immature leukocytes (white blood cells) in the bloodstream.

Etiology

The cause of leukemia is still not known, although there are interesting clues. Recently, certain animal leukemias have been proved to be of viral origin. However, a simple infectious viral cause in childhood leukemia does not seem likely at this time. Leukemia also is frequently associated with Down's syndrome and other chromosomal disorders.

Pathophysiology

Immature white cells, called blast cells, are formed in large numbers in the blood-forming tissues throughout the body, while normal white cells are progressively reduced. Leukemia in childhood is nearly always the acute type in contrast to the chronic type sometimes found in adults. About 80% of childhood leukemias are of the acute lymphoblastic type. The overall leukocyte count is normal in half the cases, but the differential count shows a predominance of immature blast cells.

Diagnosis

The diagnosis of acute leukemia is made by demonstration of leukemic blast cells in the bone marrow, blood and other tissues. Leukemia can never be positively identified except in this manner.

Incidence

The disease has its highest peak of onset between the ages of 3 and 5 years.

Clinical Manifestations

Clinical manifestations of the disease appear with surprising abruptness in many affected children, with few, if any, warning signs. Presenting manifestations are frequently lassitude, pallor and loss of appetite. Other early or presenting symptoms are fever, bone and joint pain, sore throat, or hemorrhages into the skin or the mucous membranes.

Nausea and vomiting, headache, diarrhea and abdominal pain, although seldom presenting signs, frequently occur during the course of the disease. Anemia and easy bruising are present, and enlargement of liver and spleen occur. Ulceration of the gums and throat develop due to bacterial invasion. Intracranial hemorrhages are not

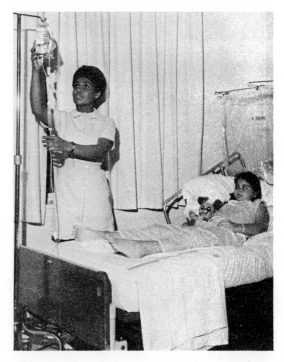

Figure 34-6. This is a child with leukemia who has been given steroids, causing the edema and the moonface features.

uncommon. Anemia becomes increasingly severe.

Treatment

In addition to symptomatic, palliative measures, certain drugs have been successful in bringing about remissions during which period the child feels and acts quite well. Remissions may last for a period of several weeks, and some children have had 2 or 3 remissions, under sustained medical therapy. About 10% to 15% of affected children respond poorly to all medical therapy, and even the children who respond favorable eventually build up resistance to the drugs and fail to respond.

Drugs being used in leukemic therapy include Methotrexate, Meticorten, Purinethol, Oncoven, Cytoxan and Myleran. These all have some toxic effects and are used under strict supervision.

At this time no confirmed cure has been found for leukemia.

Home Care for the Leukemic Child

Hospitalization for leukemic children is limited to diagnostic procedure and to the institution of therapeutic measures whenever possible. The child at home is allowed to live a normal life as much as he is able. The family needs to unite to make the home pleasant and cheerful, and should make a particular effort to keep anxiety and discouragement away from the child. Parents may need special encouragement about this, and may appreciate an understanding, sympathetic friend for support.

Over-indulgence and undue permissiveness tend to make the child anxious and confused, however, and is not in his best interest. Short periods of hospitalization for exacerbations quite possibly are going to be necessary, as well as admission for terminal care.

Nursing Care of the Critically Ill Child

Physical care for a child in the terminal stages of a wasting disease (such as leukemia) is aimed at providing all possible comfort for the patient. Frequent turning is necessary, but painful, and is dreaded by the child. Unhurried movement, a soft, gentle touch, and careful handling, helps minimize the pain. Abrupt movements should be avoided, and necessary analgesics should be used as indicated. Cleansing of bleeding, ulcerated areas in the mouth must be very gentle in order to prevent further trauma.

Emotional support for the child and his parents is of equal importance. Parents, singly or together, are allowed and encouraged, to stay with their child and to perform as much of his cares as they are able. It frequently comforts a mother to know that she is doing something for her child, rather than watching helplessly. Nurses should avoid urging parents to go away "for a little rest" at such a time. Instead, they should understand that most parents need to be with their children, and the nurse should do all she can to add to their comfort at the child's bedside. The nurse should be constantly available and as understanding and receptive to requests as possible. She may think a suggestion to call the doctor, or to perform some nursing act, useless or unnecessary, but if such acts ease things for the parents, she should cheerfully perform them. Nurses are human and may make mistakes, perhaps many; but avoiding disturbing conditions or assuming an indifferent manner should never be among them.

Idiopathic Thrombocytopenic Purpura

Purpura is a blood disorder associated with a deficit of platelets in the circulatory system. The most common type of purpura is the idiopathic thrombocytopenic purpura.

Etiology and Incidence

This condition is preceded by a viral infection in about half of the diagnosed cases.

Laboratory Data

The platelet count is reduced to below 40,000 per cu. mm. Bleeding time is prolonged and clot retraction time is abnormal. White cell count remains normal, and anemia is not present unless excessive bleeding has occurred.

Clinical Manifestations

The onset is frequently acute. Bruising and a generalized rash occur. In severe cases, hemorrhage may occur in the mucus membranes, epistaxis, which is difficult to control, or hematuria may be present. Rarely, a serious complication of intracranial hemorrhage occurs. In the majority of cases, spontaneous disappearance of symptoms occurs in a few weeks without serious hemorrhage. A few may continue in a chronic form of the disease.

Treatment and Nursing Care

Corticosteroids are useful in reducing the severity and shortening the duration of the disease in some, not all, cases. Nursing care consists in protecting the affected child from falls and trauma, regular diet and general care.

Prognosis is excellent in about 98% of cases.

Hemophilia

Hemophilia is one of the oldest hereditary diseases known to mankind. Dispensation of the rites of circumcision to the sons born subsequent to the birth of an older son who bled uncontrollably was mentioned in the Talmud.*

In modern times, a famous example of a carrier is Queen Victoria. One son, three grandsons, and six great-grandsons had the disease, while six of her female descendents were carriers. Thus the condition has occurred in several royal houses of Europe. No records of hemophilia can be found in the ancestors of Queen Victoria, and it is assumed that a mutation took place in her X chromosome. The hereditary line of Queen Elizabeth II, however, has been entirely free from this disorder.

Recent research has demonstrated hemophilia as a syndrome of several distinct inborn errors of metabolism, all resulting in the delayed coagulation of blood. Defects in the synthesis of protein give rise to deficiencies in any of the factors in the blood plasma needed for thromboplastic activity. The principle factors involved are factor viii (AHG), factor ix (PTC), and factor xi (PTA).

Mechanism of Clot Formation

The mechanism of clot formation is complex. In a simplified form, it can best be described as occurring in three stages.

1. Prothrombin is formed through plasma-platelet interaction.

2. Prothrombin is converted to thrombin.

3. Fibrinogen is converted into fibrin by thrombin.

Fibrin forms a mesh that traps red and white cells and platelets into a clot, closing the defect in an injured vessel. A deficiency of one of the thromboplastin precursors may give rise to hemophilia. This progression of events is diagrammed in Figure 34-7.

Reference to one of the specialized texts on the circulatory system is necessary for a detailed discussion and for better understanding of the clot-forming mechanism.†

Recognized Types of Hemophilia

Factor VIII deficiency (hemophilia A; AHG deficiency; classic hemophilia). Classic hemophilia is inherited as a sex-linked recessive mendelian trait with transmission to affected males by carrier females.

Hemophilia A (classic hemophilia) is the most commonly found type, and is also the most severe. It is caused by a deficiency of antihemophilic globulin (AHG)—the factor viii necessary for blood clotting.

Factor IX deficiency (hemophilia B; PTC deficiency; Christmas disease). Christmas disease was named after a five-year-old boy who was one of the first patients diagnosed as having a deficiency of factor ix.

This deficiency constitutes about 15 per cent of the hemophilias. It is a sex-linked recessive trait appearing in male offspring of carrier females, caused by a deficiency of one of the necessary thromboplastin precursors, factor ix, the plasma thromboplastin component (PTC). In either hemophilia A or hemophilia B, as many as 25 per cent or more of the affected persons can trace no family history of the disease. It is assumed that spontaneous mutations have occurred in some of these cases. Hemophilia B (Christmas disease) is indistinguishable from classic hemophilia in its clinical manifestations, particularly in its severe form. It may also exist in a mild form, probable more frequently than in hemophilia A.

Factor XI deficiency (hemophilia C; PTA deficiency). This exists as an autosomal dominant trait, appearing in both males and females. Sporadic cases may also be ob-

---

*Bearn, Alexander G.: Hemoglobin, Hemophilia and Agammaglobulinemia. p. 231. In Fishbein, Morris: Birth Defects. Philadelphia, J. B. Lippincott, 1963.

†One good source for further study is: Smith, C.: Blood Diseases of Infancy and Childhood. 2nd ed., chapter 26. St. Louis, C. V. Mosby, 1966.

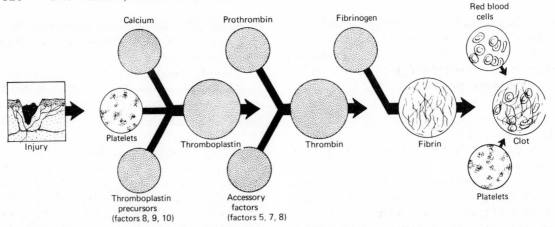

Figure 34-7. The mechanism of the formation of a blood clot is complex.

served, as in the other hemophilias. The deficient factor is plasma thromboplastin antecedent (PTA), factor xi. Bleeding is generally milder than in the AHG and the PTC deficiencies, hemorrhage usually being by trauma, and rarely spontaneous.

Von Willebrand's syndrome (vascular hemophilia; pseudohemophilia). Von Willebrand's syndrome is classified with the hemophilias. It is a mendelian dominant trait present in both sexes, and is characterized by prolonged bleeding time.

Clinical Manifestations and Diagnosis

Clinical manifestations in any type of hemophilia are similar, and are treated by transfusions to supply the deficient factor, and by measures to prevent or treat complications. In severe bleeding, the quantities of fresh blood needed may easily overload the circulatory system. It therefore becomes important to know the type of deficiency, in order that concentrated plasma containing the necessary factor may be administered when a transfusion is considered necessary.

Diagnosis of hemophilia is made by a careful examination of family history and of the type of bleeding the patient presents. Abnormal bleeding dating from infancy, in combination with a family history, suggests hemophilia. A markedly prolonged clotting time is characteristic of severe AHG or PTC deficiency, but mild conditions may have only a slightly prolonged clotting time. It must be kept in mind that in a number of

instances, no family history may be obtained.

Kinds of Treatment Available for Hemophilia

For many years the only treatment for bleeding in hemophilia was the use of fresh blood or plasma. When fresh frozen plasma came into use it became the mainstay in the management of hemophilia. Great improvements have been made possible in the treatment of hemophilia through the use of fresh frozen plasma.* It has been particularly helpful in emergency situations.

It does however have shortcomings. One major problem has been the large volumes needed to control bleeding. Another is the danger that injections of large amounts of plasma may lead to congestive heart failure.

In 1952 a method was found for separating homophilia A and B, and a suitable procedure developed for identifying the antihemolytic factor for hemophilia A.; Factor *viii*. This basic laboratory procedure known as the *partial thromboplastin time* is now commonly used for assay and diagnosis of both hemophilia A and hemophilia B.

Several factor *viii* concentrates for the treatment of hemophilia are now available. One of these, called cryo-precipitate resulted from the discovery that the precipitate remaining undissolved when frozen plasma thawed slowly could be used to stop bleeding. A procedure was developed by

---

*Brinkhous, Kenneth M.: Changing prospects for children with hemophilia. *Children*, 17:22, 1970.

which blood banks can collect this material and use it in the treatment of hemophilia A.

A newer preparation is now available which is said to supply higher potency AHG than previous preparations.* This means that only a small volume of fluid is needed for treatment, and it can be administered intravenously by syringe.

A concentrate for hemophilia B is also now available.†

These concentrates are supplied in dried form together with diluent for reconstitution. Directions for mixing and administration are included with the package. They can be given either by slow intravenous drip or injected into the vein by syringe.

Clinical Manifestations and Management

Hemophilia is characterized by prolonged bleeding, with frequent hemorrhages into the skin, the joint spaces, the intramuscular tissues and externally. Bleeding from tooth extractions, brain hemorrhages, and crippling deformities are serious complications. Death during infancy or in early childhood is not unusual in severe hemophilia, and results from a great loss of blood, intracranial bleeding, or from respiratory obstruction caused by bleeding into the neck tissues.

Excessive bleeding may follow circumcision, contraindicating circumcision if hemophilia is present. A young infant beginning to creep or walk bruises easily, and may often cause serious hemorrhages from minor lacerations. Bleeding frequently occurs from lip biting, or from sharp objects put in the mouth. Tooth eruption seldom causes bleeding, but extractions require specialized handling, and should be avoided by preventive care, if at all possible.

Topical fluoride applications to the teeth are of particular importance to these children. Particular attention should be paid

---

*Antihemophilic Factor (Human) Method Four, Dried, *Hemofil.* Hyland Division Travenol Laboratories.

†Hyland Proplex Factor Complex (Human). Factors *ii, vii, ix* and *x*. Hyland Division Travenol Laboratories.

to proper oral hygiene, well-balanced diet and to proper dental treatment. Although parents may be aware of the benefits to the teeth from a well-balanced diet and from the avoidance of in-between snacks without toothbrushing, damage frequently occurs before the patient's first visit to the dentist. Parents should be encouraged to bring their affected children to the dentist very early, in order that they may secure assistance in setting up a well-balanced diet, and in establishing good dietary habits. In this manner, the child also becomes familiar with the dental office before any care is actually needed. Parents may also appreciate any help in the selection and the use of proper equipment such as a toothbrush, tooth paste and dental floss. The parents need to use care in their selection of a dentist who understands the problems presented, and who will set up an appropriate program of preventive dentistry.

Nosebleeds in affected children are frequent, but can usually be controlled with a Gelfoam pack soaked in topical thrombin solutions and maintained by gentle pressure. Bleeding from any source in a hemophiliac, however, indicates the titer of AHG or other deficient factor is below a critical level; therefore, transfusion of whole blood, fresh frozen plasma, or plasma concentrate is necessary.

Bleeding into the joint cavities. This frequently occurs following some slight injury, and seems nearly unavoidable if the child is to be allowed to lead a normal life. Pain, caused by the pressure of the confined fluid in the narrow joint spaces, is extreme, requiring the use of sedatives or of narcotics. Prompt immobilization of the involved extremity is essential to prevent contractures of soft tissues and the destruction of the bone and joint tissues. Emergency splints are available, and should be kept in every hemophiliac's home. Ice packs should also be available for instant use. Before leaving for the hospital, a splint and cold packs should be applied, and if any great length of time is required for transportation, a transfusion of plasma should be given. (Fig. 34-8)

A bivalve plaster cast may be applied in the hospital for the immobilization of the affected part. Orthopedic surgeons disagree as to whether collected blood in the affected joint should be aspirated.

After bleeding has been stopped, the cast may be removed, and gentle traction may be applied to restore motion and alignment. Passive physiotherapy is used to help prevent the development of joint contractures. A fairly large number of patients who have had repeated hemarthroses have, however, developed functional impairment of their joints despite careful treatment.

Most children with hemophilia have their lives interrupted by frequent hospitalization. Nurses and auxillary personnel should be well informed concerning the necessary care for a hemophilia patient, as well as the care needed by a particular child.

A small child may be placed in a crib with padded sides to protect him from bruises. This, however, isolates him from the rest of the world. Coming at the same time as separation from his mother, this isolation is especially hard to bear. His choice of toys is going to be quite severely limited, because anything that could possibly cause injury must be avoided. Even if he is feeling well, he is quite possibly going to be kept in his crib, because no one will have enough time to

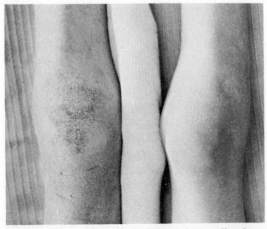

Figure 34-8. The hemophiliac may suffer from bleeding into the joints and painful swollen knees.

watch him carefully. His prospects are rather dismal, and they present a strong point in favor of allowing his mother to stay with him.

Particular attention must be paid to treatments and procedures in order to avoid pain or additional bleeding. Medication should be given orally, if possible, but if injections are ordered, care must be taken to choose and to rotate sites, avoiding bruised areas or hematomas. The medication must be injected slowly, after which manual pressure should be applied for five or more minutes. A pressure dressing and an ice pack may be used instead. Venipunctures should be done by experienced persons.

During daily hygiene, the nails should be trimmed to prevent scratching, and adequate skin care should be given to prevent irritation. Oral hygiene is important, and if a tooth brush is used, it should have very soft bristles.

If internal bleeding is present, vital signs must be watched carefully for signs of shock, and excretions should be examined for the presence of blood. If the bleeding is into the joints, the nurse should take care to avoid additional pain or injury. A bed cradle can keep the weight of the blanket off painful areas. The knee is the most commonly affected joint, and only a slight degree of motion may lead to more bleeding. Careful turning and handling are essential.

Emotional Support in the Hospital

A small child very quickly learns how to get his own way, and if his mother has been understandably apprehensive about her child's condition, he will quite possibly enter the hospital determined to get it. He does not expect any one to cross him too much, because he can always have a temper tantrum.

How, indeed, can a nurse maintain needed discipline for a child who can so easily injure himself? Freddy was an excellent example. He was allowed to play about the ward, and was completely undisciplined. If he was prevented from climbing, snatching toys from others, or from running in the corridor, he promptly responded with a full-blown temper tantrum, throwing himself on the floor and banging his head enthusiastically. The suddenness and the violence of his reactions frequently took the nurses by surprise, and it required nimbleness on their part to pick him up and carry him, kicking and screaming to his crib where he could do minimal damage to himself. Placing him in the safest possible place, and drawing the curtains around his unit seemed to be the best response to his anger. He deeply resented being watched, and could not respond to reasoning or affection when he was emotionally upset.

The nurse may frequently avoid such occasions if she uses a little forethought. If the dispute is not particularly important, as is often the case, flexibility is in order. Failure to make necessary restrictions because a child might react is not in his best interest, nor will it contribute to his emotional welfare.

For an older child, frequent hospitalizations, treatments and school absences are difficult to accept, and he needs considerable help. He can learn to understand his condition, and can learn the need for caution in his life. Occupational activities suitable for his age, and placement in the ward with others of his age and with his interests, are important adjuncts to his emotional well-being.

Home Care

A child with hemophilia is perfectly well between bleeding episodes, but the fact that bleeding may occur as the result of very slight trauma, or often without any known injury, causes considerable anxiety. For an unknown reason, bleeding episodes are more common in the spring and fall. There also appears to be some evidence that emotional stress can initiate bleeding episodes.

Parents experience continual anxiety over such questions as how much activity to allow their child, how to keep from overprotecting him, and how to help him achieve a healthy mental attitude and yet protect him from mishaps that may cause serious bleeding episodes. In some way, they must help him toward autonomy and independence within the framework of his limitations. There certainly will be times when the emotional effect of social deprivation and restrained activity must be weighed against possible physical harm.

The financial strain on the family is considerable, as is so frequently the case when a child has a long-term chronic condition. Children who have had several episodes of hemarthrosis may be crippled to the extent of needing crutches and braces, or even use of wheelchairs. Measures toward rehabilitation require hospitalization, with possible surgery, casts, and other orthopedic appliances. Rehabilitative measures have been remarkably successful when in the hands of competent orthopedists, but they take long periods of time and cannot be hurried.

A hemophilic child usually suffers much loss of school time. One college student reported an average attendance of approximately 25 days a year, with only a few weeks of home tutoring during high school. Another hemophilic boy had excessive absences but was assisted with a school-to-home telephone hookup when he was absent.* The child who must frequently interrupt his schooling, for whatever reason, suffers a considerable handicap. Each child should be considered individually, with as normal an environment as possible planned for him.

Both a child and his family must accept his limitations, and yet realize the importance of normal social experiences. School, health, and community agencies must be prepared to assist the family with counseling and encouragement, and enable them to bring up their affected child in a healthy manner, both emotionally and physically.

Rehabilitation

Extensive crippling resulting from hemophilic arthropathies presents a difficult

*Proceedings, Institutes on Hemophilia, sponsored by The National Hemophilia Foundation, Columbia University and Tulane University, 1965.

task for rehabilitation. Prompt and thorough care of any injuries as they arise helps minimize crippling. Many children, however, develop deformities severe enough to limit successful daily living.

Rehabilitation for the correction of flexion deformities requires hospitalization for periods of weeks for treatment with corrective casts. When the best possible correction has been obtained, braces usually are fitted for maintenance of the correction.

Braces are frequently needed for a period of years, during which, they must be kept in perfect repair, adusted to the patient's growth, and replaced as necessary. Rehabilitation of the severely crippled patient requires a long period under specialized orthopedic care, but the results have been eminently worthwhile.

The nurse should be aware of the resources in her community, both for family counseling and for financial assistance. State chapters of the National Hemophilia Foundation provide information, form parent groups, support the establishment of special clinics, and provide a diversity of other services.

THE CHRONICALLY ILL CHILD

We can be justly proud of the considerable progress made in reducing childhood mortality rates. When we look at children who are growing up to be self-respecting, well-integrated individuals, we know that a half-century ago, many of them would not have had this opportunity. Diphtheria and tuberculosis, to name only two conditions, all too often marked the premature end of a promising life. Today these conditions, as well as many others, are rare among the children of the United States, as well as among children in many other parts of the world. Many of the diseases that took such a heavy toll of children's lives now respond to treatment, and we owe much to those whose work has brought about this progress.

There are, however, still children who develop illnesses that respond poorly to treatment, or not at all. Cancer, in the form of leukemia and other neoplasms, is still high on the list of the major causes of childhood death. Cystic fibrosis requires careful nursing, with prognosis still poor. Childhood nephrosis has yielded only slowly to research, although the mortality rate has been markedly lowered. This is a cold comfort to the parents of the child who does not survive: for them, it still adds up to 100 per cent.

Rheumatic carditis is also a crippler of children, bringing a reduced expectancy for living a healthy, normal life. There are many other conditions for which little hope of cure can be expected at present. Research is continually seeking for a break-through, and the future appears hopeful; but in the meantime, we must care for these children with the means at our disposal.

Children with chronic illnesses are generally cared for at home, and are seen in the hospital only for diagnosis and beginning treatment, or for care during exacerbations, or, for many, terminal care.

Understanding the problems faced by these children and their parents helps make the nurse's care more effective as well as furthering her development as a teacher.

When we see a child go home from the hospital with a diagnosis of leukemia or nephrosis, we have a feeling of sadness about the difficult days ahead. Too frequently, however, we do not understand exactly what is involved in his home nursing care. As nurses, we *need* to understand this if we are to fulfill our functions as members of society.

Take a moment to consider what the role of a nurse means. As a student, the nurse may have seen herself as operating within the four walls of a hospital or a school, but she becomes increasingly aware that her influence and her responsibilities reach out much further. In her neighborhood, her community, and in her home, she does not cease to be a nurse. Perhaps as a saleswoman she could shed her identity, but as a professional woman, as a nurse, her role is an integral part of her entire life. Her advice is sought, her opinion is respected, and her influence is great; therefore, it behooves her to have a solid foundation of understanding and information. She must not be rigid, but will find her concepts ever changing as she herself grows; and she will be faithful to her principles if she understands them.

The Chronically Ill Child at Home

Sally, the third child in the family, has been petted and loved by her older brothers—her slow growth confirming her place as the baby of the family. Recently, however, she has become irritable, anorexic, and uninterested in life in general. A physical examination revealed a metabolic disorder and her mother has been obliged to assume the responsibility for a careful diet, prevention of infections, medications, treatments, and allowance for rest that is essential for such a child's care. What does this mean to Sally in terms of daily living? Her older brother is home from school with the sniffles and a slight fever. He sees no reason for staying in bed, hops in and out, and is driving his mother to distraction. Peace is finally secured when his mother finds an activity that occupies both children, with Sally a willing helper to her big brother. He throws off the infection and is back in school in a day or two; but to Sally, who has quickly picked it up, it is a major complication, perhaps sending her back to the hospital: yet it is difficult to keep the children apart.

Perhaps Sally has been invited to a neighborhood birthday party, but her diet does not allow her to eat the party foods without harm. Is Sally to be kept away from all activity? If so, what effect is this going to have on her emotional life?

Sally's diet is monotonous and uninspiring, and she lacks appetite, yet it is essential that she eat the proper foods. It is easy to suggest that the diet be made colorful and interesting, but to a busy mother, this is not quite as simple as it sounds.

Perhaps we can make suggestions that would be helpful for this mother, or for others with home care problems. In this instance, one of the major considerations is to get the uninterested child to eat. If the child is on a restricted diet, there seems little one can do to break the monotony, but the surroundings can be made more pleasant. A mother must discipline herself to make the mealtime pleasant and to avoid nagging or any other unpleasantness. Naturally, she is anxious and concerned about her child's poor appetite, but she is not going to get the child to eat by nagging. Any kind of unpleasantness at the table makes mealtime an unwelcome occasion. She must save any reprimands and discussion of unpleasant subjects for another time and place.

Colorful surroundings help make the mealtime more agreeable. A gaily decorated placemat makes the meal more exciting. The older children can crayon or paint all sorts of gay scenes on an oblong piece of shelf paper, which can easily be discarded as occasion demands. Cheap, embossed napkins lend themselves readily to decoration with crayons or paint and gaily striped drinking straws make variety. Tiny tea sets or doll dishes occasionally add charm and novelty, and do not give the impression that huge amounts of food must be eaten.

Children love flowers, and certainly a cut flower or two on the table adds charm and beauty. Common garden flowers that can be handled and sniffed are most appreciated.

Perhaps the diner would occasionally like to dress up, with a hat, a pair of high heels and a purse, for a society luncheon to which her pet doll or stuffed animal is also invited.

Eating is an aesthetic pleasure as well as a necessity for the maintenance of life. Anything that adds beauty and color to the meal may also stimulate the appetite; the food itself is more tempting if it is bright and colorful. Vegetable food coloring can change some drab-looking foods, and molds or fancy shapes can make foods more exciting.

Neighborhood parties often may be fitted into, or around, the diet of the restricted child, with decorations and prizes heavily played up while foods are kept quite simple. The excitement of partying itself means more than the kind of refreshment, especially to small children.

These seem like simple, perhaps trivial, considerations, but daily living with a chronically ill child is not kept on a high pitch of crisis; it is, largely, monotonous and wearisome.

Daily care. The child who must be kept in bed for weeks presents a most trying problem to himself and to his family. If he is suffering from one of the sequelae of streptococcal infection, such as rheumatic fever, chorea, or glomerular nephritis, he probably feels quite well after the acute phase, and deeply resents the restrictions placed upon him. If he is in a cast for the correction of a congenital anomaly, he is mechanically restrained. The long, enforced inactivity is hard for an eager, active child to accept. We must be able to keep him physically quiet to prevent heart or body damage while at the same time, prevent him from withdrawing his eager interest from living. It is not a simple task.

For the busy mother, the most important consideration is to have the bed in an easily accessible place. If the family lives on one level, this is not too difficult to achieve; if there are stairs to climb, perhaps the nurse can help the parents convert a downstairs room into a temporary sick room. A hospital bed with its added height and raised head rest is a great convenience in the home. Many communities maintain a central supply cupboard from which hospital equipment may be rented or borrowed. The nurse can find out if such is the case in her community. Many city drug stores or supply houses also maintain such a rental service, although this may become too expensive.

Hospital beds, although useful, are not imperative. Blocks can be placed under the regular bed to raise it to the desired height, and back rests can be improvised from inverted straight chairs, or made from packing cases. (Fig. 34-9)

A most important item is an over-bed table for play or eating. It can be simply supplied by placing a board across the bed, resting the ends on the backs of chairs; or a sturdy carton may be used by turning it upside down and cutting the sides down to make leg room.

A child needs diversion to keep him from complete boredom, and to prevent a loss of interest in activities for his age. This is difficult if he is allowed a minimum of activity and if his callers are restricted. Television is good in limited amounts, but is no good at all for a steady diet. The American Heart Association has source material for children's quiet activities. In the foreword to the booklet *Have Fun—Get Well!* this statement is made: "Time stretches out like a great desert for the patient who must spend a long convalescence in bed." Many quiet activities can be carried out in the home that would be difficult or impractical in a hospital setting, and the suggestions in Chapter 23—*The Play Program*—for children on bed rest, can of course be used at home as well as in the hospital.

Schoolwork at Home. Eventually, as the child progresses toward health, the doctor allows the child to resume his schoolwork at home. The nurse can help by telling the parents how to get in touch with the school authorities to arrange for home teaching or, better still, she can take care of this herself.

Before the child is allowed schoolwork, however, it is of great importance that he does not lose contact with his schoolmates. It is easy for a child to lose interest in life outside his home if he is prevented from participating in its activities, and it is equally difficult for him to step into such activities when he is again allowed to do so. The world does not stand still while he is isolated from his age mates; they will have developed skills in sports, knowledge of the world about them, and understanding of group living and cooperation. It will be difficult indeed for him to catch up, and any help we can give him along the way is essential. One way to help is to encourage his class to write letters to him, and teachers are usually happy to make this a part of their school activities. In this way, projects in which the class is interested can be extended to include the child at home.

Extracurricular Activities. If the sick child is a member of the scouts or of similar

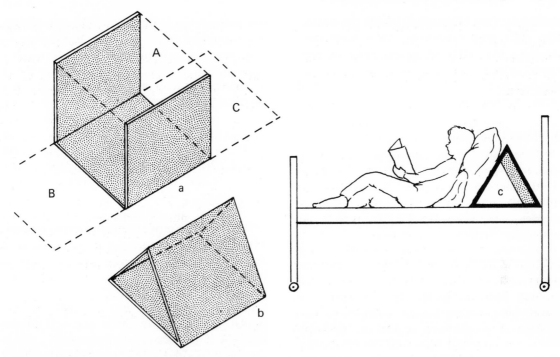

Figure 34-9. To make a triangular support for a back rest, cut a carton as illustrated.

groups, he can participate in many projects, sending and receiving information to and from the group. Perhaps eventually, when the time comes, an occasional meeting can be held in his home.

If the child is encouraged to help plan his own program, it will make more sense to him. At the start of a long convalescence, the most important thing for the nurse and the parents is to make certain that the child thoroughly understands his condition, his treatment, and his limitations. Only then can he accept his limitations and cooperate with his treatment.

Children are eager to learn and are curious about their bodies. A child with rheumatic fever can understand a simple diagram showing the heart functions. He may want to draw a diagram himself, or put together one of the plastic circulatory systems found in the toy departments. Children kept in bed for any condition can understand and profit by simple, straightforward explanations and drawings. A normal child sees no fun in illness and is willing enough to help in furthering his recovery if he understands the reasons.

Naturally, interest flags at times and cannot be kept at a continuous high level; frequent encouragement may be needed.

Resistance to Infection. Chronically ill children have poor resistance to infection, and need much more careful watching than does the healthy child. Mothers must protect them from becoming overtired, from becoming chilled, and from contact with others whose own sniffles or cough appears trivial, but which could become a serious condition in the child with low resistance. This task includes keeping the other members of the family in the best possible health, rather than making the child a person apart from the family group.

As the child becomes older, mother must then learn to relax and to let him start to take over the management of his own daily living. This is a difficult thing to do because she has protected and worried for so long. She feels that all her careful work may become undone, yet for the sake of the child's future independence and emotional stability, she must do this. It takes both patience and wisdom to help him learn to respect his limitations while keeping a cheerful and optimistic view of possibilities for the future. The child who cannot go on a week-long camping trip with his group, may become expert in some other area that contributes as much or more to his general self-respect and sense of belonging.

Grief and Mourning

Every new mother has an anxiety about her newborn child. Usually the first question is, "Is the baby all right?" Sometimes the child is not. Learning that one's child is physically or mentally handicapped is an extremely traumatic experience.

The first reaction of most parents to this tragedy is one of disbelief: this cannot be, there must be a mistake. When forced by obvious facts to accept the condition, a search for a reason begins. Sometimes the concept of punishment enters in; perhaps this pregnancy had been rejected. Probably all women have a few moments of unhappiness over their thickening figure, curtailment of previous activity, morning sickness; but if the result of pregnancy is an imperfect child, there are apt to be feelings of guilt. Many other presumed causes, frequently unrealistic, are found, because the shame of not being able to produce a perfect child must be dealt with in some manner.

Some rejection of this child is nearly inevitable, but this is also unacceptable. It may be compensated by over-protection or over-concern to the point of making the child unnecessarily helpless, with perhaps some of the anger and frustration taken out on the normal siblings.

Another method of coping with this intolerable problem is to set the child apart as someone special, someone sent to teach them love, humility and charity. If parents are to become effective, they have to face their reactions, until they can accept the child as a member of their family, to be helped, loved, disciplined and accepted just as the others.

The nurse, however, should not expect the parents to pour out their feelings to her, nor should she expect to assume the role of a professional counselor—a role for which she has neither the training nor the experience. She should be ready to listen, to observe, to help formulate a plan of care, and to use her knowledge and skills as they are desired and accepted. As she works with the family, her acceptance of them makes her an understanding partner, a partner in whom one can confide and with whom one can discuss problems. If the family and the nurse find the problems are beyond their ability, the nurse should know where they can seek expert help.

Parental adjustments. The adults in the child's life have adjustments to make as well. When a parent feels uncomfortable over a child's deformity or physical lack and tries to hide it or to keep him out of public view, she usually convinces herself that she is protecting him from pity or ridicule. Actually, it is her own pride and self-esteem that she is protecting; unfortunately, she is instilling the idea into the mind of the child that he has something of which to be ashamed. This is clearly brought out in the story of Nancy, as told by her mother. Nancy had a grotesque deformity of her legs and feet that her mother took great pains to hide. Nancy, however, was a friendly child who loved people, and who never for a moment lost faith that she could one day do all the things she wished, and who never worried about how other people saw her. Her mother writes:

"I hadn't known that I was so obviously sensitive about Nancy's body. But underneath, I realized, there was a feeling that I kept hidden and nameless even to myself. It was shame—shame that showed itself in cringing when I took Nancy out in public, in avoiding the questions in people's eyes, in being so quick to cover the deformity. Sometimes I had called it 'embarrassment' and scolded myself for it. Now I knew it was shame and despised myself for it . . . . In the unmasking of it, its power was gone. I'd never be ashamed again. Never as long as I remembered that shame is a festering kind of selfishness."*

---

*Hamilton, M.: Red Shoes for Nancy. p. 76. Philadelphia, J. B. Lippincott, 1955.

Care of the Child Whose Prognosis is Poor

We have talked about the child who has had his activity restricted, although he feels quite well. What do we do for the child who is miserable, steadily deteriorating physically, and whose interest is difficult to sustain? Children do not give up easily, but eventually even they need some hope for the future, to sustain them. There is nothing to be gained—and much to lose—by telling the child that he will never be well and able to participate in normal living, even though evidence does point in this direction. Children have great faith. They believe that adults are all-powerful, and accept their verdicts as simple truths. It is indeed a serious matter to rob a child of hope. Perhaps—who knows—next year or even next month, the breakthrough may come and research may have found a way to alleviate or even cure those conditions now believed to be incurable. Therefore, it would seem to be only good sense to keep the child in the best condition possible; emotionally, physically, and spiritually.

Morse* puts emphasis on the goals of those concerned with the care of those children for whom there is little hope for the future. She stresses the enhancement of their lives for the remaining time they have together. She states, "The ultimate purpose of medical care [is] to enhance the quality of life insofar as possible as long as life remains."

The Child with a Fatal Illness

When a child is discovered to have a disease for which we have as yet found no cure, we feel extremely helpless. The child may have been unwell and may have failed to progress normally for a period of time, or the onset of symptoms may have been very recent, as is usually the case in childhood leukemia.

The shock to the parents, on hearing that their child will not recover, is so deep that they cannot grasp the import of the information they have received. It takes time

*Morse, Joan: The goal of life enhancement for a fatally ill child. Children, *17*:63, 1970.

and a considerable emotional effort before any sort of adjustment can be made. The nurse, whether she is in a hospital situation, in public health, or just acting as a friend, will undoubtedly find herself called upon for support in such cases; and this is a difficult service for her to give.

Nursing Support of the Parents

Most nurses find it extremely difficult to face a child's impending death. It has been said that we all, both doctors and nurses, become too emotionally involved in these situations. We tend to lose perspective, to identify too much with the child, to take it all into ourselves. It becomes exceedingly hard to be the listener or to give comfort to those near to the child. We feel as one with them, and we look for comfort ourselves.

Because of this, and because the nurse cannot work with children for any length of time without being presented with this type of situation, it becomes important that she spend some time preparing herself. It is a poor time to start preparation when confronted with the actual situation.

When young nurses are asked the question "How do you answer the parents when they ask you 'Is my child going to die?'" their answers show both a need to consider this question and a reluctance to do so. The answers frequently are somewhat as follows: "I would say 'You will have to ask your doctor,' or, 'We are all going to die sometime,' or 'No one can be sure of the future.'"

These are evasive answers, and they satisfy no one. When the child asks "Nurse, is this bug I have the kind that kills people?" the nurse may say, "Why, do you think it might be?" or in some other way try to get at his thinking. This is good, but where does she go from there? She knows that he does have a disease from which he is not expected to recover, but does she tell him that, or does she say "Why don't you ask your doctor? I'm not allowed to tell you." Certainly, she does not like either choice, but what does she do?

No one has stereotyped answers for these questions, and no two situations are alike.

The point to be made here, however, is that in order to be of any help whatever, the nurse must have considered the problem very carefully before the situation arose and have formulated some ideas and convictions of her own.

After the parents have had their conference with the doctor, they quite possibly will ask you, the nurse, what is wrong with their child; or, is it true that the child has leukemia? You may be quite certain that they are not asking for a detailed explanation of the child's disease, or of the laboratory findings. Perhaps they do not ask in as pointed a manner, but talk instead about the child of a friend or neighbor who had similar symptoms. Or they may ask for your opinion about their doctor. They may want to discuss a newspaper or magazine article about some condition that seems similar to that of their child. Actually, what they are asking for is reassurance; they want you to tell them they are mistaken; that they misunderstood the doctor; or even that perhaps the doctor is mistaken.

Perhaps you can say something like this: "I think Dr. X is an excellent pediatrician. Why don't you tell me, as well as you can remember, what he told you about Michael?" This may open the way for them to recount the doctor's words as they understood them and in the process, speak of their own feelings and fears.

Although this is not the time to go into detailed explanations of symptoms or treatment, the nurse does have an opportunity to clear up gross misconceptions if they make the picture darker than it needs to be. She must be careful not to contradict anything the doctor has said, but she can suggest that the parent may have misunderstood. She never suggests that the situation is worse than the parent sees it, even though she suspects that it is not being told exactly as the doctor explained. Perhaps this was as much as the parent could absorb at the time, and it is not the function of the nurse to force her further. A physician has had much experience in dealing with people and generally can understand the parents'

reaction. Perhaps he has been aware that these people cannot take the full burden of knowledge at this time, and is giving it to them as they show that they can accept it. Again, nothing is gained by anticipating all the problems and difficulties that must eventually arise. The parents are to discover these soon enough, and need not be burdened with them unnecessarily in advance.

What we are really saying is that the nurse must be willing to listen. She cannot give out false assurance to the parents, nor should she try to impress upon them the gravity of the disease. Her warm, sympathetic manner, her undivided attention, her entire attitude toward the child and the parents are the important factors right now.

Later on, the parents will remember her understanding manner, and may feel that here is a person to whom they can turn. Then suggestions for care, as well as help in finding places and persons from whom they can receive additional help, are welcomed and acted upon.

The young nurse may feel that she is too immature or is too inexperienced to function adequately in such a situation. She is accustomed to see parents as authority figures, and who is she to give advice and comfort? If, however, she has come to understand herself, to accept her position as one of authority as well, she should find that she can handle herself well at these times. However, she should never hesitate to seek counseling herself from those more experienced.

Doctors believe that someone in the child's family must be clearly aware of the child's condition and of its ultimate outcome. If the doctor has been vague or indecisive, the parents may frantically go from place to place, seeking non-existent help. They can exhaust both their financial and emotional resources without having helped their child. They might rather conserve these resources toward making the child as comfortable and happy as possible, for as long a time as he has left. The doctor must not, of course, say that there will never be any help available; but instead present the facts as honestly as he knows how, and ought to assure the parents that should a reliable new treatment be discovered, he will be among the first to use it.

Nursing Support of the Child

The next person to be considered is the child himself. There appears to be no reason to tell a *young* child that he has a fatal illness. Taking hope away from a child robs him of all incentive, and all effort, to get what he can from life itself. A child has blind faith in his doctor; whatever he is told, he believes. If the doctor tells him that he is going to die from his disease, to the child's understanding the doctor is willing him to die; he could prevent it if he would. If a doctor takes the time to explain a particular treatment to a child, he will cooperate to the best of his ability, but he cannot understand or accept his own death.

Nature is very merciful, and as the disease progresses, the child is gradually weaned away from his strong urge to live, his perception becomes dulled, and he no longer has the acute fear and worry that he may have had earlier.

Perhaps we need to examine what death means to a young child. According to Nagy,* it is thought about mainly in terms of motor function. In a study done on a large group of children, she drew several conclusions. She found that the very young child can recognize death as a physical fact, but cannot separate it from life. Thus dead persons can still move, eat and drink, hear and feel. The only restriction comes from outside sources, such as being buried.

When a person goes out of a child's life, even temporarily, he is considered as dead, so that death means living under changed circumstances. Thus, the only painful thing about death to a small child is the fact of separation itself.

As a child grows older and begins to accept and to understand reality, Nagy concludes "he recognizes the fact of physical death but cannot separate it from life—he

---

*Nagy, M.: The child's view of death. *In* Feifel, H.: The Meaning of Death. P. 79. New York, McGraw-Hill, 1959.

considers death as gradual or temporary." Eventually, he comes to accept the definitiveness of death, first as a person who "carries people off," but eventually he begins to understand its personal nature and its universality.

The small child cannot think or reason as an adult. For example, when a child of 3 stood beside her parents at the graveside of her baby sister, an indelible picture she never forgot was engraved on her mind. Yet there were no memories of fear or despair, nor did she connect thoughts of death with herself.

Much no doubt depends upon the atmosphere in which the child has been raised. It does seem however, that it is not the thought of death itself that provokes fear in a small child. It is the thought of separation that throws the child into a panic of fear. A child is willing to face anything he can imagine if his mother is with him. She is his strength, his shield from harm, his ego. In a very real sense, his ideas of God come to him through his ideas about his parents. Therefore, separation from his parents is the greatest fear during childhood. The child who becomes separated from his mother in a crowd does not think of himself as lost; it is his mother who is lost. Perhaps he thinks that she has deserted him—he can never be entirely sure that he has not deserved this. It is the most panic-provoking situation that a child knows.

What then can the thought of death mean to a child but such a separation? Certainly his parents, the all-powerful, are letting him go, and are deserting him. It seems extremely doubtful that any amount of explanation or assurance could be effective. He is faced with the devastating fact that his parents are leaving him, and that is all that he can really understand.

An older child understands his situation a bit better and may pretty well know the outcome, but he might not ask. Any bright child has undoubtedly heard such conditions as his discussed on television or in the neighborhood. If he has normal curiosity he can readily look up the meaning in a medical book or in some other source. In this day, there is but a small chance that the average child might not have a considerable knowledge of his condition.

When such a child seems preoccupied with his own thoughts he will no doubt need help in bringing his doubts and fears out into the open where they can be discussed. One such boy gave an indication of his need for help by his (seemingly) casual questions. "Do many children here get well and go home?" And even "Do you have many children die here?"

Sometimes it appears that a young person would prefer not to have his suspicions confirmed. If so, it would seem that his wishes should be respected. With the newer drugs and treatments used today, children live many months with conditions that have no ultimate cure, and during this time, they may have periods of remission during which they feel quite well. It is difficult at such times to believe in one's own death, nor should the child be asked to do so. It seems unnecessarily cruel to destroy anyone's hope.

There is a considerable divergence of opinion about this. Some believe quite strongly that the older child certainly knows that all is not well, and may have confused and disturbing ideas from hearing and reading things that he only half understands, and can better adjust to facts that are, after all, inevitable. This is the belief held at the National Cancer Institute where children with malignancies are cared for with sympathy and understanding.

The staff personnel believe that the truth is the only answer to questions from patients about what has happened to an absent fellow patient. "The desire to protect a child from a knowledge of death", they say, "may really be a desire to protect ourselves. Though he accepts adult lies, he feels left to cope with his fears and anxieties alone, when he needs adult strength most."*

In The Story of Gabrielle,† the child and

*Truth sustains leukemic children. Medical World News, 6:62, 1965.
†Gabrielson, C.: The Story of Gabrielle. New York, World Books, 1956.

her mother were greatly supportive of each other. Gabrielle never asked about her condition, and although her mother suspected that she knew, she felt that her daughter, a courageous child who believed in frankness, would prefer not to be told. Once, when Gabrielle was in great pain, her mother's courage deserted her, whereupon Gabrielle turned to her and said severely, "I expect you to go through all these things without breaking down."

Of course the nurse must find out from the parents, and from the doctor, what they have been telling the child, and how much they wish the child to know. The nurse must respect the parents' wishes and act in accordance with them, even though she may not agree completely. The child belongs to his parents, and this may be the only way that they are able to cope with the situation. If she is greatly disturbed over their attitude, she may be able to guide them to some qualified person who can help them reach something better, but she never tries to force her own beliefs on them.

Although the nurse believes that she may need to be the person to give support to the grieving parents when a child dies, this does not mean that she should appear detached and reserved. It is supportive and comforting for a parent to know that the child was loved by his nurse, and that she, too, is grieving over his death.

BIBLIOGRAPHY

Brinkhous, Kenneth M.: Changing prospects for children with hemophila. Children 17:222, 1970.
Feifal, Herman, ed.: The Meaning of Death. New York, McGraw-Hill, 1965.
Gabrielson, C.: The Story of Gabrielle. New York, World, 1956.
Goldfogel, Linda: Working with the parent of a dying child. AJN, 70:1675, 1970.
Hamilton, Nancy: Red Shoes for Nancy. Philadelphia, J. B. Lippincott, 1955.
Hemofil—For Modern Management of Hemophilia A: Hyland Division Travenol Laboratories, Inc., Costa Mesa, California.
Morse, Joan: The goal of life enchancement for a fatally ill child. Children, 17:63, 1970.

Rabiner, S., and Telfer, Margaret: Home transfusions for patients with hemophilia a. New Eng. J. Med., *283:*1011, 1970.

Smith, C.: Blood Diseases in Infancy and Childhood. ed. 2. New York, C. V. Mosby, 1966.

Waechter, Eugenia H.: Children's awareness of fatal illness. AJN, *71:*1168, 1971.

Suggested Readings for Further Study

Geis, D.: Mothers' perception of care given their dying children. AJN, *65:*105, 1965.

Katz, Alfred H.: Hemophilia: A Study in Hope and Reality. Springfield, Ill., Charles C Thomas, 1970.

Massie, Robert K.: Nicholas and Alexandra. New York, Atheneum, 1967.

UNIT STUDY QUESTIONS

1. During the toddler age the average child exhibits which of the following maturational traits?
   a. prefers parallel play to cooperative play most of the time
   b. shows ritualistic and dawdling behavior
   c. can be reasoned with
   d. understands right from wrong and can discipline himself
   The answer is:
   1. a and d
   2. b and c
   3. a and b
   4. all of the above

2. Toddlers usually establish ritualistic behavior patterns in order to:
   a. manipulate and control adults in their environment
   b. establish learning behavior patterns
   c. feel secure among the changes and inconsistencies of their world
   d. reestablish their sense of identity

3. At this age, a child is apt to play with his food and show a distinct decrease in appetite. The mother should be advised to:
   a. remember that her child's nutritional needs are less because he is not growing as rapidly as during infancy
   b. accept his lack of appetite and do not push food at him
   c. remove his dishes quietly at the end of the meal and make no comment
   d. teach him that he has to eat the food offered him
   The answer is:
   1. a and d
   2. a, b and c
   3. all of the above
   4. none of the above

4. The best way to deal with the toddler who has a temper tantrum when kept from having his own way is to:
   a. allow him to have his own way to prevent psychic damage
   b. reason with him and show him the futility of expressing anger in this way
   c. try to avoid unnecessary frustrating situations
   d. keep him from injuring himself or others; stay nearby and make no comment
   The answer is:
   1. a and c
   2. c and d
   3. b and d
   4. none of the above

5. The accident rate is high during the toddler period because:
   a. their parents tend to neglect them
   b. their natural curiosity and activity lead them into danger
   c. they are negativistic about everything
   d. they do not comprehend warnings of danger

6. Mrs. T. finds her 3-year-old son eating aspirin tablets. She should first:
   a. induce vomiting
   b. notify the doctor
   c. take him to the emergency hospital
   d. call the poison control center

7. The first suspicion that a toddler has swallowed poison is the appearance of symptoms of toxicity such as:
   a. drowsiness
   b. coma
   c. unusual behavior
   d. nausea or diarrhea

The answer is:
1. a and d
2. b only
3. b and c
4. all of these
5. none of these

8. Young children who have developed lead poisoning usually have
a. eaten fallen plaster
b. lived in old dilapidated homes
c. inhaled fumes from burning battery cases
d. chewed paint from furniture painted with lead base paint

The answer is:
1. a, b, and c
2. b, c, and d
3. a, b, and d
4. all of the above

9. Upon testing, it was found that a child's I.Q. was around 31. According to this report, we would assume that he was
a. borderline
b. mildly deficient
c. moderately deficient
d. severely deficient

10. Of the following generalizations in regard to home care versus institutionalization for the mentally retarded child, the one that is probably the safest to make is:
a. A retarded child has the same basic needs as any other child and these are always best met in the home situation.
b. If a retarded child is living in an environment with children of his own mental age, his personality growth is likely to be fostered and feelings of self-esteem strengthened.
c. Each situation must be evaluated individually in regard to the needs of the child, the family, and the community.
d. The presence of a retarded child in the home fosters feelings of compassion for the entire family unit.

11. The mother of a mentally retarded child can be helped by:
a. showing her that this is a "special" child sent to teach her patience and humility
b. advising her to keep the child out of public view to avoid shame and ridicule for her family and the child
c. giving him special care and telling the other children in the family that his needs come first
d. treating him as one of the family who needs the same amount of affection and discipline as the others

12. Larry, who has been a patient many times because of leukemia, has been admitted in the terminal stage of his illness. How can the nurse best help the parents through this trying time?
a. The nurse can suggest, "Mrs. H., you must be tired. There is nothing you can do for Larry. Why don't you go home and get some rest?"
b. When Mrs. H. asks the nurse to call the doctor, she could say, "Mrs. H., the doctor has done everything he could. There is no use in calling him now."
c. When the nurse sees that the end is near, she can say, "Please leave the room now," because she fears they will break down.
d. The nurse can understand that these people are losing their child and let them stay.

13. The nurse can try to comfort the parents of a child who has just died in such words as:
a. "You did all you could for him. You have nothing to regret."
b. "You must think of your other children now, and forget Larry. He doesn't need you any more."
c. "We all loved him and will miss him too."

Unit Ten: The Preschool Child, Three to Six Years

Normal Growth and Development of the Preschool Child 35

There is no firm demarcation line between the toddler and the preschooler. He does not change markedly between the ages 3 and 3-1/2. There is, however, a marked difference between the ages 2 and 4. Although growth and development proceeds in a continuum from birth to adolescence, the course is nevertheless marked by plateaus and spurts of growth.

The first year of life is marked by the child's rapid physical growth. During the second year, his growth slows down a little while he perfects his muscular control and learns his identity.

By the age of 3, the average healthy child has become a fairly independent person. His weight gain continues to be slower than that of the first year, but his gain in height is somewhat faster, so that he changes from a chubby toddler to a thinner child. During this period of his life, he probably averages a gain of five pounds a year.

Physically, he is losing his baby look and is maturing into the kind of person he is going to be in later life. His incessant activity keeps him too busy to show much interest in food. His mother has no need to worry about this if he is gaining slowly, is healthy and manages somehow to get his required nutrients. His appetite will pick up as he nears school age.

The child of three has developed motor control with increasing skill in finer movements. He is less often frustrated in his efforts to control his environment, and this adds to his self-confidence.

If the child has a consistently warm, accepting relationship with his mother, he can now begin to move away from her into a larger world. No longer do objects cease to be if they are out of his sight. Now he can go away from his mother, secure in the comfortable knowledge that she will be waiting for him when he returns. At three, he should be quite secure, absorbing his world and making it a part of himself. He is friendly and cheerful, and is learning to play with others.

Three and four are interested in everything, and spend their days exploring and learning. In fact, the day is not long enough for them; they would prefer not to go to bed. Their endless calls for drinks, their numerous trips to the bathroom, the slipping downstairs to the living room to tell mother something "very important" are all evidence of their reluctance to leave the scene of living. They just might miss something!

The three- or four-year-old's appetite for living exceeds his capacity. He refuses to admit that he is tired and resists taking a nap. He frequently needs the firmness of an older person who knows that he has reached the limit of his endurance. The adult knows that he has long since reached his.

Our three-year-old, because of his increasing ability to understand is eager to learn. His eagerness ushers him into a more turbulent phase of life as he nears the age of four. At three or four, he is likely to be one big question mark. His curiosity grows as it is fed, until one thinks that he is never quiet.

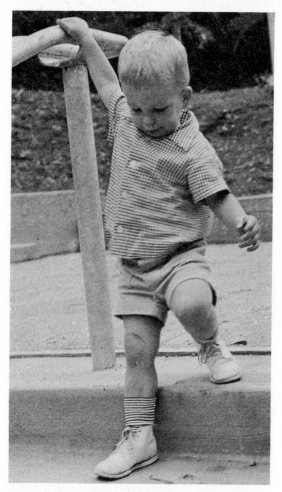

Figure 35-1. The preschool child is becoming independent. (Photograph by Carol Baldwin.)

He has the ability to construct sentences and to formulate ideas. Because he has achieved the power to vocalize, he must use this power to the limit. Not only that, but the sound of his own voice is pleasant to him. His muscles, his intellect, and his voice must all be constantly active.

His world continues to expand during kindergarten until at last, the day arrives when he can enter what to him is the truly grown-up world of the schoolboy.

AVERAGE DEVELOPMENTAL LEVEL OF THE PRESCHOOL CHILD

Three to Four Years

The three-year-old has matured in a number of ways, although he has a nearly complete ignorance of the world outside his home. Evidence of his maturing skills and perception include the following:

can go upstairs alone, alternating his feet,

can run smoothly, jump with both feet together,

is able to pedal a tricycle,

likes to feed himself and to pour from a pitcher—seldom spills,

is able to string large beads, work a very simple puzzle,

builds a tower of 9 or 10 blocks,

can build a bridge with 3 blocks,

can copy a circle,

washes and drys his hands,

can dress self with some help or supervision.

The three-year-old is developing a color sense, and loves to paint or crayon with bright colors. His perception has advanced so that now he sees you as a person, and he has developed a desire to please and to conform—usually.

He likes people, and is able to wait his turn and to share toys if he is not taxed too severely, but he still likes parallel play. He can be reasoned with, within the limits of his understanding.

At three, he is in love with words, trying out sounds for their melody or humor, and indulging in chants and soliloquies.

The three-year-old is beginning to sleep through the night without wetting, and can begin to attend to his own toilet needs. He still needs a long afternoon nap of an hour or two.

His sense of belonging to the family group is evidenced by his pleasure in doing small errands around the house, in putting silverware on the table, or perhaps in carefully drying a dish. He is indeed becoming a person.

Four to Five Years

Four-year-old has increased self-confidence. He can tell you his age, he can adapt more easily to change of routine, and has powers of generalization and abstraction.

His powers of imagination are high; so high that he cannot make a clear distinction between reality and fiction. When his father tells a remarkable story about events of the day, four-year-old will tell sociably about his adventures, which though fantastic, seem no more so to him than his father's story. He is in no way consciously "lying," and should not be told that he is. His mother may be able to help him by casually remarking "That is a good pretend story," if she is able to do so without implying criticism or rejection.

Physical and motor maturation are shown in these areas. He can walk upstairs without grasping a handrail, he can walk backward, he is able to cut out pictures, to copy a square and make a better circle than he could at three, he can dress himself, and can manage large buttons, and he may no longer take an afternoon nap, although many still do.

Intellectually, his questioning is at a peak—largely to validate his own understanding rather than to gain new information—but it seems that he never stops. At this age, he may have an imaginary companion to whom he talks and appears to treat as a real person.

The Five-Year-Old

At five, a child is about ready to join the larger world outside his family. He enjoys kindergarten and may even appreciate the short, daytime separation from home. His abilities include:

    jumping rope, skipping, good motor control,
    can brush his teeth and wash his face,
    knows primary colors, can count to ten, can copy a triangle,
    has a sense of order, likes to finish what he has started—can carry a project over from one day to the next, and his questions are now more meaningful.

The five-year-old tends to be obedient and reliable, is protective of younger children, and tries to comfort the unhappy ones. He now prefers group play and co-

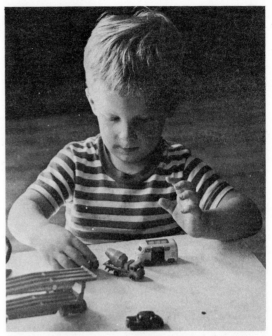

Figure 35-2. The preschool child is also becoming proficient in fine movements. (Photograph by Carol Baldwin.)

operates in projects. Playing house, dressing up, and playing at various adult roles is his specialty. He is beginning to develop an elementary conscience which has some influence in governing his actions.

LANGUAGE DEVELOPMENT

The integration of language with other kinds of behavior is a gradual process. This process begins to accelerate toward the end of the preschool period, but even then progress shows wide individual variations.

Fraiberg* likens the baby's first words to magic incantations, sounds made for pleasure and used indiscriminately to bring about a desired event. Some of the first syllables the child uses are "mama," and he soon discovers that the repetition of these sounds brings the most important person in his life to his side. He also notices that these sounds appear to cause excitement and pleasure, so that he is easily induced to make them again. Soon he tries them out for

*Fraiberg, Selma: The Magic Years. New York, Scribners, 1968.

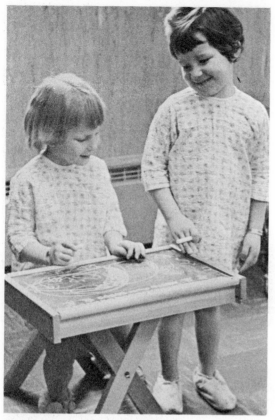

Figure 35-3. The four-year-old can play happily with others.

anything he wants; cookie or whatever. It is some time before he is able to realize that "mama" applies to one person only. Before he matures enough to understand, the syllables come to mean "someone who comforts me and takes away loneliness and pain." If one steps into a toddler's ward during a lonely part of the day, one is confronted with a number of pairs of arms beseechingly raised, while a pleading chorus of "mama, mama" makes one wonder whoever could have been callous enough to conceive of separating a sick, lonely child from his mother.

Stages of Language Development

Even after the young child has discovered that certain words usually bring about desired events, he relies more on gestures and vocal sounds. Generally those caring for him easily interpret these and

respond to the indications of his needs and wants.

As the young child matures words acquire meaning for him. He still enjoys many words for their melody or their humor, but they also begin to carry meaning for him. Dr. Gesell* states, "Jargon at 18 months, words at 2 years, sentences at 3 years." But, he states, this is an oversimplification. By the age of 3 the child starts using words meaningfully. He becomes a talker and is fascinated by words. He chants, he questions, he acts out his words. He talks to himself and to imaginary companions.

The preschooler takes in all he sees and is brimming over with ideas. But his language ability is seldom equal to his desire for expression. This frequently makes him halt and stumble in his speech and repeat sounds.

Nonfluency

Stuttering is defined as speech characterized by repetitions of syllables or words or phrases, by hesitations and tensions in speaking. In view of the fact that nonfluency is normal in many children at about 3 years of age, the question arises whether the nonfluent speech of a 3- or 4-year-old can be called "stuttering." Earlier in the child's life parents think of their child as learning to talk and disregard his lack of fluency. At about the age of 3 or 4, the average child has acquired an essential mastery of his native language. It is then that the adults in the child's life may become critical of his speech. The question arises as to whether speech problems at this age are not created by the listener who calls the child's attention to his hesitancies and repetitions.

It is the belief of speech therapists that most 3- and 4-year-olds are normally nonfluent. It is when the parent, or other adult, worries about this hesitancy and repetition, telling the child to relax, slow down, or "say that over," that trouble starts. In trying to live up to his parents' expectations, he tends to hesitate more, and begins to doubt his

*Gesell, Arnold: The First Five Years of Life. New York, Harper, 1940.

ability to speak acceptably. He tries to speak better than his age and development allow, and so is doomed to failure. Eventually, his problem can become very serious. Studies seem to indicate that when there is little or no concern over a young child's fluency, true stuttering does not occur.*

INFANTILE SEXUALITY

In the past, parents have experienced considerable confusion and misunderstanding over the role that sex plays in the life of the small child. The day when parents punished infants for playing with their bodies or put cuffs on the toddler who found pleasure in rubbing his genitals is long past, or so we hope.

Certainly the infant must do much self-exploring to develop an understanding of his own identity. The very young infant finds his attention captured by the sight of his hands waving aimlessly before his face. When his thumb accidentally comes in contact with his mouth he sucks instinctively, even before birth.

As the infant grows in awareness, he learns that those hands, that thumb, are parts of himself. He begins to explore other parts of his body. This is his way of learning where "I" leaves off and the "other" begins.

Certain regions of the body, the so-called erogenous zones, also offer opportunities for pleasure. One is the mouth; sucking is the earliest pleasure. Another is the anal region with the satisfaction provided on the expulsion of feces. A third zone is the genital area. At first the infant explores this area as he does any other. Somewhat later he finds that manipulation of his genitals gives pleasurable sensations.

The curiosity of the young child is boundless: Why does it get dark at night? Where does the sun go? Why does that bird lie so still? What is dead? Where do babies come from?

*An excellent discussion of the problem of stuttering is given in *Toward Understanding Stuttering,* by Wendell Johnson. Published by the National Easter Seal Society.

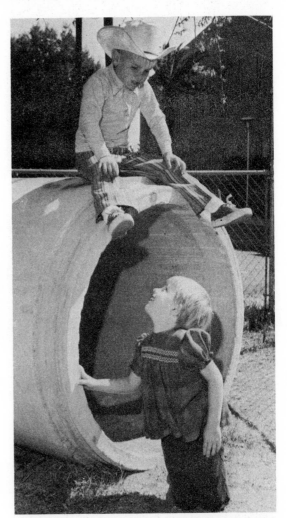

Figure 35-4. The preschool child has developed a sense of daring. (Photography by Carol Baldwin.)

The child has no more innate embarrassment about the baby's origin than he has about the sun or the dead bird. That is, until he senses the adult's embarrassment and reticence. This in turn starts him wondering what mystery the adults are keeping from him.

Sex Differences

It is probably this same curiosity that leads the small boy to wonder what has happened to his sister when he observes that her anatomy differs from his. Much has been written about penis envy and castration fears. It does not seem probable that all

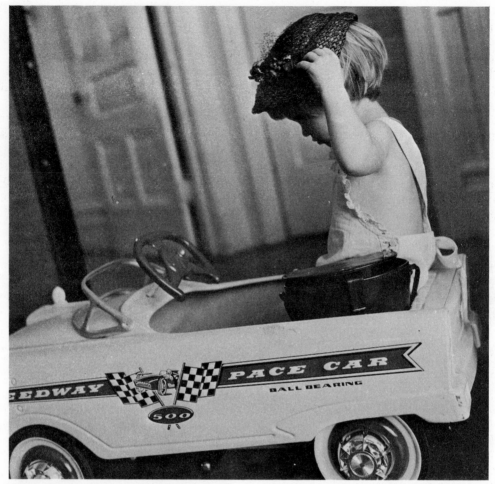

Figure 35-5.   The preschooler enjoys role playing. (Photograph by Carol Baldwin.)

young children go through these traumatic worries. Certainly there are children who willingly accept the explanation that boys and girls are made differently.

However, worry about sex differences does appear in many children at around the age of 3. The child may not—and frequently will not—ask direct questions but will show his concern in different ways.

Sex Play

It is generally curiosity that leads young children to engage in exploratory activities concerning their own bodies and those of other children. A fairly recent study in an urban community showed that out of a large group of 4 year olds, 17% engaged in sexual play at this age. No class differences were found, but there were sharp differences in parental attitudes. Apparently punishment had no more effect than any other parental attitude.*

Gagnon† writes, "The shock for adults of Freud's discoveries was not that children might be involved in sexual activity, but that this activity was not confined to a few evil children and was, in fact, an essential precursor and component of the development of the character structure of the adult."

———

*Sexuality and the Life Cycle. p. 9. SIECUS Study Guide #8, 1967.

†Gagnon, J. H.: Sexuality and Sexual Learning in the Child. Psychiatry, 28(3) August, 1965. Quoted in Sexuality and the Life Cycle, SIECUS Study Guide #8, 1967, p. 7.

Our society does not look with favor on sexual play among children. Certainly the 2- or 3-year-old is fascinated when he observes sexual differences, and the small girl may try valiantly to urinate in the same manner as her brother. But our society has a strong taboo on sex games and exploration. The older child needs to be taught that there are matters that are strictly personal. The older boy who persists in peeking in girls' toilets, or the child who shows an abnormal and persistent interest in observing the opposite sex, may well be motivated by something other than curiosity. In either case the child needs to be taught that this is not acceptable behavior and cannot be condoned. Of more importance, an effort must be made to discover the reason for his obsession and to help straighten out his problems.*

Masturbation

We need to keep in mind that it is as natural for the 2 or 3 year old to play with his genitals as it is for an infant to suck his thumb. "Self-discovery through the self-stimulation of masturbation is one of the ways by which a young child learns to perceive his body as a possible source of pleasure. These early experiences help lay the basis for future acceptance of sex as desirable and pleasurable ...."†

However, parents do have an obligation to teach their children that this is not permissable behavior in public. Every child has to learn that there are behaviors not appropriate in public.

It is not necessarily true that children who have been adequately informed about sex will not engage in sex play. Curiosity is not so easily satisfied. Fraiberg‡ writes that although sex play may be a normal

manifestation of sexual curiosity and interest in early childhood, the child may become more confused and anxious by it. Such a child needs the explanation that looking and playing sex games will not give him the answers to his questions. He needs to have confidence that his mother and father are always willing to help him by answering his questions and working along with him, helping him figure out those aspects that bother him or give him feelings of guilt. But for this assurance to be effective, his parents themselves need to understand the normal sexuality of the young child.

Several valuable, common sense books have been written on this subject. A sampling of these are included in the reference list.

Sex Education for the Young Child

Parents frequently wonder what is the right age to give the child sex information. The answer, of course, is when the child asks questions. Undoubtedly there are young children who show little curiosity in this area. Perhaps it has not occurred to them to wonder. Around the age of 3, however, children who have seen or heard of new babies in their families or those of their friends naturally wonder where they came from.

At this young age, the child's question seldom goes beyond "Where did you get it?"—perhaps with the idea in mind that it would be fun to have one in his family too. The pregnant mother can show where the new baby is living until he grows big enough to live out in the world.

Parents should avoid saying that the baby grows in the mother's "tummy." The literal-minded child will undoubtedly think that something the mother has eaten has brought this about. It is not unusual for a child to worry that something he has eaten may also grow into a baby.

One answer that seems to satisfy is that a baby grows in a special place inside his mother. Usually this is enough to satisfy the very young child. One big mistake parents

*Two exceptionally helpful guides for parents are supplied by SIECUS as study guides. Study Guide #3, Masturbation, and Study Guide #8, Sexuality and the Life Cycle.

†Masturbation, p. 8. SIECUS Study Guide #3.

‡Frailberg, Selma: The Magic Years. New York. Scribners, 1968. Chapter 7.

sometimes make is to tell the child more than he asks for. At this young age, it is best to give him only what is necessary to satisfy his curiosity at the level of his understanding.

As the child grows older, perhaps at 4 or 5, he may commence to wonder how the baby gets out, and, in fact, if it didn't come from something the mother had eaten, how did it get in?

Children normally see no reason for embarrassment or shame over such matters, but the question may come at times when it is embarrassing for the parent. If it is not a good time for a direct, frank answer, it is all right to say, "I'll tell you about it later after our guests go, or when we get home."

The important thing is to tell the child the truth. However, the truth to a small child may seem much more unrealistic than his own fantasies, and it is not at all difficult for him to put several ideas together and come up with quite strange ideas. It is well to find out what the child thinks first and then carefully help him toward reality as he appears ready for it.

For parents who are unsure about how to help the very young child there are a number of helpful books on the market. One excellent book that child and parents will enjoy looking at together is *How Babies are Made*, published by Time-Life Books. Several others are given in the reference list for this chapter.

PSYCHOSOCIAL DEVELOPMENT

In the period between infancy and school age, the young child develops increasing awareness of others. The young infant did not perceive his separateness—his "oneness." He saw himself as an extension of his mother, or mother figure. He spent much time in later infancy exploring his physical body, discovering his separateness from his environment.

As the infant matured, he developed a sense of autonomy, and with it a growing sense of power. His wishes seemed, to him, to bring about desired responses through a kind

of magic. It was no wonder, really, that he thought so. When he was hungry, food appeared, when uncomfortable, soothing arms eased his discomfort. He was a completely egocentric individual.

Now, although the child of 3 or 4 has matured, and his horizons have broadened, there is still a touch of magic in his thoughts. When he gets angry and wants to punish those who displease him, he becomes fearful that his "bad" thoughts will really do harm. In another year or so, he will commence to make the distinction. As Fraiberg says of the 5-year-old, "He explains, 'Cause if you only *think* about doing something like that it can't hurt anyone. But if you *do* it, then you can really hurt someone.'"*

Social Awareness

The preschooler is emerging as a social being, leaving behind his self-preoccupation. He is learning to share, to take turns, to have some feeling for the rights of others. This development does not come overnight, nor does it come without the cooperation and friendly assistance of his family.

The child's parents, of course, assume the responsibility for helping him to independence while at the same time recognizing his immaturity and very real dependence and his need for guidance and for firm limits. He particularly needs to feel his parents' love and enjoyment in him as he is—not as they might wish him to be. Diana Baumrind writes, "today's theories suggest that the lack of parental discipline may make a child insecure about parental love, and conversely that an unloving parent is not likely to successfully control her child's behavior."† This hypothesis and its reverse "that a combination of parental warmth and discipline produces a self-reliant, buoyant, self-controlled child" were tested in a study undertaken at the Institute of Human

---

*Fraiberg, Selma: The Magic Years. New York, Scribners, 1968.

†Baumrind, Diana: Parental control and parental love. *Children, 12:*230, 1965.

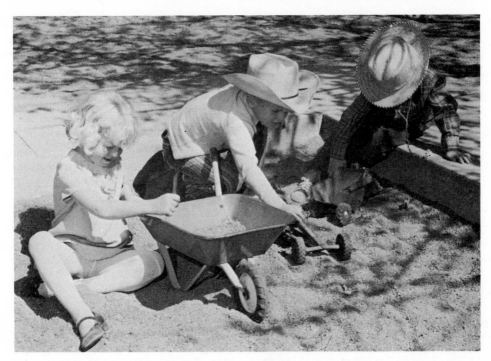

Figure 35-6.   Preschoolers learn to play together.

Development, University of California, Berkeley, in 1963. The conclusion was that "control *and* nurturance . . . are perceived by parent and child as unified manifestations of parental love."

Young children delight in "being grown-up" and feel important when they are accepted as one of the family. They enjoy dressing up in their parents' clothes, taking their "babies" out in carriages, and soberly discussing their problems with each other. There is not yet much discrimination between male and female roles unless their parents have emphasized the difference.

A group of 4-year-olds in nursery school illustrated this point. On coming in from free play outside, the teacher announced that there would be a session for making and using play dough for any who wished to join. Several children gathered around the table, but two boys looked for other activities. Joe placed a doll in a carriage and started pushing it. George asked if he could join him, whereupon Joe appeared to question the "maleness" of his activity and announced

that his child was very sick and he was rushing him to the hospital. George immediately set off an area of the playroom for the hospital and helped operate on the doll patient.

Social Interaction and Educational Experience

The experiences a young child has had in his home and immediate environment have all become a part of him before he becomes a member of the social group in nursery school or in kindergarten. Nursery school, Head Start, kindergarten, day care centers or what you will, also become a part of the child. What do we want from them?

Present day emphasis is strong on teaching reading and mathematical skills to young children. There has been considerable debate on whether very young children benefit from early teaching of such skills, or indeed, whether such early teaching is desirable. The best answer probably is that it depends on the individual child.

Certainly no child should be pushed into programmed learning before he is ready. Some children are eager for the experience and seem to absorb learning without conscious effort. As Scout says in *To Kill A Mockingbird*, "Teach me? He [her father] never taught me anything. Jem says I was . . . born reading."

Helen Heffernan* gives excellent insight into the place of nursery school and kindergarten responsibilities toward the child's development when she writes:

If in nursery school and kindergarten we can provide an environment where the child can discover things for himself through use of material and participation in experiences suited to his developmental level, we have the best chance of helping him achieve his potentialities and express his innate creativity.

---

*Heffernan, Helen: There was a child went forth—a philosophy of early education. *Child Welfare, 49:*552, 1970.

BIBLIOGRAPHY

Arnstein, Helen: Your Growing Child and Sex. New York, Avon, 1968.

Chandler, Caroline A., Lourie, Reginald S., and Peters, Anne DeHuff: Early Child Care. New York, Atherton, 1968.

Duvall, Evelyn: Family Development. ed. 4. Philadelphia, J. B. Lippincott, 1971.

Fraiberg, Selma: The Magic Years. New York, Scribners, 1968.

Gagnon, J. H.: Sexuality and sexual learning in the child. Psychiatry, *28:*3, 1965.

Gesell, Arnold; The First Five Years of Life. New York, Harper, 1940.

Ginott, Haim: Between Parent and Child. New York, Macmillan, 1970.

Heffernan, Helen: There was a child went forth—a philosophy of early education. Child Welfare, *49:*545, 1970.

Johnson, Wendell: Toward Understanding Stuttering. Chicago, National Easter Seal Society for Crippled Children and Adults, 1959.

Lee, Harper: To Kill A Mockingbird. New York, Popular Library, 1971.

Lillywhite, Herold S., Young, Norton B. and Olmsted, Richard W.: Pediatrician's Handbook of Communication Disorders. Philadelphia, Lea and Febiger, 1970.

Masturbation. Siecus Study Guide, No. 3. New York, Sex Information and Education Council (SIECUS), 1970.

Murphy, Lois: The Widening World of Childhood. New York, Basic Books, 1962.

Sexuality and the Life Cycle. Siecus Study Guide, No. 8, 1967.

Suggested Readings for Further Study

Adelson, Richard and Goldfried, Marvin R.: Modeling and the fearful child patient. Journal of Dentistry for Children, *37:*32, 1970.

Andrey, Andrew C. and Schepp, Steven: How Babies are Made. New York, Time-Life Books, 1968.

Baumrind, Diana: Parental control and parental love. Children, *12:*230, 1965.

Jeffers, Camille: Living Poor. Ann Arbor, Ann Arbor Publishers, 1967.

Communicable Diseases of Childhood *36*

DEFINITION OF SOME COMMON TERMS

Antibody. A protective substance in the body produced in response to the introduction of an antigen.

Antigen. A foreign protein that stimulates the formation of antibodies.

Antitoxin. An antibody that unites with and neutralizes a specific toxin.

Carrier. A person in apparent good health, who harbors in his body the specific organisms of a disease.

Carrier state is also a feature of the incubation period, the convalescence, and the postconvalescence of some infectious diseases.

Enanthem. An eruption upon a mucous surface.

Endemic. Habitual presence of a disease within a given area.

Epidemic. An outbreak in a community of a group of illnesses of similar nature, in excess of the normal expectancy.

Erythema. Redness of the skin produced by congestion of the capillaries.

Exanthem. An eruption appearing upon the skin during an eruptive disease.

Host. A man, an animal, or a plant that harbors or nourishes another organism.

Immunity. Passive—immunity acquired by administration of an antibody. Active—immunity acquired by an individual as the result of his own reactions to pathogens. Natural—resistance of the normal animal to infection.

Inapparent infection. Infection in a host without recognizable clinical signs.

Incubation period. The time interval between the infection and the appearance of the first symptoms of the disease.

Macule. A discolored skin spot not elevated above the surface.

Pandemic. A world-wide epidemic.

Papule. A small, circumscribed, solid elevation of the skin.

Pustule. A small elevation of the epidermis filled with pus.

Toxin. A poisonous substance elaborated by certain organisms such as bacteria.

Toxoid. A toxin that has been treated to destroy its toxicity but that retains its antigenic properties.

Vaccine. A suspension of attenuated or killed microorganisms administered for the prevention of a specific infection.

DISEASE CONDITIONS

Diphtheria

Infecting agent. Corynebacterium diphtheriae; the Klebs-Loeffler bacillus.

Source of infection. Discharges from the nose, throat, skin and other lesions of infected persons.

Mode of transmission. Direct contact with patient or carrier, indirect contact with articles contaminated by infected persons.

Immunization. Diphtheria toxoid, usually combined with tetanus toxoid and pertussis vaccine (DTP) at 2 to 3 months of age. Given in three intramuscular injections at 4 to 6 week intervals. Reinforcing dose in about 1 year. Diphtheria antitoxin if presence of the disease itself is suspected. (See Table 26-4 for immunization.)

545

Incubation period. Usually 2 to 5 days, may be longer.

Susceptibility. Infants born of immune mothers are relatively immune until about 6 months of age. Following an attack, a person may become a carrier.

Period of communicability. Variable, until 2 or 3 negative nose and throat cultures are obtained in succession, and at least 24 hours apart. Usually, communicability ceases about 2 weeks after the inception of the disease, unless the person becomes a carrier.

Clinical manifestations. A sore throat, with the formation of a grayish membrane in the tonsillar region, frequently extending into laryngeal region as disease progresses. A raw, bleeding surface is left if this membrane is peeled off. Generalized toxic symptoms of fever, headache, malaise, and body aches. Nasal diphtheria (less frequent) has lesions limited to the nose, and produces no constitutional symptoms unless it spreads to the throat. Toxins produced by the bacilli, and circulated in the bloodstream, cause paralysis, involving any muscle or group of muscles, in about 10% to 15% of all cases.

Treatment—nursing care. Immediate administration of diphtheria antitoxin if the disease is present or if it is suspected, after testing for sensitivity to horse serum, if necessary. Strict bed rest should be maintained, at least until afebrile, or longer if there is cardiac involvement. Tracheotomy may be a life saver.

Complications are many; motor and sensory nerve paralysis, myocarditis, and laryngeal stenosis, are the most common.

Treatment of carriers. Procaine penicillin intramuscularly daily for 7 days usually removes the bacilli. Two negative cultures in succession, 24 hours apart, must be obtained.

Immunity. Recovery from an attack is *usually* followed by long-lasting immunity.

Infectious Hepatitis

Infectious agent. Infectious hepatitis virus.

Source of infection. Feces and blood of infected person.

Immunization agent. None. Immune globulin may be recommended after exposure.

Incubation period. 10 to 50 days.

Susceptibility. General.

Period of communicability. Latter half of incubation period and a few days after jaundice appears.

Clinical manifestations. Abrupt onset with fever, malaise, anorexia, nausea, followed by jaundice. Cases in children are frequently mild without jaundice.

Treatment. No specific treatment. Bed rest and a high caloric diet are recommended. Sanitary disposal of feces.

Immunity. Degree and duration after attack unknown, presumably long-lasting.

Serum Hepatitis occurs following administration of infected blood or use of unsterile needles. Incidence is high among drug addicts. Course of disease same as in infectious hepatitis.

Infectious Mononucleosis

Infectious agent. A herpes-type virus.

Source of infection. Infected persons. Probably transmitted by oral route from person to person.

Immunization agent. None.

Incubation period. Probably 2 to 6 weeks.

Susceptibility. Probably general, but greatest among children and young adults.

Period of communicability. Unknown, probably before symptoms appear until end of fever and clearing of lesions.

Clinical manifestations. Sore throat, fever may be present, enlarged lymph nodes. Generally mild in children. Duration from 1 to several weeks. Isolation is not necessary.

Treatment. No specific treatment.

Immunity. One attack probably confers immunity.

Infectious Parotitis (Mumps)

Infectious agent. The virus of mumps.

Source of infection. Saliva of infected person, droplet spread, indirectly through objects freshly soiled with infected saliva.

Immunization. A live attenuated vaccine prepared in chick embryo cell culture. At present, not recommended for children under 1 year, or for egg-sensitive persons.

Incubation period. 12 to 26 days.

Susceptibility. General, but not so highly communicable as measles or chickenpox, although inapparent attacks may occur.

Period of communicability. Possibly 6 to 7 days before, and up to 9 days after the swelling appears.

Clinical manifestations. Fever, swelling and tenderness of one or both of the parotid glands. The gland becomes painful and tender, and causes difficulty in chewing.

Treatment—nursing care. Bed rest if indicated. Diet should be adjusted to patient's ability to chew.

Complications. Meningoencephalitis in children and orchitis in the adolescent and in adult males. Nerve deafness may occur.

Immunity. Immunity is apparently life-long after clinical or inapparent attacks.

Pertussis (Whooping Cough)

Infectious agent. Bordetella pertussis, the pertussis bacillus.

Source of infection. Discharges from the laryngeal and the bronchial membranes of infected persons, or indirectly by contact.

Immunization agent. Pertussis vaccine, usually given combined with diphtheria and tetanus toxoids (See Table 26-4).

Incubation period. Commonly a week or two, does not exceed 21 days.

Susceptibility. General. Many inapparent cases. Occasionally, second attacks occur.

Period of communicability. Highly communicable in early catarrhal stage. Communicability gradually decreases; after 6 weeks patients considered noninfectious.

Clinical manifestations. An acute bacterial disease involving the trachea, the bronchi and the bronchioles. The initial stage, with an irritating cough, continues for

1 or 2 weeks. The cough gradually becomes paroxysmal, with the second stage lasting from 1 to 2 months. There is a characteristic crowing or inspiratory whoop. The paroxysm is frequently followed by vomiting. Fatality in the United States is low. The majority of deaths, about 70%, occur among infants under 1 year of age.

Treatment. Antibiotics may be given to shorten the duration of symptoms. Sedation may be used to reduce vomiting and forestall convulsions. Constant nursing attendance for infants or severely affected children is essential. Suctioning to remove tenacious secretions is necessary. Nutrition and electrolyte balance should be carefully monitored. Bronchopneumonia may be a complication.

Immunity. One attack procures long-lasting immunity.

Poliomyelitis

Infectious agents. Poliovirus types 1, 2, and 3.

Source of infection. Direct contact with infected persons, feces and with pharyngeal secretions.

Immunization agent. Sabin oral or Salk vaccine for types 1, 2, and 3.

Incubation period. Three days to 3 weeks.

Susceptibility. General. Probably many inapparent infections among unprotected persons.

Period of communicability. Virus isolated from throat secretions as early as 36 hours, and from feces 72 hours after infection. The virus persists in the throat for about a week and in feces for 3 to 6 weeks, or longer.

Clinical manifestations. Fever, headache, gastrointestinal disturbance, stiffness in the neck and in the back, and paralysis in the paralytic type.

Treatment—nursing care. Bed rest, use of a hard mattress and of bed boards. Body hot packs to relax muscles. For the bulbar type, tracheotomy may be required, and a tank-type respirator for respiratory failure.

Complications. If it is the paralytic type,

muscular paralysis may be permanent, causing atrophy of the affected muscles.

Immunity. Type-specific immunity usually follows infection.

Rabies (Hydrophobia)

Infectious agent. Virus of rabies.

Source of infection. Wild and domestic rabid animals. In the United States wild bats and skunks are frequently rabid. Mode of transmission is through the bite of a rabid animal. Domestic animals may be infected by being bitten by a rabid wild animal.

Immunization agent. Pre-exposure vaccine is recommended for animal handlers and certain laboratory workers. Immunization is recommended for domestic dogs and cats.

Prevention. In areas where rabies in animals is prevalent, rabies vaccine is started immediately after the individual is bitten, unless the biting animal has been adequately immunized. Unprovoked attacks are likely to mean the animal is rabid. If the biting animal can be apprehended, it should be confined and observed for 7 to 10 days. At the first sign of symptoms in the animal, vaccination of the bitten person should start at once.

Antirabies vaccine is given daily for 14 to 21 days. Given subcutaneously in the abdomen, lower back or lateral aspect of thighs. Rabies vaccination carries a small risk of post-vaccinal encephalitis.

Incubation period. Usually 3 to 6 weeks.

Period of communicability. In rabid animals, 3 to 5 days before clinical signs are evident, and throughout the course of the disease. Isolation of bitten individual throughout course of disease.

Clinical manifestations. Onset begins with apprehension, fever, headache. Progresses to paralysis and spasms of muscles of deglutination (swallowing). Delirium and convulsions follow. Death is due to respiratory paralysis.

Prognosis. Recovery is rare.

Rubella (German Measles, 3-day Measles)

Infectious agent. Virus of rubella.

Source of infection. Direct contact, droplet, and freshly contaminated articles. It may be air-borne.

Immunization agent. Live attenuated rubella virus vaccine has been demonstrated to protect 90% to 95% of susceptibles against natural exposure. In the United States the vaccine is recommended for boys and girls between the ages of 1 and 12 years of age.

Incubation period. 14 to 21 days.

Susceptibility. Universal. The condition may be confused with other rashes.

Period of communicability. About a week before and at least 4 days after onset of rash.

Clinical manifestations. Mild catarrhal symptoms and mild fever may be present. There may be enlargement of the postauricular, the suboccipital or the postcervical lymph nodes. No Koplik spots. There is a rash resembling measles or scarlet fever. The symptoms may be mild and may go unnoticed.

Treatment—nursing care. Bed rest if febrile.

Complications. Rare, except in newborns contracting the infection in utero. (See *Congenital Rubella.*)

Immunity. One attack usually confers life-long immunity.

Rubeola (Measles)

Infectious agent. Measles virus.

Source of infection. Person to person, from nose and throat secretions, droplet spread, and from articles freshly contaminated with nose and throat secretions. These may be air-borne.

Immunizing agent. Live, attenuated vaccine.

Incubation period. 10 to 14 days.

Susceptibility. Universal.

Period of communicability. About 4 days before the rash to 5 to 6 days after the rash appears.

Clinical manifestations. Coryza, with a dry cough and a moderate fever. Photophobia. There are Koplik spots on the buccal membrane for a few hours, disappearing before the rash appears. A maculopapular rash appears on the third or fourth day, starting behind the ears, around the hair line, and spreads over the entire body.

Treatment—nursing care. Symptomatic. Protect the eyes from glare. Tepid baths and soothing lotion relieve itching. Provide a humidified atmosphere for a troublesome, harsh cough. Fluids, diet as desired and bed rest.

Complications. Pneumonia, nephritis, otitis media, and encephalitis.

Immunity. Permanent immunity is usual after an attack.

Salmonellosis

Infectious agent. Numerous serotypes of salmonellae have been found in both animals and man.

Source of infection. Feces of patients, infected animals, both domestic and wild, poultry products, some pet foods. The disease is acquired by ingestion of the organisms. Pet turtles and chicks have carried the organism. Epidemics are usually traced to commercially processed meat products, raw or lightly cooked eggs or egg products, any foods contaminated by a food handler or by the infected person or animal.

Immunization agent. None, other than proper sanitation.

Incubation period. Six to 72 hours after ingestion of contaminated food.

Susceptibility. General.

Period of communicability. Throughout course of infection.

Clinical manifestations. Acute diarrhea, nausea and vomiting, abdominal pain. Dehydration, especially in infants, may be severe. Fever is usually present.

Treatment. Temporary discontinuance of oral feeding in vomiting and diarrhea. Fluid and electrolyte replacement. (See *Diarrhea,* page 394)

Immunity. None.

Streptococcal Infections

Scarlet fever, streptococcal pharyngitis.

Infectious agent. Group A hemolytic streptococci of at least 40 distinct types. (Scarlet fever is a streptococcal sore throat with a rash.)

Source of infection. Direct contact and large droplet infection. Rarely by indirect contact.

Immunization agent. None. Patients with rheumatic fever, or who have rheumatic heart disease should be given continuous prophylaxis of penicillin or erythromycin.

Incubation period. Usually 1 to 3 days.

Susceptibility. General.

Period of communicability. Greatest during acute phase of illness. Carrier state may persist.

Clinical manifestations. In *Scarlet fever:* fever, sore throat, and rash. Rash is a fine erythema appearing most often on neck, chest, and folds of skin, rarely on face. In severe infections, nausea and vomiting may be present.

Streptococcal sore throat. Same as above but without rash.

Treatment. Penicillin, started as soon as possible and continued for at least 10 days, regardless of mildness of infection. Erythromycin is preferred as alternative to penicillin. Bed rest and treatment of specific symptoms as needed.

Immunity. None.

Streptococcal Impetigo

(See Conditions of newborn.)

Tetanus (Lockjaw)

Infectious agent. Clostridium tetani, an anaerobic organism.

Source of infection. Contaminated soil, dust, animal or human feces. Relatively rare in industrialized countries. A hazard among drug addicts using drugs parenterally.

Fatality rate is high, especially among infants. Tetanus neonatorum usually occurs through infection of the unhealed umbilicus.

Immunization agent. Tetanus toxoid (see timetable of immunizations).

Incubation period. Commonly 4 days to 3 weeks.

Susceptibility. General. Infection occurs through contaminated wounds.

Period of communicability. Not directly transmitted from man to man.

Clinical manifestations. Painful muscular contractions, especially of the masseter (mandible) and neck muscles.

Treatment. Tetanus antitoxin. Antibiotics, sedation and muscle relaxants. Nursing care in quiet surroundings is essential and tracheotomy as needed. Artificial respiration may be necessary. Intravenous fluids to maintain fluid balance. Isolation of patient not necessary.

Tetanus neonatorum treated essentially as outlined.

Immunity. Recovery from tetanus does not imply immunity.

Typhoid Fever

Infectious agent. Salmonella typhi, the typhoid bacillus.

Source of infection. Patients and carriers, through the feces and the urine of infected persons. From direct contact, contaminated water, raw food and vegetables, milk, and milk products. Flies may be sources of infection under certain conditions.

Immunization agent. Typhoid vaccine. Commonly used in areas of possible exposure. Reinforcement is recommended every 3 years.

Incubation period. Usually 1 to 3 weeks.

Susceptibility. General, with some immunity through unrecognized infections.

Period of communicability. Usually from the first week through convalescence, until three negative stool and urine cultures are obtained in succession, at least 24 hours apart. The patient may become a carrier.

Clinical manifestations. Fever, malaise, ulceration of Peyer's patches in intestines, an enlarged spleen, rose spots on the trunk, emaciation, fatigue, and anemia.

Treatment—nursing care. Bed rest, proper nutrition, and maintenance of fluid balance. Tepid sponges for the reduction of fever, and transfusions for anemia, ampicillin or chloramphenicol is used for treatment. The doors and windows of the patient's room should be screened against flies. Stools and urine should be mixed with disinfectant before being discarded. Family contacts should not be employed as food handlers during the period of contact. Carriers must register with health authorities, are not allowed to act as food handlers, and are instructed in personal hygiene. Cholecystectomy is highly effective for ending the carrier state. Carriers must have six consecutive negative cultures taken one month apart before being released from supervision.

Complications. Hemorrhage and bowel perforation is less common in children than in adults. Urinary infections and nervous complications may follow.

Immunity. A high degree of resistance to the disease usually follows an attack.

Varicella (Chickenpox)

Infectious agent. The varicella-zoster virus.

Source of infection. Respiratory secretions of infected persons (droplet). Articles soiled by discharges from the mucous membranes and from the skin of infected persons. Air-borne.

Immunizing agent. None.

Incubation period. Two to 3 weeks.

Susceptibility. Universal. Herpes zoster has been known to be an original manifestation in a few children.

Period of communicability. About 1 day before the rash to 6 days after first crop of vesicles.

Clinical manifestations. Sudden onset of a slight fever, a maculopapular skin eruption, which then becomes vesicular and leaves a granular scab. The rash appears in crops, with several stages of maturity present at the same time. There is severe itching and generalized lymphadenopathy.

Herpes zoster. This is a localized manifestation of same virus. Vesicles appear along the nerve pathways, and severe pain is usually present. It is rare in children, occurring generally in older adults.

Treatment—nursing care. Measures to relieve itching and to prevent infection from scratching include starch baths and calamine lotion. Fingernails should be kept short and mittens should be used if scratching is not controlled. The disease varies from mild to severe. Bed rest should be ordered, as well as sedation if itching cannot otherwise be relieved. Oral antihistamines reduce itching.

Complications. Secondary bacterial infection from scratching. Encephalitis and hemorrhagic complications are rare. Fatal chickenpox has occurred in patients receiving corticosteroid therapy. Such persons should be protected from exposure. If they are exposed, dosage should be reduced as rapidly as possible.

Immunity. No evidence of acquired lasting immunity. The condition may appear as herpes zoster in older people.

Variola (Smallpox)

Infectious agent. Variola virus.

Source of infection. Respiratory discharges from infected persons, from lesions of the skin and from the mucous membrane. Separated scabs may remain infectious for years.

Immunizing agent. Cowpox virus by vaccination.

Incubation period. From a week to 16 days.

Susceptibility. Universal.

Period of communicability. From 2 or 3 days prior to rash until all of the scabs disappear.

Clinical Manifestations. Sudden onset of fever, malaise, headache, severe backache, and abdominal pain, with prostration for about three to four days, followed by a rash similar to that of chickenpox. The lesions, however, are deeper.

Treatment—nursing care. Symptomatic treatment and adequate nutrition (may require tube feeding). Sedation should be given as needed.

Complications. Bacterial infections of the skin are not so common since the use of antibiotics. Bronchopneumonia is relatively common.

Immunity. Permanent immunity usually follows recovery.

*Vaccination against smallpox.** Primary vaccination procedure is recommended during the second year of life. The preferred site is the outer aspect of the upper arm. No cleansing of the skin is needed unless it is obviously dirty, in which case it can be gently wiped with water and allowed to dry. Fully potent vaccine must be used. There are three methods used. In the *multiple pressure* method a drop of vaccine is placed on the skin and a series of pressures made with a sharp needle. In the *multiple puncture* technique a forked needle is used. There is also a *jet injector* which deposits a specially prepared vaccine intradermally. No dressing should be applied.

Reactions. A "major reaction" should follow vaccination. A major reaction is one which presents a pustular or vesicular reaction 1 week after vaccination, or a definite induration surrounding the scab or ulcer remaining at the point of the vaccine insertion.

The World Health Organization's Committee on Smallpox recognizes only two responses to vaccination and revaccination: a major reaction and an equivocal reaction. The older terms of immune or vaccinoid reactions are eliminated. Revaccinations should produce major reactions in 80% to 90% of subjects. All other responses are termed equivocal and the subject should be revaccinated.†

Contraindications to vaccination for smallpox. A serious condition, called eczema

*Sources: Control of Communicable Diseases in Man, American Public Health Association, 1970, and the "Red Book" Academy of Pediatrics, 1970.
†Ibid.

vaccinatum, results when an infant with eczema is vaccinated. The eczematous skin becomes covered with vesicles resembling the primary one, and the infant becomes seriously ill. The mortality rate is as high as 40% to 50%. This reaction also takes place if the infant's exposure is to the vaccination of another person.

Other conditions that are contraindications to vaccination are leukemia, hypogammaglobulinemia, acute illnesses and corticosteroid therapy.

Vaccine immune globulin (VIG) is used in the treatment of eczema vaccinium.

ISOLATION PROCEDURE FOR COMMUNICABLE DISEASES

Definition

A separation from contact with others of a patient having a *communicable* disease. The nurses caring for the patient use aseptic medical technique; that is, they use proper measures to prevent transmission of the infection to other patients, to visitors or to personnel involved in the child's care.

Principles

Medical aseptic technique is effective in preventing cross-contamination only to the extent to which everyone caring for the child adheres to the rules.

Medical aseptic technique may be employed to protect susceptible persons from the infectious diseases of the patient, or to protect a highly susceptible patient from the hospital environment. (See *Protective Technique for Highly Susceptible Patients.*)

Protective Measures

A. Type of unit
1. The unit for the care of a child with communicable disease should be a private room, a cubicle, or a multiple-bed room admitting children with the same type of infection.
2. The unit should be equipped with running water, a wall container of liquid or powdered soap (hexachlorophene soap preferred), and wall container of paper towels.
3. Furnishings should be attractive, with eye appeal, but simple and easy to clean.
4. All utensils not necessary for the child's care should be removed from the unit before admission, i.e., the bedpan (if the patient is an infant) and similar articles.

B. Equipment in contaminated area
1. A sign saying "isolation" or some other indication that special technique must be used, and readily observable from outside the room.
2. An individual fever thermometer with its container, a solution for disinfection of thermometer (alcohol 70%, zephiran chloride, or an alcohol-iodine preparation) attached to wall out of reach of child.
3. A linen hamper with bag for used linen (covered).
4. A covered container for soiled diapers (as necessary). (A step-on can if possible, with a bag inside.)
5. Waxed paper or a plastic bag lining the wastebasket.
6. A blood pressure cuff and a stethoscope.
7. The usual equipment for the care of a child.

C. Equipment in clean area should include a stand containing
1. Laundry bags, especially marked for isolation (red tag, striped, or marked "isolation").
2. Clean waxed paper or plastic bags, and brown paper bags.
3. Clean wrapping for materials to be autoclaved. May include long boat for syringes, needles, and for instruments to be autoclaved.
4. Masks (if used).
5. Isolation gowns.

D. Additional equipment
1. A jar containing gauze flats or rags soaked in disinfecting solution for wiping off a bed-side table, a bed, and window ledges. (Microphene, alcohol.)

2. A door mat in the doorway. Two large trays lined with absorbent pads—one saturated with a phenolic solution, one dry. An alternative—clean cloth covers to be slipped over shoes when entering the room.

E. Procedure for entering unit
1. Wash hands.
2. Collect linen and equipment needed for care of the patient.
3. Remove your watch. If your watch will be needed in the care of the child, wrap in plastic and take it into the unit with the rest of the equipment.
4. Don mask (if used). Make sure the mask is securely tied, covering your nose and your mouth. Adjusting or replacing the mask while caring for a child invites the spread of infection.
5. Put on a clean gown, using care to cover the back of the uniform completely. If the gown is long-sleeved, push the sleeves back to expose the forearms.
6. Enter the unit with the understanding that all objects are considered contaminated.
7. Wash your hands and your arms for 2 to 3 minutes using friction. Use care to wash between the fingers. Clean under your nails with an orangewood stick.

Procedures Related to Patient Care

A. Care of food tray and dishes. (Children)
1. The tray may be brought to the door of the unit by a clean nurse, the dishes handed to nurse in unit, and the tray returned to the serving room.
    (Alternative—a disposable tray may be used, taken into the room, and discarded after use.)
2. Disposable dishes may be discarded after use. Attractive disposable dishes are now available and no longer make food appear unappetizing.
3. Silverware may be used in the room, washed, wrapped, and may be sent to be autoclaved with other equipment.

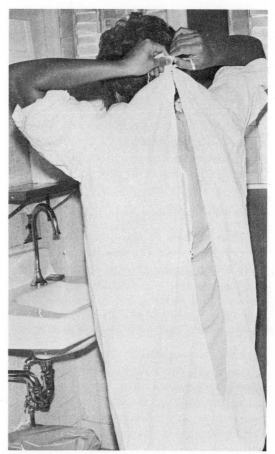

Figure 36-1. Before attending a patient in isolation the nurse puts on a clean gown, making sure to cover the back of the gown completely.

    (Alternative—plastic spoons may be used and discarded.)
4. Variation. In hospitals where facilities are available and housekeeping personnel are properly instructed, regular trays and dishes may be used, removed from a unit and put in a dishwashing machine with other dishes.

B. Care of nursing bottles. (Infants, toddlers)
1. Disposable bottles and nipples may be taken into the room and then discarded after use.
2. Glass bottles and nipples should be washed in the room, wrapped and sent to be autoclaved with other equipment.
3. Plastic bottles should be gas autoclaved (if possible) or boiled.

4. Variation. In hospitals where facilities are available and personnel are properly instructed, bottles and nipples may be washed in a unit, returned to the bottle-washing room and sterilized with other bottles.

C. Weighing child

(Infant.) The clean nurse should place the scale outside the doorway of the unit, cover the funnel with a clean sheet, and balance the scale. The nurse in the unit places the infant on the scale, and the clean nurse manipulates the weights. After weighing, the unit nurse takes the sheet and discards it in the linen hamper in the unit.

(Child.) The clean nurse brings the scale to the doorway, places paper on the platform, and manipulates the weights. The paper is disposed in a wastebasket in the unit. If the child has touched the scale, wipe it with a disinfectant solution.

D. Transporting child. (To X-ray, etc.)

Place two clean sheets on the wheelchair or on the stretcher. The nurse in the unit places the child on an inner sheet, and the clean nurse wraps the sheets around him. Personnel must be informed of the infectious nature of the child's condition. On return, both sheets are taken into the unit and are placed in the linen hamper in the unit.

E. Obtaining specimens

The clean nurse stands outside the unit, and holds the receptacle. The nurse in the unit transfers the specimen. If only one person is available and the container must be taken into a unit, the outside of the container should be thoroughly washed with an antiseptic solution.

F. Disposal of wastes

Uneaten food may be scraped into a waxed bag in the wastebasket, and liquids may be poured into the sink.

Potties and bedpans may be emptied into the disposal system. If these must be taken to a common utility room to be emptied, the following procedure is acceptable:

The nurse should remove her mask and her gown, scrub and take the bedpan or the potty in one hand, keeping the other hand clean. She should use her clean hand for opening doors, handling the flusher and similar things. Return the bedpan or the potty to the unit, scrub and change into a new gown.

Note: If the patient is a small child who urinates frequently, it may be helpful to keep a urine specimen bottle or some other container in the room, thus avoiding too frequent trips to the utility room.

G. Nursing care of child

The child in isolation has a particular need of companionship, diversion and personalized care. He needs to be held, rocked, loved, and played with. Practically any toy may be taken into the unit, including books, papers, and plastic toys, if gas autoclaving is available. If it is not available, toys should be those that can be easily cleaned by soaking in a disinfecting solution or disposable.

Visitors. The presence of the child's parents is important for his emotional well-being, and they should be encouraged to visit. They will need to be instructed about wearing the isolation gown, handwashing, and the undesirability of stepping out of the room for any purpose without taking the necessary precautions. Printed instructions are useful, but they must not take the place of demonstration and personal instruction.

H. "Scrubbing out."

Any equipment or material used in the unit must be made free from contamination before it is deemed safe for use with other patients.

Care of Used Linen

1. Place the diaper bag (closed) in the larger laundry bag in the unit. (Some hospitals may keep diapers separate.)
2. The clean nurse stands outside the doorway holding a clean isolation laundry bag open. The opening should be turned down into a cuff covering the nurse's hands.
3. The nurse in the unit closes the contaminated bag and drops it into the clean bag, using care to avoid con-

taminating the outside of the clean bag. The laundry bag in the room needs to be emptied before becoming so full that it presents difficulty when double-bagged.

4. The clean nurse turns the cuff up, closes the outer bag and makes sure that the laundry is identified as "isolation."

5. The bag is placed in the laundry chute, or in the area for the collection of soiled linen.

    Alternative. If only one nurse is available, a clean isolation bag may be hung in a laundry hamper in the doorway and the contaminated bag dropped into it. This presents the problem of leaving used linen uncovered in a clean area for the period of time it takes for the nurse to leave the unit.

Care of Wastebasket

1. The clean nurse folds the edges of a clean paper bag in a cuff, covering her hands.
2. The nurse in the unit closes the waxed bag holding wastes and drops it into the clean bag.
3. The clean nurse closes the outer bag and deposits it in a covered waste can in the utility room.

Removal of Watch from Unit

    The nurse in the unit unwraps the plastic cover, and drops the watch into the clean nurse's hand.

Treatment Trays and Equipment from Central Supply

1. The nurse in the room washes equipment, drys it and places it in a wrapper or a small bag designated for this purpose.
2. The clean nurse holds a second bag and receives the contaminated bag in same manner as for linen or for waste.
3. The outer bag is properly labeled "isolation" and designated as being for steam or for gas autoclave.
4. If the boat for instruments and syringes is used, the outside is kept clean. Tape the cover to the boat, label it, and send it to central supply to be autoclaved.

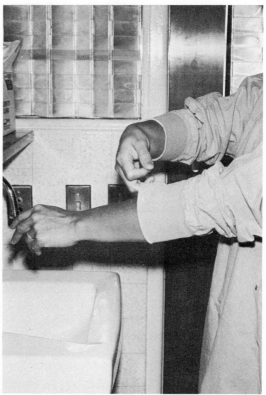

Figure 36-2. When the gown is long-sleeved, the sleeves must be pushed back to expose the forearms.

Equipment to be Returned to Pediatric Ward

1. Wash, wrap and bag as indicated above. Label it to include the ward to which the articles are to be returned.
2. Articles for steam autoclave may include bath basins, emesis basins, any monel, aluminum or stainless steel receptacles, glass bottles, rubber goods and steel or iron toys.
3. Articles for gas autoclave may include plastic utensils, paper, books, dolls, and plastic toys.
4. Materials that cannot be gas or steam autoclaved (or if gas autoclave is not available).
   a. Soak in a disinfecting solution (Dicrobe or Zephiran) if possible.
   b. Articles such as stethoscopes, blood pressure cuffs, and manometers should be aired before being used on other patients.

Leaving Unit

1. Before leaving the unit, place a fresh laundry bag on the holder and a fresh waxed bag in the wastebasket.
2. Untie the strings of the gown at the back of the waist.
3. Wash hands and arms thoroughly.
4. Untie the strings at the back of the neck.
5. Slip the right hand under the cuff of the left sleeve, and pull it over the left hand.
6. Use the left hand inside the sleeve to pull the right sleeve down.
7. Remove the gown, folding the outer side inward and avoiding touching the outer (contaminated) side.
8. Place the folded gown in the laundry bag in the unit.
9. Wash hands and arms thoroughly, using a paper towel to handle the faucets.
   Note: Reuse technique for gowns is not recommended because of the difficulty in keeping the gown free from contamination.
10. Remove mask, handling it by the strings only. Drop it into the bag for contaminated masks, or discard it if it is disposable.
11. Wash hands in clean area after leaving the unit.

Care of Room

1. The bedside table, the bedframe, the window ledges, and the shelves should be wiped off daily with microphene, alcohol, Zephiran or some other agent.
2. Floors should be wet mopped. Housekeeping personnel, if properly instructed, may clean the room.

Termination of Isolation

If isolation has been maintained only as a precaution until the communicability of disease has been determined, and until the cultures have proved negative, precautions may be discontinued and routine care may be resumed.

Removal of Patient from Isolation

When the child's condition is determined to be no longer infectious, the following procedure may be employed.

1. Collect a clean bath basin, soap, a sheet, a wash cloth and towels and a bath blanket.
2. Put on a gown, enter the unit with utensils, and wash your hands.
3. Undress the child, place him on a clean sheet, and give him a sponge bath and a shampoo.
4. Wrap the child in a clean blanket and hand him to the nurse outside the room.
5. The child should be dressed and moved to a clean unit.

Terminal Cleaning of Room

1. Bag out utensils in the routine manner for isolation.
2. Notify Housekeeping department that the room is ready for cleaning.

PROTECTIVE TECHNIQUE FOR HIGHLY SUSCEPTIBLE PATIENTS

A susceptible person is a person presumably without resistance against a particular pathogenic agent and who is therefore liable to contract the disease if exposed to it.

Certain child patients need protection against the hospital environment either because of their increased susceptibility to infection, or because of the nature of their own disease. Such patients may include the following:

Children whose leukocyte count becomes abnormally low, because of the drugs used in the treatment of their condition, or because of the nature of the disease itself.

Premature infants.

Burned children (these children will usually need both strict isolation and protective technique during the period of increased susceptibility).

Infants or children whose condition is such that any superimposed infection may have serious consequences.

Technique for Protective Measures

This technique differs from the isolation procedure in these particulars.

1. All articles going *into* the unit must be aseptically clean.
2. Articles coming out of the unit do not need to be sterilized, unless the patient has an infection.
3. Persons with infections should automatically avoid caring for sick children. If the patient is a highly susceptible child, this rule assumes paramount importance.

BIBLIOGRAPHY

Benenson, Abram, ed.: Control of Communicable Disease in Man. ed. 11. New York, American Public Health Association, 1970.
Gallagher, Richard: Diseases that Plague Modern Man. Dobbs Ferry, New York, Oceana Publications, 1969.
Report of the Committee on Infectious Diseases. (Red Book) ed. 16. Evanston, Ill., American Academy of Pediatrics, 1970.

Suggested Readings for Further Study

Smith, Margaret H. D.: Immunization: The current scene. Hospital Practice, *4:*42, 1969.

Nursing Care in Conditions Affecting the Preschool Child *37*

NEPHROTIC SYNDROME

A number of different types of nephrosis in the nephrotic syndrome have been identified. The most common in children is *lipoid nephrosis*. All forms of nephrosis have early characteristics of edema and proteinuria, so that definite clinical differentiation cannot be made early in the disease.

Lipoid nephrosis is a condition the main clinical manifestation of which is a generalized edema that becomes so great the child may double his normal weight. It has a course of remissions and exacerbations, usually lasting for months. Although the mortality rate remains high, present-day management has allowed many more children to survive until the disease disappears spontaneously than had previously been the case. Previously, before the availability of effective antibacterial agents and corticosteroid therapy, recovery rates were estimated as low as 30%. Present-day estimates place the recovery rate as high as 75% with the use of intensive steroid therapy and protection against infection.

Etiology

The cause of lipoid nephrosis is not known. It is in rare cases associated with other specific diseases. It is now generally believed that lipoid nephrosis is not a stage of acute glomerulonephritis, as other forms of nephrosis may be.

Incidence

The nephrotic syndrome is present in about 7 children per 100,000 population under 9 years of age. The lipoid form has its onset, on the average, at 2-1/2 years.

Pathophysiology

Early in the disease, only minimal changes in the glomeruli can be observed under ordinary light microscopy. With electron microscopy a characteristic lesion of the foot processes of the glomerular epithelium can be observed.

Laboratory findings include marked proteinuria, with large numbers of hyaline and granular casts in the urine. Hematuria is not usually present. Blood serum protein is reduced, and the total serum globulin level is normal or increased, with a reversed serum-globulin ratio.

Clinical Manifestations

Edema is usually the presenting symptom, appearing first around the eyes and ankles. As the swelling advances, the edema becomes generalized, with a pendulous abdomen full of fluid. Respiratory embarrassment may be severe, and edema of the scrotum is characteristic. Hydrothorax may be present. The edema shifts with change of position of the child when lying quietly or walking about. Anorexia, irritability, and loss of appetite develop. Malnutrition may become severe. The generalized edema masks the loss of body tissue, causing the child to present a chubby appearance, but after diuresis, the malnutrition becomes apparent. These children are usually susceptible to infection, and repeated acute respiratory conditions are the usual pattern.

Treatment

The management of nephrosis is a long process, with reversals and reappearance of symptoms. The use of corticosteroids has induced remissions in most cases and reduced recurrences. Corticosteroid therapy usually produces diuresis in about 7 to 14 days, but the drug is continued until a remission occurs. Prednisone is the most commonly used. Intermittent therapy is continued every other day, or for three days a week. Daily urine testing for protein is continued whether the child is at home or in the hospital.

Antibiotic therapy using a broad spectrum antibiotic such as ampicillin is used to protect the child against infection. The use of diuretics may not be necessary when diuresis can be induced with steroids. Paracentesis is rarely needed for those children who respond well to medical treatment. A general diet, appealing to the child's poor appetite, is recommended. Salt should be kept to a minimum. The parents will need encouragement and support for the long months ahead. The course of the disease is seldom less than about 18 months.

Long-Term Care

Affected children are usually hospitalized for diagnosis, a thorough evaluation of their status in regard to their general health and specific condition, and for the institution of therapy. A course of antibiotic is given to clear up any concurrent infection, and unless unforeseen complications develop, the child is discharged with complete instructions for management.

A written plan is most useful to help parents follow the program successfully. They must keep a careful record of home treatment, and bring it to the clinic or to the physician's office at regular intervals.

This home record includes the daily weight, taken at the same time each day, a daily record of urinary proteins, and a daily record of medications as to the kind, the amount, and time given.

The parents must be taught the reactions that may occur with the use of steroids, and also be made to understand the adverse effects of abrupt discontinuance of these drugs. If these things are well understood, the incidence of forgetting to give the medication, or of neglecting to refill the prescription, should be reduced or eliminated entirely. Parents also need to feel free to report promptly any symptoms that they consider caused by the medication.

Special care to keep the child in optimum health is important, and intercurrent infections must be reported promptly. Exacerbations are common, and parents need to understand that these will probably occur, and to report rapidly increasing weight, increased proteinuria or signs of infections for a possible alteration of the therapeutic regimen and the specific antibiotic agents as indicated.

An Addis count is obtained at intervals of two to three months; the parents need to know the necessary procedure to follow when making the urine collection for this test.

Caring for the child at home follows the same pattern as that for any chronically ill child. Bed rest is not indicated except in the event of an intercurrent illness. Activity is restricted only by the edema, which may slow the child down considerably, but otherwise his normal activity is beneficial. Sufficient food intake may be a problem, as it is in other types of chronic illness. Fortunately, there are usually no food restrictions, and the appetite can be tempted by attractive, appealing foods.

Complications from kidney damage necessarily alter the course of treatment. Failure to achieve satisfactory diuresis, or the necessity of discontinuing the use of steroids because of adverse reactions, will call for a reevaluation of treatment. The presence of gross hematuria suggests renal damage. Any persistence of abnormal urinary findings following diuresis presents a less hopeful outlook.

Prognosis

The course of nephrosis is generally characterized by recurrent episodes of edema of varying length. With present-day methods of treatment recovery rates have been estimated at 75%.

Test for Urine Albumin

1. Place 2 cc. urine in a test tube.
2. Add 4 drops reagent (20% sulfosalicylic acid).
3. Rotate the tube.
4. Estimation of the amount of albumin present:

0 — clear urine
Trace — slight turbidity
1 + — cloudy
2 + — quite cloudy
3 + — precipitate formed
4 + — urine becomes white, milklike

Procedure for Abdominal Paracentesis

Sterile Equipment*

1. Hypodermic syringe and needles
2. Aspiration needles
3. Cannula and rubber tubing
4. Sterile gloves
5. Sterile drapes and towels
6. Cotton balls, gauze flats

Unsterile Equipment

1. Novocain and skin antiseptic—prep tray
2. Test tubes for fluid samples
3. Pail for collection of fluid
4. Abdominal binder, safety pins

Nurse's Duties

1. Prepare child emotionally for procedure. Explain that he will feel better and be able to move about after all that water is taken out.
2. Have child void before procedure to avoid puncturing the bladder with the aspiration needle.

---

*If scalpel and sutures are to be used, these should be included. Many hospitals will have a sterile paracentesis tray available.

3. Sit child upright on edge of examining table, with legs over edge. One nurse will need to hold him in position.
4. Prepare site with skin antiseptic.
5. Help physician as necessary.
6. After procedure, apply sterile dressing, put abdominal dressing snugly around abdomen.
7. Comfort child. Hold him for a while if he desires it.

Procedure

1. The nurse or physician will prepare the site with skin antiseptic and drape with towels or sterile drape.
2. The aspiration needle is inserted by the physician.
3. Fluid is collected in test tubes, marked and sent to laboratory.
4. Needle is attached to rubber tubing and fluid allowed to drain slowly into pail.

ACUTE GLOMERULONEPHRITIS

Acute glomerulonephritis is a condition that appears to be an allergic reaction to a specific infection, most often a group A beta hemolytic streptococcal infection, as in rheumatic fever. Not all strains are nephritogenic; one type (12) appears to be the most common of nephritogenic strains, but several others have been identified.

Acute glomerulonephritis occurs most frequently in children between the ages of three and seven years. As a rule, the child is not very ill, and it is often difficult to impress on parents the seriousness of this condition.

Pathology. The kidneys are slightly enlarged and pale, with changes in the glomerular capillaries, which permit the passage of blood cells and protein into the glomerular filtrate. In a majority of cases, these changes are reversible, but there is no way to predict which cases will show complete recovery or will instead develop into chronic nephritis.

Clinical Manifestations

Presenting symptoms appear 1 to 3 weeks after the onset of a streptococcal infection. Most frequently, the presenting symptom is grossly bloody urine; periorbital edema may accompany or precede the hematuria. Fever may be as high as 103° or 104° at the onset but falls in a few days to about 100°. Slight headache and malaise are usual, and there may be vomiting. A transient hypertension appears in 60% to 70% of patients during the first 4 or 5 days, returning to normal in about a week.

Oliguria (production of a subnormal volume of urine) is usually present, and the urine has a high specific gravity and contains albumin, red and white blood cells and casts. The blood urea nitrogen level is elevated, and the serum albumin is usually low.

Complications

Cerebral symptoms occur in connection with hypertension in a small percentage of cases, consisting mainly in headache, drowsiness, convulsions and vomiting. When the blood pressure is reduced, these symptoms disappear. Cardiovascular disturbance is present in many patients, but has few clinical manifestations in the majority and is apparent only in electrocardiographic tracings. In most children, this condition is transient, but in some, it goes on into cardiac failure.

Treatment

Although the child usually feels well in a few days, it is important that he be kept in bed until clinical manifestations subside. This generally occurs 2 to 4 weeks after the onset. Penicillin during the acute stage is given to eradicate any existing infection. A fluid diet may be offered for the first few days, followed by a soft to full diet as acute symptoms subside. Low-salt or low-protein diets are not prescribed, except in the presence of edema or renal failure. The treatment for complications is symptomatic.

Nursing Care

Bed rest must be enforced until acute symptoms and gross hematuria have disappeared. The child should be protected from chill and from contact with persons with infections. When he is allowed out of

bed, he should be prevented from becoming fatigued.

Urinary output must be carefully checked and recorded every 8 hours. The amount of fluid allowed the child will be based on his output, as well as on evidence of continued hypertension and oliguria. Careful recording of the child's fluid intake is essential and careful attention paid to keep it within prescribed limits.

Blood Pressure Readings

Accurate blood pressure readings are difficult to obtain from infants and from young children. Readings are taken usually only on specific order of the physician.

Principles

1. A child should be at rest for accurate reading. Excitement or exercise may significantly raise the systolic rate.
2. Fright, discomfort, or distrust of the examiner, causes resistance and excitement.
3. The proper size cuff is essential for an accurate reading. Too wide or too narrow a cuff gives an erroneously high or low reading. The cuff should cover two-thirds of the upper arm.
4. If strict accuracy is important, use of the same cuff for each reading will be necessary.

Technique

1. Ascertain the latest reading for comparison.
2. Choose the proper size cuff. If possible, use the same cuff each time.
3. Approach the child with a gentle manner and with slow, deliberate movements. Establish good rapport. Avoid tightening the cuff beyond a necessary point.

   For an older child, prepare him with an explanation, and with an opportunity to explore the equipment. Give the reasons for the procedure.
4. Apply the cuff to arm. Raise the manometer gradually to a point above the obliteration of the radial pulse.

5. Deflate the cuff slowly. The *systolic* pressure reading is made when the first sound is heard with each heart beat. The *diastolic* pressure reading is made when the sound suddenly diminishes in volume. A sudden muffling of the sound denotes a pressure equal to the diastole.

6. Compare this reading with previous readings. If there is a significant discrepancy, have the pressure checked by second person.

7. Remove the cuff. Reassure and console the child as it seems necessary.

8. Report any significant variation from the previous reading.

9. Record the time and the reading on the patient's chart.

AVERAGE BLOOD PRESSURES*

Age	Systolic	Diastolic
4 years	85	60
6 years	90	60
8 years	95	62
10 years	100	65
12 years	108	67
14 years	112	70
16 years	118	75

Blood pressure readings in infancy and in early childhood are essentially the same as those of a four-year-old.

If hypertension becomes a problem, a diuretic such as reserpine may help reduce the pressure to normal levels. Apresoline may be added if needed. A diastolic level of 100 or over is an indication for the administration of hypertensive drugs. Specific gravity of the voided urine, as well as tests for any urinary protein are also part of nursing procedure. Tests such as the Addis count or urine concentration require preparation.

Specific Gravity Determination

Fill the cylinder with urine to within 1 inch of the top (25 cc.). Grasp the float at the tip and insert slowly until it is immersed in

*Adapted from Nelson, W., ed.: Textbook of Pediatrics. ed. 9. Philadelphia, W. B. Saunders, 1969.

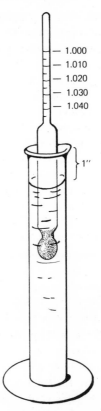

Figure 37-1. A urinometer is used for determining the specific gravity of urine.

the urine to near the top of the graduation marks. Give the float a slight twirl, and note the reading as it comes to rest. While reading, keep the float away from the sides of the container. Avoid wetting the stem above the water line because this gives an inaccurate reading. A normal specific gravity is 1.015-1.025. (Fig. 37-1)

Addis Sediment Count

Purpose: To estimate the concentration power of the kidney.

Preparation: (For children)

4 P.M.	Give the child his usual evening meal, include fluids up to a quantity of 200 cc.
4 P.M. to 8 A.M.	No fluids allowed.
8 P.M.	Child voids, urine discarded.

8 P.M. to 8 A.M. Save all urine as a single specimen; 0.5 cc. of 40% formaldehyde may be added to the collecting bottle as a preservative. Send the entire specimen to laboratory.

The normal values of formed elements in concentrated urine after a period of fluid restriction:

R.B.C. upper normal 1,000,000
W.B.C. upper normal 1,000,000
Casts upper normal   10,000
Protein upper normal   35 mg.

In inflammatory renal disease, there is a sharp rise in formed elements and in the quantity of albumin.

Continuing Care

Traces of protein in the urine may persist for months after the acute symptoms disappear, and an elevated Addis count, indicating urinary red cells, persists as well. Parents are taught to test for urinary protein routinely, and to collect the urine for an Addis count about every 3 months, until all evidence of kidney damage disappears. If the urinary signs persist for more than a year, the disease has probably assumed a chronic form.

Prognosis for recovery. In spite of such grave implications, a recovery rate of 82% or higher is reported. In an additional, small number of children, the condition progresses into chronic nephritis. Mortality rate figures for the acute condition are about 2%.

HANDICAPPED CHILDREN

Hearing Problems

It has been estimated that of the 40 million school children in the United States, 200,000 have a serious hearing loss. A hearing loss presents a definite handicap to a child, a handicap that has a profound effect on his development, on his emotional stability and on his vocational ability as he grows older.

An explanation of some of the terms used to describe hearing difficulties may permit a better understanding of the problem.

A hard of hearing child is one who has had a loss of hearing acuity, but his hearing has been sufficient to enable him to learn speech and language by imitation of sounds.

A deaf child is one who has no serviceable hearing.

The failure of an infant or a young child to react to sounds does not necessarily mean that simple deafness is the cause. A child may fail to respond to sound or may fail to develop speech for several different reasons. Some of these are mentioned here.

1. Conductive hearing loss. In a conductive hearing impairment, the middle ear structures fail to carry sound waves to the inner ear.

2. Sensory-neural (or perceptive hearing loss). This may be caused by damage to the nerve endings in the cochlea, or to the nerve pathways leading to the brain.

3. Central auditory disorders. This child may have normal hearing, but because of damage or faulty development of the proper brain centers, he is unable to use the auditory information he receives.

4. Mental retardation. This condition or a severe emotional disturbance may prevent the child from responding to auditory stimulation. His hearing may not be impaired, however.

The discussion in this section is limited to true hearing loss, whether it is partial or complete.

Causes of Deafness

Conductive hearing impairment is most commonly the result of otitis media of long standing. Serous otitis media is a condition in which fluid is present in the middle ear, possibly because of an allergy or as the result of a protracted ear infection that has not been completely treated. The child complains of "fullness in his ear," but has no real pain or fever. Drainage relieves the symptoms and improves his hearing, but repeated recurrences, if they are not treated, may cause a permanent hearing loss. Long standing middle ear infections that have destroyed part of the ear drum or the ossicles

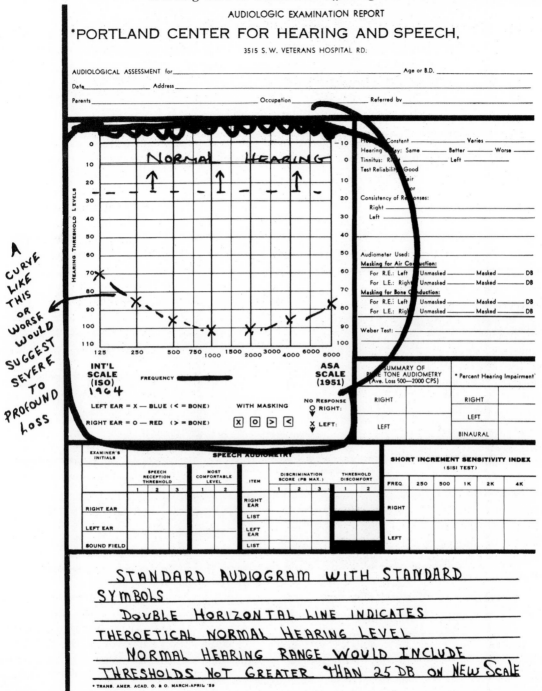

Figure 37-2. Audiogram showing severe or profound hearing loss.

lead to conductive deafness. (Other causes may include congenital ear deformities.) Deafness is seldom complete, and improvement through treatment is frequently possible.

Perceptive, or sensory-neural losses are generally severe and unresponsive to medical treatment. Diseases such as meningitis or encephalitis, hereditary or congenital factors, or toxic reactions to certain drugs (such

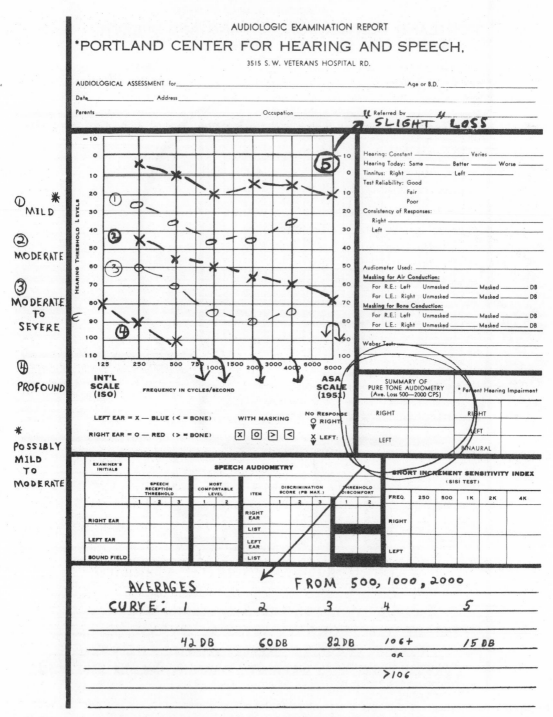

Figure 37-3. Audiogram showing curves for mild to profound hearing loss.

as streptomycin) may cause perceptive hearing losses. It is believed that maternal rubella may be the largest single cause of perceptive nerve deafness in children.

Discovering the Defect

A child should not have to wait until he is in difficulty at school before anyone

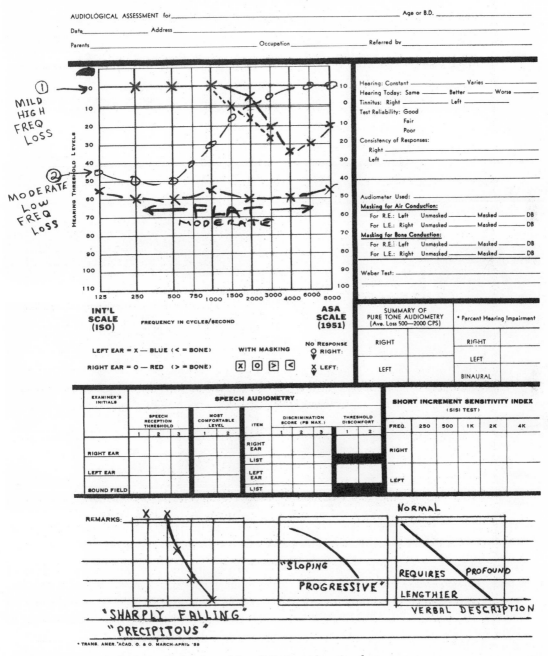

Figure 37-4. Audiogram for high and low frequency hearing loss.

discovers his poor hearing—yet this happens to many children. He may have had a gradual hearing loss, and yet have been so skillful at lip reading that neither he nor his family have become aware of his partial deafness. His teacher is frequently the first person to recognize the child's trouble. She may not be alert to this possibility, however,

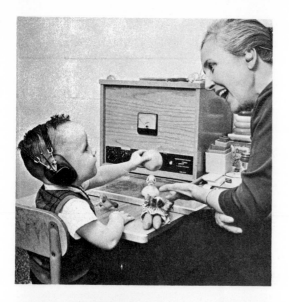
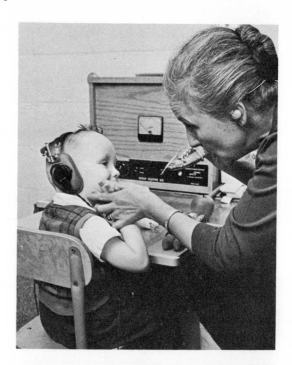
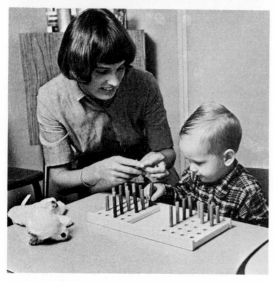
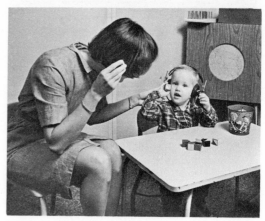

Figure 37-5. The child is taught to talk with the use of visual aids. He learns the sound apple (*A*), the sound shoe (*B*), color and form (*C*). And he is helped to make use of his residual hearing (*D*).

and may scold him for inattention. Children who are noisy or who create a disturbance in class may be expressing resentment over their inability to understand, but may not realize that they are not hearing correctly.

Certain reactions and mannerisms should alert the parent, a teacher or a school nurse to the possibility that the child is not hearing well. He may not be able to localize sound. He may turn his head to one side when listening; he may fail to comprehend when

spoken to, or he may appear inattentive or give inappropriate answers. A child who has never heard may also go undetected until his parents realize that he is not responding to sounds or learning to talk.

Diagnosis and Evaluation of Hearing Problems

The child who is suspected of having a hearing loss is entitled to an audiological assessment. This includes pure tone audiometry testing, speech reception loss and speech discrimination tests. Persons with perceptive nerve impairment have, as a rule, a greater loss of hearing acuity in the high pitched tones. The loss may vary from slight to complete. Persons with a conductive loss are more apt to have equal losses over a wide range of frequencies (pitches). (Figs. 37-2, 37-3, 37-4)

A child's hearing level should be tested at all frequencies in a soundproof room by a pure tone audiometer. Speech reception and speech discrimination tests measure the amount of hearing impairment for both speech and communication. Accurate measurements can usually be obtained from children of five years old or more.

Infants and very young children must be tested differently. An infant with normal hearing should be able to localize a sound at 28 weeks, be able to imitate sounds at 36 weeks, and associate sounds with people or objects at one year. A commonly used screening test employs noisemakers of varying intensity and pitch. The examiner stands to the side or to the back of the child who has been given a plaything of interest. As the examiner produces sounds with a rattle, a buzzer, a bell, or with some other noisemaker, a hearing child is usually distracted from his play, and turns to discover the source of the new sound, whereas the deaf child pays no heed. More discriminating tests help to distinguish the deaf child from an autistic, a brain damaged or from a retarded child.

The Child Who has Never Heard

The deaf infant not only does not hear, but if he has never heard, he has no language concept. One has only to consider the amount of time it takes a hearing child to learn to communicate with language, to get some idea of a deaf child's handicap. Although persons feel and experience emotion, they *think* in words, and a congenitally deaf child has no words. A deaf child has to learn to communicate and to use the language if he is to develop a well-adjusted personality or if he is to share his

thoughts and his feelings with others. It is a terrific problem, but deaf children can and do acquire language. This is not saying that a deaf child does not have ideas and concepts: he simply lacks the words to express them. The child who has heard and has learned to talk has an immense advantage—even if he should lose all hearing—because he has learned expression.

The children who learn sign language rather than lip reading and speech suffer a communication disadvantage because this is a talking world. His parents must be their child's first teachers until he is old enough to venture away from home. The parents need to be aware of all phases of a child's development—physical, emotional, social, intellectual and communicative, and then to seek ways to aid this development if a lack of hearing impedes his progress.

For a deaf child, sight and not hearing is the main "way in" by which words can reach his brain. Because the first five years of life are the years of learning and perfecting speech, these are the years when speech reading (lip reading) can most readily be learned.

Personnel who work with preschool deaf children advise parents to "talk-talk-talk" to a young child. Of course a deaf child can not understand all or perhaps any of what is said, but neither does a hearing baby understand his mother's words until he is able to make a connection between what is done and what is said. A deaf baby learns to lip read in the same way, only it takes him much longer. His mother's interaction with him, as she directs his attention to the movements of her mouth, to her facial expressions, and to the way she moves and acts, all are part of his training.

Sense perception training (in matching colors and shapes and later figures) is another basis of any readiness program. Training in the use of all his senses, sight, smell, taste, heat, and vibration, make him better able to make use of whatever hearing he may have, and it is believed that most children do have *some*.

Preschool classes for deaf children seek to create an environment in which a deaf child can have the same experiences and activities that normal preschoolers have. Children are generally enrolled at the age of two-and-a-half years and are expected to attend all sessions. Enrollment in the Preschool Deaf Classes at the Portland, Oregon Center for Hearing and Speech carries the requirement that the child have a hearing loss significant enough to preclude normal speech and language development, and that he have the mental and physical capacity to benefit from the program.

The John Tracy Clinic* in Los Angeles is concerned with the young child who has been born with a severe hearing loss or who has lost his hearing through illness before he has acquired speech and language. The clinic's purpose is "to find, encourage, guide and train the parents of deaf and hard of hearing children—first in order to reach and help the children, and second—to help the parents themselves."

All services to parents and children are given without charge. The clinic exists to help all deaf children. Consulting service, a nursery school and weekly clinic hours are offered. Of particular interest is the correspondence course available to parents of children 5 years old and under anywhere in the world. This is a 12-month course which includes first lessons in sense training, lip reading, language, auditory training and speech preparation. The clinic also suggests ways in which parents can help a younger child until he reaches the age of 20 months. Parent education films are also available for group viewing. Information concerning the many services offered by this clinic is available on request to the John Tracy Clinic.

Education for the School-Age Deaf Child

There are certain advantages for the deaf child who can attend day school. He is not segregated from people who can hear and talk, but can go home each afternoon to a normal home setting, where he can participate in the activities of his home and his neighborhood. Some public school systems have established such day classes. If these classes are held adjacent to the regular school, the children may participate in certain activities with the hearing children, particularly in the higher grades.

For many children, such opportunities are not available, however, and placement in a residential school is necessary. School education continues to provide speech therapy, lip reading and auditory training. Group hearing aids with individual earphones are used in classes, and various types of visual aids are utilized as well. One class of five-year-olds in a public day school had been prepared for a visit from a group of student nurses by a picture of a nurse in uniform cut out and posted on a placard. Most of the children had been in a hospital at some time, so identification was not difficult, although the student nurses were not in uniform. One mischievous little boy—rather bored perhaps with the obvious—identified the picture readily enough, but when he was asked to name it, he replied, with a sparkle in his eye, "witch!" (Perhaps he was remembering those "shots.")

Vision Defects

Definition of Blindness

The legal definition of blindness is a visual acuity of 20/200 or less in the better eye after correction. It has been found, however, that many children with a visual acuity of less than 20/200 can see well enough to use equipment and special educational media provided for the partially sighted.†

Partially sighted children. These are children with a visual acuity between 20/70 and 20/200 in the better eye after all necessary medical or surgical correction.

---

*John Tracy Clinic, 806 West Adams Blvd., Los Angeles, California, 90007.

†Hathaway, W.: Education and Health of Partially Seeing Children. P. 17. ed. 4. New York, Columbia University Press, 1959.

The Child with a Visual Defect

"There are still many problems. She is going to have to learn to be helped a little, to have people give her a hand crossing streets and show her around in new places. She'll have to learn to fight the pity and vain hope that sighted people too often extend to the blind. She will have to convince teachers and employers that being blind does not necessarily mean being helpless, sad or stupid.

"In my mind I can see her walking confidently into that world with a smile on her face."*

No one, certainly, has to be convinced that blindness is a severe handicap, and that to have been blind from birth is to miss all of the light and the color, the beauty and the majesty of the world about us. Yet, to quote again from *Our Daughter is Blind:* "We began to think about her blindness in a clearer way: We've never heard a dog whistle. There must be a whole universe of sounds above and below what we can hear. And there are myriads we will never know. Yet we never grieve for these lost sounds and colors. She knows nothing of what we see, so why assume she will feel any loss?

"This was the first step in our emancipation. We began to forget that we were the parents of a *blind* baby. We were parents of a happy, bouncy little girl, who was, incidentally, blind."

*Johnson, M.: Our Daughter is Blind. McCalls, Dec., 1953.

Sighted children with eye problems. Such children have a visual acuity of 20/20 or more after any necessary correction.

Causes of Eye Problems

Myopia (nearsightedness). Among sighted children with eye problems, errors of refraction are the most common. This appears in the early school years and progresses until the early twenties, after which it may remain stationary. The common belief that eye strain causes nearsightedness or increases its progression is a fallacy. When proper lenses are fitted, vision is corrected to normal. This is a type of defect that may label a school child as being inattentive or retarded, simply because he cannot decipher blackboard writing or distinguish objects at a distance.

Hyperopia (farsightedness). Farsightedness is a common condition of young children, and frequently persists into the first grade of school, or even longer. Whether corrective lenses are needed must be decided on an individual basis by the specialist examining the child. His teachers and his parents should be aware of the considerable eye fatigue that may result from efforts at accommodation for close work.

Astigmatism. Here there is a difference in the refractive power of the various meridians of the eye that results in a distorted image. Astigmatism is usually combined with myopia or hyperopia. Slight degrees often do not require any correction; moderate degrees usually require glasses for reading, television and movies; severe degrees require that glasses be worn constantly.

Partially sighted children also have a high incidence of refractive errors, particularly myopia. Eye injuries are also responsible for the loss of vision, as well as those conditions that can be improved by treatment but result in diminished sight, as is the case in many instances of cataract. Nemir* states that about one in 500 school-age children needs special attention because of defective vision—children whose vision cannot be improved with glasses.

The causes for *blindness* have been brought under control in those areas in which medical and surgical care have been adequate, and readily available for those who need it. We still have children in our schools for the blind who are blind by legal definition, however, and we will continue to have them for a long time to come.

Case Finding and Visual Testing

Behavior patterns such as squinting and frowning while trying to read a blackboard, holding work too close to the eyes while reading or writing, and rubbing the eyes to

*Nemir, A.: The School Health Program. P. 73. ed. 3. Philadelphia, W. B. Saunders, 1970.

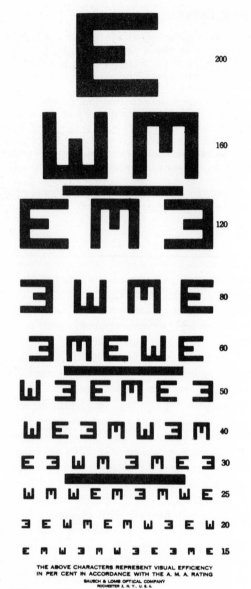

THE ABOVE CHARACTERS REPRESENT VISUAL EFFICIENCY IN PER CENT IN ACCORDANCE WITH THE A. M. A. RATING
BAUSCH & LOMB OPTICAL COMPANY
ROCHESTER 1, N. Y., U. S. A.

Figure 37-6. The Snellen E chart is used for sight-testing small children.

see better are all possible signs of visual difficulty. Simple screening tests are routine in many schools and can be performed by either a teacher or a school nurse. The *Snellen test* is commonly used for children who can read, and the *Snellen E test* is used for younger children who have not yet learned to read.

The Snellen chart. This is the familiar one on which the letters in each line are smaller than those in the preceding line. If the child can read the lines when standing 20 feet away from the chart, his visual acuity is stated as 20/20. If he can read only the line marked 100, his acuity is given as 20/100. The chart should be placed at eye level, with good lighting, and in a room free from distractions. One eye is tested at a time, with the other eye covered. A child should be allowed to take his time reading the letters.

The Snellen E chart. This chart has a series of E letters, with their "fingers" pointing in various directions. The child first learns what is expected of him by placing his fingers over the letter on the chart in the same direction. He then takes his stand at 20 feet, and indicates in which direction the E points by extending his own fingers in the same direction. Some children are apt to become confused, in which case a child may find it easier to hold a large E, and turn that letter in the appropriate direction. Some young children who have a poorly developed sense of direction, or who are confused about what is expected, profit from a little practice at home. One little boy could not make up his mind about which direction he wanted, so a motherly girl his own age promptly took him in charge, and a few days later he passed the test with no difficulty. Such practice does not alter results of the test. (Fig. 37-6)

Picture charts for identification may be used, but are not considered to be so accurate. It is quite easy for a bright child to memorize the pictures and to guess from the general shape without seeing distinctly.

Long-Term Planning

A child able to associate with normally sighted children is at an advantage, whether he has poor sight or has none at all. The trend is to provide the special education needed by a child with a visual handicap within the context of a regular school. This may be by means of a special class plan, in which a special classroom is his base, and from which he goes out to join the normally seeing children for activities not requiring intensive use of his eyes. A specially prepared teacher directs the work done in the special classroom.

A second plan enrolls a partially sighted child in a regular classroom. He leaves this classroom for concentrated eye work in a specially equipped classroom with a specially prepared teacher.

Another plan, called an *Itinerant Teacher Plan* provides a specially prepared teacher, who acts as consultant for the regular classroom teacher. Together, they work and plan to meet the child's needs. This latter plan is especially useful in small communities where a special room and a teacher would be impractical.

Special equipment for the use of children with sight impairment includes printed material with larger type, pencils with large leads for darker lines, cream colored writing paper, tape recordings (which the entire class can enjoy), magnifying glasses and typewriters. The class is inclined to think of these as special privileges rather than in terms of any handicap.

For the children who have a serious impairment and whose participation in regular activities is sharply curtailed, talking books, raised maps and braille equipment is needed as well. Such programs prevent a child from being isolated from the community and do much to minimize his differences from the rest of the children.

Residential schools have played an important part in the education and adjustment of children with severe visual handicaps, and their value should not be minimized. Although it is desirable to keep children in their own homes and in their own community, this is not always possible—or in the child's best interest.

A *blind child*, particularly a child who has never seen, may profit greatly from close contact with sighted children. Children are normally attracted to everything they see about them, and are quite vocal in their enthusiasm. Their spontaneous observations can do much to enrich the life of a blind child, who sees through the eyes of the others. These children can learn to develop their other senses to a degree where they learn to take their place quite confidently among their friends.

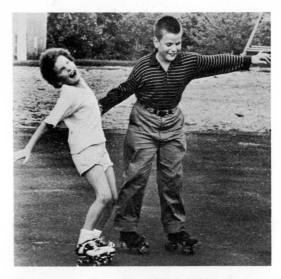

Figure 37-7. Partially sighted children can participate in such active sports as roller skating. (Courtesy of American Foundation for the Blind; Oak Hill School.)

In localities in which facilities are available, the same kind of program described for the partially sighted child may be used to advantage. Residential school personnel also realize the disadvantages of isolation from sighted persons, and promote opportunities for community experiences.

Cerebral Palsy

Cerebral palsy is a term used to denote a group of disorders arising from a malfunction of motor centers and nerve pathways in the brain. A difficulty in controlling voluntary muscle movements is one manifestation of this organic brain damage, and other manifestations occurring in conjunction with the motor defect may include seizures, mental retardation, various sensory defects and behavior disorders. The condition may be very mild, moderate, or perhaps severe enough to be totally disabling. Training and individual therapy help an affected child to take advantage of every bit of his residual ability, but there is no cure, and some children are too severely affected to respond to treatment. Cerebral palsy may have its origin in the prenatal, the natal, or in the postnatal period. Heredity is

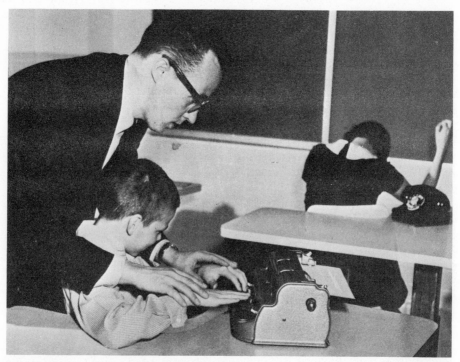

Figure 37-8. Multiple handicapped children. (Courtesy of American Foundation for the Blind; the Hope School for the Blind.)

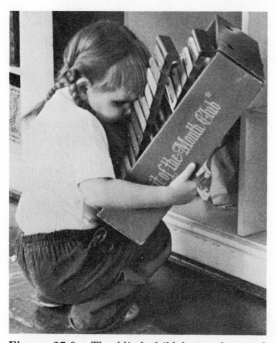

Figure 37-9. The blind child learns by touch and should be encouraged to do things for himself. (Courtesy of American Foundation for the Blind; Charles Schuler, Dallas Services for Blind Children.)

a factor in some cases, as are prenatal infections in others. Adverse factors at birth can be traced in many affected children. Anoxia caused by respiratory obstruction, atelectasis, placenta praevia and breech delivery with a delay of the aftercoming head are frequently cited causes. Maternal toxemia, dystocia, and premature separation of the placenta are mentioned as well.

Postnatal causes include trauma, infections of the central nervous system, kernicterus, and a variety of other nervous system affections.

The most common types of cerebral palsy are:

1. Athetoid. Athetosis is marked by involuntary incoordinate motion with varying degrees of muscle tension. These are the cerebral palsied children who are constantly in motion, described as the whole body being in a state of slow, writhing, muscular contractions whenever voluntary movement is attempted.

2. Spastic. This is the most frequent type. There is a hyperactive stretch reflex in

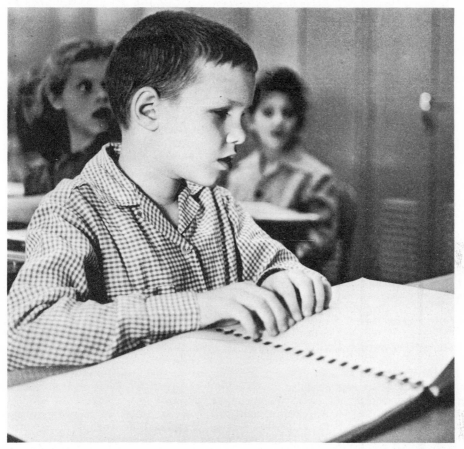

Figure 37-10. The blind child follows his Braille textbook in class. (Courtesy of American Foundation for the Blind.)

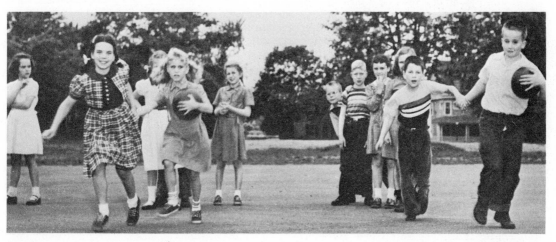

Figure 37-11. Blind and sighted children play together. (Courtesy of American Foundation for the Blind.)

associated muscle groups, an increased activity of the deep tendon reflexes, clonus, and contractures affecting the antigravity muscles and scissoring. When *scissoring* is present, the child crosses his legs and points his toes when he is set on his feet.

3. Ataxia. This is essentially a lack of coordination caused by disturbances of the kinesthetic and the balance senses.

4. Rigidity. This type is characterized by rigid postural attitudes.

5. Mixed types. These are seen, but one form usually predominates.

Treatment

Treatment is directed toward helping the child make the most complete use of his residual abilities, and toward helping him achieve satisfaction and enrichment to the full limit of his capacities.

Three Children with Cerebral Palsy

The first child, whom we shall call Mary L., is a petite, blue-eyed 5-year-old with a sweet smile and happy, friendly disposition. Mary has severe athetosis. She has two sturdy, active brothers of six and three years of age, and understanding, loving parents.

Case 1. Mary was born about two weeks after the expected date, with a birth weight of 6 pounds, 8 ounces. There was no history of any hereditary condition, maternal infection or birth injury. Mary's mother noted that at about the age of one to two months that her baby smiled, cooed, and followed objects with her eyes, but did not kick or use her arms freely as her brother had.

At 13 months of age, she was examined in the crippled children's division at a medical center. At that time she was unable to sit, to hold her head erect, or to roll over. Her babbling and her vocal play was limited — she echoed some vowel sounds but had no true words. She appeared to be alert, reacting differently to various words, and responding visually with facial expressions. At this time a diagnosis of cerebral palsy, athetoid type, was made.

At the age of five, Mary is an appealing little girl, shows an interest in the world about her, and adapts well to functional situations. She has no speech, and no functional use of her arms or her legs. Her "yes" response is a smile, and her "no" is a crying response or puckered lips.

With the aid of short leg braces and a walker, Mary is able to attain an upright position. She loves to be with people, especially with other children, and appears content to watch their play. Because of her severe physical handicaps an accurate assessment of her intellectual ability is impossible. Swallowing presents some difficulties, but she is progressing from strained to solid foods. She is partially toilet trained, and functions adequately if placed on the toilet, but she is not always able to make her needs known.

Mrs. L. states that the diagnosis of her daughter's condition was difficult for her to accept. She feels that her husband's strongly supportive role has helped her greatly, and she has learned to accept Mary as she is, and has learned to appreciate her gentle, lovable personality. The relaxed, accepting attitude of the family is quite apparent, and undoubtedly plays a considerable role in the child's own adjustment. Mrs. L. is concerned about Mary's future, and is anxious for her to have speech therapy. Mary is thought to be too immature, however, to accept a planned program of instruction at this time.

Case 2. Louise C. is a 7-year-old with severe spastic diplegia. No maternal infection or other difficulties were apparent at birth, but she was cyanotic at birth, and stained amniotic fluid gave evidence of fetal distress. She received oxygen during the first 24 hours after her birth, and was kept in the hospital for two weeks. Thereafter she had an uneventful postnatal course.

Her mother became aware of her slow development, when, at the age of six months, she did not coo, did not grasp objects and was unable to sit with support. A diagnosis of cerebral palsy, spastic type, was made at the age of eight months. At the age of one year, Louise commenced having grand mal seizures that ultimately became frequent. At the present time, her seizures occur less frequently now that she takes Dilantin and Mebaral.

Louise commenced therapy at a crippled children's center at the age of two years. She had an increased tonus with stretch reflexes of the spastic condition, with an evaluation of a motor quotient of six or seven month level. Her mother was taught methods of speech therapy to carry out at home in conjunction with therapy at her regular sessions at the center.

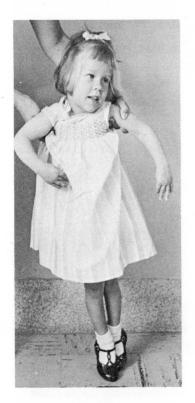

Figure 37-12. A five-year-old girl with athetosis uses a walker. She cannot stand alone and does not talk. Two healthy brothers (shown below) accept her naturally. Although heredity may be a factor in this condition, note that the posture and general appearance of the siblings indicate normal muscular control.

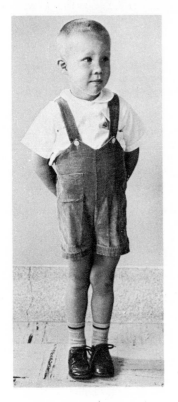

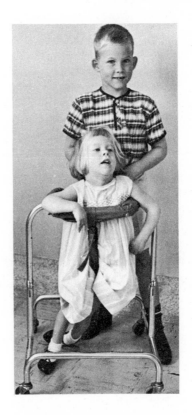

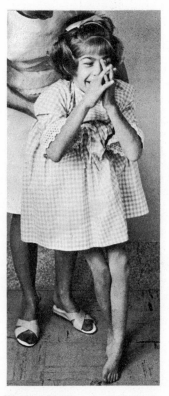
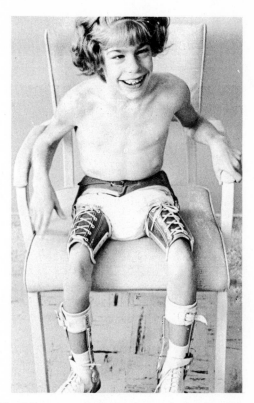

Figure 37-13. In this cerebral palsied seven-year-old with severe diplegia the typical scissoring without braces and the forward thrust of the head are evident (left). The child wears hip and leg braces (right).

At the age of six years, surgery was performed for a right hip flexor release, and long leg casts were applied. At present she wears hip and leg braces to help her maintain an upright position and to help her place her feet squarely on the floor. She does not stand unsupported, but must use a wheelchair instead.

Louise is the second child in the family, with both older and younger brothers. Her parents give her support and understanding care, and have been able to adjust to her disabilities. She attends a special day school three times weekly, and has a moderate mental deficiency. Her voice has a hypernasal quality. She rarely initiates speech, using a few words but not in connected sentences.

Case 3. Sharon H. is an 11-year-old girl in a family of six children, a beautiful collie, a cat, and a litter of kittens. She has brothers aged thirteen, nine, seven and four, and a busy sister of toddler age.

Sharon has cerebral palsy, athetoid type. She was born prematurely (caused by placenta abruptia) was lethargic and had postnatal breathing difficulties. She was given oxygen and intravenous fluids for a few days, but appeared to be in good condition at discharge.

Mrs. H. states that she was told she might expect Sharon to show some brain damage, but she did not know how this would be manifested and feared that the term meant severe mental deficiency. A diagnosis of athetosis was made at the age of nine months. Mrs. H. found it is not easy to accept a handicap in one's child, even when one has been alerted to the possibility. Both of Sharon's parents set about with faith and persistence, however, to help her develop to the limit of her potential.

Sharon had difficulty sucking and taking baby foods because of the reverse tongue thrust common in athetosis. She eventually achieved control, but her drooling is a problem, and she has to make a conscious effort to swallow.

As Sharon grew older, her parents wished to enroll her in a school for handicapped children, but psychological testing gave indecisive and conflicting results, and the question was raised as to her ability to profit from such schooling. This was very discouraging to Mrs. H., who believed that Sharon's ability was not accurately reflected in her test scores. A teacher was obtained to teach her

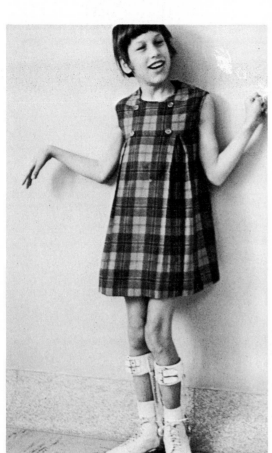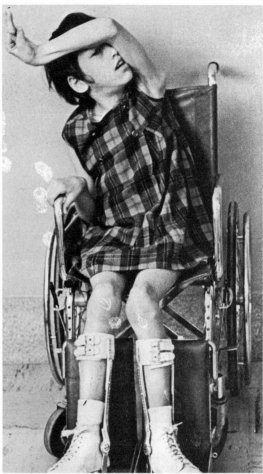

Figure 37-14. This eleven-year-old with athetosis wears short leg braces and special shoes to keep her feet fairly flat on the floor (left). The child shows the random movements of athetosis (right).

at home for two years, after which she was accepted at school where she has shown remarkable progress. Testing now reveals her intelligence to be within normal range.

Sharon is a girl of great determination, with a strong desire to be independent. She has consistently accepted challenges, achieving beyond the predictions of her probable ability. She is able to stand alone momentarily with the use of braces, can take several steps with crutches, and she frequently succeeds in turning herself around. She achieved fair control of her random movements, dresses herself except for buttons and zippers, and takes care of her own toilet needs with the aid of specially built appliances.

Sharon was greatly pleased to be interviewed at home with her family, because, as she said, "I want to help other children." Speech is difficult for her because an effort may produce a spasm, but she is persistent and very patient. The family atmosphere is casual; Sharon realizes her difficulties and no one glosses over them or hides them. They are accepted the same way any disability might be. She is hard to understand, but this does not deter her from talking. Her mother may say, "I didn't get any of that," and Sharon will try again—and again; beaming with pride when things get across. Sometimes, when things are too difficult, she goes to her typewriter and types out the message.

The family loves camping, and Sharon joins in with zest, although her mobility is considerably more difficult than in the atmosphere at home or in school. She attends Easter Seal camp and wishes it lasted longer. Her greatest interest is school, however, and she "can hardly wait for school to start," for the fall term.

She became somewhat excited during the evening, but when the interviewer remarked that an entire evening of being talked about was hard to take, she giggled and relaxed. When she was asked about how she felt about her difficulties she said wistfully, "I would like to be able to walk," but in other respects, she has accepted herself as she is and lets nothing interfere with her enjoyment of life.

Mrs. H. worries somewhat about the future as Sharon matures, and is rather apprehensive about the problems that face this severely handicapped girl. Sharon, with her stubborn determination, may still have some surprises for everyone.

General Discussion

These three girls have several points of similarity. They all have severely handicapped speech and motor abilities, and they all have parents who show tenderness and affection toward them. The outstanding factor, however, is the manner in which they are simply accepted as a part of the family unit, each with her own unique problems, but not someone who is "different" or an outsider. They differ in their personalities as any persons do; Sharon, with her intense drive to succeed, and Mary, with her quiet acceptance of a passive role.

Each child exemplifies some reaction that frequently appears among children with cerebral palsy. One author mentions the "occasional abnormal fears," that are found in many children with cerebral palsy. Sharon's parents were somewhat puzzled by the existence of totally unreasonable fears in an otherwise well-adjusted child, until they were informed that they are not uncommon. As a small child, Sharon was thrown off balance by the exuberant greeting of a large puppy. Her subsequent fear of dogs grew into fear of furry toy animals, and then into a fear of music boxes! Her parents reason that the inability of a handicapped child to run away from a fear-provoking object may help account for this persistent conditioning.

Mary appears to be the sort of child who accepts her limitations and finds her satisfaction from the affection of her family. Her active brothers, absorbed in the normal pursuits of their age, certainly show no indications of rejection.

The manner in which each set of parents has met the problem has undoubtedly been the basis for the total family integration and adjustment. The parents who had been able to attend parent-group meetings and who had been able to talk over their mutual problems had felt they profited considerably.

Treatment and Special Aids

The control of the body, needed to carry out physical activities, is learned automatically by a normal child, but must be consciously learned by a physically handicapped child. Physical therapy attempts to teach such a child to carry out an activity that he has not previously been able to accomplish. The methods must be suited to the needs of the individual child, as well as to the general needs arising from his condition. Such methods are based on principles such as conditioning, relaxation, utilization of residual patterns, stimulation of contraction and relaxation of antagonistic muscles, and on other pertinent principles.

Braces are used as supportive and control measures to facilitate muscle training, to reinforce weak or paralyzed muscles, or to counteract the pull of antagonistic muscles. They are of various types, designed for specific purposes. Orthopedic surgery may improve function and correct deformities in many instances. (The release of contractures and the lengthening of tight heel cords are just two examples.)

Helpful appliances for home care and training. A child who has had difficulty maintaining balance while he sits may need a high backed chair, with side pieces and a foot platform. If a child has serious difficulty, straps may be needed to help hold him in place. The addition of casters or wheels behind the back legs make it possible to move the chair about. Specially constructed toilet seats also help the child achieve independence.

Feeding aids include spoons with enlarged handles for easy grasping, or with bent handles allowing the bowl of the spoon to be brought easily to the mouth. Plates with high rims and suction devices to prevent slipping (such as those used for infants) enable a child to feed himself. Covered cups, set in holders, with a hole in the lid to admit a plastic drinking tube, help a child who does not have hand control.

An improvement in manual skill can be aided by games such as peg boards, or by cards that must be manipulated. The ability to use a typewriter is an enormous morale booster for a child whose handicap is too severe to permit him to write legibly. A shield placed over the keyboard, with round holes over each key, allows the child to strike the desired letter key with a rubber-tipped stick. This has even been successful for those children with poor hand coordination and has proved valuable as a means of self-expression.

Prognosis

The basic defect is a fact that must be accepted. The child's future is dependent on so many variables that no flat statements can be made about his future. Some children, given the amount and type of help necessary, and the important emotional support they need, are able to achieve a satisfactory degree of independence. Vocational training with employment in a sheltered workshop may furnish an opportunity to many who otherwise might never achieve independence. Some of them will always need a significant amount of nursing care, with the possibility of residential care in an institution when their parents can no longer care for them.

When the significant advances that have been made and the present interest in these children are taken into consideration, the future for the children presents a more optimistic picture than formerly.

BIBLIOGRAPHY

Gellis, S. and Kagen, B. M. eds.: Current Pediatric Therapy. Philadelphia, W. B. Saunders, 1970.

Illingworth, R., ed.: Recent Advances in Cerebral Palsy. Boston, Little, Brown, 1958.

Lillywhite, H. S., Young, N. B., and Olmsted, R. W.: Pediatrician's Handbook of Communication Disorders. Philadelphia, Lea and Febiger, 1970.

McConnell, F.: A new approach to the management of childhood deafness. Ped. Clin. N. Amer., *17:*347, 1970.

McCrory, W. W. and Shibuya, Madoka: Poststreptococcal glomerulonephritis in children. Ped. Clin. N. Amer., *11:*633, 1964.

Nemir, A.: The School Health Program. ed. 3. Philadelphia, W. B. Saunders, 1970.

Payne, P. D. and Payne, R. L.: Behavior manifestations of children with hearing loss. AJN, *70:*1718, 1970.

Tracy, Mrs. Spencer: The role of parents in the education of young deaf children. (pamphlet) Los Angeles, John Tracy Clinic.

The Child with Congenital Heart Disease *38*

It is a great shock to parents when the discovery is made that their child has a heart abnormality. The heart is *the* vital organ; one can live without a number of other organs and appendages, but life itself depends on the heart. To know that an infant is starting life with an imperfect heart is a matter of great concern. Naturally, the question is: "How serious is it?" People have heard about "innocent" heart mumurs. Is there a chance that he can outgrow the condition? And, finally, can it be fixed?

It is a difficult task for a doctor or a nurse to try to answer questions about a child's heart condition. In the first place, a definite answer may not be known. Second, how do you answer, encouraging optimism and hope, without giving false assurances and without encouraging unfounded hopes? For example: a mother mourned and upset the ward because her child was on his way to heart catheterization. She was sure he would not survive this procedure, and was not helped at all by the assurance that children don't die from heart catheterization. Her child *did* die during the procedure. The mother was understandably bitter, and the nurse learned an unforgettable lesson.

A brief discussion of the development and functioning of the embryonic heart is useful for the understanding of malformations that occur during embryonic development of the heart.

PATHOPHYSIOLOGY

Embryonic Development of the Heart and Circulatory System

The heart of the embryo has been beating since early in the first month of intrauterine life. The heart when first formed is a simple tube receiving blood from the placenta and pumping it out into its developing body. During this period it rapidly develops into the complicated four-chambered heart with which we are familiar.

Adjustments in circulation must be made at birth. During fetal life, the lungs were inactive, requiring only a small amount of blood to nourish their tissues. Blood was circulated through the umbilical artery to the placenta, where waste products and carbon dioxide were exchanged for oxygen and nutrients. The blood was then returned to the fetus through the umbilical vein.

At birth, the umbilical cord is cut, and the infant establishes his own independent system. Certain circulatory bypasses, such as the *ductus arteriosus,* the *foramen ovale,* the *ductus venosus* are no longer necessary. They close and atrophy after birth, although probably more gradually than had formerly been supposed. (See Fig. 38-1)

During the period of complex development, any error in formation can be the cause of serious circulatory difficulty. The in-

583

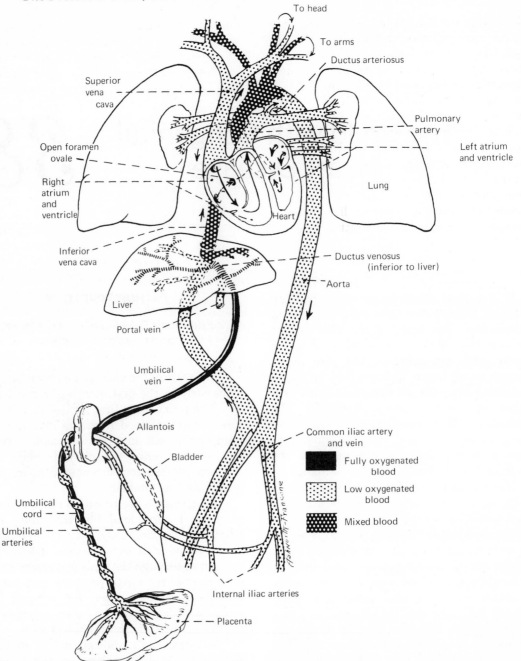

To head

To arms

Ductus arteriosus

Superior
vena
cava

Pulmonary
artery

Left atrium
and ventricle

Open foramen
ovale

Right
atrium
and
ventricle

Lung

Heart

Inferior
vena
cava

Ductus venosus
(inferior to liver)

Aorta

Liver

Portal vein

Umbilical
vein

Allantois

Bladder

Common iliac artery
and vein

Fully oxygenated
blood

Low oxygenated
blood

Mixed blood

Umbilical
cord

Umbilical
arteries

Internal iliac arteries

Placenta

Figure 38-1. Diagram of fetal circulation.

cidence of cardiovascular malformations is about 6 per 1,000 births.

Etiology

Rubella in the expectant mother during the first trimester of pregnancy is a common cause of cardiac malformation. Irradiation or ingestion of certain drugs during pregnancy may be a cause. The drug *thalidomide* has had a high association with congenital heart disease. Maternal malnutrition and heredity are assumed to play a role also.

The newborn with a severe abnormality, such as a transposition of the great vessels, is blue from the start of his life, and requires oxygen and special treatment from the beginning. A less seriously affected child, whose heart is able to compensate to some degree for the impaired circulation, may not have symptoms severe enough to call attention to his difficulty until he starts to walk. Others may live a fairly normal life and not be aware of any heart trouble until a murmur or an enlarged heart is discovered on physical examination in later childhood. Some abnormalities are slight, and allow the person to lead a normal life without correction. Some may cause little apparent difficulty but need correction to improve the chance for a longer life and for optimum health during the adult years. Some severe anomalies are incompatible with life for more than a very short time, and others may be helped but not cured by surgery. For still others there may be no treatment as yet.

Early Indications of Cardiac Difficulty

A cardiac murmur discovered early in life is an indication for frequent physical examinations. This may be a functional, "innocent" murmur that may disappear as the child grows older, or it may be the chief manifestation of an abnormal heart or an abnormal circulatory system. The most frequent parental complaint is of feeding difficulties. Infants with cardiac anomalies severe enough to cause circulatory difficulties have a history of being poor eaters, tiring easily from the effort to suck, and fail to grow or to thrive normally.

Manifestations of congestive heart failure may appear the first year of life in infants with such conditions as transposition of the great vessels, large ventricular septal defects, and with other serious defects. One indication of congestive heart failure in infancy is easy fatigability, manifested by feeding problems. The baby tires, breathes hard, refuses a bottle after one or two ounces but soon becomes hungry again. He has greater difficulty lying flat, and appears to be more comfortable if held upright over an adult's shoulder.

Other signs are failure to gain weight, a pale, mottled or cyanotic color, a hoarse or weak cry, and tachycardia. Rapid respiration (with an expiratory grunt), flaring of the alae nasi, and the use of accessory respiratory muscles with retractions at the diaphragmatic and the suprasternal level are other clinical manifestations of congestive heart failure. Edema is a factor, and the heart generally shows enlargement. Anoxic attacks (fainting spells) are common.

Treatment for congestive failure includes digitalization, diuretics to reduce any edema, oxygen, and the use of morphine for relaxation. The infant should be placed in a slanting position with the head elevated. The example below illustrates the care and treatment of infants in failure.

Because surgery carries less danger for an older child than for an infant, whenever possible affected children should be maintained on medical treatment until the optimal time for surgical procedure.

SURGICAL CORRECTION

The Child at Home Before Surgery

A child with congenital heart disease may show easy fatigability and retarded growth. If he has a cyanotic type of heart disease with clubbing of his fingers or toes, periods

---

Baby C, at the age of 28 days, had a history of atelectasis at birth with continuing respiratory difficulties for several days. He was moderately dusky, becoming increasingly cyanotic with feeding, and had been in an isolette with oxygen since birth. A loud, systolic murmur was present. At four weeks of age, he showed no undue respiratory distress, but he had experienced two anoxic spells. He held his breath, became stiff and rolled his eyes. His color became deep red. Cardiac catheterization showed a transposition of the great vessels, with a large patent ductus and an atrial septal defect. He was given a course of digoxin intramuscularly, followed by a maintenance dosage. A diuretic was given for diuresis, and morphine was given for anoxic episodes. Improvement was noted. His color was less dusky, even when he was out of oxygen, and his feeding pattern improved. Because of the patent ductus and the atrial septal defect allowing the mixture of saturated and unsaturated blood, maintenance on medical treatment may be possible for the present.

of cyanosis and reduced exercise tolerance are evident. This young child assumes a squatting position when he is tired from play. Specific manifestations in several heart conditions are given in the section describing the various types.

Such a child should be allowed to lead as normal as possible a life. Parents are naturally apprehensive and find it difficult not to over-protect the child. They frequently increase their child's anxiety and make him fearful about participating in normal activities. Children are rather sensible about finding their own limitations, and will usually limit their activities to their capacity if they are not made unduly apprehensive.

Some parents are able to adjust well and provide guidance and security for their sick child. Others may become confused and frightened, and show hostility, disinterest or neglect, and stand in great need of guidance and counseling for themselves. Some children have had several periods of hospitalization for respiratory infections, cardiac difficulties or for other reasons.

Routine visits to a clinic or to a doctor's office become a way of life, and the child may come to see himself set apart from others. Doctors and nurses have a responsibility to both the parents and the child to give clear explanations of the defect, using readily understandable terms and illustrating their explanations with appropriate diagrams, pictures or models. A child can accept much and can continue with the business of living if he understands what it is all about.

Hospital Preparation for Surgery

When a child enters the hospital for cardiac surgery, it seldom is his first admission. Generally, it has been preceded by cardiac catheterization or perhaps by other hospitalizations. Admission is scheduled to precede surgery by a few days, in order to give time for adequate preparation. Parents should understand that blood may be drawn for typing and cross-matching and for other determinations as ordered. Possibly additional X-rays may be made, and the child may be photographed.

Apparatus to be used after surgery should be described with drawings and pictures. If possible, the parents and their child should be taken to a cardiac recovery room and should be shown chest tubes, an oxygen tent, and the general appearance of the unit. Judgment should be shown about the timing and the extent of such arousing additional anxiety with premature or excessively graphic descriptions. A young child can become familiar with the surgical dress worn by personnel, with the oxygen tent, and perhaps listen to his own heart beat. He should practice coughing, and should understand that he will be asked to cough after surgery, even though it will hurt a little. The preparation described in the nursing care study at the end of the section clearly illustrates what can be done for a young child in order to minimize the strangeness and fearfulness of this type of surgery.

Cardiac Surgery

Open heart surgery, using the heart-lung machine, has made extensive heart correction possible for many children who would have been otherwise hopelessly doomed to invalidism and a short life span not many years ago. Machines are now available for infants and small children, although the mortality rate among infants undergoing open heart surgery is still high. If a choice is possible, surgery should be postponed until later childhood.

Hypothermia is a useful technique for providing a bloodless field for the surgeon. The preferred method for inducing hypothermia at present is to cool the blood by the use of cooling agents in the by-pass machine, rather than by packing the child's body in ice.

At the end of surgery, thoracotomy tubes are left in the pleural space so that any collections of fluid or air may be removed by suction, and the blood loss is replaced. The child is taken to the intensive care unit to be skillfully nursed by specially trained personnel for 72 hours, or longer if necessary. Children who have had closed chest surgery need the same careful nursing.

Postoperative Care

On admission to the intensive care unit, the chest tubes are attached to the closed suction bottles, and the child is placed in a croupette or in an oxygen tent. Attachment of a cardioscope to the patient enables the nurse to monitor the heart rate constantly, as well as the rhythm, and the electrocardiogram. (Fig. 38-2)

Nursing care for a patient following open heart surgery is highly specialized, and requires specially trained personnel. Intravenous blood and fluids are monitored, because great care must be taken not to overload the heart. Chest drainage should be observed for its color and its amount, and recorded. The patient should be turned every hour and helped to cough. Daily chest X-rays should be taken, and the urine output should be recorded. The patient is carefully observed for any signs of hemorrhage, shock, infection or cardiac arrest. With all this, the patient must be kept as relaxed and as free from apprehension as possible. Sedation is sometimes ordered for this purpose. Because of the specialized training necessary to care for a child immediately following open heart surgery, no attempt is made here to detail the care given in the recovery or in the intensive care units.

By the time the child returns to the ward, his chest drainage tubes have been removed, he has started taking oral fluids and is ready to sit up in bed or up in a chair. He probably feels rather weak and helpless after his experience, and needs encouragement and reassurance. As he recovers, however, a child is usually quite ready for activity. His improved health provides the incentive. Mothers usually need to reorient themselves and to accept their child's new status—an attitude that is not easy to acquire after years of anxious watching.

The surgeon and his staff evaluate the results of the surgery and make any necessary recommendations regarding the resumption of the child's activities. Plans should be made for both follow-up and supervision, as well as for counseling and guidance, as the parents need it.

The American Heart Association has established standards for centers caring for patients with congenital heart disease, together with recommendations for their use. In general, the facilities needed for this type of cardiac surgery are not readily available

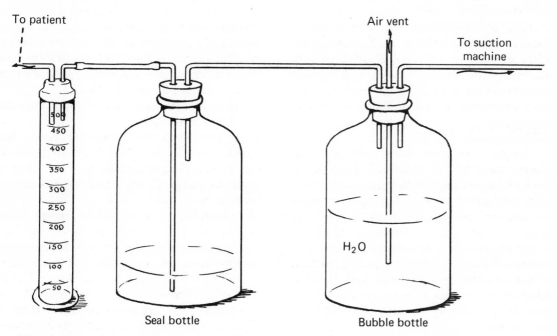

Figure 38-2. After cardiac surgery, water seal chest drainage apparatus is used.

outside of medical centers. Crippled children's centers include diagnosis, surgery and follow-up care in their programs. In addition, regional centers for the diagnosis and treatment of children's congenital heart conditions have been established in certain areas with the help of a special grant from the Children's Bureau of the Federal Government.

Open heart surgery requires complicated, highly specialized apparatus that is fantastically expensive. In addition, many hours of service by a large number of professionally trained persons are required. It is with help provided by such programs that an average family is able to take advantage of these professional services.

Diagnostic Tests

Electrocardiography

Electrocardiography is of relatively less importance in the diagnosis of congenital heart anomalies than it is in acquired heart disease. Nevertheless, it is still a useful, convenient tool in pediatric cardiology, especially if it is used together with data obtained from clinical and X-ray examination.

Cardiac Catheterization

Cardiac catheterization assists greatly in the evaluation of difficult cases of congenital heart defects. It should be used in conjunction with all of the other diagnostic procedures, such as physical examinations, an assessment of the clinical evidence, roentgenographic examinations and electrocardiographic studies.

Cardiac catheterization has been employed as a diagnostic device for a number of years. It is not entirely benign, a fact that must be kept in mind when giving assurance to anxious parents. The mortality rate, however, is very low. An extremely ill child is at risk regardless of any procedure—or even at rest in his crib. A nurse may feel that the mother is unduly disturbed and may be tempted to give her false assurance, an act that she may deeply regret if the child does not survive.

The patient must be relaxed and without apprehension, but care must be taken to avoid medications that depress respiration. General anesthesia may be employed for very small children, but generally sedation is sufficient.

Right Heart Catheterization

The cardiac catheter is inserted into an exposed vein, frequently the saphenous vein in infants and small children, or perhaps the median basilic vein in older children. The catheter is advanced through the median basilic, the axillary, the subclavian, and the innominate veins, into the superior vena cava, the right atrium, the right ventricle, the pulmonary artery, and from there, usually out into one of the smaller pulmonary branches.

This procedure takes place under intermittent fluoroscopy, with spot films or cine strips taken at particular locations. Blood pressure is recorded and blood samples are taken while the catheter is in the various arteries and heart chambers.

Left Heart Catheterization

If a more complete study is necessary, left heart catheterization is performed. In small children, it is frequently possible to enter the left atrium and the left ventricle by passing the catheter from the right atrium across the foramen ovale. When it is not possible to enter the left ventricle by this route, or, when disease of the aortic valve is suspected, a catheter is passed retrograde from the femoral artery to the aortic arch and the left ventricle.

When left heart catheterization is performed on children over 9 or 10 years of age, a trans-septal needle may be used to puncture the atrial septum, and the catheter may then be passed through into the left chambers. Some centers use the trans-septal needle on small children as well.

Angiocardiography and cinefluorography are used as necessary during catheterization.

Angiocardiography

Angiocardiography is the term used to describe roentgenography of the heart and the great vessels following the injection of an opaque material. In venous angiocardiography, a radiopaque catheter is inserted (under fluoroscopy) into a peripheral vein, contrast material is injected, and then films are taken.

Although venous angiocardiography has been largely superseded by selective angiocardiography, it is still useful for the diagnosis of certain anomalies of the systemic veins, and in certain very sick infants who can stand little trauma.

Selective angiocardiography has proved to be a more satisfactory method of diagnosing specific heart lesions. The radiopaque catheter is introduced into the heart cavities and the contrast material is injected. Modern equipment permits roentgenograms to be taken rapidly, reproducing quite faithfully the structural changes in the heart.

Cinefluorography

This term describes the taking of motion picture records of successive images appearing on a fluoroscopic screen. This has some advantages over serial angiocardiography. There is less radiation, and it provides a demonstration of pathophysiology, as well as being a useful monitoring system. Cinefluorography and serial angiocardiography complement each other in the diagnosis of particular conditions.

THE COMMON TYPES OF CONGENITAL HEART DISEASE

In order to be able to give a child entering the hospital for cardiac surgery intelligent care, the nurse should understand the nature of the defect involved. The more common types of congenital heart disease are briefly outlined here. Several excellent texts are available for more precise and detailed information.

Congenital heart defects are commonly described as cyanotic or acyanotic conditions. Cyanotic heart disease implies an oxygen saturation of the peripheral arterial blood of 85 per cent or less. This condition occurs when a heart defect allows any appreciable amount of oxygen-poor blood in the right side of the heart to mix with the oxygenated blood in the left side of the heart. Defects that permit right-to-left shunting can occur at the atrial, the ventricular or at the aortic level.

Many defects occur in combination, giving rise to complex situations. Many of the complex defects, and most of the rare, isolated defects may never be seen by the average nurse. The only conditions discussed here are common enough to obligate the pediatric nurse to be familiar with their diagnosis and treatment.

Conditions that Ordinarily do not Cause Cyanosis

Ventricular Septal Defect

This is the most common intracardiac defect. It consists of an abnormal opening in the septum between the two ventricles, allowing blood to pass directly from the left to the right ventricle. There is no leakage of unoxygenated blood into the left ventricle, and thus no cyanosis. (Fig. 38-3)

Small, isolated defects are usually without symptoms, and are frequently discovered during a routine physical

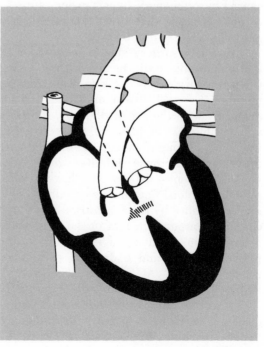

Figure 38-3. The ventricular septal defect is the most common intracardiac defect.

examination. A characteristic loud, harsh murmur, associated with a systolic thrill, is occasionally heard on examination. There may be a history of frequent respiratory infections during infancy, but growth and development are not affected. The child leads a normal life.

This type of defect, known as *maladie de Roger,* appears to be compatible with a normal life span. It is usually treated conservatively under medical supervision, but without curtailment of ordinary activity.

In the presence of a large defect, overloading of the left side of the heart, an increased work load for both ventricles, and pulmonary engorgement appear. Congestive heart failure during infancy frequently occurs. Dyspnea, easy fatigability, failure to thrive, and frequent respiratory infections are common. The shunt may eventually be converted into a bi-directional or a right-to-left shunt, as in the Eisenmenger's Complex, making this a cyanotic condition.

Treatment of ventricular septal defects. Surgery is indicated for the repair of large ventricular septal defects with left-to-right shunts. When a shunt reversal has been caused by pulmonary hypertension, surgery is not recommended because the surgical mortality rate is prohibitive.

Corrective surgery should be postponed, if at all possible, until the age of three years, when the surgical risk is less than that for infants. A very ill infant may be cared for medically with the use of digitalis, diuretics and antibiotics. A banding procedure has frequently brought about a marked improvement in those infants with large ventricular septal defects who have a large pulmonary blood flow and heart failure. This is accomplished by the application of a nylon cloth band around the root of the pulmonary arterial trunk, causing a reduction in the pulmonary flow and a drop in pulmonary artery pressure. At subsequent corrective surgery, the band is removed.

Corrective surgery of ventricular septal defects is carried out in a dry field, using a bypass machine. The defect is closed by direct suturing, or, if necessary, with a nylon patch.

Atrial Septal Defects

In general, left-to-right shunting occurs in all true atrial septal defects. A patent foramen ovale, which is situated in the atrial septum, however, is present in a large number of healthy persons, and normally causes no problems. This is because the valve of the foramen ovale is anatomically structured to withstand left chamber pressure, and makes the patent foramen ovale functionally closed. (Fig. 38-4)

True atrial septal defects are common heart anomalies and may occur as isolated defects or in combination with other heart anomalies.

Atrial septal defect—secundum type. Early in embryonic life, septal structures form to partition the single chambered atrium into both right and left chambers. The ostium primum rises to form a partial partition, followed by the ostium secundum, which completes the atrial partitioning. The secundum defect is in the nature of a hole high in the atrial septum. The child with such a defect is usually symptom-free. Cardiac enlargement and hypertension may appear in later life, however, and bring on the possibility of congestive heart failure. Without surgical repair, the expected life span may be significantly reduced.

Atrial septal defect—primum type. The ostium primum atrial septal defect is a serious, but fortunately less common, anomaly. The defect is in the lower portion of the atrial septum, and is frequently associated with a deformity of the mitral or the tricuspid valve, or both. It is often found in persons with Down's syndrome.

Treatment of atrial septal defects. The ostium secundum defect is amenable to surgery, with a low surgical mortality risk. Since the advent of the heart-lung bypass machine, this repair can be performed in a dry field, replacing the older "blind" technique. The opening is either sutured or is closed with a nylon patch. The optimum age for surgery is between five and ten years, before irreparable damage has been caused by prolonged pulmonary hypertension.

The repair of the ostium primum defect is now feasible, with good results possible.

Patent Ductus Arteriosus

The ductus arteriosus is a vascular channel between the left main pulmonary artery and the descending aorta. In fetal life, this allows blood to bypass the nonfunctioning lungs and go directly into the systemic circuit. After birth, the duct normally closes, eventually becoming obliterated and forming the ligamentum arteriosum. If, however, the ductus remains patent, blood continues to be shunted from the aorta into the pulmonary artery. This results in an overflooding of the lungs and in an overloading of the left heart chambers.

Normally the ductus arteriosus is nonpatent after the first or second week of life, and should be obliterated by the fourth month. Why it fails to close is not known at the present time. Patent ductus arteriosus is common in infants who exhibit the rubella syndrome, but most of the infants with this anomaly give no history of exposure to rubella during fetal life.

Clinical manifestations. Symptoms are frequently absent during childhood. Growth and development may be retarded in some children, with an easy fatigability and dyspnea on exertion.

Diagnosis. This can be based on a characteristic, machinery-like murmur over the pulmonary area, a wide pulse pressure, and a bounding pulse. Cardiac catheterization is diagnostic but is not required in the presence of classical clinical features.

Treatment. Surgery is indicated in all diagnosed cases, even if they are asymptomatic. Some persons may possibly live a normal life span without correction, but the risks involved far outweigh the surgical ones.

The most serious complication to be considered in patent ductus arteriosus is pulmonary hypertension, resulting from the

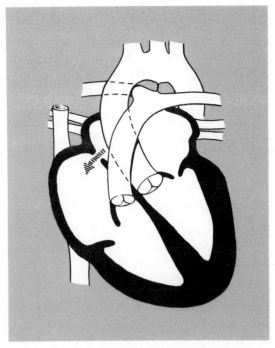

Figure 38-4. The true atrial septal defect may occur as an isolated defect or in combination with other heart anomalies.

excessive pulmonary blood flow (and which may lead to cardiac failure). Other complications may include subacute bacterial endoarteritis and pulmonary or systemic emboli. Uncorrected patent ductus arteriosus is believed to be responsible for a sharp reduction in the life expectancy of an average affected person.

Surgical procedures. Surgical correction consists of closure of the defect by ligation or by division of the ductus. Division is the method of choice if the child's condition permits, because the ductus occasionally reopens after ligation. Optimal age for surgery is between two and five years, with earlier surgery for severely affected infants. Prognosis is excellent following a successful repair.

Coarctation of the Aorta

This is a congenital cardiovascular anomaly consisting of a constriction or

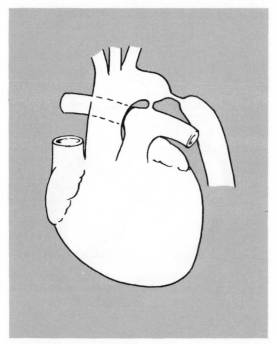

Figure 38-5. Coarctation of the aorta is a congenital cardiovascular anomaly consisting of a constriction or narrowing of the aortic arch usually adjacent to the ligamentum arteriosum.

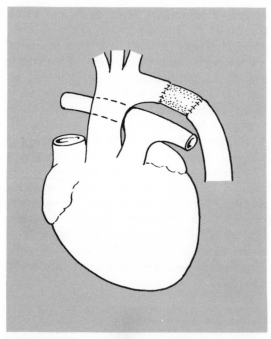

Figure 38-6. A coarctation of the aorta is shown resected and a graft applied.

narrowing of the aortic arch, or of the descending aorta, usually adjacent to the ligamentum arteriosum. (Figs. 38-5 and 38-6)

A majority of children with this condition are asymptomatic until later childhood or young adulthood. A few infants have severe symptoms in their first year of life showing dyspnea, tachycardia and cyanosis, these are signs of developing congestive heart failure.

The condition is easily diagnosed from hypertension present in the upper extremities, and from hypotension in the lower extremities. The radial pulse is readily palpable but the femoral pulses are weak or even impalpable. Blood pressure is normal or elevated in the arms and is low or undetectable in the legs. A high-pitched systolic murmur is usually present, heard over the base of the heart and over the interscapular area of the back. Diagnosis can be confirmed by aortography.

Obstruction to blood flow caused by the constricted portion of the aorta does not cause early difficulty in an average child because the blood bypasses the obstruction by way of the collateral circulation. The bypass is chiefly from the branches of the subclavian and the carotid arteries which arise from the arch of the aorta. Eventually, the enlarged collateral arteries erode the rib margins, and the rib notching can be visualized by roentgen examination.

The uncorrected coarctation may cause hypertension and cardiac failure later in life. The optimal age for surgery is probably between the ages of five to ten or twelve years. Early surgery may be necessary for a gravely ill infant if medical measures fail, but the mortality rate is high.

Surgery consists of resection of the coarcted area with an end-to-end anastomosis of the proximal and the distal ends of the aorta. Occasionally a long defect may necessitate an end-to-end graft, using tubes of dacron or similar material. Prognosis is excellent for the restoration of normal functions after surgery.

A Boy with Coarctation of the Aorta*

Melvin G. was born prematurely and weighed five pounds at birth. His mother gave a history of exposure to rubella during the first trimester of her pregnancy, but a careful examination of the newborn infant revealed no abnormalities. He was discharged on a Similac formula.

When he was two months of age, his mother reported that he was a poor eater and had gained weight slowly. A chest roentgenogram revealed cardiomegaly, but no murmur or other evidence of an abnormal heart condition was noted on physical examination. He was sent home with instructions to visit a pediatric clinic.

At the age of nine months, Melvin was hospitalized for an acute upper respiratory infection. Pallor and difficult breathing were noted, and a soft mid-systolic murmur could be heard. Chest films revealed both right and left ventricular enlargement and engorged pulmonary vascular markings. He was judged to be in congestive heart failure, with possible pneumonitis.

Treatment included digitalization, oxygen with mist, and antibiotic therapy for the respiratory infection. Further investigation of his cardiac status revealed hypertension in the upper extremities—a blood pressure reading in the right arm of 110/60, and a systolic reading in the right leg of 50. Tentative diagnosis was coarctation of the aorta, possibly infantile, with patent ductus arteriosus. In view of his good response to treatment, however, it was decided to treat him medically, and to send him to a cardiac clinic. He was discharged on a daily maintenance dose of Lanoxin.

Melvin continued to eat poorly, remaining in the 10th to the 25th percentile in weight. His height was average, and his developmental progress was within normal limits. His appearance was described as that of an active, but chronically ill infant.

Examination at 18 months revealed a long systolic murmur over the left sternal border and a longer systolic murmur at the apex, but no third sound. Electrocardiography indicated moderate left ventricular hypertrophy. Radial pulses were bounding, and femoral pulses were barely palpable. He appeared to compensate adequately for the cardiac defect on a regimen of low sodium diet and digoxin (Lanoxin).

At the age of two and a half years, an electrocardiogram was essentially within normal limits. Pulses and blood pressure continued in the previous pattern; a systolic murmur could be heard over the precordium, and a venous hum was heard on the right side, but no diastolic murmur could be heard. Recommendations were to continue with the Lanoxin and with the low sodium diet. A prophylactic course of penicillin was suggested in connection with a proposed tooth extraction.

During his fourth year, Melvin's mother reported that he had leg pains at night severe enough to waken him. Shortly after his fifth birthday, he was admitted to the hospital for cardiac catheterization. Cineangiocardiography revealed a short segment coarctation of the aorta, adult type, but no patent ductus arteriosus. A decision was made to correct the defect surgically, and he was scheduled for surgery one month later.

On his admission for cardiac surgery, he was chosen for the subject of a nursing care study by one of the student nurses. She found him to be a likable, well mannered boy, apparently well adjusted and showing no signs of undisciplined or overprotected behavior. Excellent rapport was established. Melvin was cooperative and calm, accepting the impending surgery with a casual "I had surgery before"; meaning the cardiac catheterization.

On the afternoon before the day of surgery, Janice, his nurse, read him stories, played games with him, and casually discussed the sequence of events for the next day. They talked about Mommy coming early, and the fact that he would not have breakfast. Melvin asked if he would "get a shot"; Janice said he would, and that his mother could hold him afterward until he became sleepy. They talked about the elevator ride, and about the queer operating room garb, which he remembered from the cardiac catheterization. Janice assured him that she would be with him all of the time, which pleased him greatly.

Because he appeared to show no anxiety about surgery itself, Janice talked about what he would see in the cardiac recovery room. She told him about the oxygen tent, and drew a picture of the chest drainage tubes, which interested him. He was quite intrigued with the idea of a little machine that would go "beep" every time his heart beat, and listened to his own heart through a stethoscope, saying "beep" with each beat. He was also interested to know that he would get

*Condensed from an original study made by Janice O'Sullivan, junior student nurse at University of Oregon School of Nursing. Patient's real name has not been used.

"food" through a tube in one of his veins. Janice thought that he might be disturbed over his incision, so she drew a picture, explaining to him that it would heal just like a cut finger. Melvin appeared interested and talked freely, but he exhibited no real anxiety.

The physical preparation for surgery included a pHisoHex bath and shampoo, blood determinations and crossmatching, and urinalysis. He received staphcillin, penicillin and streptomycin on the evening and the morning preceding surgery. Preoperative sedation consisted of intramuscular injections of Demerol 30 mgm., atropine 0.2 mgm. and Nembutal 60 mgm. Melvin relaxed and was asleep on admission to surgery.

In the operating room Melvin was positioned in a lateral position with his left side up, was given general endotracheal anesthesia, and had skin preparation with Virac and alcohol. The fifth intercostal space was entered, and a short, narrow coarctation of the aorta found directly proximal to the ligamentum arteriosum. The coarctation was excised, and the aortic ends anastomosed without difficulty. A blood loss of 300 cc. was replaced, chest tubes were inserted, and the incision was closed.

In the cardiac recovery room, the chest tubes were connected to closed suction bottles, and Melvin was placed in a croupette with mist. His heart action was monitored, his vital signs carefully watched and intravenous blood and fluids were given as indicated. Antibiotics and digoxin were continued by intramuscular injection, and morphine was given in sufficient quantity to keep him sedated as ordered. His parents visited him, content to be able to hold his hand through the tent opening.

His vital signs remained stable, his skin was warm to the touch, and his recovery was uneventful. Chest films were taken daily. Melvin was turned and made to cough. On the third day, he was allowed to sit up in bed. Oral fluids were started, the chest tubes were removed, and the oxygen tent was no longer required. On the fourth day, he was returned to the pediatric ward.

Melvin was pleased to be back on the ward, showed Janice his new toys and displayed his incision which was healing "just like a cut." He gradually returned to full activity, and, on the tenth postoperative day, he was discharged. He was to continue with a low sodium diet and with daily Lanoxin, until his return to the clinic in four weeks.

On his return to the clinic, his parents reported that he had been quite active and was feeling well. His weight was still in the 10th to the 25th percentile, but his appetite was improving. A systolic ejection murmur was still audible in the aortic area, but no ventricular overactivity was evident. His blood pressure was 130/80 in the upper extremities, with a systolic reading of 110 in the lower extremities. He was considered to be making good progress. The salt restriction was removed, and digoxin was discontinued. He was to return to the cardiac clinic in six months for further evaluation.

Cyanotic Congenital Heart Defects

Eisenmenger's Syndrome

This term is used to denote a condition in which pulmonary hypertension is present in combination with a ventricular septal defect. The shunting of blood through the defect is reversed, causing a right-to-left flow.

It is believed that the pulmonary hypertension may be a physiological abnormality by itself. The normal newborn has a high pulmonary vascular resistance that falls to adult levels within a few months. In Eisenmenger's syndrome, the pulmonary resistance remains high, and this resistance has probably been present from birth.

Clinical manifestations. These infants show signs of severe heart disease early in life. Feeding difficulties, failure to thrive, recurrent respiratory infections and dyspnea are all associated with this condition. Cyanosis, which increases as the child grows older, is associated with clubbing of the fingers and the toes and with polycythemia. The child may assume a squatting position to relieve fatigue.

Cardiac catheterization and selective angiocardiography are useful for locating the site of the shunt.

Treatment. Attempts to correct this anomaly have been unsuccessful to date. Medical treatment to make the child as comfortable as possible, and perhaps to prolong his life, constitutes the only treatment at the present time.

Tetralogy of Fallot

Tetralogy of Fallot is a fairly common congenital heart defect, involving 50 to 70 per cent of all cyanotic congenital heart diseases. It consists of a grouping of heart defects, the term "tetralogy" denoting four abnormal conditions. These are *pulmonary stenosis, ventricular septal defect, overriding aorta,* and *right ventricular hypertrophy.*

The pulmonary stenosis is usually of the infundibular type, in which there is a narrowing of the upper portion of the right ventricle. It may include, however, stenosis of the valve cusps. Pulmonary stenosis results, in turn, in right ventricular hypertrophy.

The aorta appears to straddle the ventricular septum, overriding the ventricular septal defect. This defect allows a shunt of unsaturated blood from the right ventricle into the aorta, or into the left ventricle. (Fig. 38-7)

Clinical manifestations. The child may be precyanotic in early infancy with the cyanotic phase starting at from four to six months. Some severely affected infants, however, may show cyanosis earlier. It is believed that as long as the ductus arteriosus remains open, enough blood passes through the lungs to prevent cyanosis.

The infant presents feeding difficulties and poor weight gain with retarded growth and development. Dyspnea and easy fatigability become evident, especially when the child begins to walk. Cyanosis becomes grossly severe after the first year, even when the child is at rest.

Exercise tolerance depends somewhat on the severity of the disease, some children becoming fatigued after very little exertion. As the child experiences fatigue, breathlessness and increased cyanosis, he usually assumes a squatting posture for relief. Squatting apparently increases the systemic oxygen saturation.

Attacks of paroxysmal dyspnea are common during infancy and early childhood. An anoxic spell is heralded by sudden restlessness, gasping respiration, and increased cyanosis, leading into a loss of consciousness and possibly into convulsions. These attacks last from a few minutes in length to several hours and appear to be

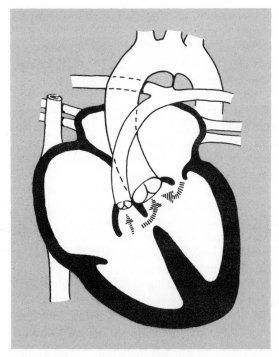

Figure 38-7. Tetralogy of Fallot is a congenital heart defect involving 50 to 70 per cent of all cyanotic congenital heart diseases.

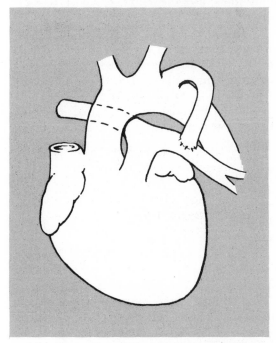

Figure 38-8. The Blalock-Taussig procedure is an end-to-end anastomosis of a vessel arising from the aorta to the corresponding right or left pulmonary artery.

unpredictable, although stress does seem to trigger some episodes.

Iron-deficiency anemia is a common complication caused by the poor food intake. Polycythemia is usually also present.

Diagnosis. Diagnosis is made by utilizing all available techniques. Roentgen examination reveals a boot-shaped heart contour and a concave pulmonary conus. Cardiac catheterization, using angiocardiography and cine recording, helps present a clear picture of the anomalies involved.

Treatment. Treatment is aimed at medical management until the child can tolerate surgery. The constant aim, of course, is to keep the child in the best possible physical condition.

An infant suffering an anoxic spell should be placed in a knee-chest position for the greatest possible relief. Oxygen is administered, and morphine is given to relax any child suffering an anoxic episode. Intravenous sodium bicarbonate has also been proved useful in severe spells. As the child grows older, however, he learns his physical limitations, and the anoxic episodes become fewer.

Anemia, if present, is treated with iron therapy. Surgery on the nose, the throat or on the ears carries the danger of subacute bacterial endocarditis. Therefore, antibiotic therapy is utilized if such surgery is necessary. Fevers, vomiting and diarrhea diminish the fluid component of the blood, aggravating the existing polycythemia.

Surgical relief is imperative for these children as early as possible. The average age span for uncorrected cases is not over ten years. Heart surgery does carry a risk, and thus it is necessary for the child to be in the best possible physical condition.

Surgical procedures. Palliative surgery has been in use for several years. Dr. Taussig observed that the infant with tetralogy of Fallot thrived much better as long as the ductus arteriosus remained open. Together with Dr. Blalock, she devised an operation creating an artificial shunt between the pulmonary and the aortic systems. Later, Dr. Potts and his associates devised a similar shunt.

1. Blalock-Taussig procedure. This is an end-to-end anastomosis of a vessel arising from the aorta, usually the subclavian, to the corresponding right or left pulmonary artery. (Fig. 38-8)

2. Potts procedure. This is a side-to-side anastomosis between the aorta and the left pulmonary artery. (Fig. 38-9)

These procedures do nothing to correct the anatomical defects, but they do relieve the cyanosis and the dyspnea by increasing the flow of blood to the lungs. As the child grows, these shunts tend to become ineffective, but they are useful for carrying the child along in relatively good health until he is a candidate for total correction.

Total surgical correction. This procedure can only be carried out in a dry field, necessitating the use of a cardiopulmonary bypass machine. The heart is opened, and extensive resection is done. The septal defect is closed by use of an Ivalon patch and the valvular stenosis and infundibular chamber are resected.

Total correction is delayed, if possible, until after the age of three to five years. Palliative surgery carries the young child along and does not interfere with later correction. Because of the high surgical risk involved if correction is attempted in infancy, most surgeons prefer the sequence of palliative surgery at an early age, followed by total correction. Some surgeons have attempted total correction on selected infants with reported good results, but the risk for an average infant is still too high.

Successful total correction transforms a grossly abnormal heart into a functionally normal one, as far as we can tell from present knowledge. Most of these children are left without a pulmonary valve, however. Whether this will prove harmful with age we cannot tell as yet.

Transposition of the Great Vessels

In this condition the aorta arises from the right ventricle, and the pulmonary artery arises from the left ventricle, forming two independent, closed circuits. Thus the aortic circuit carries unoxygenated blood to the systemic system, while the pulmonary circuit carries oxygenated blood back to the lungs. This condition is only compatible with life if an associated defect allowing mixing of blood is present, such as an atrial or a ventricular septal defect, or a patent ductus arteriosus.

Clinical manifestations. Extreme cyanosis and dyspnea are present at birth or shortly following. Progressive congestive heart failure appears in most cases, with survival beyond six months uncommon except in instances when there is a good mixture of saturated and unsaturated blood. Growth retardation, with marked clubbing of the fingers and the toes, together with severe cyanosis, is the rule for those who survive.

Diagnosis. Laboratory findings include polycythemia and an elevated hematocrit. Definitive diagnosis is made by cardiac catheterization, with the use of angiocardiography and cineangiograms.

Treatment. A number of surgical procedures have been devised, some of which are palliative, and some of which attempt reconstruction of the atrial septum.

Palliative procedures, designed to create an artificial atrial-septal defect have been used early in infancy. The Blalock-Hanlon procedure involves the creation of an artificial defect in the atrial septum, allowing the mixture of saturated and unsaturated blood. Mortality rate has been about 15% to 35% under palliative surgery.

A newer nonsurgical procedure is being used which gives temporary relief without the trauma of open heart surgery. This procedure, the balloon atrial septostomy technique designed by Dr. Rashkind in 1965, is performed during cardiac catheterization. A balloon catheter is passed through the foramen ovale and inflated. It is then pulled back to tear a larger opening, thus creating an artificial atrial-septal defect. This method usually results in temporary but rapid improvement, the infant becoming pink almost immediately. This procedure has been performed in infants between the ages of 1 day and 3 months.

About 75% to 80% of the infants so treated survive to undergo open heart correction, which is carried out when the

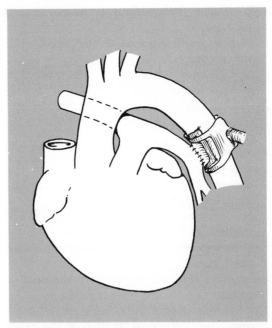

Figure 38-9. The Potts procedure is a side-to-side anastomosis between the aorta and the left pulmonary artery.

child is between 2 and 5 years of age. The Mustard procedure is the surgical corrective of choice at present. It involves removal of the atrial septum, as in the Blalock-Henlon procedure, and use of the pericardium to channel blood from the pulmonary veins into the right ventricle.

GLOSSARY

Atelectasis. Incomplete expansion of the lungs at birth.

Basilic vein. A superficial vein that passes up the forearm and joins with the brachial veins to form the axillary vein.

Bypass machine. A mechanical lung machine used in open heart surgery.

Collateral circulation. Secondary or accessory branch of a blood vessel.

Conus. A term used to designate a structure resembling a cone in shape.

Dyspnea. Difficult or labored breathing.

Heart-lung machine. See bypass machine.

Hypertrophy. Enlargement or overgrowth of an organ or part.

Hypothermia. Induced low body temperature. Used in some surgical procedures, especially on the heart.

Infundibular. Resembling a funnel-shaped passage.

Palliative procedure. Affording relief, but not a cure.

Patent foramen ovale. A foramen ovale that has not closed after birth.

Peripheral. Situated at or near the surface.

Polycythemia. Excessive red corpuscles in the blood.

Pulmonary conus. See conus.

Pulmonary stenosis. Narrowing of the opening between the pulmonary artery and the right ventricle.

Pulse pressure. The difference between the systolic and diastolic pressures.

Saphenous vein. A large superficial vein of the leg.

Stenosis. Narrowing or stricture of a duct or canal.

Tachycardia. Rapid pulse rate.

Thoracotomy. Surgical incision of the chest wall.

BIBLIOGRAPHY

Barnes, C.: Working with parents of young children undergoing heart surgery. Nursing Clinics of North America, 4:11, 1969.

Belling, D.: Complications of open heart surgery. Nursing Clinics of North America, 4:123, 1969.

Betson, C., Valoon, P., and Soika, C.: Cardiac surgery in neonates: a chance for life. AJN, 69:69, 1969.

Goldring, David, Hernandez, Antonio, and Hartman, Alexis F., Jr.: The critically ill child: care of the infant in cardiac failure. Pediatrics, 47:1056, 1971.

Waldhausen, J. A. et al.: Total correction of transposition of the great arteries following balloon atrioseptostomy. Circulation [Suppl.], 51:II, 1970.

Suggested Readings for Further Study

Altschuler, Anne: Complete transposition of the great arteries. AJN, 71:96, 1971.

Blake, Florence G.: Open heart surgery in children—a study in nursing care. U. S. Department of Health, Education and Welfare, Children's Bureau, 1964.

UNIT STUDY QUESTIONS

1. Preschool children show their increasing maturity in which of the following ways?
   a. learning to take turns and to respect the rights of others
   b. showing full understanding of their male or female roles
   c. have now lost their belief in magic
   d. like to feel part of the family by doing errands around the house
   The answer is:
     1. a and b
     2. b and c
     3. a and d
     4. c and d

2. Sammy, age 4, first showed some hesitation in speech, then later began to "stutter" with a few words. His parents and other family members can help him most by:
   a. saying the word for him when he stutters
   b. not calling special attention to his speech hesitation
   c. ignoring his requests until he can speak without stuttering
   d. reminding him to think through his words before uttering them

3. Sammy's parents can help him develop into a self-reliant, confident being in which of the following ways:
   a. accepting him as he is, and respecting him as a person
   b. giving him freedom to learn while setting up limits
   c. giving him top priority while subordinating their own wishes
   d. maintaining strict control and demanding instant obedience
   The answer is:
     1. a and b
     2. b and d
     3. b and c
     4. a and d

4. This is an age when communicable diseases are prevalent. The disease rubella is also known as:

a. red measles
b. German measles
c. streptococcal infection
d. 3-day measles
The answer is:
   1. a and c
   2. a and b
   3. b and d
   4. a and d

5. A mother sees no reason for having her child vaccinated against measles, as "it is just a simple childhood disease." The nurse can:

a. point out that measles can have serious complications
b. agree that the child may as well have the disease and get it over
c. agree, because there is no reliable immunizing agent

6. In working with a blind child, one must be careful to:

a. not embarrass the child by using the words "see" and "look" when talking with him
b. practice extreme caution, lest he should injure himself
c. provide stimulation and opportunities for learning from infancy on up
d. provide a verbal explanation of a new environment and location of facilities
The answer is:
   1. a, b, and d
   2. a and d
   3. a and c
   4. c and d
   5. all of these

7. The mother of a deaf child does not talk to him because, she says, "He cannot hear." She should be taught that:

a. nothing can be done for him until he is of school age
b. he will do his best if he is sent to a residential school for the deaf where he will be with others like him
c. she should talk, talk, talk to him just as if he had normal hearing

8. Some types of congenital heart disease are not due to structural malformation of the heart, but are due to persistence of normal fetal openings which fail to close after birth such as:

a. coarctation of the aorta
b. ventricular septal defect
c. tetralogy of Fallot
d. patent ductus arteriosus

9. The hematuria seen in glomerulonephritis is due to:

a. cells escaping through the walls of capillaries of glomeruli
b. kidney tubule damage
c. invasion of glomeruli by streptococcal organisms
d. sulfonamide crystal damage

10. The cause of nephrosis in children is:

a. previous kidney infection
b. respiratory infections
c. degeneration of renal tubules
d. unknown

11. The characteristic symptoms of nephrosis are:

a. edema, albuminuria, hematuria, hypertension
b. hyperlipemia, hypoalbuminemia, hypoproteinemia, albuminuria
c. hypolipemia, hyperalbuminemia, hyperproteinuria, albuminuria
d. dyspnea, edema, weakness, weight loss

12. Jenny had been in the hospital many times with nephrosis, but in spite of all treatment her condition steadily worsened. In her last illness she was restless and irritable, and no one could please her. She constantly asked for things, only to turn away and cry when they were brought her. The nurse decided that:

a. Jenny had been "spoiled rotten" at home
b. if Jenny had not been disciplined at home, it should be done now
c. what Jenny was really saying was "Why can't you take away this pain and make me feel better?"

Normal Growth and Development of the School-age Child

39

PHYSICAL DEVELOPMENT

Growth

The healthy child shows relatively steady growth between the ages of 6 and 12 years. Average gain in weight is about 7 pounds (3 to 3.5 kg.) a year. Growth in height is about 2-1/2 inches (6 cm.) per year. This period ends in the preadolescent growth spurt—in girls at about the age of 10, and in boys at about 12. (Fig. 39-1 and Fig. 39-2)

Dentition

At about the age of 6, the child starts to lose his baby, or deciduous, teeth. The first to come out are usually the incisors. At about the same time, his first permanent teeth, the 6-year molars, appear directly behind the deciduous molars. (Fig. 39-3)

These 6-year molars are of the utmost importance and merit some discussion. Because they appear in the spaces behind the deciduous teeth, they are often mistaken for deciduous teeth. This is unfortunate because they are the key or pivot teeth which help to shape the jaw and affect the alignment of the permanent teeth. If they are allowed to decay to the point where they must be removed, the child suffers a handicap that may give him trouble later. Education for the care of the teeth, with particular attention to the 6-year molars, is important. It is disturbing to inspect young children's teeth and see such a large number with decaying 6-year molars.

Dental hygiene for children includes a routine inspection, with cleaning and ap-plication of a fluoride at least twice a year and conscientious brushing after meals. A well balanced diet is important for healthy teeth. Sweets should be limited to mealtimes.

Health of the School-age Child

In general, this is a healthy age for most children. Very few major diseases have their onset during these years. Minor respiratory diseases spread among children in the close proximity of the schoolroom, although the incidence tends to decrease after the age of 5 or 6.

Children with head colds, or coughs or sore throats should be kept home from school, kept indoors during cold weather and encouraged to rest as much as possible. With adequate care, a healthy child can throw off these infections easily enough. Un-fortunately, the younger brother or sister whom he infects may not come off so lightly, but may instead become seriously ill.

Communicable diseases also make the rounds of the schoolroom among those children who were not immunized during their earlier years, either by inoculation or by the disease itself. Most children, with proper care, recover promptly, but encephalitis and pneumonia may cause severe after-effects.

Skin diseases, such as ringworm or scabies, as well as pinworm infestations, are also easily spread, although present day school health supervision and teaching has reduced their incidence.

Schoolchildren need their full amount of sleep, even though they consider it a waste of

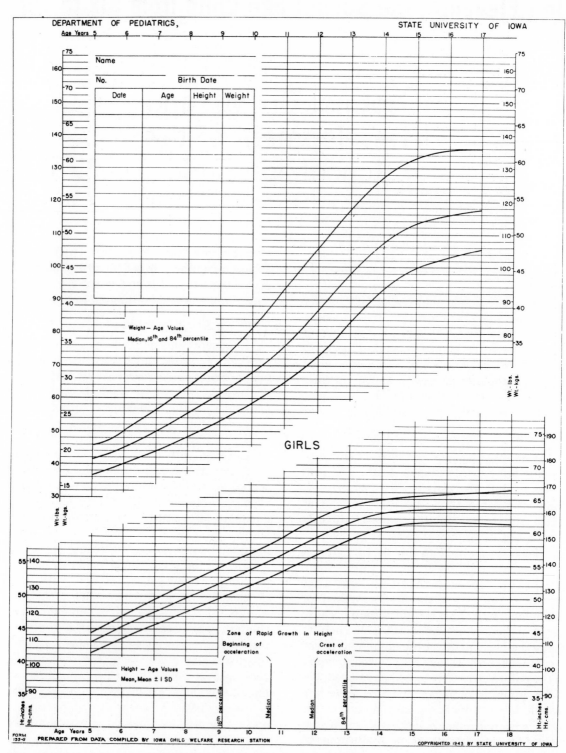

Figure 39-1. Iowa growth chart for girls (University of Iowa).

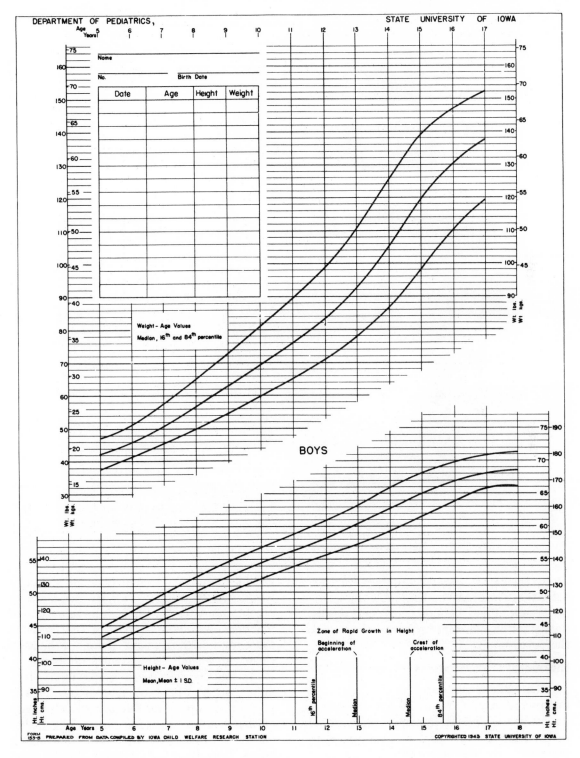

Figure 39-2. Iowa growth chart for boys (University of Iowa).

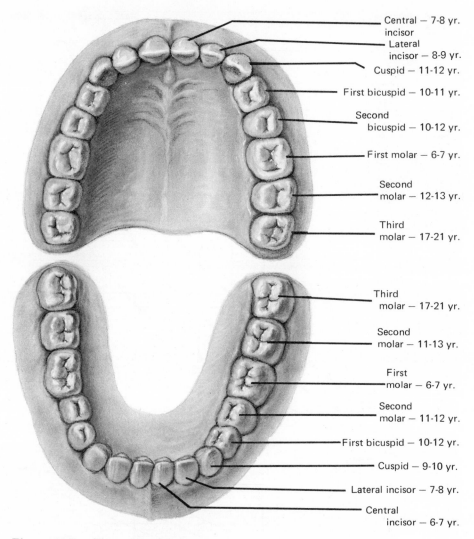

Central — 7-8 yr. incisor
Lateral incisor — 8-9 yr.
Cuspid — 11-12 yr.
First bicuspid — 10-11 yr.
Second bicuspid — 10-12 yr.
First molar — 6-7 yr.
Second molar — 12-13 yr.
Third molar — 17-21 yr.

Third molar — 17-21 yr.
Second molar — 11-13 yr.
First molar — 6-7 yr.
Second molar — 11-12 yr.
First bicuspid — 10-12 yr.
Cuspid — 9-10 yr.
Lateral incisor — 7-8 yr.
Central incisor — 6-7 yr.

Figure 39-3. Chart showing sequence of eruption of permanent teeth.

time—the day is already too short for their activities. Ten or eleven hours of sleep is still necessary. Rest periods may be needed during the day for the six-, and perhaps even the seven-year-olds.

Nutritional Considerations

The child's appetite should start to improve at 5 or 6 years of age. Certainly an adequate diet is important, but other factors, including a pleasant mealtime atmosphere, are also important.

Mealtime should never be used for nagging, fault finding, or for correcting a child's manners. A child lives in a child's world, not an adult world. He can learn to accept more readily the adult valuation of manners, soft voices, and all the customs associated with gracious living, if he sees them carried out, consistently, at home.

Indeed he does learn by example. Jimmy's father does not like string beans; everyone knows this, but tonight, Jimmy's mother has served string beans. The father says,"Now Bess, you know I don't like string beans. Here Jimmy, have some, they're good for you." Naturally, Jimmy does not like string beans either, and passes them on.

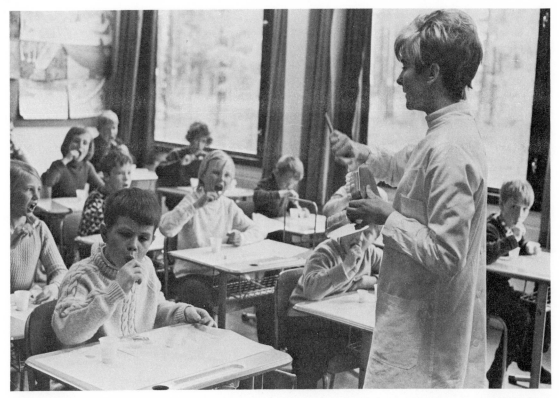

Figure 39-4. Good habits of dental care must be learned early. (Courtesy of the World Health Organization.)

Children frequently go on food "jags," wishing the same food day after day. This soon passes and is unimportant if the child generally gets the necessary nutrients. It does not matter greatly if a child dislikes or refuses a certain food; he is apt to learn to like it later if too much emphasis is not placed on his dislikes. He would have a greater inclination to eat most foods, however, if everyone else accepted them in a matter-of-fact way.

Children like simple, plain foods, are good judges of their own needs if their appetites have not been perverted by coaxing, nagging, bribes or rewards. Even in sickness, an average child knows enough not to eat more than is good for him. A long, debilitating disease may affect him so that he loses his appetite, and strong emotions may cause him to lose interest in food, but force helps little and may have harmful effects.

A child may easily fall into the habit of running into the house frequently and grabbing a handful of cookies or crackers, and then showing a conspicuous lack of appetite at mealtime. Strict curtailment of such snacks may be needed, with only a mid-morning or after-school snack allowed, with perhaps a possible something at bedtime.

A healthy child, full of energy, and generally properly nourished, undoubtedly eats as much as he needs, even though his weight may remain stationary for a time, or show only a very slight gain. Preschool children have sometimes fallen into the habit of dawdling, or of interrupting their meals with play, so the school entrance age may be a good time to start afresh. A small child does not have a clear concept of time and may dawdle, until it is too late to eat a good breakfast if he has to clean his teeth, use the bathroom, and get to school on time. He needs a clearly planned schedule, and no

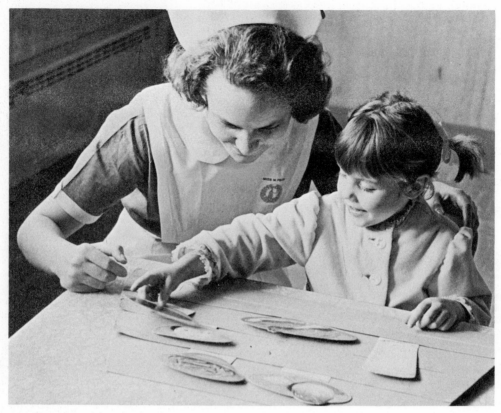

Figure 39-5.   It is important that a child learn the principles of nutrition.

doubt plenty of help to keep it. (Fig. 39-5)

The health teaching in school reinforces a mother's teaching, sometimes more than she expects, or even likes. Children, at least in the early grades, are greatly impressed by what their teacher has to say. One small boy accused his mother of not serving as many vegetables daily as he thought his teacher had said were necessary; for days, he counted them suspiciously to make sure that he got the right number.*

As a child grows and becomes absorbed in his own private life, he needs direction and discipline in both standards of hygiene and in acceptable table manners—all administered in a cheerful, matter-of-fact way. If he comes to the table with dirt-encrusted hands, he has to be sent back to wash, and may even need to go back a second time to

---

*Your Child from six to twelve. P. 113. U.S. Department of Health, Education and Welfare. Children's Bureau, publication no. 324, 1964.

spread the clean area a little further. He expects this, even if he feels it his duty to mumble and to grumble.

CHARACTERISTICS OF SIX- AND SEVEN-YEAR-OLDS

His temporary teeth are now beginning to loosen, and he looks forward to the time when one comes out—nor is he above helping this event along by wriggling the loose tooth with his tongue or his fingers. He is quite willing to believe that the coin he finds under his pillow, in place of the tooth he left, was really left by a good fairy.

His belief in magic is real. Usually he still believes in Santa Claus, although this may be from choice rather than conviction. Because his imagination is still keen, he has fears, especially at night, concerning remote, fanciful or imaginary events.

He may lie to escape punishment, or to make himself important, because his ability to distinguish reality from imagination has usually not yet developed fully.

He enjoys group play, but his groups frequently break down into smaller ones of only two or three children. He loves parties, but to him "party manners" are of little importance. His delight in learning is real, and his interest in everything he encounters is intense. Sometimes, to the dismay of his parents, he still shows a lack of discretion. Name calling and the use of vulgar words is common. He can rapidly alternate between good and bad behavior.

Physically, this is an age of great activity. He cannot sit still for long. Running, jumping and tumbling are enjoyed for their own sake. He is able to ride a bicycle, and can hop, skip, and gallop at about the sixth or seventh year, and he can keep time to music. (Fig. 39-6)

CHARACTERISTICS OF SEVEN- TO TEN-YEAR-OLDS

The six-year-old is moving into a new world, because now a well adjusted school age child has developed sufficiently to move easily from the small confines of his home into the larger community. He frequently seems to use his home simply as a place of departure. Nevertheless, it is still very much his source of security and strength.

After the age of seven or eight, he tends to shake off his acceptance of parental standards as the ultimate authority in all matters, and is somewhat more impressed by the behavior of his peers.

Physically, his permanent teeth continue to erupt, requiring the same care needed by his temporary teeth. A child has so many absorbing interests at this point, however, that he needs frequent reminders to brush his teeth or to tend to other hygienic matters such as washing his hands, bathing and changing his clothes.

His interest in group play increases, with acceptance into the group or the gang of great importance. These become either boy groups or girl groups. Formed at first mainly for their own sake, they become increasingly project-oriented. Interest in organizations,

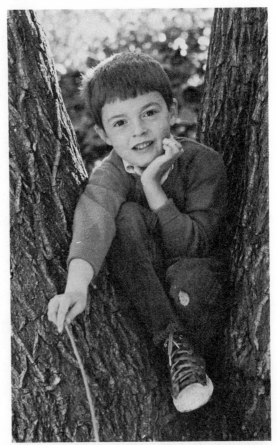

Figure 39-6. The healthy child enjoys climbing. (Carol Baldwin)

such as the Scouts and athletic groups, is usually high.

Secret codes and secret language are popular. Individual friendships are formed as well, and they are apt to become quite intense.

Table games, and arts and crafts requiring skill and dexterity are popular, as well as more active pursuits. (Fig. 39-8)

Although acceptance by his peers is extremely important, a child will have incorporated into his own personality the normal standards of his parents. He may, under stress, cheat, lie or steal, but he suffers considerable guilt if he has learned that these are unacceptable values. With understanding guidance at home, a let-up of pressures if necessary, and acceptance of him as a person, he should not wander too far from acceptable behavior.

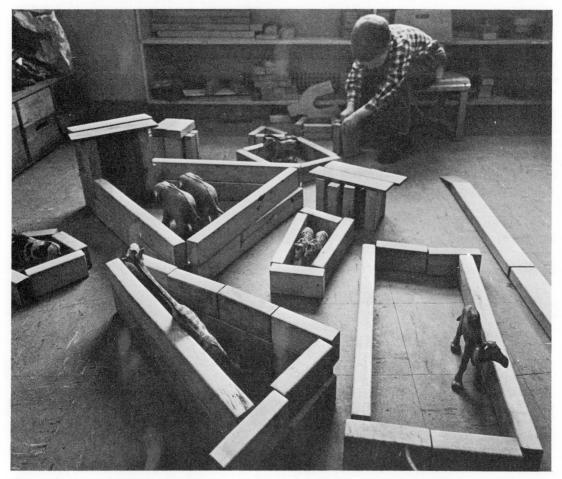

Figure 39-7.   Imaginative play is part of the growing process. (Carol Baldwin)

SCHOOL DAYS

A six-year-old is indeed moving into a new world, that of the schoolroom. Perhaps he has attended nursery school or kindergarten and may feel himself to be an "old pro," but he knows that this was not "real" school.

Six-year-old Ruthie dressed up in her new and prettiest school dress and started off with confidence for her first day in the first grade. At noon, an important young lady called home. "Mother, will you pick me up at school and take me to the store? I must buy some school supplies right away. No; I had better not come home first. The supplies might be all gone." So her mother picked up Ruthie in the car and took her to the ten cent

store where she carefully selected some crayons, a ruler, an eraser and a pencil. "We have started to study jography," she said. "The teacher asked us where we had spent our vacations, and I told her Pennsylvania. Then I found Pennsylvania on the globe." Ruthie seemed to be off to a good start.

Most children appear eager to start school and go willingly enough. If they have maturational readiness for this experience, are physically healthy and emotionally secure, this eagerness should help them get off to a good start and keep them interested as time goes on.

A child is entitled to an adequate physical examination before entering school, either by a private pediatrician, a child clinic,

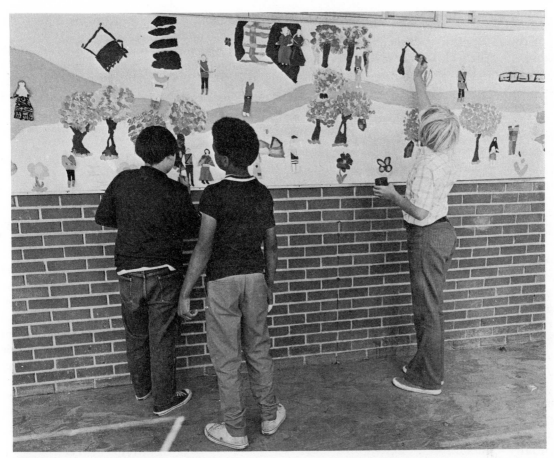

Figure 39-8. Cooperation and creativity can work together. (Carol Baldwin)

or by a school physician. Hearing and sight should be checked, defects should be corrected whenever possible, teeth examined, and the general health should be checked. His immunizations should be brought up to date. (See immunization schedule in Chap. 26.)

Readiness for school is more than physical, however. He should understand certain safety rules, and practice them until they are routine. He should know his full name, his father's name, his street address and his telephone number. It would be extremely helpful if he has met and has become acquainted with policemen, so that he understands one of their duties is to help small children, not to punish them.

He should have learned the function of traffic lights and, hopefully, has watched his family obeying them as a matter of course.

Readiness also includes being able to go to the toilet alone, and to be able to manage his own clothing, with perhaps a little help with the really hard parts of his outdoor wear.

If a child has already attended nursery school, kindergarten or Head Start program, entering the first grade should be pleasing, exciting, and not unduly disturbing. If he has not had that privilege, any preparation should include one, or perhaps several visits to school, a proven ability to accept separation from his home and his mother during the day, and some experience in getting along with other children. He must be able to sit still for short periods of time, and learn to take his turn. Some children who have not matured sufficiently for this experience will do poorly and will dislike school.

DEVELOPMENTAL TASKS

Erikson speaks of this developmental phase of a child's life as the need to develop a sense of *industry* versus *inferiority*. His new status as a school-age child has opened up wide fields of experience. In his desire to find a place among those of his own age, he directs all his energies toward mastering problems as they arise. Yet he knows that he is still a child and is not capable of taking an equal part in the adult world. This tends to give him a feeling of inferiority and spurs him on to learn and experiment more diligently.

The sense of duty and accomplishment, which quite logically grows out of the preceding levels, occupies the years from 6 to 12. This is the period of *industry*, during which the child is interested in engaging in "real" tasks and is capable of seeing them through to completion. His developmental learning includes how to cooperate, to lead, to follow, and to observe the rudiments of fair play. He must, however, have his accomplishments noted and rewarded if he is to develop a sense of achievement and to be able to evaluate himself realistically. If he continually encounters defeat or disparagement—"Bobby does that much better"—he will eventually give up and no longer try.

EMOTIONAL SUPPORT FOR THE CHILD

An adult can never fully enter into the world of a child. When we say "What makes him act this way?" or when we try to put ourselves in his place, we can do so only to a degree. We know something about how and why a child, under certain circumstances, reacts as he does, because we have studied child reaction and child behavior and because we can also remember our own childhood. We cannot know all of the particular factors that influence any particular child's behavior. Neither does the child. He is not good or bad because of any innate goodness or badness, but rather because of the impact of his heredity, his environment, his un-

derstanding, and, to a surprising extent, his physical condition.

A child is born with a need to be loved and accepted. When his parents are entirely satisfied with him as he is, he can take his place as a member of the family, with all of the rights and privileges (as well as the restrictions suitable to his age) that such a place provides.

As he grows, his home should be a place where he is accepted for himself. He is expected to make mistakes; if he makes no mistakes, he cannot be learning to be self-reliant. He must be able to turn to his parents when mistakes do occur, and expect to receive direction and advice.

His parents should also make him feel that they think he is the finest child in the world. Not that he can do no wrong; they should recognize that he has to grow and develop. Therefore, they should praise him for his efforts, but should not shame him for his failures or compare him to others to his own detriment. They should help him to build confidence in himself. A child thrives on praise and will work to make himself worthy of still more praise.

THE DEPRIVED CHILD

Discussions of normal growth and development assume that the child comes from a secure, well-adjusted home in which there is an ample opportunity for cultural enrichment. Unfortunately, that assumption ignores a sizeable portion of the population which, for a number of reasons, does not have such a background.

Society seems to be awakening to its responsibilities to such children, if only in terms of its own preservation. Enriched nursery school and kindergarten experiences are important ways of preparing for a satisfactory school adjustment for those children whose home life cannot do this for them.

Children who have not been able to achieve a sense of security and trust, because of placement in foster homes, inadequate parents, or because of broken homes, need special understanding, warm acceptance from someone, and intelligent guidance in order to grow into self-accepting individuals.

Head Start Programs

Recognition that environmental enrichment is frequently not available in families of limited social, cultural and economic resources, has led to the establishment of Head Start programs. Children in such programs have an opportunity to broaden their horizons through varied experiences. Their understanding of the world they live in is increased, and they are better prepared for a successful entry into the schoolroom. Parent participation is encouraged, although this is frequently difficult for working parents.

SEX EDUCATION FOR THE SCHOOL-AGE CHILD

Dr. Mary Calderone writes, "The sex education of the small child should begin in kindergarten and continue into college."*

What is sex education? It certainly includes education about reproduction, but it must be much broader if the child is to grow up to learn how to understand himself and develop into a sexually mature person. It means helping the child develop desirable attitudes toward his own body, his sex and his sexual role, in order to develop optimum satisfaction in being a boy or in being a girl.

The child has been learning about femininity and masculinity since birth. His mother's gentle touch and handling, her soft voice, the smell of her body and breasts, will help him associate these qualities with being a female. His father's actions toward him, and his parents' respect and love for each other, all enter into the child's sex education and prepare him for his future role. Conversely, downgrading of the male or female role may make him hate and fear his sex and cause him confusion about his sexual role.

Dr. Calderone points out that during the

*Calderone, Mary: Goodbye to The Birds and The Bees. Reprinted from American Education, Nov. 1966 and distributed by Sex Information and Education Council of the U.S. (SIECUS), New York.

"latency" period (roughly between 5 and 10 years of age), there is an enormous broadening of the child's range of interest. However, his sexual interests are still there, although somewhat masked by his involvement in the wider world.

Explicit sex information should be taught in the home, in the schools, and in the churches, with competent, well informed teachers. This is of particular importance in today's society, where the child is exposed on every side to superficial and misleading views of sex. In today's world, so much emphasis is placed on the importance of truthful explanations that mothers at times become over-anxious. It is obvious that the best teaching can be done by parents who are relaxed and natural and who fit their teaching into a context of daily living. This is not always easy, however, and many parents feel quite at a loss as to how to work this out.

Intellectually, a mother can accept quite wholeheartedly the concept that she should answer the child's questions frankly and simply. Matters become rather more complicated, however, when Sonny chooses the Sunday mother has guests for dinner to ask, "Mommy, where do babies come from?" For parents who are rather insecure about this, there are excellent booklets that serve as guides for helping children from the preschool age up through young adulthood.

As school-age children near puberty, they should be told about the physical changes they should expect, well in advance. A girl who has her first menstrual period at 9 or 10 stands a chance of receiving a considerable shock if she has not been prepared. No doubt she has heard various tales from her schoolmates, which admittedly leave much to be desired as a source of information.

In general, girls accept sex teaching best from their mothers, and boys from their fathers. Unfortunately, there are many homes in which either the mother or the father is absent. When a single parent feels inadequate to this task, the various printed aids offer a valuable source of support. These aids are recommended as support for parents, and provide them with a clearer understanding, allowing them to assume a relaxed attitude. They should not be a substitute for parental guidance. They are valuable, however, as a supplement to parental counseling.

DISCIPLINE IN THE HOME

Much has been written about the effects of overpermissiveness. Parents have at times acted as though they were afraid to discipline their children. Perhaps a closer examination of the terms *permissiveness* and *discipline* would be helpful.

Haim Ginott defines permissiveness as "an attitude of accepting the childishness of children."* This means that parents do not expect the child to have the judgment or knowledge of an adult, but they do respect the child as a person in his own right. Discipline can be thought of as a means by which a child is helped to learn socially acceptable behavior. Discipline at its best is preventive discipline—its goal the achievement of self-discipline and a reduction in the need for later punishment.

Respecting the child as a person means that he has the rights and privileges of his age, maturational status and understanding. The parent's role is to set standards, to indicate necessary limits, to allow the child to accept the consequences of his acts while still protecting him from physical or emotional injury. Children need, and indeed desire, to be protected from the harmful effects of their actions. Parents' rights need to be respected also. How can a child learn to respect the rights of others if he has never learned in his own home?

A child needs to feel his parent's disapproval when he misbehaves. When his place in the home is secure and he knows he is loved, being temporarily out of favor will help him try harder to act in a responsible manner.

When a child abuses his privileges, the logical consequence is deprivation of those

*Ginott, Haim: Between Parent and Child, p. 93. New York, Macmillan, 1970.

privileges, else how will he learn? Fraiberg writes that punishment should teach a useful lesson or correct. In other words, punishment is only useful when the child learns constructively from it. It is not useful when a child learns to conceal his acts to avoid punishment or when he learns to invite it to clear his conscience.

Punishment should come as a logical effect of the misdoing. A child who has disobeyed safety rules and plays baseball in the street, can have the privilege of playing baseball taken away from him for a day or two. This makes sense to him, but he will see no logic in having other privileges, such as watching his favorite television program, taken away for an unrelated offense.

Bettelheim writes: "Some homes have been geared mainly to the rhythm and interests of the children as though there were no adults present.... The resultant insecurity is great, since the protectors a child needs are absent, and the child is properly confused ...."†

---

†Bettelheim, Bruno: Love is Not Enough, p. 24. New York, Macmillan, 1970.

BIBLIOGRAPHY

Arnstein, Helene S.: Your Growing Child and Sex. New York, Avon, 1968.
Bettelheim, Bruno: Love is Not Enough. New York, Macmillan, 1970.
Erikson, Erik H.: Childhood and Society. ed. 2. New York, Norton, 1963.
Ginott, Haim: Between Parent and Child. New York, Macmillan, 1970.
Johnson, Eric: Love and Sex in Plain Language. Philadelphia, J. B. Lippincott, 1967.
Lerrigo, Marion and Southard, Helen: A Story About You. Sex Education Series, (distributed by the American Medical Association and the National Education Association), 1966.
Maier, Henry W.: Three Theories of Child Development. New York, Harper and Row, 1969.
Your Child from 6 to 12. U. S. Department of Health, Education and Welfare, Children's Bureau, 1966.

Nursing Care of the Child with Diabetes 40

"When it comes to diabetes, the child must not be regarded as a little adult. The cause of his diabetes is different. Treatment is different, more complicated."*

An average student nurse has spent considerable class and study time learning about diabetes mellitus and its effects on adults. Perhaps she has done some patient teaching about this. Thus it sometimes happens that she feels this is one area that she knows well enough so that she can spend her pediatric classtime more profitably in other ways. This train of thought is unfortunate, because the study of diabetes mellitus in children needs a fresh approach. The condition is somewhat the same, but its manifestations are greatly modified by certain factors peculiar to children.

CLASSIFICATION OF DIABETES

Diabetes mellitus appearing before the age of 15 years is termed juvenile diabetes to distinguish it from the type of diabetes mellitus that has its onset in later life. The condition called *diabetes insipidus* is a disease of the pituitary or the hypothalamus gland, and has no relationship to diabetes mellitus. Diabetes insipidus is a relatively rare condition, however, and is designated by the entire name. Diabetes mellitus, therefore, is usually simply called diabetes, or juvenile diabetes if the onset occurs during childhood.

---

*Jackson, Robert L.: The child with diabetes. *Nutrition Today*, 6:2, 1971.

INCIDENCE

It is estimated that there are perhaps 120,000 children under 15 years of age in the United States who have diabetes. This in itself is important enough to justify spending additional time learning about its manifestations and its treatment.

Diabetes is now known to be an hereditary disease, probably of a recessive gene character. The widespread variability in the manifestation of diabetes mellitus (that is, clinical severity and wide range of age at onset) complicates the study of the genetic pattern. In childhood, the presence of an acute infection may, it is believed, be the trigger mechanism activating a latent diabetes.

True diabetes is very rare in the newborn but it does occur. A transient type of diabetes may be found that clears up shortly after birth and probably does not recur. True diabetes may occur, however, as early as 6 months of age, although the onset of presenting clinical symptoms is more often in the 4 to 12 year age group.

PATHOGENESIS OF DIABETES MELLITUS

Normally, the sugar derived from digestion and assimilation of foods is burned to provide energy for the body's activities. Excess sugar is converted into fat or glycogen and stored in the body tissues. A substance secreted by the pancreas, called insulin, is responsible for the burning and storing of sugar. In diabetes mellitus, because of a deficiency of insulin, sugar accumulates in the bloodstream and spills over into the urine. In the child, there is an abrupt, pronounced decrease in insulin production, thus resulting in decreased ability to use the food he eats. It may be this combination of failure to gain weight and lack of energy that prompts the parents to bring the child to the doctor or pediatric outpatient department for a check-up.

More frequently, however, a child is brought to the physician in a state of acidosis, often in a semicomatose state, and sometimes actually in coma. It is, of course, possible that this condition has not appeared so suddenly as it would seem. This is an area in which the nurse in the community has an important role to play. A mother may comment that her baby never seems to be dry, and appears to need diaper changes more frequently than he did formerly. Another mother may find it extremely difficult to toilet-train her toddler; he just won't stay dry long enough. She may also notice, as one mother did, that the child always seems thirsty and wanting a drink. Other children who have been toilet-trained may go back to bedwetting.

EARLY DETECTION—THE NURSE'S ROLE

Children of families in which diabetes is or has been present should be tested routinely. This is particularly important whenever a child in such a family has an infectious disease. Dr. Robert Jackson, an authority on juvenile diabetes, states*: "there is a growing body of evidence that, even in children, the (glucose) tolerance test may be abnormal for many years before clinical diabetes itself becomes evident."

Whenever a nurse has knowledge of a family history of diabetes, she has an obligation to all members of that family. She needs to be alert to suggestive symptoms in any member, regardless of age. The public in general is not sufficiently aware of the high incidence of diabetes in children, so that the

*Ibid

parents may not connect the difficulty in toilet training or the child's unusual thirst with physical abnormality.

The nurse's obligation extends beyond her ability to recognize potential danger signals, however. In her role as educator, she should make the parents aware of their own obligations. All relatives of diabetics should be considered a suspect group, and should have periodic testing for diabetes.

A nurse need not be an alarmist, but should present the facts in an orderly manner. She should explain the hereditary aspect of the disease, its incidence of onset during childhood among the diabetic population, and the importance of regularly scheduled screening tests.

It is well established that early detection and control are of extreme importance in postponing or minimizing complications later in life. For reasons not yet clear, the diabetic's need for insulin increases during the stress of an infection. Acute infections do appear to frequently activate a latent or chemical diabetes† into a clinically active state.

Tests for Detection of Diabetes

Children in diabetic families can have their urine tested by their parents. Although presence of sugar in the urine does not of necessity indicate a diabetic state, it should be reported to the physician. The physician will probably follow up with a glucose tolerance test. The presence of sugar in the urine or an elevated blood sugar is indicative of diabetes, but occasionally is due to other causes. A postprandial blood specimen is often ordered for the determination of glucose metabolism. However, only a full scale glucose tolerance test can give a definite diagnosis of diabetes mellitus.‡

---

†Chemical diabetes is a term used to denote a state in which no overt symptoms of diabetes are present but the glucose tolerance curve is in the diabetic range.

‡Tests for glycosuria and hyperglycemia are described later in this section on diabetes.

TREATMENT AND FAMILY TEACHING

After it has been determined that a child is diabetic, he is usually hospitalized for a period of time, to stabilize his condition under supervision. The nurse must remember that this is a trying time for the parents as well as for the child, especially if he is old enough to understand its significance. The parent sees his child as someone who "will always be different," and who will need to take special care of himself all his life. The idea of giving insulin injections is in itself appalling. The combination of giving insulin, checking daily urine and calculating diets must appear overwhelming, especially to parents with other children.

Insulin was discovered as recently as 1922. Before that time it was a rare diabetic child who lived to grow up. The parents of a present-day diabetic child almost certainly have heard terrifying stories from friends and from relatives about childhood diabetes. Many of these parents may remember some member of the family, alive at that time, who suffered from all the frequent complications before the advent of insulin.

A child enters the hospital not only for the treatment of his illness and for the regulation of his diet and insulin. He and his parents are there to *learn*. The teaching program in a hospital is concerned primarily with a sound, basic concept of the disease itself. A child can assimilate facts and concepts only as much as his maturational level permits him to. As time goes on, his parents must be his principal teachers; therefore, they must have a satisfactory understanding of the condition. The success of any subsequent teaching about diet, insulin, exercise and control depends largely on the degree in which the parents grasp the entire picture, as well as the older child mature enough to take the responsibility for some of his own management.

If the hospital does not have a regular instruction program outlined for the patient and for his parents, the nurse should be able to find a number of books and articles to assist her in her teaching, and that would also be valuable for the family to read.

Principles of Diet

Before diagnosis has been made, the diabetic child's nutritional stores have been depleted. In the initial phase of management he needs additional calories and nutrients to rebuild his body's tissues and stores. He will also need larger doses of insulin to take care of the additional calories. This is one of the important reasons for putting him in the hospital under the care of a dietician.

Understanding the principles of a diabetic diet is an important aspect of the teaching program in the hospital. The dietician should be principally responsible for this, but the nurse is the person who ultimately is going to have the task of reinforcing this information, as well as the possibility of having to interpret it.

The present tendency with respect to diet is to put the child on a diet best suited to his nutritional needs for his weight and for his age. Weighed diets are not used so frequently as they were in the past, because many physicians prefer a measured diet, or even a free diet. The measured diet provides a nutritionally adequate diet with the emphasis on protein and vitamin-rich foods. Exchange foods lists are used with this diet, and the standard measuring cups and spoons can usually be used. A child on a free diet should have his nutritional needs considered. The only restriction on the types of food taken is to limit his intake of excessive carbohydrates, such as candy, pastries and cake.

Whether the diet is a measured one with food exchanges, or a so-called free diet, it is especially important that it be nutritionally well-balanced. It is necessary to find out how much the family understands about basic nutrition and to fill in the gaps when necessary. A diabetic child needs a liberal amount of protein in his diet, as well as vitamin-rich foods. All this the family must learn and understand.

There are demonstration food trays on the market that are excellent for helping the child and his family learn the basic principles of a well-balanced diet. These trays are of heavy cardboard with slots cut into the tray for the various cardboard food dishes. All the basic dishes are available in cut-out form with the nutritional value of the food given on the back of each item. It is as much fun as any game to set up various well-balanced meals on this tray.*

Urine Reductions

The parents, as well as the child, need instruction in urine reduction. A child of five or six years is not too young to learn, under supervision, the mechanics of urine testing. The parents must be reminded that the tablets, if they are used, are corrosive and harmful, if by chance they are swallowed. The color may be attractive to the child who might want to investigate further. Perhaps the parents should feel the test tube while the tablet is dissolving to discover how hot the solution actually becomes. Any reagent, of whatever type, should be stored away when it is not in use, in order to keep it out of the hands of small children.

A young child in the hospital can watch the nurse while she does the test, and he can help count the drops of urine as they are added. He will be proud of his ability to count, and fascinated over the change of color. Soon he should be able to do it himself under the watchful eye of his mother and should be able to keep his own chart by coloring-in the correct color change.

A child of three or four very quickly learns that there is a relationship between voiding and urine testing, and accepts this as a way of life.

Juvenile diabetes is extremely labile, making it important that urine be tested before each meal, at least until control is established. A second specimen, voided 20 to 30 minutes after the first, will be more ac-

curate and should be obtained, if at all possible. It does present a problem to little tots who have only recently been toilet-trained. When asked to "go potty" they are apt to protest, "But I did go potty," and to feel quite injured that they are not considered to have performed satisfactorily. Usually, it is best to test a toddler's urine every time he voids, because it is entirely unpredictable as to whether he will go at the designated times. After the child leaves the hospital, urine reductions are usually continued three or four times daily.

Many physicians prefer to regulate the insulin so that a small amount of sugar will appear in the urine (one plus or trace). They consider the slight spill-over of sugar in the urine to have a less dangerous potential than the possibility of frequent insulin reactions from lowered blood sugar. The physicians who treat in this manner ask to have repeated reductions showing negative results reported for a possible decrease in insulin. Tests for acetone, using acetest tablets, are made at the same time as a blood sugar monitoring device. Any appearance of acetone in the urine should be reported immediately.

A school-age child may have difficulty, or may experience embarrassment over noon-time urine reductions. If he does not go home at noon, the physician may allow him to skip the noon test, or a child may go to the school nurse's office to do the test. One girl collected urine in a tightly corked test tube, carried it in her purse and tested it at home after school.

A child should be taught to keep a record of urine reductions, making a color chart or using one of the prepared charts. Some supervision from the parents is necessary, particularly if the chart is repeatedly negative. Children frequently get bored or angry over the whole thing, and the testing of tap water in place of urine is not unheard of. Charts have even been made up neatly for a week in advance. Parents need to understand the child's emotions, however. Probably some scheme of a routine check—perhaps a weekly test—would be more ac-

---

*Food models and display piece obtainable from the National Dairy Council, 111 N. Canal, Chicago, Ill., 60606. A catalog of educational materials is available on request.

ceptable than a check based on doubt or suspicion.

Insulin: Type and Method of Injection

Because diabetic children have no residual ability to produce insulin, it is probable (according to our present knowledge) that he will always need to take insulin. Oral medications are frequently useful in maintaining a satisfactory blood sugar level for an adult who has developed diabetes late in life. The child, however, must have insulin supplied to him, and to date, insulin is only effective when given by injection. The type of insulin ordered is determined by the individual child's needs. After stabilization, many children can be maintained on an intermediate or long-acting type of insulin.

It is important that all children receiving long-acting insulin in the morning have a bedtime snack in the evening, in order to avoid an insulin reaction during the night.

Frequently, children on long-lasting insulin go into shock during the early morning hours. The night nurse must observe the child at least every two hours, note the tossed bedding that would indicate restlessness, note any excessive perspiration, and if necessary, try to arouse him. As the child becomes regulated and observes a careful diet at home, his parents need not watch him so closely, but they should have a thorough understanding of all aspects of the disease.

An example of the sort of thing that can happen in a hospital concerns a six-year-old boy, who, after being put to bed at 9 PM, slept soundly all night. His night nurse became suspicious of a possible reaction at about 4 AM when she found him quite wet with perspiration and discovered his bedding tossed about. She was able to awaken him enough to get a urine specimen, which upon testing showed a strong positive reaction for sugar. Not satisfied, however, she asked advice, but the decision was made that the high sugar ruled out insulin shock, so nothing was done. At 7 AM the child could not be roused. A blood sugar determination revealed hypoglycemia, and intravenous glucose had to be administered to bring the child out of coma. Why did he show glycosuria at 4 AM? The answer is simple; he had last urinated at 9 PM, and sugar-containing urine had been collecting in his bladder all night.

Insulin reactions. Because diabetes in children is extremely labile, the child is subject to insulin reactions. A nurse should

Varieties of Insulin*

Type	Onset of Action	Peak of Action	Duration of Action
Rapid Acting			
1 Regular	1/2 hr.	2-4 hrs.	6-8 hrs.
2 Semi-Lente	1/2 hr.	2-4 hrs.	10-12 hrs.
Intermediate Acting			
1 N.P.H. (isophane)	2 hrs.	8-10 hrs.	28-30 hrs.
2 Lente	2 hrs.	8-10 hrs.	20-26 hrs.
3 Globin	2 hrs.	8-16 hrs.	Up to 24 hrs.
Long Acting			
1 PZI (protamine zinc)	4-8 hrs.	14-20 hrs.	24-36 hrs.
2 Ultra-Lente	4-8 hrs.	14-24 hrs.	36 hrs. or more

*Adapted from Nelson, W., Vaughn, V. C., and McKay, R. James: Textbook of Pediatrics, p. 1161. Philadelphia, W. B. Saunders, 1969.

Insulin reactions in children may be difficult to recognize. Two-year-old Donald was hospitalized for the regulation of his diabetic condition. He had entered the hospital in deep coma and now, two weeks later, he was still having some difficulty in adjusting satisfactorily to his diet and his insulin dosage. One day at naptime, he went to sleep in his usual manner, and it did not occur to his nurse that anything was wrong, yet he went into insulin shock during his sleep. When a nurse found him perspiring deeply, and had great difficulty arousing him from his nap, she realized that these children present somewhat different problems from those of the diabetic adult.

take note that a child may not recognize an impending reaction, particularly if he is young. She should also recognize that both she and the parents may have some difficulty recognizing reactions.

Some of the symptoms of impending insulin shock in children are—any type of odd, unusual or antisocial behavior; headache and malaise; blurred vision and faintness, and undue fatigue or hunger. One small child complained of hunger just before evening tray time, and before the nurse could bring her supper tray, she went into a convulsion. After two such episodes, the nurse learned to have orange juice readily available for the child whenever she complained of hunger. One older child, however, worked a system for obtaining a little extra juice. Every afternoon, he regularly complained of faintness and was convincing enough to get his juice. After a few such episodes, blood sugar determination revealed that his blood level was at the highest at this time of day. He was an intelligent child, and after the tests and their significance were explained to him, he cooperated, and his afternoon reactions ceased.

Most newly diagnosed diabetic children show a decreased need for insulin during the first weeks or months after control is established. This is a natural reaction, and it should be explained to avoid the false hope that the diabetic is "getting better." As the child grows, his need for insulin increases and continues to do so until he reaches full growth. Again, this needs to be explained; the child's condition is not "getting worse."

Another matter that merits discussion is the use of insulin during illness or an infection in a diabetic child. When an ill child is unable to eat his prescribed diet, his mother rather naturally assumes that his insulin dose should be reduced. This is not the case, however; his insulin may actually need to be increased during this period

In actual fact, this all points up the importance of close supervision by the physician. Parents need to understand this, and should have no hesitancy about reporting any change in the child's health, any recurring insulin reactions, the persistence of more than a small amount of urine sugar, and, in particular, any positive urine acetone reaction.

Methods of giving insulin. The child will not be able to take over the management of his insulin dose as early as he learned to test his urine, but he can watch the preparation of the syringe, and learn the technique for drawing up the dosage. If he can watch until it becomes routine, it might be helpful. By the time he is eight or nine, he should be thinking out his dose and getting the feel of the syringe. He should be drawing up his own dosage and preparing for the time when he will be caring for himself. Just when that comes cannot be stated arbitrarily. No two children mature at the same rate; some may be able to do this quite early. For others, this may be an act of love on the mother's part, showing her concern and care for him. A child should be encouraged, however, to take over the management of his therapy as soon as he is ready. *He can learn the importance of the routine and accept the restrictions his disease imposes if he has helped to make the decisions.* (Fig. 40-1)

Manner of injection. The child and his parents should be taught the correct way to give insulin, and supervised until it is certain that they are injecting the insulin subcutaneously rather than intradermally.

Rotating injection sites is also a matter of considerable importance. If insulin is given frequently in the same location, the area is apt to become indurated and is eventually fibrosed, hindering proper insulin absorption. The atrophic hollows in the skin, or the lumps of hypertrophied tissue, are unsightly as well. Some people, however, appear to have a greater skin sensitivity than others.

Definite instruction should be given concerning the importance of rotating sites. Areas on both the upper arms and the upper thighs can be used, allowing several weeks between the use of the same site, if a plan is carefully mapped out. Starting from the inner, upper corner of the area, each injection is given one-half inch below the preceding one, going down in a vertical line, with the next series starting one-half inch outward at the upper level. The lower abdomen may also be used if necessary. If there is any sign of induration, the local site should be carefully avoided for a period of weeks after all signs of irritation have disappeared.

Exercise in the Hospital

It would be unrealistic to attempt to regulate a child's diet and insulin dosage if we insist on keeping him unduly quiet in the hospital. We want him to be a normal, active child at home, and thus we teach him that he can resume all normal activities. He needs an opportunity to be active, at the same time learning how to handle his condition. If possible, a child should be allowed to play outside. If conditions do not permit this, he should be able to obtain activity within the hospital, with an opportunity for active exercise, such as bicycle riding, in the physical therapy department and in the playroom.

Continuing Home Care

A diabetic child should carry some form of sugar with him at all times. Candy is useful, although perhaps it presents more temptation to the child than does pure sugar. In cases of doubtful insulin reactions, it is undoubtedly better to give sugar than to

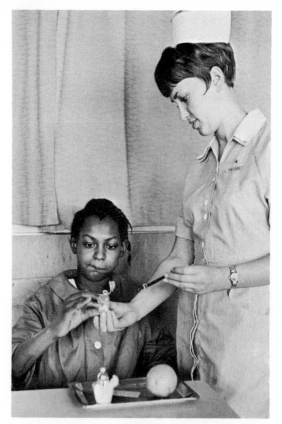

Figure 40-1. An adolescent learns to prepare insulin.

withhold it, but frequent reactions indicate a need for a physician's attention.

It is extremely important that a child wear an identification medal or a bracelet, with information about his diabetic status.* Identification cards, such as those carried by many adult diabetics, are seldom practical for a child diabetic.

Some of the difficulty encountered in regulating blood sugar stability stems from the variations in an average child's activity. His school day contains many hours of sitting still, interspersed with sports or gymnastics, whereas on weekends and vacation periods, he may be much more active. Theoretically, his greatest periods of activity should come at the time of day when

*Medic Alert, An International Nonprofit Organization, supplies these bracelets at a nominal price.

his blood sugar is highest; in practice, this is not always possible for a school child. Many physicians advocate a diet increase for those days when the child is more active physically. This calls for good judgement and understanding on the part of the child's parents.

A diabetic child should participate in normal activities for his age, and should consider himself a normal child. He should, however, make his diabetic condition known to at least one friend, and should not go swimming or hiking without a responsible individual nearby, who knows what to look for and who knows what to do if the child should have a reaction.

Some older children are quite sensitive about their condition, and fear that they seem "different" from their friends. Even with the best of instruction and preparation they may feel this way, and wish to keep their condition secret. They must understand that a teacher or some other adult in their environment should be acquainted with their condition. Classroom teachers should know which of their students have such a condition, and should understand the signs of an impending reaction. Any unexplained inattention, blurring of vision, or other unusual behavior, should alert the teacher to this possibility.

Diabetic children under good control need not be kept from such activities as camp-outs, overnight trips with the school band, or other, similar activities away from home. Of course, a child must be capable of measuring his insulin and giving his own injections. Some young people report that a desire to participate in such an activity was the factor that overcame their reluctance to take over this responsibility.

The disposable insulin syringes and needles now on the market simplify traveling for the diabetic. They come several to a package, and are relatively inexpensive. A diabetic must keep in mind, however, that a number of states sell insulin syringes and needles only on prescription—a fact that a young person might not realize if his syringes have been bought in one drug store.

When he travels, he should take a prescription with him for presentation if, for any reason, he needs to buy equipment. He must also make sure that a responsible person on the trip knows that he has diabetes, has a knowledge of the symptoms of insulin reaction and diabetic acidosis, and knows what to do. The family with whom he stays on week ends must also have this information.

The Treatment of Insulin Shock

Any indication of an insulin reaction should be treated immediately by allowing the child to take sugar, candy, or orange juice, even if the parents suspect the child of faking. Any normal child breaks the rules once in a while. Repeated reactions, or impending reactions, either real or fancied, call for a checkup by a physician.

Because reactions are apt to progress rapidly, every adult responsible for a diabetic child should clearly understand the procedure to be followed if the child is unable to take any form of sugar orally. Glucagon is a substance that can be administered subcutaneously, brings about a prompt rise in blood sugar, and is invaluable for use as an emergency measure. All parents, school teachers or nurses, and other adults, even temporarily in charge of diabetic children, should have access to this drug and should understand its use.

Glucagon is a hormone produced by the pancreatic islets that also produce insulin. Whereas an elevation of blood glucose results in an insulin release (in a normal person) a fall in blood sugar stimulates glucagon release. The released glucagon in the blood stream acts on the liver to promote glycogen breakdown and glucose release.*

Glucagon is now available as a pharmaceutical product, packaged as a powder in individual dose units. A person preparing the dosage need only add the diluent, which comes with the powdered drug, by the use of

*Jacob, S., and Francone, C.: Structure and Function in Man. P. 476. Philadelphia, W. B. Saunders, ed. 2, 1970.

a sterile syringe and needle, draw up the solution, and administer it in the same manner as insulin.

Glucagon acts within minutes to restore a child to consciousness, after which he can take candy or sugar. This treatment prevents the long delay occasioned by waiting for a doctor to come and administer glucose intravenously, or waiting for an ambulance trip to the hospital emergency department. It is, however, a form of emergency treatment, and not a substitute for proper medical supervision.

ADOLESCENCE

Adolescence is an extremely trying period for many diabetics, as it is for other young people. Because a normal child has to work through from dependence to independence, so does the diabetic child. Even when a child has accepted much of his own care, he may rebel against the control that this condition places on him. Frequently he becomes impatient, and seems to convince himself that he really does not care about his future health. He may skip meals or drop controls over his diet, or he may neglect urine reductions. It can be a difficult time for both the parents and their child. The parents naturally become concerned, and are apt to give the child more controls to rebel against. Special care should be taken by the family, the teachers, the nurses and the doctors to see that these young people find enough maturing satisfaction in other areas, and do not need to rebel in this vital area.

If a child completely understands all aspects of his condition (especially if he has been allowed to assume control of his treatment previously) he should be allowed to continue. Should he run into difficulty, this is a time when an adolescent clinic can be of great value. Here he can discuss his own problems with understanding people who treat him with dignity and listen to him.

FUTURE HEALTH

According to present knowledge, a person who develops diabetes during childhood will always have diabetes. No way has been found to stimulate the nonfunctioning Isles of Langerhans in the pancreas to the production of insulin. Since the discovery of a chemical method of producing insulin, however, the lack can be overcome, and a young person can look forward to a life of normal activity.

BABIES OF DIABETIC MOTHERS

Babies born to diabetic mothers are among the "high-risk" babies, with a high percentage of stillbirths or early death. These babies tend to be large and plump, with a puffiness resembling a "cushingoid" appearance. They frequently are hypoglycemic and hypocalcemic, and the respiratory distress syndrome appears more commonly than in other full-term infants.

A diabetic prospective mother who places herself early under adequate medical supervision and who adheres conscientiously to her diabetic regime, affords herself and the infant the best chance for a healthy life.

DIABETIC ACIDOSIS

Diabetic acidosis needs to be clearly distinguished from *insulin shock. Diabetic acidosis* occurs in untreated diabetics. Due to the inadequate production of insulin by the pancreas, carbohydrates are not converted into fuel for energy production. Fats are then mobilized for energy but in the absence of glucose are oxidized incompletely. Ketone bodies (acetone, diacetic acid and oxybutyric acid) accumulate. They are readily excreted in the urine, but in the process the acid-base balance of body fluids is upset and acidosis results.

Symptoms of Diabetic Acidosis

A child developing diabetic acidosis presents the classical symptoms: drowsiness, a dry skin, flushed cheeks and cherry-red lips, acetone breath with a fruity smell and hyperpnea (abnormal increase in the depth and rate of the respiratory movements). There may be nausea and vomiting. If untreated, a child lapses into coma and exhibits the characteristic Kussmaul breathing*, rapid pulse, and subnormal temperature and blood pressure.

Treatment

The patient should be kept warm but not excessively so. Blood chemistries and urine studies are done to evaluate the degree of acidosis. If the child is unable to urinate, a catheter will be put in place. Gastric lavage may be done to relieve abdominal distention. Regular insulin is given subcutaneously or intramuscularly. Intravenous fluids will be given.

INSULIN SHOCK

Insulin shock occurs due to an overdose of insulin. This may be due to a change in the body's requirement, carelessness in diet such as failure to eat proper amounts of food, or perhaps from an error in insulin measurement.

Symptoms of Insulin Shock

Symptoms of insulin shock are: unusual hunger or fatigue; unusual or antisocial behavior; blurred vision; headache; malaise; faintness; dilated pupils; pallor; and sweating. If untreated, the child may have generalized convulsions or become unconscious.

Treatment

Give the child orange juice, sugar or a piece of candy. If the child is unconscious, glucagon can be given subcutaneously, followed by sugar by mouth when the child responds. If the child does not respond, he should be seen by a physician. Intravenous glucose may be needed.

TESTS FOR BLOOD SUGAR

Normally, circulating blood contains enough glucose to take care of the body's needs. Normal fasting blood glucose readings are 70 to 100 mg. per 100 cc. of blood.

*Kussmaul breathing—a distressing dyspnea occurring in paroxysms, often forerunning an attack of diabetic coma.

Postprandial Glucose Test

The patient eats a regular meal with an emphasis on carbohydrates and desserts. Two hours after the meal, blood is drawn and tested for glucose. If blood sugar is above 200 mg. per 100 cc., a tentative diagnosis of diabetes is made, but a glucose tolerance test is necessary for a conclusive diagnosis.

Glucose Tolerance Test†

Preparation:

1. Give regular diet for 4 to 5 days before test.
2. Fasting period directly preceding test: children for 12 hours, young infants for a maximum of 9 hours, and newborn and premature infants for 7 hours.
3. On the morning of the test, a capillary blood specimen is taken (fasting).
4. A urine specimen is obtained (fasting).
5. A glucose solution is given orally. It may be flavored with a few drops of lemon juice. The amount of solution is determined by body weight.
6. Capillary blood is taken 1/2, 1, 1-1/2, 2 and 3 hours after the ingestion of glucose.
7. Urine is collected 1 to 2 hours after the ingestion of glucose.

Average normal response is a rise in blood sugar of 30 to 40 mg. per 100 cc., reaching a peak 30 to 45 minutes after the ingestion of glucose. The blood sugar level returns to normal within 2 to 2-1/2 hours.

URINE SUGAR TESTS

Under normal circumstances, the urine is usually sugar free. However, the presence of sugar in the urine is not conclusive evidence of diabetes. Repeated findings of glycosuria, together with an elevated blood sugar, is a positive sign. For a definitive diagnosis, a glucose tolerance test is needed.

†Adapted from Behrendt, H.: Diagnostic Tests in Infants and Children, ed. 2. Philadelphia, Lea & Febiger, 1962 (and from other sources).

Benedict's Solution Urine Test

1. Place 5 cc. of Benedict's solution in a test tube.
2. Add 8 drops of urine.
3. Place test tube upright in a pan of water and boil for 5 minutes.
4. Remove from pan, wait for a few seconds, shake tube gently. Compare color with color chart.

(Benedict's has largely been replaced by the simpler Clinitest tablets or reagent strips.)

Urine Sugar Test (Clinitest)

1. Put five drops of urine in a test tube, and add 10 drops of water.
2. Add a Clinitest reagent tablet.
3. The solution will then "boil." After the boiling stops, wait 15 seconds, shake the tube and compare it with color chart.
   Negative — no change
   Trace — blue green
   1+ — light green
   2+ — yellow green
   3+ — yellow or orange green
   4+ — orange
   Do not use if tablets have commenced to change color.
   Caution: Clinitest tablets are caustic and should be kept away from small children.

TesTape (urine sugar analysis paper, Lilly)*

1. Collect urine specimen (only a small amount needed).
2. Holding a strip of TesTape in your hand, dip the end of the tape in the urine.
3. Remove; wait for one minute. Hold dry end of tape in hand to prevent contamination.
4. Compare darkest area on test strip with color chart. Color ranges from yellow (negative) to dark green (4+).

Reagent strips should be stored out of direct light, moisture and heat to be assured of correct results.

Do not use after expiration date.

---

*Other reagent strips are Diastix (for urine glucose) and Keto-Diastix (for urine glucose and ketones). Ames Company, Division of Miles Laboratories.

BIBLIOGRAPHY

Behrendt, H.: Diagnostic Tests in Infants and Children ed. 2. Philadelphia, Lea & Febiger, 1962.

Jackson, Robert L.: The child with diabetes. Nutrition Today, 6:2, 1971.

Jacob, S. and Francone, C.: Structure and Function in Man. ed. 2. Philadelphia, W. B. Saunders, 1970.

Nelson, Waldo *et al.*, eds.: Textbook of Pediatrics. ed. 9. Philadelphia, W. B. Saunders, 1969.

Nursing Care of the Child with Other Conditions

41

APPENDICITIS

Appendicitis is rare in infancy. Most cases in childhood occur after the fourth year. In young children the symptoms may be difficult to evaluate.

Etiology

Obstruction of the lumen of the appendix is the primary cause. The obstruction may follow a generalized infection or on occasion an infestation of pinworms may be the cause.

Clinical Manifestation

In the older child symptoms may be the same as in an adult. These are pain and tenderness in the right lower quadrant of the abdomen, nausea and vomiting, fever and constipation. These presenting symptoms are infrequent in young children, many of whom have a ruptured appendix when first seen by the physician. The young child has difficulty localizing pain. He may act restless and irritable, have a slight fever with flushed face and rapid pulse. The white cell count is usually mildly elevated. It may take several hours to rule out other conditions and make a positive diagnosis.

Treatment

Surgical removal of the appendix is the necessary procedure and should be performed as soon as possible after diagnosis.

If the appendix has not ruptured previous to surgery, the operative risk is nearly negligible. Even after perforation has occurred, mortality rate is less than 1%.

Preparation for Surgery

Food and fluids by mouth are withheld prior to surgery. If the child is dehydrated, intravenous fluids will be ordered. If fever is present, temperature should be reduced to below 102° F.

Recovery is rapid and usually uneventful. The child is ambulated early and is able to leave the hospital a few days after surgery. In the unusual case where peritonitis or a localized abscess is a complication, gastric suction, parenteral fluids, and antibiotics may be ordered.

SCOLIOSIS

Scoliosis is most commonly of the functional type, usually caused by unequal length of the legs. It may also be caused by muscle spasm due to trauma. Functional scoliosis may be overcorrectable by using a lift under the short leg and by keeping the spine flexible by doing daily stretching exercises. Scoliosis of this kind is most frequent among young girls during the rapid growth period before puberty.

Fixed scoliosis is a structural scoliosis not correctable by the above means. The curvature may be due to congenital deformities or some infection such as Pott's disease. However, most cases are idiopathic. Treatment is by application of braces and spinal fusion. The brace most commonly used is the Milwaukee brace, which exerts pressure on certain areas to maintain correct posture. It may also be used after spinal fusion for immobilization. Other kinds of devices used are the turnbuckle cast and the newer Risser jacket. Detail concerning these orthopedic appliances may be found in the orthopedic texts.

SYNOVITIS

Synovitis of the hip is a condition not infrequently found in boys of early school age. It is a relatively benign condition most frequently caused by trauma to the hip. Symptoms are pain in the hip or knee and a limp. The joint later becomes full of fluid. Bed rest and avoidance of weight bearing will usually clear up the condition within a week or two, followed by gradually increased activity. If pain and spasm persist, Buck's traction may be applied.

LEGG-CALVÉ PERTHE'S DISEASE

Legg-Calvé Perthe's disease is an aseptic necrosis of the head of the femur. It occurs most frequently in young boys, and may possibly be caused by trauma to the hip although the cause is generally unknown. Symptoms similar to synovitis make immediate diagnosis difficult. After a few weeks, x-ray studies reveal opacity of the epiphysis; this is followed by a stage in which the epiphysis becomes mottled and fragmented. During the third stage, reossification takes place. Each stage lasts approximately 9 months.

The most important treatment is the avoidance of weight bearing. Immobilization of the hip is essential for recovery without deformity. Several methods are used to achieve this. Use of braces and crutches, bed rest with traction for a period, or possibly casts for a while may be used.

The time needed for recovery is counted in years, which may be from 2 to 5. Complete recovery without difficulty later in life is dependent on the age of the child at time of onset, the amount of involvement and the cooperation of the child.

BONE INFECTIONS

Osteomyelitis

Osteomyelitis is an infection of the bone usually caused by the hemolytic staphylococcus aureus. Acute osteomyelitis results from a primary infection such as staphyloccocal skin infection. The bacteria enter the blood stream and are carried to the metaphysis of a bone. Here an abscess forms, ruptures, and the infection spreads along the bone under the periosteum.

Symptoms usually begin abruptly with fever, malaise, pain and localized tenderness over the metaphysis of the affected bone. There is limitation of joint motion.

Diagnosis is made on laboratory findings of leukocytosis of 15,000 to 25,000 cells or more, and on positive blood cultures. X-ray examination does not reveal the process until 5 to 10 days after the onset.

Treatment. Acute osteomyelitis requires immediate treatment. Antibiotic therapy is started at once, and surgical drainage of the involved metaphysis is performed. If the abscess has ruptured into subperiosteal space, chronic osteomyelitis follows.

Prognosis. Prompt specific antibiotic treatment, vigorously employed, brings acute osteomyelitis under rapid control and prevents the extensive bone destruction of chronic osteomyelitis. Relief of pain and immobilization of the affected joint are other aspects of treatment. If extensive destruction of bone has occurred before treatment has begun, surgical removal of necrotic bone becomes necessary.

There are many orthopedic conditions occurring infrequently among children and young people. The student is referred to one of the orthopedic texts available in medical libraries.

MUSCULAR DYSTROPHY

The most common form of muscular dystrophy is the condition called *pseudohypertrophic muscular dystrophy*. It is found more frequently in boys than in girls. It is a sex-linked recessive hereditary disease.

First signs are noted in childhood or infancy, when the child finds it difficult to stand or walk. Later trunk muscle weakness develops. The child has an inability to rise readily to an upright position from a sitting position on the floor. He rises by "climbing up" his lower extremities with his hands.* Weakness of leg, arm and shoulder muscles progresses gradually. The victim becomes progressively weak, and usually succumbs to some intercurrent infection in early adult life.

The patient is encouraged to be as active as possible to delay muscle atrophy. Physiotherapy, diet to avoid obesity and parental encouragement aid in keeping the child active. It is helpful to approximate a normal life for the child, keeping him ambulatory and in school as long as possible. No effective treatment has as yet been found.

CRYPTORCHIDISM

The male gonads, or testes, lie in the abdominal cavity in fetal life. Shortly before or soon after birth the testes descend to their normal position in the scrotum. Occasionally one or both of the testes do not descend. The testes are usually normal in size but remain in the abdomen or the inguinal canal. The cause for the nondescent is not well understood; the condition is called cryptorchidism.

The testes may descend any time before puberty. However, a testis that has not descended before puberty will start to degenerate and become nonfunctioning. If both testes remain in the abdomen or inguinal canal, the person will be sterile.

A surgical procedure called *orchidopexy* is used before puberty to bring the testis down into the scrotum and anchor it there. Some physicians prefer to try medical treatment before doing surgery. This consists of administration of a gonadotropic hormone, usually given during the preschool period. If this is not successful in bringing the testis down, orchidopexy will be done. Surgeons differ in their opinion as to when this operation should be performed, some preferring to wait until the child is 10 or 11 years old.

---

*See Nelson, Textbook of Pediatrics. ed. 9. Philadelphia, W. B. Saunders, 1969. Fig. 21-4, p. 1362, for illustration.

Care of the Child After Surgery

The testis will be held in position in the scrotum by a suture placed there during surgery. This suture will be attached to a rubber band which has been secured to the child's thigh with adhesive tape. This attachment will be removed 5 to 7 days after surgery. However, the child is encouraged to resume normal activity on recovery from anesthesia. Prognosis for a normal functioning testicle is good if no degenerative action has taken place before treatment.

ENURESIS

Enuresis is a term used for involuntary urination beyond the age when control of urination should have been acquired. Many children do not acquire complete nighttime control before 5 to 7 years of age, and an occasional bed wetting may be seen in children as late as 9 or 10 years of age. Boys have more difficulty than girls, and in some cases enuresis may persist into the adult years.

Persistent bed wetting in a child of 5 or 6 is often due to too vigorous toilet training before the child is physiologically ready. Neurotic enuresis in the older child may express resentment toward parents or a desire to regress to an earlier level in order to receive more care and attention. Occasionally persistent bed wetting may have a physiological cause. The child should have an examination to rule out any abnormality.

Nagging and punishment will only increase the child's anxiety. Efforts should be made to discover the cause of emotional stress. If the child is interested in achieving control, as for instance in order to go to camp or visit friends overnight, waking him during the night to go to the toilet, or limiting fluids before retiring may be helpful. These measures should not be used as a replacement for searching for the cause, however. In deeply disturbed persons, help from a psychiatrist may be needed.

ENCOPRESIS

Encopresis is the involuntary defecation of feces beyond the age when control is expected. Speech and learning disabilities may be concomitant. It is evidence of a deep seated emotional problem, and is an indication for psychiatric help. Examination should be made to rule out physical abnormalities before the disorder is diagnosed as true encopresis.

ALLERGIC REACTIONS IN CHILDREN

Allergic Rhinitis (hay fever, rose fever)

Hay fever in children is most often due to sensitization to house dust, pollens and molds. Pollen allergy seldom appears before the age of 4 or 5 years.

Symptoms. Sneezing, watery nasal discharge, postnasal drip, and an allergic conjunctivitis are the usual symptoms.

Treatment consists in removing offending allergens from the environment if this is possible. Desensitization may be carried out as in asthma.

Asthma

Asthma is an allergic response to allergens involving the bronchial system.

Etiology. House dust is an important cause of asthma in children as in adults. In young children, asthma may be the response to certain foods to which the child is allergic. Pollens and molds are important trigger mechanisms in older children. In children who have asthmatic tendencies, emotional experiences may start an attack.

Pathology and Clinical Manifestations. There is a narrowing of the lumina of the bronchi and bronchioles due to spasms of the smooth muscles. Edema of the mucous membrane lining these bronchial branches and thick mucus within their lumina, in combination with the spasms, are responsible for the signs of respiratory obstruction.

The onset of an attack is usually abrupt. There is a hacking cough, wheezing, and difficult breathing. Asthmatic attacks frequently occur at night, waking the child from his sleep. The child has to sit up and is totally preoccupied with his efforts to breathe. Attacks may last for only a short time or the difficult breathing may extend for several days. Thick, tenacious mucus may be coughed up. A long period of difficulty may be followed by a period of bronchitis.

Treatment. Ephedrine combined with a sedative, such as in Tedral, may be given by mouth and has a prolonged action. Pseudoephedrine is available in liquid form and does not have the cardiovascular effects of ephedrine. Ephedrine accelerates the heartbeat and elevates the blood pressure. A sedative such as phenobarbital given with ephedrine reduces the undesirable effects.

Adrenalin by subcutaneous injection or given in inhalant form gives quick relief but is not as long-lasting. In severe attacks aminophylline is given by rectal suppository or in an oral preparation such as elixophyllin. Care must be taken when giving one of the phylline derivatives as some children become agitated and restless. If the child is dehydrated and feverish, the physician should be notified before the prescribed dose is given. Steroids are also used to terminate attacks and to prevent recurrence.

Allergic Skin Testing and Therapy

Intradermal testing using the allergens in solution may be useful in determining the offending material. A positive skin reaction is measured by the size of the weal at the point of injection. Skin testing is generally done when removal of obvious inhalants is not possible or has not brought relief.

Desensitization is carried out for those allergens that produced a positive reaction on skin testing. The allergist sets up a schedule for giving injections in gradually incremental doses, until a maintenance dose is reached. The patient should remain in the doctor's office for 20 to 30 minutes in case any reaction occurs. Reactions are treated with adrenalin. Severe reactions in children are uncommon, and desensitization is considered a safe procedure. Some children benefit considerably through desensitization measures.

CONVULSIVE DISORDERS

Convulsive disorders are not uncommon in children; they are estimated to occur in about 5% of children under 5 years of age. Convulsive seizures may occur from a variety of causes. A common form of seizure is the febrile convulsion that occurs in association with fevers and acute infections.

Epileptic Seizures

Organic epileptic seizures (recurrent convulsive disorders) may be caused by injuries or infections of the meninges and of the brain, or they may be the result of organic or degenerative changes.

Idiopathic epilepsy is the more common form. Onset of seizures of unknown cause is usually between the ages of 4 and 8 years of age. It is considered probable that some genetic defect is responsible in many of these children.

Clinical manifestations: Epileptic convulsions are classified as grand mal, petit mal, psychomotor, focal and myoclonic.

Grand mal seizures may be preceded by an aura, although children may have difficulty describing it. The attack consists of a sudden loss of consciousness, with generalized tonic and clonic movements. The initial tonic rigidity changes rapidly to generalized jerking movements of the muscles (clonic phase). The child may bite his tongue or lose control of his urine and his bowel functions. The jerking movements gradually diminish, then disappear, and the patient relaxes. The seizure may be brief, lasting less than a minute, or it may last 30 minutes or longer. Following the attack, some children return rapidly to an alert state, while others go into a prolonged period of stupor.

Petit mal seizures last for only a few seconds, rarely longer than 20. The child loses consciousness and stares straight ahead but does not fall. He becomes immediately alert following the seizure and continues conversation, but does not know what was said or done during the attack. Petit mal attacks have a high frequency of recurrence, which may be as high as 50 to 100 in a single day. Petit mal seizures usually decrease or stop entirely at adolescence, but

they may develop into grand mal attacks that may persist into adult life.

Psychomotor seizures are difficult to recognize. They consist of purposeful but inappropriate, repetitive motor acts. The child gradually loses postural tone and falls to the floor. After a few minutes of unconsciousness he may sleep or he may resume his former activity.

Focal seizures may be motor or sensory in type. Involuntary, unilateral convulsive movements begin in the extremities, such as the fingers, and progress up through the limb to the body. These are of short duration and consciousness may not be disturbed. However, a generalized typical grand mal seizure may at times follow, if the spread has been rapid and extensive.

Akinetic seizures. The child has a brief loss of consciousness and muscle tone. There are no tonic or clonic movements. The child may sleep following the seizure.

Diagnosis. Differentiation between the types of seizures may frequently be made through the use of electroencephalograms. However, some individuals who have never had seizures may have abnormal tracings. It is also true that others who do have seizures may not show abnormal readings. Roentgenograms (x-rays) of the skull may also be helpful in locating the disorder.

Treatment

Complete control of seizures is the main goal, and this is achieved through the use of anticonvulsant therapy. A number of anticonvulsant drugs are available and are used according to their effectiveness in controlling seizures and their degree of toxicity. Phenobarbital, Mebaral and Dilantin given singly, or in combination, have a relatively low toxicity. Mysoline may offer control if these have been unsatisfactory. Approximately 60% of patients gain complete control of grand mal and focal seizures with the use of these medications.[*]

Phenobarbital or Milontin, or the two in combination, may control petit mal seizures.

---

[*]Farmer, T., ed.: Pediatric Neurology. New York, Harper and Row, 1964.

Other drugs of choice are Celontin, Tridione and Paradione. Zarontin is effective in minor seizures when the child does not respond to phenobarbital. Other drugs used are Valium and Diamox.

Many of these drugs have an adverse effect on the hemopoietic, hepatic or genitourinary systems. Periodic tests and examinations are made when these drugs are used, with the drug in question immediately discontinued and replaced by another at the first sign of reaction.

Nursing care consists in protecting the child from injury during a seizure. Care is as described in febrile convulsions.

Antiepileptic Drugs in Current Use

Celontin (methsuximide) oral
Initial dose 0.3 gm./24 hrs.
Dilantin (diphenylhydantoin) oral, I.M., I.V., slowly
3 to 8 mg./kg./24 hrs. Single or divided doses
Gemonil (metharbital) oral
Initial dose 50 to 100 mg. One to three times daily
Mebarol (mephobarbital) oral
Under 2 years 32 mg./t.i.d.
2 to 4 yrs. 32 mg./q.i.d.
4 to 6 yrs. 50 mg./q.i.d.
6 to over 100 mg./t.i.d.
Mesantoin (mephenytoin) oral
3 to 15 mg./kg./24 hrs. Divided doses
Milontin (phensuximide) oral
1 to 3 gm./24 hrs. Divided doses
Mysoline (primidone) oral
Initial dose 125 mg./24 hrs. for children under 8
Initial dose 250 mg./24 hrs. for children over 8
Given in weekly increments. Dose not to exceed 2 gm./24 hrs.
Paradione (paramethadione) oral
Under 2 yrs. 0.3 gm./24 hrs. In divided doses
2 to 6 yrs. 0.6 gm./24 hrs.
6 yrs. and over 0.9 gm./24 hrs.

Phenobarbital (luminal)
Anticonvulsant dosage. Oral or I.M.
Under 2 years   16 mg. 3 times daily
2 to 4 years   16 mg. 4 times daily
4 to 6 years   32 mg. 3 times daily
Over 6 years   32 mg. 4 times daily
Tridione (trimethadione) oral
Under 6 yrs. 150 mg. 2 times daily
Over 6 yrs. 300 mg. 2 times daily
Valium (diazepam) oral
Not given to infants under 6 months.
Effective dosage differs considerably from patient to patient.
Zarontin (ethosuximide) oral
Under 6 years. 0.25 gm./24 hrs. Divided doses
Over 6 years. 0.5 gm./24 hrs.

All anticonvulsants are increased or decreased according to the patient's tolerance. Doses here given are suggested starting doses.

Phenobarbital is the least toxic of any of these drugs. Hyperactivity in young children sometimes results, but is reversible. All of the other anticonvulsants have numerous side effects such as skin rashes and behavior changes. Toxic effects include gastrointestinal and central nervous system symptoms, blood dyscrasia, liver damage. All children on these medications need to be followed carefully by a physician.

Long-Term Management

Although no accurate figures are available, epilepsy is a common disease. Because of the stigma attached to the condition, some victims make great efforts to conceal their condition. It is probably wiser not to use the term epilepsy when explaining the diagnosis to young children. Livingston recounts the instance of a very young child who told his playmates he had epilepsy.* The playmates told their parents, who in turn forbade their children to play with the child,

*Livingston, S.: Living With Epileptic Seizures. P. 202. Springfield, Illinois, Charles C. Thomas, 1963.

saying that epileptics were crazy and insane.

Epileptic children should be given the same opportunity to receive an education as that provided for other children. In the past, schools have often been reluctant to accept these children; they were given home instruction or else got no opportunity for education. With better understanding, attitudes have changed, and most epileptic children now attend regular classes. Problems still exist, however, mainly because of the lack of understanding of the condition by the general public and because of the notion, still prevalent among many parents, that epilepsy is shameful. Also, many still believe that nothing can be done.

The following narrative of the experiences of two epileptics illustrates the difficulties experienced by many. Attitudes are slowly changing, but much education concerning the nature and treatment of this disorder is still needed.

A Child Who Desperately Needed Help

Helen S., a senior student nurse receiving her public health experience in a small suburban town, had the responsibility for visiting the elementary school in her area. While she was still getting acquainted, the school principal asked her to stop in his office for a conference.

"We have a little girl in the second grade whom we are probably going to ask to leave school," he said. "She so disrupts the entire grade that the teacher can't handle the situation any longer. Part of the time she is sweet and loving—too loving in fact. She rushes up to to her teacher, regardless of what is going on, kisses and hugs her fiercely, and upsets order and discipline completely. At other times, she is sullen and uncooperative, refusing to take part in the schedule. She hits the other children and has even hit the teacher—for no reason at all. She is an epileptic and has had several seizures in school, frightening the rest of the children. Parents are starting to object, and the teacher says she must go."

The principal said that he had talked with Susie's mother, who said that her daughter was getting medicine and that nothing more could be done for her. He was reluctant to accept such a defeatist attitude and wondered if the student nurse could help in any way.

Helen made a visit to Susie's home, where she met the child's mother, a pleasant woman who seemed to have accepted the situation as something the family had to live with. The other children went their own way, ignoring Susie as much as she would let them. The child was definitely resented in the neighborhood, and the tale of her misdemeanors was long.

Susie's mother admitted that she "was so wild she climbed the wall," and that she had no control over the child. Susie frequently had "staring" episodes during the day as well as frequent generalized convulsions. Questioning revealed that she had been examined two years before at a seizure center, and had been started on medication, although her mother did not know the name of the medicine—"two kinds of pills," she said. Shortly afterward, the family had moved to another state. Susie had not been examined in the meantime. Her mother continued to give Susie the original pills, but she said they did her no good. She had taken Susie to a doctor once, but nothing came of it, and after the pills were used up, she did nothing more

Helen discussed the situation with her, strongly urging that Susie be taken to the seizure center in the city for an evaluation. Mrs. S. felt, however, that her husband earned too much for them to be eligible for this kind of service, and yet with a household of children, they could not afford to pay a specialist. She seemed to feel that because Susie did have epilepsy and because the examination two years ago had done nothing more than confirm this, that there was nothing more to be done. She was willing, however, to let Helen make inquiries at the center in the city as to whether they would work with Susie.

Helen did visit the seizure center, which had been opened a short time previously, and after describing the situation, she was able to arrange for Susie's acceptance. Susie was given a complete physical and neurological examination, including an electroencephalogram and psychological testing, and started on a combination of Dilantin and phenobarbital.

Back at school again she became quite manageable, and no more seizures were noted. She was, however, thought to be drowsy and rather slow to respond, and medications were adjusted in an effort to meet her needs. Her parents now began to realize that this was not a hopeless situation, and they were now much more inclined to continue the treatment. Susie's mother was no longer afraid to discipline her and risk another attack. A better understanding of her daughter's condition made her realize that Susie's unacceptable behavior was not the result of her physical condition, as she had supposed. It was rather an expression of her child's deep-seated resentment of the rejection she had received, and of bewilderment over the complete lack of discipline and restraint despite the fact that the other children in the family had to behave. The entire atmosphere was improving, and it seemed likely that this little girl could eventually be helped to achieve a more normal and satisfying life.

Mary T. was a young woman with a somewhat different background. She was an attractive teenager, and worked in the housekeeping department of a hospital. Her sympathetic, cooperative manner made her well liked by both patients and nurses, although they wondered why an intelligent young person was content to spend her days dusting and cleaning. Mary explained this by saying that she had dropped out of high school and had an insufficient education or training for any other sort of employment.

One day, however, the entire unit on which Mary worked was shocked when she had a severe generalized convulsion. The housekeeping supervisor was angry that Mary had concealed her epileptic condition, and thus her dismissal was imminent. Mary tearfully confided to her nursing friends that her life had been miserable. She had not been accepted at school, and had found high school so traumatic she had dropped out. Her seizures, although infrequent, were completely uncontrolled, and she dared not accept dates, or participate in any social life. She had neither close friends, nor any family to help her.

Mary also believed that her condition was hopeless, and she was close to complete despair. Now that she had been forced by this most recent seizure to acknowledge her difficulty, the interested nursing personnel were able to persuade her to seek medical help, and the housekeeping department agreed to keep her on as an employee if she would accept the treatment.

The physician who examined her assured her that she could be helped. His confident, optimistic attitude gave her the first hope she had ever known. Drugs were found to control her seizures completely. After two years without a seizure, Mary had adjusted to the normal social life of any young person, and shortly thereafter was married. She became a well-adjusted member of society, with just a little more sympathy and understanding of the problems of young people than an average person.

The Epileptic in the Community

Parents and older children are entitled to receive complete and accurate information concerning their disorder. The advances in medical understanding, and the ability to control seizures with newer medications take away the hopelessness of the situation and provide the possibility of a normal, well-adjusted life for a majority of affected persons. They also need to understand that epilepsy does not inevitably lead to mental retardation. Studies indicate that continued and uncontrolled seizures increase the possibility of mental retardation, and that the longer the epilepsy is uncontrolled, the greater the possibility of mental retardation. The data point up the importance of the early discovery and control of seizures.

Although the general outlook is optimistic, there is no point in concealing the nature of the restrictions with which the epileptic is presented. The likelihood is that an epileptic will be forbidden by law to drive a motor vehicle in many, but not all, states. Most states lift the restriction for a person whose seizures are completely controlled, but some do not.

A person whose seizures are under control should be able to obtain employment and perform the work normally expected of any employee, but he may find that he is not accepted. There are also some occupations from which he will find himself excluded by state law or by social custom.

Marriage for an epileptic is still forbidden in certain states, some of which designate marriage by an epileptic, granting a license to marry, or performing the marriage of an epileptic, as a crime.* These laws should be considered archaic, because there seems no reason for an epileptic to forego marriage,

*Livingston, Samuel: Living with Epileptic Seizures. p. 227. Springfield, Ill., Charles C Thomas, 1963.

provided he and his partner understand the nature of his disorder, and accept it.

Whether an epileptic should have children is difficult to answer until a genetic mode of transmission is established. The general opinion is that this decision must be an individual matter, with the consideration that the risks of transmission do not appear, at this time, to be much greater than in the normal population.

RHEUMATIC FEVER AND RHEUMATIC CARDITIS

Rheumatic fever is a chronic disease of childhood, occurring as one of the sequelae of Group A beta hemolytic streptococcal infections. It occurs throughout the world, particularly in the temperate zones, but recent studies show it to be more prevalent in the tropics than had previously been reported. For approximately the past 20 years, its incidence has shown a marked decline in the United States, but it is still the leading cause of acquired heart disease in children. The condition is rare before the age of 5, occurring primarily between the ages of 6 and 12 years.

Clinical Aspects

Etiology

Rheumatic fever appears to be a sensitivity reaction precipitated by streptococci. The initial streptococcal infection may be inapparent or unrecognized, and the resultant rheumatic fever manifestation may be the first indication of trouble. An elevation of antistreptococcal antibodies, indicative of recent streptococcal infection, however, can be demonstrated in about 95 per cent of the rheumatic fever patients tested within the first two months of onset. An hereditary influence is also recognized.

Clinical Manifestations

Following the initial infection, a latent period of 1 to 5 weeks ensues; in certain cases, such as chorea, the period may be longer. The onset is frequently insidious. The child may be listless, anorexic, pale, and may lose weight. He may complain of vague muscle and joint, or of abdominal pains. Frequently a low grade, late afternoon fever may be the noticeable symptom. None of these are diagnostic in themselves, but if such signs persist, the child merits a medical examination.

Major manifestations of rheumatic fever are polyarthritis, chorea, and carditis. The onset may be acute rather than insidious, with severe carditis or arthritis as the presenting symptom. Chorea, if it is present, generally has an insidious onset.

Polyarthritis. This is an arthritis of the migratory type, moving from one major joint to another; to the ankles, the knees, the hips, the wrists, to the elbows and to the shoulders. The joint becomes hot, swollen, and painful to either touch or movement. Body temperature is moderately elevated, sedimentation rate is increased. Although extremely painful, this type of arthritis does not lead to the crippling deformities that occur in rheumatoid arthritis.

Chorea (Sydenham's chorea). In this manifestation, the affected portion of the body is the central nervous system. Emotional instability, purposeless movements and muscular weakness are characteristic. The onset is gradual, with increasing incoordination, facial grimaces and repetitive involuntary movements. Movements may be mild and remain so, or they may become increasingly violent. Active arthritis is rarely present when chorea is the major manifestation. Carditis occurs, although less frequently than when polyarthritis is the major condition. Attacks tend to be recurrent and prolonged, but they become rare after puberty. It is seldom possible to demonstrate an antistreptococcal antibody rise, because of the generally prolonged latency period, and because of the length of time after the onset before the condition may be recognized.

Carditis. Carditis is a serious manifestation because it is the major cause of death or of permanent disability among children with rheumatic fever. Carditis may occur singly, or it may occur as a complication of either arthritis or chorea. Presenting symptoms may be vague enough to be missed. A child may have a poor appetite or pallor, perhaps have a low grade fever, appear listless and show a moderate degree of anemia. If observed carefully, a slight dyspnea on exertion may be noted. Physical examination reveals a soft systolic murmur over the apex of the heart. Unfortunately, such a child may have been under par physically for some time before the murmur is discovered.

Acute carditis. This may, however, be the presenting symptom, particularly in young children. An abrupt onset of high fever, perhaps as high as 104°, tachycardia, pallor, poor pulse quality, and a rapid fall in hemoglobin are characteristic. Weakness, prostration, cyanosis and intense precordial pain are frequently present. Cardiac dilatation usually occurs. The pericardium, the myocardium, or the endocardium may be affected.

Other rheumatic fever manifestations. *Epistaxis* is common, and may be severe. *Subcutaneous nodules* are shot-like, hard bodies felt on the extensor surface of certain joints, particularly on the elbows, the knees and the wrists. They are painless and do not occur in every case, but if they are noted, they provide one criterion for diagnosis. *Erythema marginatum* is another useful diagnostic aid, when it is present. It consists of a recurrent, pink, characteristic rash, which appears on the trunk or on the extremities, and migrates from place to place. It never appears on the face.

Diagnostic Criteria

Rheumatic fever is difficult to diagnose, and it is sometimes impossible to differentiate it from other diseases. The possible serious effect of the disease demands early and conscientious medical treatment. It is unfortunate, however, to cause apprehension and disrupt the patient's life if the condition proves to be something less serious. The nurse should naturally not attempt a diagnosis, but she should understand the criteria on which a presumptive diagnosis is based.

The Jones criteria (modified), a guide based on criteria formulated in 1944, is generally accepted as a useful rule for guidance when making a decision as to whether to treat the patient for rheumatic fever. The list is divided into major and minor categories.*

The presence of two major, or one major and two minor criteria, is accepted as an indication of a high probability of rheumatic fever if supported by evidence of a preceding streptococcal infection. It is not infallible, because no one criterion is specific for the disease, and other additional manifestations are helpful aids toward a substantiation of the diagnosis.

Laboratory Tests and Treatment

The chief concern while caring for a patient with rheumatic fever is the

*The American Heart Association has issued the Jones Criteria (revised) 1965. It retains the diagnostic criteria and lists other manifestations that may support the diagnosis.

JONES CRITERIA (MODIFIED) FOR DIAGNOSIS OF RHEUMATIC FEVER

Major Criteria	Minor Criteria
Carditis	Fever
Polyarthritis	Arthralgia
Chorea	Prolonged P—R interval in the ECG
Subcutaneous nodules	Increased ESR, WBC, or presence of C—reactive protein
Erythema Marginatum	Preceding beta hemolytic streptococcal infection
	Previous rheumatic fever or inactive heart disease

prevention of residual heart disease. As long as the rheumatic process is active, progressive heart damage is possible. Bed rest, therefore, is essential in order to reduce the work load of the heart. How long the period of bed rest should last cannot be arbitrarily stated. It is generally agreed that a child should be kept in bed until both laboratory and clinical evidence of the acute stage of the disease have disappeared.

Laboratory appraisal tests, although they are nonspecific, are useful for an evaluation of the activity of the disease. Two commonly used indicators are the *erythrocyte sedimentation rate*, and the presence of *C-reactive protein*. The erythrocyte sedimentation rate (ESR) is elevated in the presence of an inflammatory process, and is nearly always raised in the polyarthritis or in the carditis manifestations of rheumatic fever. It remains elevated until after any clinical manifestations have ceased, and after any subclinical activity has subsided. It seldom rises in uncomplicated chorea. Therefore, ESR elevation in a choreic patient may point toward cardiac involvement.

C-reactive protein. This is not normally present in the blood of healthy persons, but it does appear in the serum of acutely ill persons, including those ill with rheumatic fever. As the patient improves, C-reactive protein disappears.

Leukocytosis. This also is an indication of an inflammatory process. Until the leukocyte count returns to a normal level, the disease probably is still active.

Medical Treatment

Medications used in the treatment of rheumatic fever include salicylates and corticosteroids. Salicylates are given in the form of acetylsalicylic acid (aspirin) to children, with the daily dosage calculated according to the child's weight. Remarkable relief from polyarthritis is afforded by the use of this drug. The continued administration of a relatively large dosage may cause toxic effects, because individual tolerance differs greatly. The child's nurse must assume the responsibility for noting any signs of toxicity and must report them promptly. Tinnitus, nausea, vomiting, and headache are all signs of toxicity. Salicylates tend to interfere with the synthesis of prothrombin. Purpura, ecchymotic skin manifestations or frank hemorrhage may be the result. Of particular importance is the toxic reaction of hyperpnea, which may lead to respiratory alkalosis and to metabolic acidosis.

In the presence of mild or severe carditis, corticosteroids appear to be the drug of choice because of their prompt, dramatic action. Neither drug is expected to alter the course of the disease, but the control of the toxic manifestations of this disease contributes to the patient's comfort and to his sense of well-being, and help to reduce the burden on his heart. This is of particular importance in acute carditis with congestive failure. Because a premature withdrawal of a steroid drug is likely to cause a relapse, its use is continued until any evidence of activity has subsided. It is then gradually discontinued. Toxic reactions are naturally to be watched for and reported as well.

Because the presence of group A streptococci prolongs the rheumatic activity, a course of penicillin should be given to eliminate these organisms from the child's body.

Corticosteroids and salicylates are of little value in the treatment of uncomplicated chorea. Sedation with phenobarbital for relaxation, or the use of a tranquilizer such as chlorpromazine (Thorazine) helps to relax the child. Bed rest is necessary, and with protection such as padding the bed sides if the movements are severe. When the chorea is complicated by a heart condition, the treatment should include therapy for that condition too.

Bed rest. Prolonged strict bed rest is no longer considered necessary for every patient with rheumatic fever. The psychological trauma that so many children suffered from such a program brought about a careful study of the effects of controlled activity. It was concluded that many children were being needlessly restricted.

Bed rest is essential during the acute stage. Strict bed rest, including feeding the child by the nurse or mother, is essential for patients with cardiac enlargement or congestive failure. Gradual ambulation may be started when the clinical and laboratory signs of the acute stage have subsided. This may be as early as 7 to 10 days where there is no evidence of cardiac disease. Bed rest from 3 weeks to 3 months may be prescribed for patients with cardiac involvement. Residual heart disease is treated in accordance with its severity and its type with digitalis, restricted activities, diuretics and a low sodium diet as indicated.

Recurrences

Recurrences were formerly considered to be nearly inevitable, with the possibility of additional heart damage with each attack. Understanding that attacks recur as responses to fresh streptococcal infections has resulted in a strict adherence to a prophylactic regimen of penicillin, with a resultant marked decrease in recurrent attacks.

The American Heart Association recommends the administration of penicillin or streptomycin for an indefinite number of years to all persons who have had one or more attacks of rheumatic fever. Specifically, recommendations include prophylactic medication for all patients who have a *well-documented history* of rheumatic fever or of chorea, or who show a *definite evidence* of rheumatic heart disease.

They state that the safest procedure is that of continuing the prophylaxis indefinitely, particularly in the presence of rheumatic heart disease. It is recognized, however, that some physicians may wish to terminate prophylaxis in certain adult patients who have been free of attacks for several years and who have no present involvement. Adolescents, who are generally negligent in regard to prophylactic medications, are urged to continue protection.

Prophylactic Program

Initially, a full therapeutic course of penicillin is given to eradicate the streptococci, regardless of whether their presence is detected by culture tests. Prophylactic therapy is maintained by the use of benzathine penicillin G, oral penicillin, or oral sulfadiazine. The public health nurse in the community should encourage adherence to the prophylactic program. She should be aware of the merits and of the disadvantages of each type of program in her support of the physician and his patient.

Intramuscular injections of benzathine penicillin G have given the most consistently reliable results. Benzathine penicillin G (marketed as Bicillin) is injected in a dosage of 1,200,000 units once a month. The physician is thus assured that his patient is receiving the proper medication. Oral penicillin is equally as effective, but is too often omitted or taken haphazardly by a patient in good health.

A careful history of allergic reactions to penicillin should be obtained before the program is started. Sulfadiazine may be substituted if penicillin intolerance is present.

Oral penicillin is given in dosages of 200,000 to 500,000 units daily. Reactions from this administration probably occur less frequently than do those from intramuscular penicillin, but similar precautions are necessary. The temptation to be careless about continuing medication for a well child is great, especially if there is a financial problem once the home supply has been used up.

Oral sulfadiazine is cheaper than oral penicillin and is as effective. Reactions are infrequent, but they should be watched for. Chief reactions are skin eruptions, an associated sore throat or fever, and leukopenia. Weekly white blood cell counts are recommended for the first two months of prophylaxis with this drug, after which the occurrence of leukopenia with agranulocytosis is extremely rare. Erythromycin may be used for penicillin-sensitive patients.

Nursing Care

Home Care

A child who has developed rheumatic fever may be hospitalized for diagnosis and beginning therapy, and may then be returned home for continuing care, depending on the particular circumstances.

The severity of the condition, the home circumstances, and the availability of care outside the home should all be considered. If the family is able to provide adequate physical care and emotional support, and if medical supervision is obtainable, home care would appear to be the best method of meeting the child's needs.

The nurse involved in helping the family to prepare for their child's care as well as the other family members, must have a clear understanding of the physician's definition of strict bed rest. Must the patient be positioned with pillows, turned and fed by others and not allowed to hold books or toys? Is he to be lifted onto the bedpan, and is the urinal to be held for him? Consideration of the various gradations of meaning in the terms strict bed rest or bed rest with bathroom privileges is outlined in an article in Nursing Research.*

A child may be willing to accept total dependency when he is in pain and is acutely ill, but any prohibition of all activity when he feels better may be extremely traumatic emotionally—with the trauma possibly outweighing the adverse physical effects. Not only the nurse and the family need to understand the physical limitations imposed, but a child patient must have the need for any limitations clearly explained to him in terms suited to his understanding and his ability to accept.

Preparation for home care includes the selection of a room for the temporarily bed-ridden child. If at all possible, he should have his own room, within easy accessibility by his mother. If a hospital bed cannot be rented, blocks placed under the bed legs will raise it to permit easier care, and a back rest can be improvised. Although an ill child needs quiet, his surroundings should be cheerful, with colorful objects of interest spread about the room. Limits for watching television, reading, and for visits from other persons, as well as the resumption of his schoolwork are set by the physician in accordance with the child's condition.

The tendency to overindulge a chronically ill child and to relax discipline is quite understandable. It is not in the child's best interest. He would shortly become a serious burden to his family, and to himself, if guidance is withheld from him and if discipline is not enforced as necessary.

If schoolwork is permitted, homebound teachers are available in most communities. Some communities have two-way closed television circuits that allow the child to participate in classroom instruction from his bed.

Preventive Health Services for School-Age Children

Because rheumatic fever is a condition that has its peak of onset in school-age children, health services for this age group assume an added importance. The overall approach is one of the promotion of continuous health supervision for all children, including the school-age child. The establishment of well child conferences or clinics, with an encouragement among the general population for their use is one opportunity of which more advantage should be taken. Well infant and child conferences are quite well established throughout the United States with attendance fairly evenly divided between infants and preschool children. An expansion of these services to include school-age children is viewed by many health authorities as the most satisfactory method of providing a continuity of care.

School nurses, public school teachers and public health nurses now have the responsibility for health teaching, for observation, and for case finding and referral of children for diagnostic services. The streptococcal infection that precedes rheumatic activity is

*Roose, J. Interpretation of bed rest by doctors and nurses. Nursing Research, *12:*111, 1963.

transferred much more easily in densely populated areas. Typically, studies have shown that children who migrated from Puerto Rico to New York City were particularly susceptible to rheumatic fever, although the disease was rare in the tropical climate of their homes. Socio-economic factors, hygienic practices and vigorous campaigns directed toward case finding and prophylaxis have played a significant role. One can scarcely claim, however, that overcrowding no longer exists, or that a majority of children live under optimal sanitary conditions.

Clinic services in the area of prevention and treatment are available from several sources. Crippled children's agencies funtion with the support of the Children's Bureau. Public health agencies and the Heart Association, through its state associations, are also sources of support.

Registration with a state heart association is a helpful way of keeping in touch with persons who have had one or more attacks of rheumatic fever. Through the association, prophylactic drugs may be purchased at wholesale prices, a service that also makes possible guidance and encouragement during the continuation of self-care.

Prognosis

Prognosis is related primarily to the presence or absence of heart disease. Most chronic disabilities and most deaths occur in the presence of repeated attacks. Supportive prophylactic therapy has greatly reduced the incidence of death and chronic disability. Patients with rheumatic heart disease are susceptible to subacute bacterial endocarditis. Adequate protection with penicillin or erythromycin should be given during surgical or dental procedures.

What is the Meaning of this Type of Illness to a Child?

Six-year-old Billy was home with a cold, with a fever and a cough, a moderately sore throat. His mother worried, but Billy was not too ill, and, in two or three days he appeared to be quite well again. It was not until several weeks later that his mother worried again—Billy was so irritable and touchy, and had developed a strange, repetitive head jerking. A visit to the pediatrician provided a considerable shock when a "probable chorea" was the verdict.

Billy was put to bed and was placed on elixir of phenobarbital twice daily. All of the well-developed theories concerning the needs of such children are excellent, but fall somewhat short of being adequate when the family is desperately poor, and when the mother must work full time outside the home. Well-intentioned neighbors helped, but Billy was alone a great deal, and received a minimum of support from a mother who desired only to come home to peace and quiet.

Eventually Billy progressed to full activity, but a few months later, a second attack of considerably greater severity made such haphazard care entirely inadequate, and Billy entered a children's convalescent home. Here the hours and the days stretched endlessly. Eventually some degree of ambulation was attained, but the development of a rapid pulse and a suggestive heart murmur put an end to all activity for months to come.

No residual heart condition developed, however, and Billy was beginning to find his place in the community when a third attack of lessened intensity sent him back to bed. This was the final recurrence, and eventually the time came when Billy was sent back to school with no restrictions placed on his activities. No restrictions imposed—so they said. What restrictions are imposed on a child by the effect of two years of nearly total exclusion from the healthful activities of his peers? Especially for a boy, who is expected to compete in physical activities at school and on the playground. Billy could not swim, and his coordination was poor. He did not know how to throw a ball or how to perform any athletic feats. His schoolmates laughed at his clumsy attempts, and his physical education directors were impatient. Billy's efforts became almost totally concentrated on academic study and on means for avoiding all physical recreational pursuits. His self-consciousness and previously enforced isolation made him excessively shy, and greatly multiplied his adolescent problems.

Billy's situation was not unique. Rheumatic fever is declining in incidence and in severity, but our pediatric wards have large numbers of children who are repeatedly admitted for treatment of the exacerbations of chronic illnesses that keep them from participating in activities appropriate for their age group. Larry, the six-year-old whose recurrent laryngeal papillomas necessitate a permanent tracheotomy and frequent excisions of the recurring growths; Ruthie, whose nephrosis fails to respond to treatment; the children with hydronephrosis who are chronically ill; these are a few who, without outward deformities, are still unable to live the full life of childhood. Nursing these children must mean much more than giving them bedside care.

INTESTINAL PARASITES

Enterobiasis (Oxyuriasis, Pinworm Infection)

Etiology. The pinworm, *Enterobius vermicularis*, is a white, threadlike worm which invades the cecum and may enter the appendix.

Epidemiology. Pinworms are spread from person to person by articles contaminated with pinworm eggs. The infestation is common among children.

Infestation occurs when the pinworm eggs are swallowed. The eggs hatch in the intestinal tract and grow to maturity in the cecum. The female worm, when ready to lay her eggs, crawls out of the anus and lays the eggs on the child's perineum.

Itching around the anus causes the child to scratch and trap new eggs under his fingernails, where frequently he reinfects himself when he puts his fingers in his mouth. Clothing, bedding, food and other articles become infected, and the infestation spreads to other members of the family.

The life cycle of these worms is from 6 to 8 weeks, after which reinfestation commonly occurs unless treated. The condition appears most frequently in school-age children, next highest in the preschool age. Mothers of children with pinworm infestation are also susceptible.

Identification. Capturing the eggs from around the anus by the use of scotch tape, and examining under a microscope is the usual method. Adult worms may also be seen when the child is lying quietly or sleeping, as they emerge from the anus.

The Scotch-tape test for identifying worms is carried out as follows:
1. Wind Scotch tape around the end of a tongue blade, sticky side outward.
2. Spread the child's buttocks and press the tape against the anus, rolling from side to side.

3. Transfer the tape to a microscope slide and cover with a clean slide to send to the laboratory.
4. Tape is examined microscopically in the laboratory for eggs.

The most favorable time for finding pinworms or their eggs is in the early morning before the child wakens.

Prevention and Treatment. The child should be taught to wash his hands after bowel movements and before eating, and to observe other hygienic measures such as regular bathing and frequent change of underclothing. Bedding should also be changed frequently to avoid reinfestation.

Treatment consists in the use of vermifuge medications. Povan and Antepar are most commonly used (see Medication table in Appendix).

Roundworms

Ascaris lumbricoides is a large intestinal worm found only in humans. Infestation is from the feces of infested persons. It is usually found in areas where sanitary facilities are lacking and human excreta is deposited on the ground.

The adult worm is pink and from 9 to 12 inches in length. The eggs hatch in the intestinal tract and the larvae migrate to the liver and lungs. The larvae reaching the lungs ascend up through the bronchi, are swallowed and reach the intestines where they grow to maturity and mate. Eggs are then discharged into the feces. Full development requires about 2 months. In tropical countries where infestation may be heavy, bowel obstructions may present serious problems. Generally, however, no symptoms are present in ordinary infestations.

Identification. Microscopic examination of feces for eggs.

Treatment. Antepar is the specific medication. Improved hygienic conditions to prevent infestation.

Hookworm Infestation

Etiology. The hookworm lives in the human intestinal tract where it attaches itself to the wall of the small intestine. Eggs are discharged in the feces of the host.

These parasites are prevalent in areas where infected human excreta is deposited on the ground and the soil, moisture and temperature are favorable for the development of infective larvae of the worm. In the southeastern United States and tropical West Africa the prevailing species is *Necator americanus*. In other parts of the world both this species and *Ancylostoma duodenale* are present.

Epidemiology. After feces containing eggs are deposited on the ground, larvae hatch. Usually they penetrate the skin of barefoot persons. They produce an itching dermatitis (ground itch). The larvae pass through the bloodstream to the lungs and into the pharynx where they are swallowed and reach the small intestine where they attach themselves to the intestinal wall. Heavy infestation may cause anemia through loss of blood to the worms. Chronic infestation produces listlessness, fatigue and malnutrition.

Identification is made by examination of the stool under the microscope.

Treatment. An antihelmintic drug called alcopar has been successful in treating hookworm infection caused by *Ancylostoma Duodenale*. Tetrachlorethylene appears more effective for *Necator americanus*. The drug may have toxic effects and must be administered carefully according to directions. The infected child will need a well balanced diet with additional protein and iron. Transfusions are rarely necessary.

FUNGOUS INFECTIONS OF THE SKIN

Tinea or Ringworm of the Scalp

This infection is called tinea capitus or tinea tonsurans. The most common cause is *Microsporum*, transmitted from animal to child. A less common type, *Microsporum*

audoiuni, is transmitted from person to person.

Tinea capitus begins as a small papule on the scalp and spreads, leaving scaly patches of baldness. The hairs become brittle and break off easily. Examination under ultraviolet light (Wood's light) is helpful for diagnosis. Griseofulvin, an antifungal antibiotic, is the medication of choice. As treatment may be prolonged, it is not recommended that children who are being properly treated be kept out of school.

Ringworm of the Body

The lesions of tinea corporis occur on any part of the body and resemble the lesions of scalp ringworm. Whitfield's Ointment applied to the area relieves the itching. Griseofulvin is also used in this condition.

Ringworm of the Feet (Tinea Pedis)

Tinea pedis is the scaling or cracking of the skin between the toes commonly known as athlete's foot. Examination under a microscope of scrapings from the lesions is necessary for diagnosis. Transmission is by direct or indirect contact with skin lesions from infected persons. Contaminated sidewalks, floors and shower stalls spread the condition to those who walk with bare feet.

Treatment. The feet should be washed with soap and water, scabs and crusts removed, and a topical agent applied. Tinactin is useful after the acute inflammatory stage begins to subside. Griseofulvin by mouth is also useful. During the chronic phase, Whitfield's ointment, scrupulous foot hygiene, and frequent change of socks is helpful. Desenex foot powder may also be useful.

PEDICULOSIS

Lice are a common infestation of the scalp, or of the hairy parts of the body. The most common condition seen in children is infestation with head lice. The infesting agent is *Pediculus capitis*. Animal lice are not transferred to man.

Head lice are passed around from child to child by direct contact or indirectly by contact with combs and other headgear. Lice lay their eggs, called nits, on the head, attaching them to strands of hair. The nits hatch in about a week, and the lice become sexually mature in approximately 2 weeks.

Clinical Manifestations. Severe itching of the scalp is the most obvious symptom. Combing the hair with a fine-toothed comb will remove lice, but nits are difficult to remove.

Treatment. Use of Kwell shampoo gives the most satisfactory results. After wetting the hair with warm water, the Kwell is applied like any ordinary shampoo. About one ounce is used. The head should be lathered for 4 minutes, rinsed thoroughly and dried. Shampooing may be repeated if necessary in 24 hours, but should not be used more than twice a week. Care must be taken to avoid getting Kwell in eyes or on mucous membranes.

BIBLIOGRAPHY

Gamstorf, I.: Pediatric Neurology. New York, Appleton-Century-Crofts, 1970.
Livingston, S.: Drug Therapy for Epilepsy. Springfield, Ill., Charles C Thomas, 1966.
———: Living with Epileptic Seizures. Springfield, Ill., Charles C Thomas, 1963.
———: What hope for the child with epilepsy. Children, *12:*9, 1965.
Markowitz, M.: Eradication of rheumatic fever— an unfulfilled hope. Circulation, *41:*1077, 1970.

Suggested Readings for Further Study

Lennox, W. G.: Epilepsy and Related Disorders. Boston, Little, Brown, 1960.
Scott, D.: About Epilepsy. New York, International Universities Press, 1969.

UNIT STUDY QUESTIONS

1. The first permanent teeth to erupt are the:
   a. bicuspids
   b. central incisors
   c. six-year molars
   d. lateral incisors

2. The child entering school should have an adequate physical examination. Which of the following parts of the examination is least important and can be omitted?
   a. general health check
   b. sight and hearing check
   c. examination of teeth
   d. history of immunizations
   e. booster shot of DTP and polio vaccine
   f. revaccination against smallpox
   The answer is:
   1. b, c, and f
   2. c, d, and e
   3. f only
   4. none of them

3. Erikson speaks of the development phase of the school age child as one of the need to develop a sense of industry versus inferiority. Which of the following will best help the child master this development?
   a. an opportunity to engage in real life tasks and encouragement to see them through to completion
   b. comparison with his peers or siblings, such as "Bobby does that much better"
   c. reward and praise for his accomplishments
   d. acceptance of his accomplishments as something to be expected for his age
   The answer is:
   1. a and c
   2. a and b
   3. b and d
   4. c and d

4. For his emotional health the child's parents should show which of the following attitudes?
   a. entire satisfaction with him as a person
   b. that they expect him to make mistakes
   c. praise for his doing well
   d. willingness to give him unrestricted freedom to make his own mistakes
   The answer is:
   1. a, b, and c
   2. a, b, and d
   3. b, c, and d
   4. b and d

5. What is meant by sex education?
   a. teaching the child about pubertal changes
   b. teaching the child the anatomy and physiology of reproduction

c. giving him an example in the home of satisfaction in the male or female role

d. avoidance of downgrading the female role to the girl, the male role to the boy

The answer is:
1. a, b, c
2. a and b
3. c and d
4. all of the above

6. Which of the following is *not* proper discipline for a child?
a. respecting the child as a person
b. setting standards and defining limits
c. giving punishment for misdeeds that is a logical consequence for the wrongdoing
d. taking away the child's allowance

7. In the hospital, the nurse's responsibilities in caring for a child prior to surgery for appendicitis are:
a. N.P.O., check his vital signs, check laboratory tests, apply ice bag
b. N.P.O., give cleansing enema, give preoperative medications
c. give ice chips, shave operative site, give preoperative medications
d. N.P.O., have him empty bladder, record vital signs, check lab findings and operative permit

8. Rheumatic fever has often been unrecognized as a sequel of a streptococcal infection. Which of the following is *not* a possible clinical manifestation of rheumatic fever?
a. listlessness, vague muscle, joint or abdominal pains
b. Syndenham's chorea
c. a red, raw sore throat
d. a pink, migratory erythema, appearing on any part of the body except the face
e. cardiac involvement

9. The epileptic child should be treated in the following manner:
a. kept out of school and tutored at home
b. be made to understand that he will not be well accepted in society
c. given a thorough physical examination and placed on anticonvulsants

d. be placed under the care of a physician because of the need to adjust medications

The answer is:
1. a, b, and d
2. c only
3. a and c
4. c and d

10. Diabetes in children has the following characteristics:
a. insidious onset with loss of weight, polyuria, and polydipsia
b. more difficult to control than in the adult because of child's changing needs
c. insulin required for control—oral medications do not give satisfactory control
d. need to continue his normal activities

The answer is:
1. a, b, and d
2. b and c
3. none of the above
4. all of the above

11. A definitive diagnosis for diabetes can be made by which of the following?
a. a postprandial glucose test
b. a urine glucose test
c. a glucose tolerance test
d. clinical manifestations

The answer is:
1. a and b
2. b only
3. c only
4. d only
5. any of the above

12. Diabetic acidosis exhibits some of the following:
a. drowsiness, flushed cheeks and dry skin
b. fruity, acetone breath
c. Kussmaul breathing
d. lack of treatment or inadequate treatment
e. overdose of insulin

The answer is:
1. a, b, c, and d
2. a, b, c, and e
3. e only
4. d only

Normal Growth and Development During Adolescence

42

A child moving from middle childhood into adolescence moves from a climate of security into a new sphere. This is a transition period in which physiological changes, as well as society's expectations, bring about uncertainty in his mind as to the role he should play. This uncertainty frequently extends to the adults in his environment as well. Quite literally, the rapid changes in his physical development make him a stranger to himself.

SOME DESCRIPTIVE TERMS FOR THIS AGE GROUP

Some clarification of terms is necessary. The pubescent period denotes the time from the onset of the adolescent changes and ends in puberty itself. It is marked by a spurt in physical growth, changes in body proportions and by the maturation of the secondary sex characteristics. This period, lasting approximately 2 years, may be called the prepubescent or the preadolescent period, although the latter term is not strictly accurate.

Puberty. This is the point at which the biological changes reach a climax; it marks the termination of the pubescent period. It is marked by the appearance of the menarche in girls and the production of spermatozoa in boys.

Adolescence. This period begins with a growth spurt and ends when the individual has reached his full physical and social maturity.

Menarche is the term used for the first menses.

PHYSICAL DEVELOPMENT IN THE PUBESCENT PERIOD

Development during this period differs in timing and in degree between boys and girls. It becomes necessary to consider physical development separately.

Pubertal Changes

The growth spurt commences in the average girl at about the age of 9, marking the start of the prepubertal period. This occurs, on the average, about 2 years earlier than it does in boys, thereby accounting for the fact that girls of this age generally appear taller and larger than many of their male classmates.

Changes begin with an increase in the width of the pelvis and with the start of breast development. This is followed by the appearance of pubic hair, and a little later, by axillary hair. Because of the wide variance between individuals in their rate of growth and maturation during this period, one may see children of the same age in all stages of development. Within a group of thirteen-year-old girls there are some who are small and thin, with flat breasts and narrow hips. Others may show quite womanly figures with developing breasts, widened hips and tall stature.

A young girl may become embarrassed about her budding breasts, but she is secretly often pleased about this evidence of her femininity. Sometimes, however, she may really resent that she is a girl and may try to resist development. Similarly, a girl experiencing delayed puberty may feel left

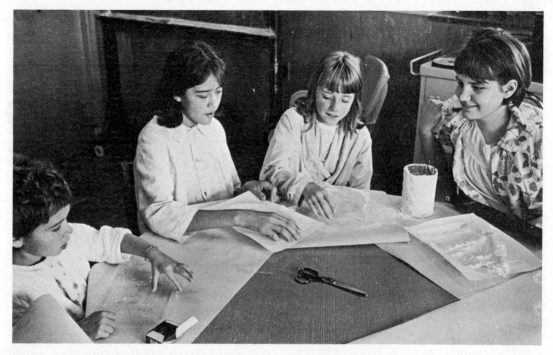

Figure 42-1.   Note the different degrees of development of these adolescent girls, ages 11 to 13. (The small girl is 11.)

out among her more rapidly maturing peers. She is apt to feel that she is not normal and that something has gone wrong. She may ask for a bra to fill out her figure, and there appears to be no reason to deny her this help to her ego.

Boys start their pubescent period, on the average, 2 years later than girls. The earliest secondary sex change is the increase in size of the external genitalia, followed by the appearance of public hair, then axillary and facial hair. Rapid growth in muscular strength and coordination appears on the average after the 13th year. Change of voice occurs gradually, beginning in the early pubescent stage. Nocturnal emissions commence about a year after the appearance of secondary changes.

A review of epiphyseal centers shows that ossification of bones begins at about the fifth month of intrauterine life and is completed during adolescence. This closure of the epiphyseal centers marks the end of growth in height. Late maturing young people, particularly boys, can take some

comfort in the knowledge that they still have an opportunity to grow taller.

A boy, however, suffers most keenly over his delayed development. His ideal is to become manly, and in our culture, short stature in the male (or any "feminine" characteristics) are traits ridiculed or disapproved of by the majority. A virile looking male is the ideal. Therefore, the despair of a boy is very real if he believes that he is not developing the appropriate characteristics.

DEVELOPMENTAL PROBLEMS

The Adolescent's Need for Assurance

These young people need someone to listen to their fears and somone to be sympathetic to them. They need to be reassured that many people are slow to develop and that in but a few years, they will have achieved normal growth. As a matter of fact, the late developers have the best possibility for becoming tall because an early closure of the epiphyses also marks the end of bone growth. Perhaps the father could show that he too was slow in maturing. Some parents need to be reassured, however, and may need to have pointed out to them that their concern is only fixing the idea more firmly in their boy's mind that something is wrong.

A young person grows and develops with great rapidity after pubescence has started. He may grow unevenly, perhaps one arm may be temporarily shorter than the other, or his legs may be growing out of proportion to the rest of his body. A girl may develop breasts that are large in proportion to her size. Many boys develop "feminine" breasts because of an increase in hormones and suffer agonies because they feel they are abnormal. They need to be assured that this, too, is normal, and, in nearly every instance, is no cause for concern. Some boys ask for surgery if this period is prolonged, but unless the boy's emotional life is seriously disturbed, his breasts are better left alone.

Self Image

Because of the rapid changes in body development, a young person has difficulty in forming a clear image of himself. This accounts for much of his seeming awkwardness. Actually, adolescents can be very graceful and well coordinated, as are figure skaters and athletes.

An adolescent's glandular changes make him seem like a new person to himself as well. He must learn to be an effective person all over again, and the developmental demands of this period are unique. These include achieving an emotional independence from adults, establishing satisfying relations with both boys and girls, choosing and preparing for a vocation, building social, ethical and spiritual values, developing socially responsible behavior, and reaching forward to maturity.

Need for Parental Guidance

As he leaves his childish self behind him and tries on his new adult role, he naturally wishes to be considered by others as adult. The transition cannot be as abrupt as this,

however. These new forces appearing are so powerful and so little understood by him that often he is secretly terrified by them, even though he strongly desires to act as an adult. He sometimes is desperately afraid that he cannot control these forces within himself. Although he almost certainly grumbles and rebels, he is often relieved when his parents put the weight of their authority behind his own inadequate control, in much the same manner as when he was a toddler exploring his strange, bewildering universe.

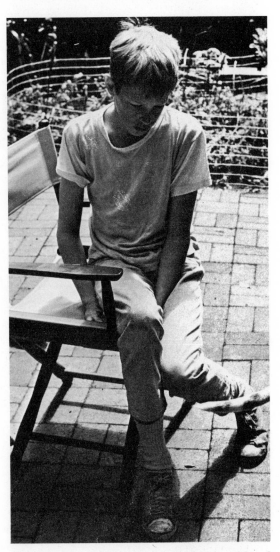

Figure 42-2. The adolescent is often bewildered by the changes going on in his body. (Photograph by Carol Baldwin.)

Indeed, in spite of his maturation and his changing status, he is the same person he was at 2 or 3. Unquestionably, the foundations laid down during early childhood are the factors that can help either to smooth or trouble his present development. This realization is extremely important in child-rearing practices, but it brings cold comfort to both the parents and their offspring when, because of any number of circumstances, the child's early environment was somewhat less than ideal. Parents are human and make mistakes just as anyone else does. It seems to make little sense to say to a troubled parent, "This is the result of your rejection, or your possessiveness, or your over-

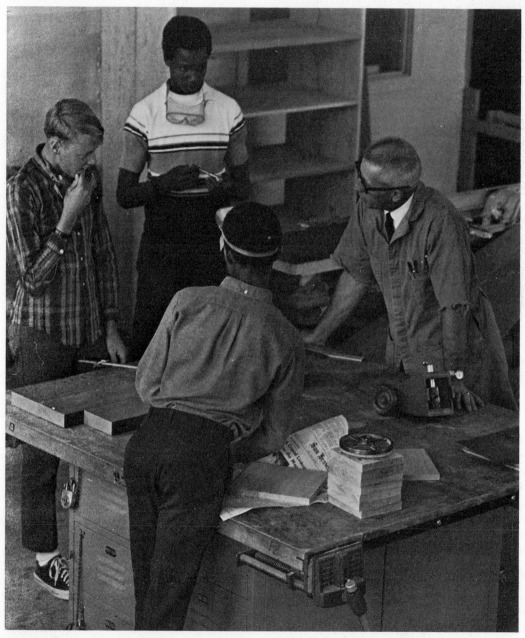

Figure 42-3. To the adolescent learning can be challenging. (Photograph by Peter Whitney.)

protection." If the parent is at all intelligent or sensitive, he already has some awareness of his own failure, and a confirmation does not ease his sense of guilt or help him face the present situation. Also, for a maturing child, the sense of failure on the part of his parent may become a rationalization of his own inadequacies, and, in a very real way, prevent him from facing and conquering his problems.

Need for Independence

What are the problems and tasks of this period? The most important is finding oneself and discovering what sort of person one is. The youth is actually "trying on for size" different types of personalities in an effort to discover one that fits his present idea of himself. As his self-concept is constantly changing, his conscious personality is changing with it. He can discard last week's concept easily and expects you to do the same.

If he is to develop an individuality, he must have independence and the freedom to *be* independent. Hence his intense, fierce rebellion against parental restraint even while, secretly, he would like to be back in that simpler period when he could conform without question. Although he would be relieved if he could occasionally surrender his independence, his need to achieve status with his peer group forbids it.

PUBERTY

The onset of puberty in a girl is marked by the *menarche,* or first menstrual period. Menarche is commonly preceded for several months by a recurrent, clear vaginal discharge. The average age for the first menstrual period of American girls is 11.5 years of age. However, there is a wide variation among individuals. Menarche may appear as early as the age of 9, or it may be delayed as late as the age of 17 or 18.

During the first year following menarche, menstrual periods are irregular in many girls. A girl who has had menstruation properly explained to her should experience little difficulty in accepting it. She will, in fact, no doubt feel a sense of pride in her approaching womanhood. Young women today have a freedom during their periods not known to their elders during their adolescence.

Nutritional Needs

In response to the rapid growth of this period, there is a corresponding increase in appetite and an increase in daily energy requirements.

The revised Recommended Daily Dietary Allowances* gives the daily caloric requirement for boys from 10 to 14 years of age as 2500-2700 calories. From the period of 14 to 18 years this increases to 3000 calories per day. Caloric requirements for girls are given as 2300 to 2400 calories per day for the 12 to 16 year period, and 2300 for the 16-18 year period. It must be remembered that these are only average allowances for young people of average height and weight. The very rapidly growing or active person, or the smaller child, may need an adjustment. Protein needs are from 50 to 55 g. per day for boys and girls.

Health Care

Although many pediatricians will continue to treat the adolescent, many young people resist going to a "baby doctor." Physicians who specialize in the care of the adolescent are available in many areas. Adolescent clinics, completely geared to adolescent needs, are increasing throughout the country. The adolescent is comfortable in such a facility, where the physician is interested in the total adolescent and his problems, whether they are physical, emotional or social.

DEVELOPMENT TASKS OF ADOLESCENCE

Erikson's developmental chart speaks of the puberty and adolescent period as the stage of *identity versus role confusion.* During this period, the young person

---

*Prepared by the Food and Nutrition Board of the National Research Council. Reported in *Nutrition Today, 3:* 18, 1968.

needs to question and to clarify the roles and skills which he has learned earlier. Because of his own physiological changes and his approaching maturity, he has to "refight many of the battles of earlier years, even though to do so [he] must artifically appoint perfectly well-meaning people to play the role of adversaries; and [he is] ever ready to install lasting idols and ideals as guardians of a final identity."*

The danger of this stage is confusion of the role he is to play. To avoid complete confusion, the adolescent is prone to identify with certain leaders, cliques or crowds. The adolescent mind is essentially in a psychosocial stage between childhood and adulthood. It is confused by the disparity

---

*Erickson, Erik: Childhood and Society. ed. 2. p. 261. New York, Norton, 1963.

between the moral code taught him as a child, and the practices he sees in the everyday life of adults.

Erikson sees this stage followed by a phase of intimacy versus isolation as the adolescent moves into young adulthood. He is ready and eager for the intimacy of close affiliations and friendships. Avoidance of such experiences may lead to a deep sense of isolation. These developmental phases are discussed again later in the section concerning adolescent problems.

Adolescence is said to be the state between childhood and adulthood in which there is accelerated physical and psychological growth. At the start of adolescence the child is dependent on his parents. During the adolescent period his task is to move toward independence, both social and emotional.

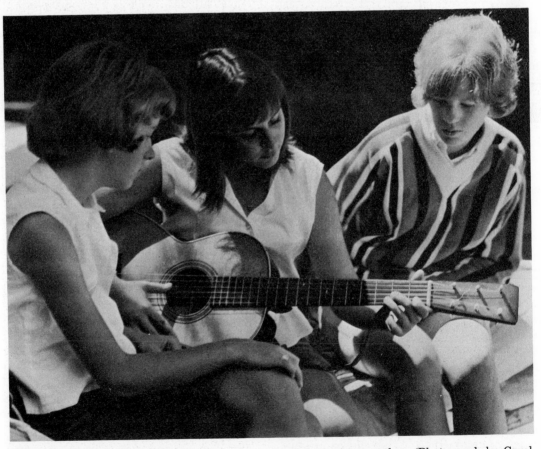

Figure 42-4. Youth are interested in music and enjoy singing together. (Photograph by Carol Baldwin.)

This may be a difficult period for parents who still see him as a child and mistrust his judgment. Yet in order for the adolescent to discover what kind of person he is, what values and mode of living he will adopt for his own, he must have the freedom to experiment, to test out his own insights and abilities. Parents need to realize that their role in the life of their child is coming to be that of advisor and counselor.

Parents need to accept the moods and turmoil of adolescence. Adolescence is a time of shaking loose from the dependency of childhood, of re-examining naive beliefs that his parents were all-powerful, all-knowing. Until he again can function on an even keel, the adolescent may go to the extreme of questioning all his parents' values.

The young person who has been a member of a warm, loving family and has been respected as a person is likely to be a person who is interested in the world around him. He sees the world with fresh eyes and is eager to try out all of the intriguing things he sees around him. Like the young child who stood in awe in the big public library and determined that when he could read he would read "all the books there are," the young person is eager to try out everything.

He is fortunate if his family and school are willing to provide opportunities for him to make decisions of his own, to ex-

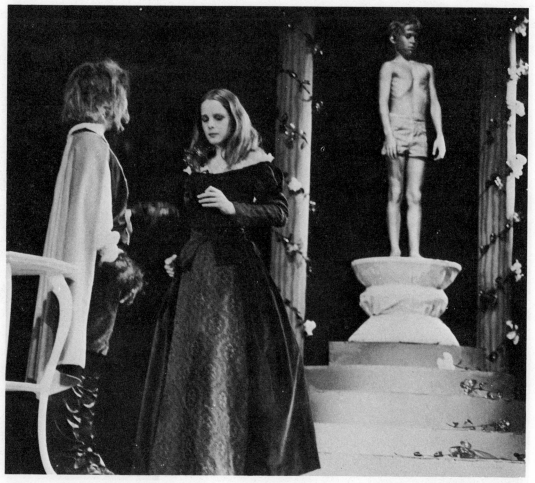

Figure 42-5. Grace and charm and talent are displayed in theatrical productions by young people. (Photograph by Carol Baldwin.)

periment, to apply his own common sense. He is most fortunate if he has an opportunity to get involved with his companions in interesting projects. Whether it is an impromptu music group, an amateur theater group, or just "rapping" sessions, he can find his life worthwhile and interesting. He will have little need for asocial actions.

Adjustment to Society

The adolescent of today is facing a society of changing values. The values taken for granted by the parents and grandparents are up for close scrutiny and evaluation. Too often it seems to the young person that his elders are saying "do as I say, not as I do."

"We have come to a turning point in history which we must all try to understand .... Its [the new culture's] values are not to be ignored or despised."* Canham further writes: "To argue for understanding is not to argue for tolerance of evil. That's what the youth culture says, too."

No doubt the rapid changes in technology and science of the 20th century have brought confusion to both adult and adolescent. The

*Canham, Erwin D.: Campus Crisis. Reprint from Christian Science Monitor.) Boston, Christian Science Publishing Society, 1971.

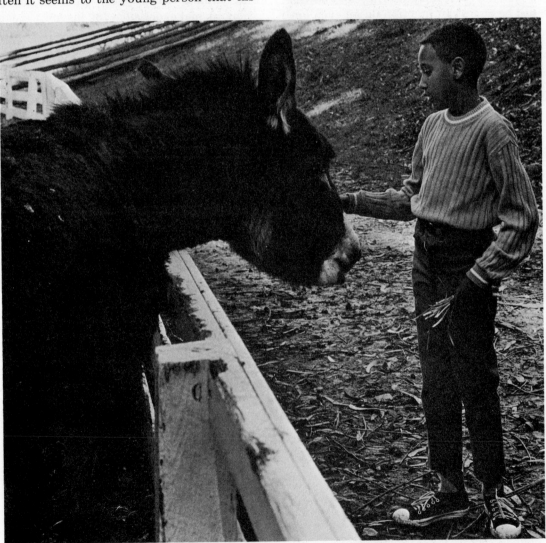

Figure 42-6.   Young people are often very fond of animals. (Photograph by Peter Whitney.)

standards of the older generation are questioned at every turn. Indeed, they are geared to a different way of living, a quieter pace. The adults of the present time need to rethink their accepted norms and way of life.

BIBLIOGRAPHY

Canham, Erwin D.: Campus Crisis. Reprint from Christian Science Monitor. Boston, Christian Science Publishing Society, 1971.

Duvall, Evelyn Millis: Family Development. ed. 4. Philadelphia, J. B. Lippincott, 1971.

Erikson, Erik: Childhood and Society. New York, Norton, 1963.

Gesell, Arnold, Ilg, Frances L., and Ames, Louise Bates: Youth—The Years From Ten to Sixteen. New York, Harper, 1956.

Lerrigo, Marion O. and Southard, Helen: Finding yourself. Sex Education Series, distributed by American Medical Association and National Education Association, 1968.

Suggested Readings for Further Study

Ginott, Haim: Between Parent and Teenager. New York, Macmillan, 1969.

Johnson, Eric: Love and Sex in Plain Language. Philadelphia, J. B. Lippincott, 1967.

McCandless, Boyd R.: Adolescent Behavior and Development. Hinsdale, Ill., Dryden Press, 1970.

Physical Problems and Diseases of Adolescence 43

ACNE VULGARIS

Acne is a condition that is so common among young people that it may be considered as one of the hallmarks of adolescence. This does not make it popular, nor does it diminish the seriousness with which teen-agers regard it. Young people wish to be popular and need to be attractive. An unsightly skin condition can decrease their self-confidence and can cause shyness and social withdrawal. A young person with acne may consider the blemish to be much more severe than do others, which causes a disproportionate amount of anxiety. This trait of concentrating on one defect, to the extent of ignoring one's own assets, is not, however, limited to adolescents.

Acne vulgaris is characterized by the appearance of blackheads, whiteheads, papules or pustules on the face and, to a lesser extent, on the back and the chest. The sites of these changes are the follicles into which the sebaceous glands empty sebum, the lubricant they secrete. The inflammatory lesions appear to be a result of the irritant action of sebum, and impaction of these follicles causes the comedones (or blackheads) of acne.

Predisposing Causes

Adolescent acne is primarily an expression of the endocrine imbalance that occurs at this time of life—but a variety of factors contribute to its production. Hereditary factors seem to be involved, as well as emotional conflicts, infection, poor hygiene and diet. The acne may be mild, characterized by an oily skin and by blackheads; it may be a severe type with ropelike cystic lesions and scarring a common feature. Because the condition may become severe, it is good to give it early attention.

Local Treatment

Washing and cleansing of the skin two or three times a day makes the face feel drier and more comfortable. Vigorous scrubbing causing irritation should be avoided. A soap substitute containing sulfur and salicylic acid (Fostex) may be more effective than soap.

Comedones should not be squeezed, but should be removed by a comedo extractor—generally by a physician. Lotions containing sulfur and resorcin are useful for drying the skin.

Severe acne that does not respond to these measures may be treated by the dermatologist with systemic antibiotic therapy. Ultraviolet light therapy has also brought improvement. Roentgen therapy and dermabrasion are generally not recommended during adolescence.

General Management

Sufficient sleep and exercise, recreation and social activities are all beneficial. The role of diet is inconsistent, but certain foods such as chocolate, nuts, fried foods and sea foods may aggravate the condition. A young person may have fantasies about the cause of his condition, and encouragement to discuss it with a physician or the school nurse may help him understand the nature of this skin infection. Of even more importance, the understanding, interested manner of a nurse or a physician may give him the courage to discuss some of his anxieties. Young people frequently find it difficult to discuss personal, emotionally charged matters with their parents because they need to be emancipated from their role of childhood dependency. An adult who listens objectively, with the emphasis on *listen,* may be able to give the most help, whether this is a nurse, a teacher, a counselor or a physician.

OBESITY

Obesity is another condition that can have an adverse effect on an adolescent's self-image. Obesity means, quite simply, an excessive accumulation of fatty subcutaneous tissue. It is a common problem in adolescence—a particularly unwelcome problem to girls in American culture—where to be fat is to be unattractive.

Obesity undoubtedly is caused mainly by overeating, but the problem cannot be solved by commanding a young person to use will power and to eat less food. Many factors enter into the problem and should be considered.

Activity is of major importance in controlling adolescent obesity. An active adolescent may eat large amounts and still not gain weight, while his sedentary counterpart may have a relatively low caloric intake but remain fat. Many obese young people do not eat excessively, but instead lack enough activity to burn up the food they eat.

Excessive food intake does necessarily need correction, but correction usually means something more than following a low calorie diet. Why does this person eat too much? Does he turn to food for emotional relief, because of unpopularity, low self-esteem, or because he is unsuccessful? Unless he can be helped in these areas, a dietary restriction may take away his only source of satisfaction and may only make his emotional difficulties worse.

Some shy, anxious adolescents retreat into obesity as a way of avoiding the world's competitive challenges. Other factors may, of course, enter into the causes of obesity.

Heredity may be one, and a nurse or a physician should be careful not to make a young person feel that his obesity makes him unacceptable. Heredity does not mean that the condition is untreatable, but an obese person is not inclined to cooperate if he feels that he is being rejected because of a condition for which he had little responsibility.

Regulation of Diet

An adolescent may be getting the greater amount of his caloric intake from carbohydrates and fats, with a low intake of proteins and minerals. A record of his total food intake for a few days may be important in determining whether he should change his eating habits. He may be well versed in the "basic four," but not until he can relate it to his own problems will it mean much to him.

MENSTRUAL DISTURBANCES

Delayed menarche. Menarche appears within a range of 9 to 17 years in the United States. Age differences are attributed to general health, nutrition, heredity, climate and psychosocial development. Delay beyond the 16th year should warrant a diagnostic survey for genetic abnormalities.

Dysmenorrhea is a common problem among teenage girls. It is characterized by cramping abdominal pain, leg pain and backache. Rarely, a pelvic abnormality is present. The specific cause of primary dysmenorrhea is unknown, but tension, anxiety or emotional states can aggravate the condition.

When no abnormality is present a simple, frank explanation of the physiology of maturation will help clear up any misunderstanding of the process. In addition, encouragement to participate in regular activities, and to practice good hygiene will help.

Irregular Menstruation is very common during the first year after menarche. Eventually a regular cycle appears.

Menorrhagia. Excessive, irregular, or protracted vaginal bleeding is frequently due to an imbalance in the secretion of hormones. It may take a period of months to achieve hormonal balance. These cycles are usually anovulatory (not accompanied with the discharge of an ovum). Anovulatory cycles may be considered normal for the first 1 to 3 years after menarche, but complete physical examination should be made to rule out organic causes. If no lesions are found, the adolescent girl should be put on a high protein diet with iron and vitamin supplements.

PULMONARY TUBERCULOSIS

Tuberculosis is present in all parts of the world, although many countries have shown a downward trend of mortality for several years. Prevalence of infection has declined rapidly in certain countries, as for example, in the United States and Japan.

Infectious agent. The predominant cause of pulmonary tuberculosis is the human tubercle bacillus, *Mycobacterium tuberculosis.* The bovine type, caused by *M. bovis* in cattle and communicated to man through dairy products, is now rare in the United States and a number of other countries.

Mode of transmission is contact with bacilli in the sputum of infected persons. The bacillus is predominantly airborne.

Incubation period is about 4 to 6 weeks between exposure and a primary lesion. Relapse of a latent infection accounts for many of the active cases.

Susceptibility is highest in children under 3 years of age and in adolescents and young adults.

Period of communicability. As long as sputum contains infectious tubercle bacilli, antimicrobial medications generally terminate the period of communicability in a few weeks.

Clinical manifestation. In children, pulmonary tuberculosis usually gives general symptoms of chronic infection, such as fatigue and irritability. Some malnutrition may be present. Primary lesions in children generally go unrecognized.

Secondary lesions are more apt to occur in the adolescent period and symptoms resemble those in an adult. Cough with expectoration, fever, loss of weight,

malaise and night sweats may be present.

Treatment of active pulmonary tuberculosis. Medical treatment includes administration of isoniazid (INH) and para-aminosalicylic acid (PAS), orally. A newer drug, ethambutol, also given orally, is said to be effective. Bed rest for children is usually not indicated unless the child appears ill, and physical activity is not restricted. A well balanced diet is important, but forced feedings are not indicated.

Prevention requires correction of such undesirable social conditions as overcrowding and poverty. Health education, availability of medical, laboratory and x-ray facilities for examination and control of contacts and suspects are all needed.

Identification and preventive treatment. Children who demonstrate active tubercular lesions anywhere in the body and children under the age of 4 years who have tuberculin-positive reactions are generally given a course of isoniazid for about a year. Older children who have recently become tuberculin-positive and who have been exposed to tuberculosis are treated in like manner whether or not they have a demonstrable infection.

Diagnostic tests include the intradermal Mantoux test using measured quantities of old tuberculin (O.T.). A commonly used test injects purified protein derivative (P.P.D.) into the skin by use of the tine method. In the tine test P.P.D. is inserted into four small puncture holes made in the upper arm with a four-pronged instrument.

Tuberculin testing is recommended when the child starts school and at adolescence. A positive reaction gives presumptive evidence but not proof of an active lesion. X-ray screening of tuberculin-positive persons gives further evidence. Positive proof is obtained when tubercle bacilli are found in the sputum. For infants who swallow their sputum gastric washings are indicated.

A vaccine called BCG is used in countries where the incidence of tuberculosis is high. It is given to tuberculin-negative persons, and is said to be effective for 12 years or longer. Mass vaccination is not deemed necessary in parts of the world where the incidence of tuberculosis is low.

Other Tuberculous Lesions

About 90 per cent of tuberculous lesions in children are of the pulmonary type. Tuberculosis can also affect the meninges, causing tubercular meningitis, the glandular system, or the vertibrae, as in Pott's disease.

Pott's disease is seen rather infrequently, since the methods for early diagnosis and treatment of tubercular infection are available for early use. Treatment for Pott's disease is the same as for general tuberculosis if the lesion is recognized early. If destruction of the bony structure is advanced or if nerves are affected, immobilization on a Bradford frame is necessary to facilitate healing. Spinal fusion may be necessary.

Although tubercle bacilli may attack other body tissues, such cases are rare among children.

The Hospitalized Adolescent

What does all this have to do with nursing an adolescent? We find here too that we cannot function in a situation that we do not understand, or that we only partially comprehend.

When an adolescent enters the hospital, he brings his own personality structure with him. It may be quite difficult for a young nurse, who is too near this age herself, to feel comfortable or to function effectively under these circumstances. She may become too involved, and find any objectivity very nearly impossible.

An adolescent may also find the situation difficult when the nurse is so near his age level. Because of his increased self-consciousness, his body becomes a source of embarrassment. Although the adolescent depends on his peers for approval and acceptance, he senses that a mature adult is the kind of person he needs when he is made dependent by an illness. He can now dare to indulge his need for "mothering" because of the imposed dependency.

The authority and status conferred by the nurse's uniform and by the title of Nurse may help a young nurse or a student nurse to achieve this role of authority figure, both for herself and for her patient.

If a nurse is functioning in the situation that still prevails in a majority of hospitals, she will not have much choice as to whether she cares for adolescent patients. Practices vary, but a large number of hospitals set the upper age for patients in their pediatric departments as anywhere between 12 and 14 years. In such situations, adolescent patients are scattered throughout the hospital, on the adult wards. While this may seem unrealistic in terms of development, it is often necessary in terms of the hospital's facilities which may not be geared to handle an adolescent in the pediatric department.

A newer trend, which is becoming increasingly popular, is to establish adolescent wards. These may consist of a few rooms set aside at one end of the pediatric department or, more probably, an entire adolescent wing. Because of the fascinating possibilities for the improved care of teen-agers in such an arrangement, this idea is dealt with in some detail later in this chapter.

To return to the patient himself, and to the problems that illness and hospitalization bring, we find that because of his absorption in his body image and in its changes, illnesses also have an increased interest for him. He is apt to have a large fund of information, much of which is incorrect or distorted. He probably has many fears about the effect of his illness on his appearance or on his future adequacy.

This intensified interest, as well as the alert and curious nature of a teen-ager provides a wealth of opportunity for the nurse, if she can recognize it. The way is open for some sound health teaching.

The adolescent, of course, is experiencing a renewed interest in sex, and is trying to chart a course for himself in an area in which he finds very little guidance. Often he is quiet about this and gives little indication of any need for help. On the other hand, he frequently does throw out clues. One fourteen-year-old boy repeatedly attempted

Miss Brown was busy behind the bed-side curtains while she was caring for a twelve-year-old boy, while four other boys in the ward were discussing life in general. Ignoring her presence, they were busily discussing menstruation. They were honestly puzzled, especially as to the effects of "all that bleeding." Finally Johnny suggested, "Why don't we ask Miss Brown?" which they promptly did. Startled, but rallying bravely, Miss Brown gave an elementary lesson in the physiology of menstruation, which satisfied the boys. One needs to be prepared for all eventualities when working with young people.

---

physical intimacies while receiving his morning care (which included a bed bath) from the student nurse. The nurse was confused and troubled. She knew that Jerry was from a deprived, broken home, and she fancied that she would be showing him more "rejection" if she refused the kiss he demanded. She began to dread her clinical experience. When she was asked why she had not sought advice, she admitted a reluctance to do so for fear that she would be considered "squeamish," or unable to work out her own problems. In this case, both the patient and his nurse were confused. A student should be willing to accept her own inexperience and lack of background. This young woman simply did not have the maturity to handle the situation alone, and should have sought help from someone competent to give it to her. Undoubtedly Jerry had been a rejected child, but the student could not undo the years of environmental deprivation in a matter of days, nor did she have the experience to try. A young nurse should have a very clear idea of her role. She is not a psychiatrist, a medical doctor, a social service specialist, nor is she a priest. She is a nurse, and does all that she can to bring a child back to health, and undoubtedly draws on all these resources. She should also know her limitations very clearly.

It would seem that at this point Jerry needed firmness. He probably needed an older person for his nurse, because a young woman giving him intimate care confused him.

Adolescent Clinics

An adolescent has worries and fears that may seem childish to an adult, and because an adolescent fears that he may seem childish, he often keeps his troubles to himself. Gallagher, commenting on a youth's reluctance to discuss his problems with his parents, says, "For this reason if the physician will present as a strong, warm, interested person—non-authoritarian, neither approving or disapproving—he will gain their confidence and he can be of great help."*

Adolescent clinics seem to provide the ideal setting for an exploration of the needs and the anxieties of adolescents. There are a number of these unique clinics in the United States, and they are proving to be very successful. An adolescent clinic is a place set apart for young persons only. Personnel and doctors are sympathetic to their problems. The young person has reached a phase of his life in which he has an intense interest in his own body. This is also an age at which his desire to identify with his peers is paramount. This is all preparation for his maturity and should thus be respected.

One great difficulty that an adolescent seems to experience is that no one appears to want to listen to him. He may talk, worry and question, but it seems to him that adults are not really listening. The attitude strikes him as one of, "These things do not mean anything. You will soon get over them. This is just a phase you are going through."

An adolescent clinic is a place in which they can be heard, in which their worries are respected, and in which they and their doctors together can try to work out problems. Adolescent patients make their own appointments and go unaccompanied to the clinic, where they find all the other patients are of their own age group.

One girl has acne, which worries her greatly, but she hesitates to talk to her mother about it because she boasts about the

*Gallagher, J. R.: Medical Care of the Adolescent. New York, Appleton-Century-Crofts, 1960.

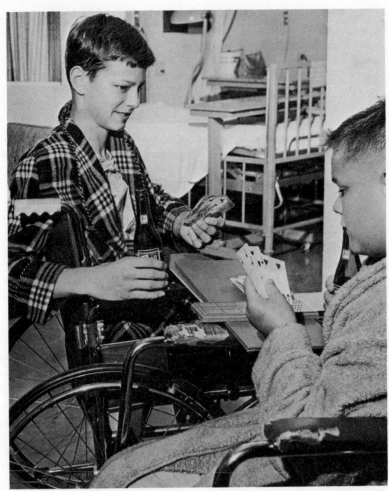

Figure 43-1.   The adolescent ward provides a suitable atmosphere for these young people.

beautiful complexion she had when she was young. A boy is concerned about his slow development, while another worries over a functional heart murmur that has convinced his mother that he should not play football. Still another is puzzled about his severe headaches which are worse during the sports season (in which he is active) but at which time his grades "are not so good."†

All of these persons need and must receive consideration, not only of their ailments, but also of their confusing personal problems. At the clinic they have careful physical examinations, and are shown their X-rays and the results of laboratory tests.

───────────

†From the film *Medical Care for the Adolescent*, 16 mm., sound (color) 30 min. Philadelphia, Merck, Sharp and Dohme.

The entire setting is geared to a consideration of a young person's problems.

Adolescent In-Patient Care

For a young person who must be hospitalized, a separate adolescent unit seems so right that one wonders why it has taken so long to get them started. Virtually any hospital should be able to set aside at least a small unit for this purpose. (Figs. 43-1 and 43-2)

Some hospitals that have done so have found the experiment very successful. The director of one hospital had his attention drawn to the unhapply situation of teen-age patients scattered throughout the hospital, by the experience of his own son. Here, as in

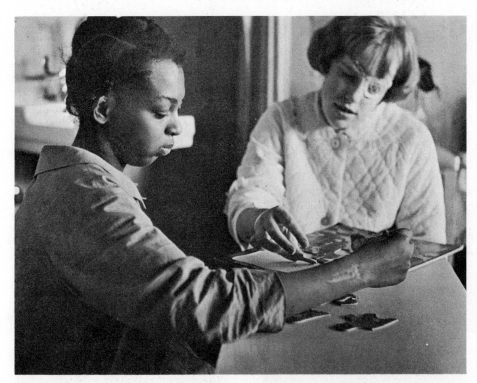

Figure 43-2. Companions and activity in the adolescent ward help speed recovery.

many hospitals, teen-agers were assigned to adult wards according to the nature of their ailments. A young boy in a ward with older men found them quite free with unwholesome stories. A young girl had for roommates senile, withdrawn patients; another was in a room with women suffering from gynecological troubles, who freely discussed their ailments. To the administrator, this did not seem to be the best setting for learning "the facts of life." In fact, he was shocked by the situation and resolved to do something about it.

The "doing something about it" took the form of a unit of care just for teen-agers. A wing adjacent to the children's ward was utilized, and it has been an outstanding success.

In such a setting, enthusiastic young visitors do not annoy older, sick persons. The patients are sympathetic and understanding toward each other. Their interests are similar, their school work is shared, and the staff is chosen from among those who have a sympathetic understanding of this age group. Rules are enforced, of course—but

they are written with this age group in mind. Meals are nutritious, and the food is plentiful, geared to adolescent appetites. The unit has now passed the experimental stage and is an integral part of the hospital.

Young nurses may gain both insight and competence if they are assigned to care for patients in an adolescent ward, but some caution is indicated. Most young males feel embarrassed about having personal services performed by someone near their own age, and they may occasionally show this by aggressive behavior. They may also attach too much personal meaning to the attention given them. Girls in this period of development are also very shy about their bodies and may prefer an older, motherly person to care for them, or perhaps an older, impersonal woman.

A student or a young nurse should be quite secure in her own role. She can do much to put a patient at ease, in any situation, with her professional manner and her impersonal ministrations, and thus the experience can have great value for both the nurse and her patient.

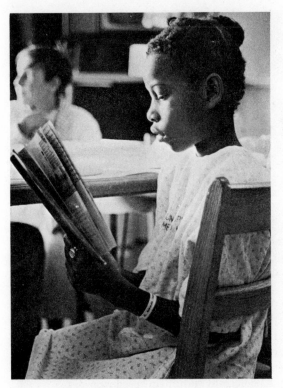

Figure 43-3. Recuperation in the adolescent ward affords time for reading.

BIBLIOGRAPHY

Blattner, R. J.: Isoniazed prophylaxis in tuberculin reactors. Journal of Pediatrics, *72:*191, 1968.

Chapman, A. H.: Management of Emotional Problems of Children and Adolescents. Philadelphia, J. B. Lippincott, 1965.

Domonkos, Anthony N.: Acne Vulgaris. In Cohn, Howard F.: Current Therapy 1972. p. 558. Philadelphia, W. B. Saunders, 1972.

Gallagher, J. R.: Medical Care of the Adolescent. ed. 2. New York, Appleton-Century-Crofts, 1966.

Schowalter, John and Lord, Ruth D.: The hospitalized adolescent. Children, *18:*127, 1971.

Suggested Readings for Further Study

Meyer, Herbert L.: Predictable problems of hospitalized adolescents. AJN, *69:*525, 1969.

Rosenburg, Morris and Gottleib, Ruth P.: Current approach to tuberculosis in childhood. Pediatric Clinics of North America, *15:*513, 1968.

Social Problems of Adolescence 44

DELINQUENCY

Up until the 20th century no distinction was made between children and adults accused of criminal acts. Punishment was the only legal consequence of acts against society. Children were put in overcrowded jails with hardened criminals, where no attempt was made to understand the "why" behind their behavior. Society's need to be protected had first priority.

Juvenile courts came into being in America at the turn of the 20th century, largely as a result of Jane Addams' concern for more compassionate treatment for all children. Juvenile courts sprang up all over the nation, with rehabilitation of the delinquent child as their goal. Unfortunately, Lisa Richette writes, "communities have used the juvenile courts as dumping grounds for *all* unruly children,"* rather than as constructive forces.

What makes a child delinquent? One important factor to be considered is the sense of worthlessness, low self esteem. Children who have been shifted from one foster home to another, for example, eventually develop a very low opinion of their own worth.

Many children in foster care go through the traumatic experience of being moved from one home to another, often many times. A most moving look into a little girl's heart has been portrayed in the story of one such child. She had gathered into herself all of the hurt and the criticism that she had received

---

*Richette, Lisa Aversa: The Throwaway Children, p. 291. New York, Dell, 1969.

in her moves from one home to another, until she was afraid to respond naturally to anyone. Always she was the outsider. "In this home, do they want me to make my bed as soon as I get up, or will I be scolded for not letting it air? Should I offer to help with breakfast, or will I be in the way?" It took long, patient understanding and acceptance in a home where she was really wanted before her barriers could finally come down. For some children, it is too late.

Billy was a child whom no one wanted. A slight congenital deformity appeared to make him rejected everywhere he went, and he had been in and out of hospitals and foster homes since early infancy. At last a social worker thought she had found him a home. A mature couple agreed to take Billy with adoption in mind. They visited him and told him of the good home he would have with them.

Finally the time came for Billy's placement, and he went with hope in his eyes. Two weeks later he was back, "We just don't feel that we can go through with this." This seemed the last chance for Billy. One can speculate about what his future would hold, but none of it looks pleasant.

The causes of delinquency, writes Howard James, in *Children in Trouble*, are multiple. Large numbers are children of alcoholic or unstable parents. Millions grow up in destructive slums; others are the products of inadequate schools. Still others are neglected children of wealthy parents. Many children sent to detention homes or reform schools have their futures as social misfits set for them. Sending children to reform school can do them more harm than good.

Helping to Prevent Delinquency

Undoubtedly the most important step is to become personally involved. There are many ways to help a child know that someone believes he is worth saving. Tutoring a disadvantaged child may give him a new impetus toward a brighter future. Many children of Mexican, Puerto Rican, or other cultural groups need help to feel at home in a society where they are poorly accepted.

Student organizations have a wonderful opportunity to work with their peers, "rapping" with them, exchanging ideas and discussing social values. Needing a purpose for existing, such organizations have assisted in many socially oriented endeavors. When the society seems hypocritical, materialistic, and unheeding, the group can provide solid support and inspiration.

This is not saying that violence and riots are an accepted method of protest. Peaceful revolution, "friendly persuasion" still brings more converts, while angry aggression antagonizes.

DRUG ABUSE

Another area in which some young people express their reaction to the changing scene of today's world is in the use of addicting drugs. Many adolescents and children have experimented with such drugs out of curiosity, as boys once did in Grandfather's time with making and smoking cornsilk cigarettes. The young person who is merely curious and has other less dangerous interests to absorb his mind may go no further. But unfortunately too many children today lack means for coping with problems of growing up in a changing society, and they turn to drugs for a way out, not realizing that they are greatly compounding their difficulties.

In all honesty, it is necessary to state that the problem is not strictly confined to young people. However, it is most saddening to see young people with their great potential risking their emotional, mental, and physical capabilities following such a futile course.

A listing of terms used when speaking of drug abuse may be helpful.

Drug. A chemical substance given with the intention of preventing or curing disease or otherwise enhancing the physical or mental welfare of men or animals. *Habit-forming drugs.* Drugs which tend to cause addiction.

Drug abuse. Use of a drug to excess, or in a way not sanctioned medically, socially, or culturally.

Drug dependence. Dependence may be psychological, physical, or both. Psychological dependence denotes a compulsive need to use an agent for its satisfying or pleasurable effects. Physical dependence is the result of drug-induced changes in body tissue functioning that make the presence of the drug necessary for a normal state of activity. Magnitude of physical dependence or severity of withdrawal symptoms varies directly with the amount, frequency, and duration of drug use.

Drug tolerance. Development of ability of body tissues to endure and adapt to continued or increased use of a drug.

Withdrawal symptoms. A characteristic pattern of signs and symptoms when a drug is discontinued or withdrawn. The drug-adapted body cells lose their ability to function normally, and must go through the process of adjusting to the absence of the drug.

Management of Drug Poisoning or Overdose

There are many substances which have abuse potential. An outline of the most commonly used substances, their effects, and their antidotes is given here.

Volatile Solvents

Toluene, zylene, benzene, gasoline, alcohol. Used as solvents in paint and lacquer removers, ingredients of some types of glue, lighter fluid, cleaner fluids, hair spray, and others. Volatile hydrocarbons used as propellents in aerosol spray.

Mode of use. "Sniffed"—inhaled. Used mainly by young children.

Effects. Feeling of euphoria and mild hallucinations, dizziness, slurred speech, blurred vision. Nausea may be present. There may be a feeling of reckless abandon, aggressiveness, breakdown of inhibitions.

Dangers. May lead to permanent brain, kidney, liver, and bone marrow damage. Fumes inhaled from spray can products from a plastic bag can freeze the esophagus and congest the lungs, causing asphyxiation. Many deaths have been reported.

Treatment. Artificial respiration.

Hypnotics—Sedatives, Barbiturates

Nembutal, Seconal, Amytol, Butisol, Doriden, and others.

Mode of use. By mouth in pill or capsule form, injected in muscle or vein.

Effects. General nervous system depressant. In overdose effects resemble drunkenness. Coma and death frequently result from overdose.

Dangers. Physical addiction, with severe withdrawal symptoms. Sudden withdrawal may cause convulsions, mental disturbances, death.

Treatment. Artificial respiration, gavage. Withdrawal should be gradual under medical supervision.

Slang names for hypnotics. Barbs, goof balls, yellow-jackets, red devils, many others.

Amphetamines and Other Stimulants

Methedrine, Dexadrine, Benzedrine, Amphetamine.

Mode of use. Same as hypnotics.

Effects. Heavy doses can cause hallucinations leading to mental derangement. Abnormal heart rate, psychotic states, personality disorders. Unaccustomed high doses can cause death. Body acquires tolerance, making progressively larger doses necessary to feel effects.

Antidote. Thorazine, Mellaril.

Slang names. Pep, speed, bennies, dexies, many others.

Hallucinogens—Psychedelic Drugs

LSD, DMT, DOM, morning glory seeds, peyote, mescaline.

Mode of use. Oral.

Effects. Alter perception. Mystical and religious experiences, sensory perception affected, such as tasting, color sense, synesthesia, perception of supranatural powers, e.g., that one can fly.

Dangers. Bad trips: panic, paranoia, acute anxiety, may last 8 to 18 hours. Flashbacks of bad trips may occur after single dose and sometimes lead to suicide. LSD does produce chromosomal aberrations, but its capacity to cause congenital malformations in offspring is not well established. High incidence of spontaneous abortions and stillbirths in pregnant LSD users.

Antidote. User on a "high" or a bad trip should be talked down slowly. Avoid stimulation, keep in quiet room, offer comforting and closeness.

Marijuana

Mode of use. Commonly smoked as marijuana cigarettes.

Effects. Few physical symptoms. Mood changes can range from depression to exhilaration. Sense of time and distance may be distorted.

Dangers. May interfere with clear thinking and retard concentration. Psychological dependence may occur. Legal penalties are heavy for possession or use of marijuana.

Slang names. Pot, grass, weed, reefers, joints.

Narcotics

Heroin, morphine, codeine, Demerol, opium. Heroin is the narcotic most abused in America.

Mode of use. Injected under skin (popping), into vein (mainlining), or into muscle.

Effects. Euphoria, relief from all anxieties, followed by stupor. Slows down body organ functions, reduces hunger, thirst, sex drive.

Dangers. Tolerance develops quickly, physical and psychological dependence is marked. Hepatitis is frequent as a result of using unsterile needles. Most heroin sold to addicts is diluted with other substances in themselves poisonous. Death can occur after doses above the user's tolerance level, or as a result of substances mixed with heroin. Addicted users need to have a "fix" three or four times daily. Heroin is extremely expensive; addiction leads to robbery, prostitution, mugging, to get money to support habit.

Withdrawal and Treatment

Methadone is a synthetic opiate which gives relief from an addict's craving for heroin and also blocks the euphoric effects of heroin if it has been taken. Methadone is itself addicting but does not cause the harmful effects of hard drugs. The addict who takes methadone as prescribed has his heroin craving removed and is able to live normally, attending school or holding a job. He will, however, need to keep taking methadone.

At clinics where methadone is distributed, the patient must take his dosage under supervision and furnish a urine specimen. Some addicts who are not sincere about getting off heroin will save up tablets, taking a large dose at one time to produce a high. Some who cannot give up the habit will deny taking heroin while collecting the methadone to hoard or to sell. Heroin, however, shows up in the user's urine, therefore specimens are given at the clinic rather then having them brought in from home where they could be faked.

An addict must be totally sincere in his desire to break the habit before he can find the strength to try to do so. Some people are against the use of methadone, as it substitutes the use of one habit-forming drug for another. As it is nearly impossible for most addicts to break their habit, the argument is that a benign habit replacing such a harmful one as hard drug addiction is far superior to the sort of life the confirmed addict must lead to support his habit.

The use of methadone to replace heroin aims to return the addict to legitimate employment and impetus for living.

Methadone needs to be used in combination with a rehabilitation program. Treatment properly conducted suggests a 2 in 3 chance of success with voluntary patients.

Therapeutic communities. The patient lives in the community for a period of 1 to 2 years. Sudden, complete, "cold turkey" withdrawal is used, although some communities will allow use of methadone for a few days after admission.

Patients are gathered into a close, concerned community, kept busy with household chores. Treatment consists of acting out games, encounter groups, meditation. It is said that with such support and encouragement, withdrawal symptoms are mild. However, only about one in ten applicants is deemed suitable for the program.

Preventive Measures

Basic reasons for drug abuse among youths. Reasons given are poor self-concept, social pressures from peers, escape from problems, boredom, experimentation, curiosity.

Education about the misuse of drugs is certainly a step in the right direction, but only a step. Scare techniques are worse than useless, serving mainly to arouse aggression, disbelief and not infrequently furnishing an added fillip of danger and thrill to experimentation. Yet there are much more satisfying and fulfilling ways to meet the needs of young people.

Action programs can engross a person, make use of abilities, stretch his capacities, provide thrills and excitement, and give him pride and self respect. A "natural high" is much more satisfying and real than a synthetic high from drugs.

Interest in social and political causes brings a young person out of boredom and introspection. The recent political action of giving the vote to 18-year-olds offers enormous opportunities for participation in correcting abuses, providing equal opportunities for all, fighting pollution, and raising the standard of living for deprived people. Such exciting participation is fulfilling; it also calls for clear and realistic thinking.

VENEREAL DISEASE AMONG YOUNG PEOPLE

Venereal disease has become widespread throughout the world, gonorrhea having reached epidemic proportions. Although formerly teenagers had been the highest risk group, this is no longer true, as the highest rate of syphilis is found in the 20-34 age group. Gonorrhea has its most rapid increase in the 20-24 year group.*

However, venereal disease is increasing rapidly among adolescents in spite of the availability of antibiotics.

Although venereal diseases have been considered diseases found principally among depraved and delinquent persons, this is no longer true. They are showing alarming increases among the middle and upper class population, particularly among young people of both sexes. Although both syphilis and gonorrhea are reportable diseases, it is estimated that for every case reported, at least three go undetected.

However one may feel about the changing society and sexual permissiveness, it is true that the relaxation of sexual controls has been indicted as the principal cause of the rise in venereal disease. A significant number of cases occur among homosexuals.

Besides being a serious and ugly disease, venereal disease still carries a stigma. Many teenagers fear to tell their parents, and as doctors are still legally barred in many states from treating minors without their parent's consent, they have nowhere to go for treatment. A movement to remove this ban is currently being pushed with good results: in a number of states doctors may now legally treat minors with gonorrhea or syphilis without parental consent.

Syphilis still responds to penicillin therapy when it is carried through. A course

of injections takes about 2 weeks. The treatment of choice for gonorrhea has also been penicillin, but recently the gonococcus has developed a number of penicillin-resistant strains. In some areas, doctors give penicillin only a 50-50 chance of curing gonorrhea. The fact that often both gonorrhea and syphilis show mild primary symptoms and go undetected adds to the difficulty of detection and treatment.

In view of the above facts, the urgent problem is one of prevention. Massive educational programs, especially among young people, are urgently needed. Also more research on the nature of venereal disease, search for better preventive methods (possibly a vaccine) and better methods of treatment and control are high on the list.

Here is a resume of information currently being circulated.†

Syphilis

A disease caused by a spirochete which can involve every part of the body.

Communicability. Through intimate, personal contact with an infected person.

Signs and symptoms. Painless sore at point of entry of the spirochete, appearing 10 to 90 days after exposure.

Secondary stage. Rash, sore throat, fever, appearing in 2 to 6 months after original infection. Signs of both 1st and 2nd stage will disappear without treatment, but the spirochete remains in the body, eventually causing severe nervous system disorders in later life, unless early, adequate treatment has been given.

Gonorrhea

Caused by the gonococcus. Caught at the time of intimate physical contact with the sex organs or rectum of an affected person.

In the female, infection may progress to serious pelvic disorders. It may render the male sterile. Neither condition gives any immunity after one or more attacks.

*Faigel, H. C.: Reported patterns of venereal disease in adolescents. *Clinical Pediatrics*, 8:620, 1969.

†Adapted from "Do You Know About the Most Commonly Reported Communicable Disease?" Pamphlet distributed by Pfizer Laboratories, containing information adapted from material issued by the California State Dept. of Public Health.

THE UNMARRIED TEENAGE MOTHER

The conflict in today's culture about the acceptance of sex as a basic drive, and the disapproval of pregnancy out of wedlock, is most confusing to teenagers, as it is to the older members of our society who attempt to meet their responsibilities to these younger people. As one writer put it: "There seems to be widespread tolerance of extramarital sexual intercourse—as long as there is no baby."*

Consider the extent of the problem. In 1960, there were 91,700 illegitimate births to teenage girls, of whom 48,300 were girls of school age.† Contrary to popular belief, however, the highest rate of pregnancy out of marriage is not among teenagers, but among women in the 20 to 30 age group.

Why illegitimacy? There have been many attempts to pinpoint the reason, but the truth is that there is no one answer. Social and emotional immaturity, faulty child-parent relationships, and weak, confused moral standards no doubt contribute. A feeling of rejection, and of never having been accepted may lead a girl to seek affection and acceptance in relationships outside of her home. She becomes involved in highly emotional romantic relationships that have little contact with reality. It may not seem to her to be immoral as long as affection is involved. To have sexual relationships may seem the thing to do: the others tell about their experiences—she just happened to be "unlucky." There is little understanding or social maturity.

Other generalizations, such as membership in a socioeconomic class or ethnic group, a broken home, and dependency needs are offered as reasons for behavior unacceptable to the prevailing culture, but no one theory gives the entire answer. We must study this problem a great deal more. Those who make studies must first free themselves from stereotyped ideas and from bias, and give consideration to individuals rather than to general groups, or social classes.

Prenatal Care for the Teenager

An adolescent girl does not have the motivation to seek antepartal medical care that is normal for an older, married woman. Pregnancy means being excluded from school, rejection from her family, and a strange, frightening, immediate future. She thinks of herself as a young girl, not as an expectant mother. She may even deny her pregnancy. Small wonder then that she lacks enthusiasm for traveling across the city to an impersonal prenatal clinic, to join a group of patients with whom she feels no bond whatever.

The lack of prenatal care that many (but not all) unmarried teenagers receive accounts for much of the high rate of prematurity and infant mortality found in this group. A greater effort must be made to reach these young people and provide them with the necessary medical care as well as with counseling and guidance. A school nurse may be a person with a real opportunity to initiate a sound course of action. If she has established a good relationship with the students, a troubled girl is very likely to take this problem to her as she has done with other problems. The nurse, the teacher, the social worker, and the girl herself, may work as a team to arrange for physical care, for an emotional adjustment, as well as for continuing education.

A Nurse's Role in Counseling

A young nurse may have difficulty relating to a young unmarried patient in the postpartum department, unless she has been able to resolve her own feelings. Her understanding of her professional role will help her; her need to be of service and her desire to assist her patient in achieving physical and emotional health should provide the necessary stability.

An adolescent mother must choose whether she keeps her baby or gives him up for adoption. The position that adoption is the best answer has been widely held. A

---

*Garland, P.: The community's part in preventing illegitimacy. Children, *10:*71, 1963.
†Adams, H., and Gallagher, U.: Some facts and observations about illegitimacy. Children, *10:*43, 1963.

normal home life for an infant and a healthy future are more likely than with the uncertainties of life with a mother who is herself immature. A girl may put an end to this unfortunate phase, complete her schooling and later make a successful life for herself.

The question is now being asked as to whether this is inevitably the right solution. Again, we have been dealing in generalities. Many mothers have kept their children and have been able to provide them with satisfactory lives. These mothers need services and support from the community in greater measure than they have received in the past.

An unmarried adolescent father needs counseling and guidance as well. Those who have worked with teenage fathers have found that they feel more responsibility and concern than had been thought. Someone is greatly needed to help them work out their confused, troubled feelings.

Educational Programs for Pregnant Girls of School Age

Traditionally, if a schoolgirl became pregnant she was obliged to drop out of school as soon as her pregnancy became known. This applied to married as well as unmarried girls. In many school systems, married students, pregnant or not, have also been discharged from school or have been allowed to continue but denied participation in extra-curricular activities.* Eventually it became evident that this was essentially a "throwaway" policy. It was seen as contributing to a girl's lack of belief in her own worth and value to society. As long as her baby was taken from her and she herself became an outcast, society took little interest in what did become of her.

The maternity homes set up for salvaging these girls unwanted by society attempt to meet the emotional and educational needs of the pregnant unmarried adolescent. Regular scholastic classes are held in many of these homes, with credit for work done applied to the girl's school record. These girls are usually prepared to resume their regular classes after delivery. Unfortunately, only a minority of pregnant girls are reached through these maternity homes.

Public school boards began experimenting with means for providing continuing education for these girls. As one school system puts it, they provide help for girls "with the temporary problem of being pregnant."† Various programs were created to meet the needs of girls who had to leave school because of pregnancy. These programs vary from strict, restrictive rules concerning school attendance to rules permissive enough to allow a pregnant girl to remain in her own class if she so desires.

Illustrations of kinds of programs for pregnant school girls:

Traditional rules still maintained in many school districts.

A pregnant girl, married or unmarried, must leave school immediately. If the girl wishes to return to school after delivery, she must attend a different school. An unmarried student who has had more than one child cannot return to regular school. Unmarried fathers may not be welcomed in school, may be counseled to attend evening school. Other policies stipulate that a pregnant schoolgirl continue her education at home through correspondance courses.

A More Insightful Program

This type of program consists of setting up special schools, usually within the public school program. One such program was created in a rural area with the help of a federal grant.‡ This is a program for middle class, average girls, whose ages range from 14 to 18 years. Most of the girls are 16 or 17 years of age, in the 11th or 12th grade. A house in a residential section was obtained for the schoolroom. A full range of high school subjects is offered, including vocational as well as educational subjects.

---

*McMurray, Georgia A.: Community action on behalf of pregnant schoolage girls, educational policies and beyond. *Child Welfare, 49:*342, 1970.

†Ibid.

‡Zober, Edith: The pregnant schoolgirl. *Child Welfare, 48:*362, 1969.

A number of city school boards have adopted similar plans. In most of these, the student may attend on a regular school basis as long as she feels able to do so before delivery. She is allowed to resume classes at the special school after delivery until her doctor allows her to return to her regular class. Grades and credits earned are sent to her regular school. Some of these schools provide nurseries for the babies while their mothers attend classes.

The question remains, however, whether even this is the best way of helping the pregnant schoolgirl. Some schools are now allowing pregnant girls to stay in their regular classes. Convincing arguments are given for both solutions. It is not necessarily easier for a girl to leave the school environment with which she is familiar. Too often she may view this as a form of punishment or of nonacceptance. Arguments for the special schools consist of her ability to adjust in a warm, friendly atmosphere. Perhaps there is need for both.

BIBLIOGRAPHY

Cohen, Allan Y.: The journey beyond trips: alternatives to drugs. Journal of Psychedelic Drugs, *3:*16, 1971.

Godenne, Ghislaine D.: Adolescent crisis today. Clinical Proceedings of the Children's Hospital of the District of Columbia, *26:*317, 1970.

Irwin, Samuel: Drugs of abuse: an introduction to their actions and potential hazards. Journal of Psychedelic Drugs, *3:*5, 1971.

James, Howard: Children in Trouble: a national scandal. Christian Science Publishing Society, 1969.

Richette, Lisa Aversa: The Throwaway Children. New York, Dell, 1969.

Senay, Edward C. and Renault, Pierre F.: Treatment methods for heroin addicts: a review. Journal of Psychedelic Drugs, *3:*47, 1971.

Shiller, Alice: Drug Abuse and Your Child. New York, Public Affairs Comm., 1970.

Suggested Readings for Further Study

Barnard, Janice E.: Peer group instruction for primigravid adolescents. Nursing Outlook, *18:*42, 1970.

Canham, Erwin D.: Campus Crisis. Boston, The Christian Science Monitor, [reprint]. Boston, Christian Science Publishing Society, 1971.

Fisher, Rona C. and Austen, Simon L.: Juvenile drug abuse. Clinical Proceedings of the Children's Hospital of the District of Columbia, *25:*80, 1969.

Herzog, Elizabeth, Sudea, Cecelia E. and Harwood, Jane: Youth Reporters Discuss "Problem" Drugs. U. S. Department of HEW, Children's Bureau, 1970.

Hughes, John: The Junk Merchants. Christian Science Monitor Reprint Series. Boston, Christian Science Publishing Society, 1971.

Keniston, Kenneth: The adolescent in 1970. Clinical Proceedings of the Children's Hospital of the District of Columbia, *26:*1, 1970.

Rueveni, Uri: Using sensitivity training with junior high school students. Children, *18:*69, 1971.

Scott, Max L.: Small groups—an effective treatment approach in residential programs for adolescents. Child Welfare, *49:*161, 1970.

Washington, Bennetta B.: Cultural deprivation and the high school dropout. Clinical proceedings of the Children's Hospital of the District of Columbia, *24:*35, 1970.

Yolles, Stanley F.: The drug scene. Nursing Outlook, *18:*24, 1970.

UNIT STUDY QUESTIONS

1. Skeletal growth is completed when:
   a. epiphyses close
   b. pelvic girdle widens
   c. cranial fusion occurs
   d. greater trocanteric growth finishes

2. Children who begin maturation early may be expected to:
   a. become larger than the average child
   b. develop undesirable traits of behavior
   c. attain full growth later than the average child
   d. attain full growth earlier than the average child

3. All of the following are common adolescent fears or worries *except:*
   a. sexual maturity
   b. making a good adjustment
   c. marital adjustment
   d. personal appearance

4. Usually the strictest behavioral control over the early adolescent is exerted by his:
   a. parents
   b. peers
   c. church
   d. school

5. Acne is a condition primarily due to:
   a. an allergy to certain foods
   b. lack of cleanliness
   c. poor diet, insufficient sleep
   d. skin changes that occur in adolescence

6. Drug abuse is a present-day problem. Some of the reasons thought to be the cause are:
   a. inability to cope with everyday problems
   b. a need to be accepted by one's peers
   c. curiosity
   d. boredom
   The answer is:
   1. a and b
   2. b and d
   3. none of the above
   4. all of the above

7. Those who turn to the use of drugs today are mainly:
   a. young people from deprived areas
   b. delinquent young persons
   c. people of all ages and walks of life
   d. the misfits of society

8. Hard-core drug addicts find the habit nearly impossible to break. Society is best advised to do the following:
   a. write off these people and concentrate on prevention
   b. enact legislation requiring compulsory treatment for all addicts
   c. employ scare tactics and heavy punishment for the use of drugs
   d. by research and experimentation, seek ways for prevention and treatment of drug addiction

APPENDIX

DRUGS USED MOST FREQUENTLY IN MATERNAL AND CHILD NURSING*

This listing of drugs, used in the care of maternity patients and sick children, gives average doses, major side effects, and cautions for use. The adult dose is given in terms of average usage. For the child, however, different criteria must be used.

Doses of most potent medications are calculated by the physician according to the individual child's age, weight, and general physical condition. The nurse will do well to check the dosage according to the formula *dosage per kilogram of body weight, divided into x doses.* This is written as

mg. (or g.)/kg./no. of doses or
mg. (or g.)/kg./in 24 hours. Divide in x doses.

Example. An infant weighing 6 kg. has an order for Dilantin 15 mg. given 2 times daily.†

Average dosage of Dilantin is 3–8 mg./kg./24 hr. To check dose, divide 15 mg. by 6 kg. = 2.5 mg./kg. given twice daily. This equals 5 mg./kg./24 hrs. which is within the average range of 3–8 mg.

Anticonvulsants (see table in Chapter 41 on Recurrent Convulsions)

---

*Material in this list comes from several sources. Much of the material concerning children's medications comes from the 1971 Pediatric Dosage Handbook, published by the American Pharmaceutical Association. This material is reprinted with the permission of the copyright owner.

†To convert child's weight in pounds to kilograms multiply pounds by 0.454.

Apresoline hydrochloride (hydralazine hydrochloride)
Uses in pregnancy. Hypertension associated with toxemias of pregnancy.
Dosage. Usual dose is 20–40 mg. I.M., I.V. or orally.
In *toxemia* 40 mg. daily (10 mg./4 id.), increase by 40–50 mg. daily until desired result obtained. Do not increase daily dose beyond 400 mg. May be given by infusion.
Uses in children. Hypertension in glomerulonephritis. Use cautiously in advanced renal damage.
Dosage. 0.75 mg./kg./24 hr. Tablet form, divided doses.
Adverse reactions. Headache, palpitations, anorexia, nausea, vomiting, diarrhea, tachycardia, angina pectoris.

Aspirin (acetylsalicylic acid). Analgesic
Children's dosage. 65 mg./kg./24 hr. divided 4–6 i.d. or gr. I for each year of life q. 4 hr. p.r.n. up to age of 5 years.
Caution. Salicylism—especially in infants.

A and D ointment. Contains vitamins A and D in lanolin base. Soothing, healing, for diaper rash.

Atarax (hydroxyzine hydrochloride). Tranquilizer.
Uses in pregnancy and labor. Antiemetic, produces calming effect. Potentiates action of a narcotic.
Dosage. Pre- and postpartum. 25–100 mg. I.M. q. 4–6 hrs. p.r.n.
Uses in children. Behavior problems, antiemetic.
Dosage. 2 mg./kg./24 hr. orally, divide in 4 doses.

Adverse reactions. Drowsiness, dryness of mouth, convulsions. Do not give S.C. or I.V.

Atropine sulfate. As preanesthetic in children.
Dosage. 0.01 mg./kg. dose. S.C.
Caution. May cause such side effects as dryness of mouth, restlessness, hypersensitivity rash.
Toxic effects. Tachycardia, dilated pupils, delirium, urinary retention.

BAL (dimercaprol). Heavy metal antidote.
Uses in children. Acute and chronic poisoning by arsenic, gold and mercury.
Dosage. Usually 2.5 mg./kg./I.M. q. 4–12 hrs.
Warnings. May produce hypertension, nausea, vomiting, severe headache, constriction in chest. Symptoms subside within about 1 hour. *Not to be used in lead or cadmium poisoning.*

Bicillin (Benzathine Penicillin G). Long-acting penicillin.
Uses in children. Rheumatic fever prophylaxis.
Dosage. 1.2 units once a month. I.M.
Caution. Same as for penicillin.

Carbocaine HCl. (mepivacaine HCl.). 1% and 2% solutions.
Uses in labor. Produces rapid, marked and prolonged anesthesia, lasting for several hours. Some people who are allergic to procaine anesthetics show no allergy to carbocaine. Used in caudal and paracervical blocks and in epidural anesthesia.
Dosage. For paracervical plus pudendal block, up to 40 cc. of 1% solution.
Pudendal block 5–20 cc. of 1 or 2% solution.
Caudal and epidural anesthesia
  15–30 cc. of 1% solution
  10–25 cc. of 1½% solution
  10–20 cc. of 2% solution
  In pudendal and paracervical blocks, ½ of total amount of solution is injected in each side.
Warning. Oxytoxic drugs should not be used with carbocaine. May cause persistent hypertension in the postpartum period.
Adverse reactions
  1. Intoxication due to intolerance and overdosage.
  2. Allergic reaction such as anaphylaxis (circulatory collapse) (antigen-antibody response) urticaria or bronchospasm.

Codeine phosphate. Addictive analgesic.
Uses in adults and children. Pain reliever.
Dosage in adults. 15–30 mg. oral or S.C.
Dosage in children. 3 mg./kg./in 24 hr. 0.3–1.5 mg./kg./single dose.
Adverse reactions. Constipation. May cause excitement in overdose. Addictive, but less so than morphine.

Cyclopropane. General anesthetic.
Use for maternity patients. Does not interfere with uterine contractions or with the breathing of the mother or the baby.
Administration. Cyclopropane with oxygen mixtures is given by closed circuit method. Should be given by an experienced anesthesiologist.
Adverse reaction. Can produce cardiac arrhythmias.
Caution. Highly explosive.

Darvon (propoxyphene HCl). Non-narcotic analgesic.
Darvon compound, Darvon 65 (propoxyphane HCl with aspirin, phenacetin and caffeine).
Uses in adults. Synthetic analgesic for relief of mild to moderate pain.
Dosage. 65 mg. 3 to 4 times daily.
Adverse reactions. Dizziness, headache, somnolence, insomnia, skin rashes, gastrointestinal disturbances, constipation.
Drug dependence. Tolerance, psychological and physical dependence have been reported, similar to codeine.

Deladumone OB (Testosterone Enanthate 360 mg. and Estradiol 16 mg.). I.M.
Postpartum use. Long-acting preparation for the prevention of lactation. A balanced

combination of testicular and follicular hormones.

Dosage. 2 cc. in oil. Single injection. Give deep into the gluteal muscles in upper outer quadrant.

Contraindications. History of established or suspected mammary or genital malignancy or hepatic dysfunction or disease.

Action. Inhibits release of lactogenic hormone from pituitary gland.

Optimal time for administration. Just prior to the onset of the second stage of labor.

Demerol HCl (Meperidine HCl). Addictive analgesic.

Use in adults. Relief of pain, especially smooth muscle pain.

Dosage. Average adult dose 100 mg.

Range. 25–100 mg. I.M. or I.V.

Use in children. Frequently used as preoperative medication for children of one year of age or older.

Dosage for children. I.M. or S.C.

For preoperative medication 1.0–2.0 mg./kg./dose.

For pain relief. 6.0 mg./kg./24 hr. Divide in 6 doses.

Antidote for overdose. Nalline

Diethylstilbestrol (stilbestrol). Synthetic estrogen.

Use in maternity patients. Prevention of painful engorgement of breasts postpartum.

Dosage. Orally 1–5 mg. t.i.d. for a total of 30 mg.

Digoxin (Lanoxin). The form of digitalis most frequently used for newborn infants and children with cardiac problems. It has a relatively rapid course of action and is fully excreted in 48 to 72 hours. The elixir form makes digoxin useful for oral administration. Also available in ampules for I.M. and I.V. use.

Dosage. Digoxin is given in carefully calculated digitalizing and maintenance doses for the premature, newborn infant and child. The nurse should consult a reference such as the PDR* for average dosage at various ages and weights of children.

Toxic effects of digitalis. Anorexia, vomiting, diarrhea, visual symptoms, dizziness, and irregularity or slowing of heart beat. Reporting of any such symptoms is important, with withholding of additional dosage until child has been examined by the physician.

Diuril (chlorothiazine). Diuretic and antihypertensive.

Uses in pregnancy. For all types of edema.

Dosage: 0.5–1.0 gm. once or twice daily.

Uses for children. May be used in cardiac decompensation. Available in syrup for oral use; vials for I.V. administration.

Dosage for children. 20 mg./kg./24 hr.

Precautions. A careful check of the patient's fluid and electrolyte balance should be done as hypokalemia may develop.

Dulcolax (Bisacodyl). Laxative. Tablets and suppositories.

Action. Contact laxative acting directly on the colonic mucosa.

Use in preparation for delivery. To replace the use of enemas if given 2 hours prior to the second stage of labor. No contraindications for its use in nursing mothers.

Adult dosage. 2 to 3 tablets or one suppository.

Child's dose. 0.3 mg./kg. orally about 6 hours before desired action.

Caution. Tablets enteric coated; avoid chewing. Avoid rectal suppositories if rectal fissures or ulceration.

Ephedrine Sulfate. Adrenergic and nasal decongestant.

In maternity use. To raise the blood pressure in hypotension from caudal or saddle block anesthesia.

Dosage. 50 mg./cc. in injectable solution.

*PDR–Physician's Desk Reference. Published annually by Medical Economics, Inc., Oradell, N.J. and readily available.

For children. Syrup or injectable. Used in asthmatic attacks, usually combined with a mild sedative. *Pseudoephredine,* an isomer of ephedrine, gives fewer side effects.

Dosage. 3 mg./kg./in 24 hr. Divide into 4–6 doses.

Side effects. Headache, insomnia, nervousness, palpitation, precordial pain, nausea, sweating, urinary retention.

Ergotrate maleate (ergonovine). Oxytocic. Oral, I.M. and I.V.

Action postpartum. Causes uterus to contract within a few minutes after administration. Effective for 1/2 to 3 hours after injection.

Use. To prevent and treat postpartum and postabortion hemorrhage.

Dosage. 0.2 mg. I.M. 0.2 mg. x 3 daily (oral) for 48 hrs.

Precautions. Should not be given until after delivery of placenta.

Contraindications. Should not be used for induction of labor or in spontaneous, threatened abortion.

Adverse reactions. Nausea and vomiting, elevated blood pressure.

Erythromycin. See Ilosone.

Esidrix (hydrochlorothiazide). Diuretic.

Uses in pregnancy. Edema and hypertension.

Dosage. 50–100 mg. once or twice daily for several days, followed by maintenance dose of 25–100 mg. daily or intermittently.

Caution. Crosses the placental barrier and may result in fetal hyperbilirubinemia or thrombocytopenia.

Precautions. Observe for signs of fluid or electrolyte imbalance.

Fluothane (halothane). General anesthetic.

Uses in delivery. Pleasant induction without increasing secretions. Fast recovery without nausea and vomiting. Should be given by anesthesiologist. May produce uterine relaxation and subsequent postpartum hemorrhage.

Gantrisin (sulfisoxazole). Urinary antiseptic. Oral in tablet or suspension.

Uses for children and infants. In treatment of urinary infections.

Dosage. 180 mg./kg./24 hr. Given in divided doses.

Contraindications. Same as for sulfadiazine. May cause many organic symptoms if not carefully monitered.

Glucagon. Hyperglycemic. Given S.C. or I.M. to raise blood sugar in patients having hypoglycemic reactions from overdose of insulin.

Dosage. 0.5 to 1 mg. may be repeated in 20 minutes; generally given when patient has lost consciousness and is unable to take some form of sugar by mouth.

Side effects. None noted.

Griseofulvin. Antifungal.

Used orally in many common dermatological fungus infections, particularly ringworm of the scalp.

Dosage for children. 10 mg./kg./24 hr. Divide into 2–4 dosages.

Contraindications. Sensitivity to the drug.

Caution. Prolonged therapy requires blood cell counts at regular intervals.

Ilosone (erythromycin estolate). Oral antibiotic in chewable tablets, suspension, pediatric drops. Broad spectrum antibiotic.

Dosage. For children under 11 kg. weight —40 mg./kg./24 hrs. In divided doses. 11–23 kg.—500 mg./24 hr. 23 kg. and over—1 gm./24 hr.

Contraindications. Sensitivity to the drug, or pre-existing liver disease.

Caution. Gastrointestinal and allergic reactions.

Ipecac syrup. Emetic. To induce vomiting in poison ingestion as an emergency measure. One-ounce bottles are now permitted to be sold without prescription for this purpose.

Dosage. 15 cc., followed by water. May repeat once in 20 minutes. If child does not vomit, the dose should be recovered by lavage.

For use in croup. To help the child cough up thick secretions.

Dosage. 2 to 4 cc. (or ½ teaspoonful).

Caution. Be sure ipecac *syrup* is used. Fluid extract of ipecac is several times stronger and has proved poisonous when given in place of syrup.

Lorfan (levallorphan tartrate). Narcotic antagonist. (See Nalline)

Lytren. Oral electrolyte formula to supply maintenance electrolyte therapy. Give according to physician's calculation of individual need.

Caution. Do not mix with milk, fruit juices or other electrolyte fluids.

Magnesium sulfate. Sedative, anticonvulsant, and diuretic.

Action. Central nervous system depressant.

Dosage. 10 to 20 cc. of a 50% solution every 6 hours deep intramuscularly. Often given with a special 3-inch needle with 1 to 2 cc. of 1% procaine added to minimize discomfort.

Precautions. Have a physician check the knee jerk reflex before administering. The nurse should check the respirations (if they are below 12 per minute do not give) and the urine output prior to giving the medication.

Antidote. Calcium (calcium gluconate) is given to offset the action of magnesium sulfate.

Masse Breast Cream. Used for prevention and treatment of cracked nipples in postpartum period and for preparing nipples for nursing during the antepartum period.

Dosage. Apply ¼-inch of cream twice daily beginning early in the sixth month of pregnancy. Massage gently into the nipple at the same time pulling the nipple outward.

Postpartum. Gently massage around the nipple and areola after the breast has been cleansed following each nursing period.

Methergine (methylergonovine). Oxytocic

Use for maternity patients. To contract the uterus, prevent postpartum atony and hemorrhage, and subinvolution.

Dose. 0.2 mg. (1/320 gr.) orally, I.M. or I.V. May be repeated in 2 to 4 hours. Given after delivery of the placenta, or with the birth of the anterior shoulder, or during the puerperium.

Adverse reactions. Nausea, vomiting, transient hypertension, dizziness, or headache.

Mucomist Spray (acetylcysteine). For use in chronic bronchopulmonary disease to liquefy viscid secretions. Used in nebulizer and by face mask or mouth piece; or in tracheostomy care.

Dosage. 1–10 ml. of 20% solution, or 2–20 ml. of 10% solution.

Adverse effects. A few people have a sensitivity to mucomist. Asthmatics may not be able to tolerate drug.

Mycostatin. (nystatin)

Action. Antibiotic with antifungal activity against a wide range of yeasts and yeast fungi. For oral use in thrush, and in intestinal and vaginal infections.

Dosage for pregnant women with monilia infection. To prevent thrush in newborn— 1 to 2 tablets daily for 3 to 6 weeks before term.

Use for infants with thrush. Suspension of 100,000 units per cc. swabbed inside mouth 3 or 4 times daily.

Nalline (Nalorphine HCl). Narcotic antagonist. I.V. or I.M.

Uses in maternity. Reverses respiratory depression of the fetus.

Dosage. 5–10 mg. I.V. to the mother. Dose may be repeated two times at intervals of 10–15 minutes.

Dosage to newborn. 0.2 mg. by umbilical vein.

Children's dosage. 0.1 mg./kg./dose. May repeat in 15 minutes. (See package insert.)

Nembutal (pentobarbital sodium)

Use in obstetrics. 30–60 mg. for sedation. 200 to 300 mg. may be given in a single dose, orally.

Use for children. Sodium pentobarbital injectable used for preoperative sedation in children over the age of 6 years. Dosage calculated on child's age, weight and condition. 3.0–4.0 mg./kg. – maximum dose 120 mg.

Neo-Synephrine (phenylephrine HCl). Antihypotensive drug (vasoconstrictor)
Use in maternity. To prevent or overcome hypotensive reactions during spinal and inhalation anesthesia.
Dosage. 2–5 mg. of a 1% solution, S.C., I.M. or I.V.
Caution. Do not use for patients who have hypertension, hyperthyroidism, diabetes, or heart disease.

Nesacaine (chloroprocaine). Local anesthetic resembling procaine. Used for local infiltration and pudendal block in childbirth.

Nitrous Oxide. Gas anesthetic. Used intermittently during second stage of labor.
Disadvantage. Poor relaxation.

Pancreatic granules. An enzyme used to aid in digestion of starchy and protein foods. Given to children with cystic fibrosis. Granules given with meals, tasteless; may be sprinkled on cereal or other foods.
Dosage ¼–½ tsp. with meals.

Penicillin G. Antibiotic. Supplied in many forms, as oral or injectable.
Dosage for children. 25,000–50,000 units/kg./24 hrs.

Phenergan (promethazine). Use in obstetrics. As a sedative in early stages of labor. Used in combination with meperidine to provide analgesia and control nausea and vomiting during labor. Also used to control nausea and vomiting of pregnancy.
Dosage. For nausea and vomiting of pregnancy – 25 mg. on retiring, followed by 12.5 to 25 mg. on rising if necessary.
In labor. 50 mg. for sedation and to relieve apprehension in early labor.
Use for children. Preoperative sedation, antihistamine, motion sickness, nausea,

and vomiting. Supplied in syrup, tablets or injectable.

Phenobarbital (Luminal). Barbiturate and hypnotic. As compared with other barbiturates, action develops slowly and persists a relatively long time.
Use in pregnancy. In toxemia or for sedation for temporary calming effect when something has gone wrong with infant, as in stillbirth.
Dosage. 100–200 mg. daily in divided doses.
Use for children. Effective in preventing epileptic seizures. Used also in chorea, and febrile convulsions. For dosage see Chapter 41.

Piperazine (Antepar). Used in treatment of pinworms and round worms. Oral administration.
Dosage. 0.250–1.0 gm. once daily for 7 days.

Pitocin (oxytocin injection synthetic). For induction of labor; also for prevention and treatment of postpartum hemorrhage.
Dosage for induction of labor. 10 units added to 1,000 cc. of 5% dextrose solution, administered by slow intravenous infusion. Rate of drip adjusted in accordance with uterine response and fetal condition. Given 10–15 drops per minute, up to a maximum of 40 drops if necessary. Infusion discontinued if sustained contractions occur or changes in fetal heart rate indicate fetal distress.

Povan (pyrvinium pamoate). Used as single dose treatment for pinworms. Oral.
Dosage. 5 mg./kg./single dose.
Caution. Colors stools red. Occasionally nausea and vomiting.

Scopolamine Hydrobromide (hyoscine). Sedative.
Use in obstetrics. To produce amnesia and sedation.
Used alone or in combination with narcotic analgesics.
Dosage. 0.3–0.6 mg. S.C.
Warning. May cause marked depression.

Use in children. May be used for preanesthetic sedation in children over one year of age.

Dosage. 0.006 mg./kg./single dose.

Silver Nitrate. Preventive eye treatment (see page 175)

Sulfadiazine. Sulfonamide. Given orally, I.M., I.V.

Use for children. Systemic infections, particularly in meningitis. Useful in urinary infections caused by *E. coli.* Prophylactic in rheumatic fever.

Dosage for children. 150 mg./kg./24 hr. orally.

In rheumatic fever prophylaxis: 0.5 gm.–1.0 gm./24 hr. orally.

Contraindiction. Sensitivity to sulfonamides under 2–3 months of age.

Synkayvite (synthetic vitamin K)

Use. Antihemorrhagic in newborn infants.

Dosage. 1 mg. I.M. in anterior aspect of the thigh.

Adverse reactions. May cause hyperbilirubinemia.

Tace (chlorotrianisene). Synthetic estrogen.

Use. Postpartum breast engorgement.

Dosage. One 12 mg. capsule 4 times daily for 7 days, or two 25-mg. capsules q. 6 hours x 6 doses.

For immediate postpartum use to suppress lactation first dose should be given within 8 hours after delivery.

Adverse reactions. Prolonged administration can result in breakthrough bleeding.

Tempra (acetaminophen). Nonaddictive analgesic and antipyretic. Available in syrup, tablet and pediatric drops.

Dosage. Under 1 year 60 mg.

   1–3 yr.   60–120 mg.

   3–6 yr.   120 mg.
   6–12 yr.   240 mg.

Tenlap (acetaminophen). Same as Tempra. Label carries warning "Do not give to children under 3 years of age or use for more than 10 days unless directed by a physician." (nonprescription drug)

Triline (Trichloroethylene). Self-administered anesthetic.

Use in maternity. Produces anesthesia adequate to relieve labor contractions without complete loss of consciousness.

Caution. Tends to produce cardiac arrhythmias. Cannot use closed circuit methods of anesthesia with soda lime following its use.

Tylenol (acetaminophen). Same as Tempra. Label carries this note: "Consult a physician for use by children under 6 or for use longer than 10 days."

Vistaril (hydroxyzine HCl)

Use in maternity. Calming effect in labor, antiemetic, potentiates the action of narcotics. (Dosage of narcotic should be reduced by 50%.)

Side effects. Drowsiness, dryness of the mouth.

Dosage. 25–100 mg. I.M.

Caution. For *intramuscular* administration *only.*

Xylocaine (lidocaine). Local or regional anesthetic

Uses in maternity. Caudal, pudendal, or local anesthesia.

Dosage. Pudendal block—using 1% solution, 10 cc. on each side—Total dose: 100 mg.

Caudal anesthesia—using 1% solution, 20 to 30 cc.—Total dose: 200–300 mg.

ABBREVIATIONS COMMONLY USED

ABBREVIATIONS	MEANING	DERIVATION
aa	of each	ana (Greek)
a.c.	before meals	ante cibum (Latin)
ad lib	as desired	ad libitum (Latin)
A.P.	apical pulse	
b.i.d. (or 2 i.d.)	two times daily	bis in die (Latin)
B.P.	blood pressure	
C.	centigrade	
c̄	with	
cc	cubic centimeter	
cm.	centimeter	
D.C.	discontinue	
F.	Fahrenheit	
fl.	fluid	
Gm.	gram	
gtt.	drop, drops	guttae (Latin)
(H)	hypodermically	
h.s.	at hour of sleep	hora somni (Latin)
I.M.	intramuscularly	
I.V.	intravenously	
kg.	kilogram	
L.	liter (1000 cc., or 1 qt. approx.)	
mg.	milligram	
mm.	millimeter	
O.D.	right eye	oculus dexter (Latin)
O.S.	left eye	oculus sinister (Latin)
O.U.	both eyes	oculus unitas (Latin)
oz., or ℥.	ounce	
p̄	after	
p.c.	after eating	post cibum (Latin)
P.O.	by mouth	per os (Latin)
p.r.n.	as necessary	pro re nata (Latin)
q.	every	
q.i.d. (or 4 i.d.)	four times daily	quater in die (Latin)
q.s.	as much as necessary	quantum satis (Latin)
R.B.C.	red blood count	
s̄	without	
s̄s̄	one-half	
t.i.d. (or 3 i.d.)	three times daily	tres in die (Latin)
W.B.C.	white cell count	
X	times	
ℨ.	dram	

METRIC DOSES WITH APPROXIMATE APOTHECARY EQUIVALENTS*

LIQUID MEASURE

Metric		Apothecary
4000	ml.	1 gallon
1000	ml.	1 quart
500	ml.	1 pint
30	ml.	1 fluid ounce
4	ml.	1 fluid dram
0.06	ml.	1 minum

Note: a milliliter (ml.) is the approximate equivalent of a cubic centimeter (cc.).

---

*When prepared dosage forms such as tablets, capsules, and pills are prescribed in the metric system, the pharmacist may dispense the corresponding approximate equivalent in the apothecary system, and vice versa.

EQUIVALENT WEIGHTS IN METRIC AND IN APOTHECARY SCALES

Metric		Apothecary
30	Gm.	1 ounce
15	Gm.	4 drams
1	Gm.	15 grains
60	mg.	1 grain
30	mg.	1/2 grain
15	mg.	1/4 grain
1	mg.	1/60 grain
0.4	mg.	1/150 grain
0.25	mg.	1/250 grain
0.2	mg.	1/300 grain
0.12	mg.	1/500 grain

CONVERSION OF AVOIRDUPOIS BODY WEIGHT TO METRIC EQUIVALENTS

lb.	kg.	kg.	lb.
10	4.5	10	22
20	9.1	20	44
30	13.6	30	66
40	18.2	40	88
50	22.7	50	110
60	27.3		
70	31.8		
80	36.4		
90	40.9		
100	45.4		

One pound = 0.454 kilograms
One kilogram = 2.2 pounds

CONVERSION OF HEIGHT TO METRIC EQUIVALENTS

Inches	Centimeters
18	46
24	61
30	76
36	91
42	107
48	122
54	137
60	152
66	168

One inch = 2.54 cm.
One cm. = 0.3937 inch

EQUIVALENT CENTIGRADE AND FAHRENHEIT TEMPERATURE READINGS

Centigrade	Fahrenheit
35	95.0
36	96.8
37	98.6
38	100.4
39	102.2
40	104.0
41	105.8

To convert Centigrade readings to Fahrenheit, multiply by 1.8 and add 32.
To convert Fahrenheit readings to Centigrade, subtract 32 and divide by 1.8.

Answer Key for Study Questions

Unit Two

1. a
2. d
3. d
4. b
5. c
6. d
7. b
8. d
9. d
10. c
11. b
12. c
13. a
14. d
15. c
16. a
17. a
18. d
19. b
20. d
21. d
22. c
23. d
24. a
25. a

Unit Three

1. a
2. c
3. b
4. b
5. d
6. a
7. b
8. b
9. d
10. c
11. d
12. b
13. c
14. a
15. c
16. b
17. a
18. d

19. c
20. a
21. b
22. a
23. a
24. d
25. d

Unit Four

1. d
2. a
3. d
4. b
5. c
6. d
7. c
8. a
9. d
10. c
11. a
12. c
13. b
14. c
15. d
16. a
17. c

Matching

9
8
11
10
4
1
7
3

Unit Five

1. 4
2. d
3. c
4. b
5. 3
6. c

7. b
8. d
9. d

Unit Six

1. a
2. d
3. b

Unit Eight

1. 1
2. 3
3. 1
4. c
5. d
6. d
7. d
8. d
9. a
10. a
11. a
12. d
13. d
14. 1

Unit Nine

1. 3
2. c
3. 2
4. 2
5. b
6. a
7. 4
8. 3
9. c
10. c
11. d
12. d
13. c

Unit Ten

1. 3
2. b

3. 1
4. 3
5. a
6. 4
7. c
8. d
9. a
10. d
11. b
12. c

Unit Eleven

1. c
2. 4
3. 1
4. 1
5. 4
6. d
7. d
8. c
9. 4
10. 4
11. 3
12. 1

Unit Twelve

1. a
2. d
3. c
4. b
5. d
6. 4
7. c
8. d

Index

Numerals in italics indicate illustrations or tabular material.

683